# POULTRY DISEASES
## A Guide for Farmers and
## Poultry Professionals

# POULTRY DISEASES
## A Guide for Farmers and Poultry Professionals

### (Second Revised and Enlarged Edition)

**J.L. VEGAD**

Adviser
Phoenix Group
201/15, Ratan Colony,
P. B. 75, Gorakhpur,
Jabalpur - 482001

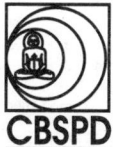

**CBSPD**

## CBS Publishers & Distributors Pvt Ltd

New Delhi • Bengaluru • Chennai • Kochi • Kolkata • Lucknow • Mumbai
Hyderabad • Jharkhand • Nagpur • Patna • Pune • Uttarakhand

## Poultry Diseases

**ISBN:** 978-81-239-2789-3

Copyright © Publisher

**First CBS Reprint:** 2015
Reprint: 2018, 2020, 2022, **2025**

Published by **Satish Kumar Jain** and produced by **Varun Jain** for

## CBS Publishers & Distributors Pvt Ltd

4819/XI Prahlad Street, 24 Ansari Road, Daryaganj, New Delhi 110 002, India.
Ph: 011-23266838, 23289259          Website: www.cbspd.com
                                    e-mail: delhi@cbspd.com

*Corporate Office:* 204 FIE, Industrial Area, Patparganj, Delhi 110 092
Ph: 011-4934 4934          Fax: 011-4934 4935
                          e-mail: publishing@cbspd.com; publicity@cbspd.com

### Branches

- **Bengaluru:** Seema House 2975, 17th Cross, KR Road, Banasankari 2nd Stage, Bengaluru 560 070, Karnataka, India
  Ph: +91-80-26771678/79          Fax: +91-80-26771680          e-mail: bangalore@cbspd.com
- **Chennai:** 7, Subbaraya Street, Shenoy Nagar, Chennai 600 030, Tamil Nadu, India
  Ph: +91-44-26680620, 26681266          Fax: +91-44-42032115          e-mail: chennai@cbspd.com
- **Kochi:** 42/1325, 1326, Power House Road, Opp KSEB, Power House, Ernakulum Kochi 682 018, Kerala, India
  Ph: +91-484-4059061-65,67          Fax: +91-484-4059065          e-mail: kochi@cbspd.com
- **Kolkata:** 147, Hind Ceramics Compound, 1st Floor, Nilgunj Road, Belghoria, Kolkata-700056, West Bengal, India
  Ph: +033-25633055, 033-25633056          e-mail: kolkata@cbspd.com
- **Lucknow:** Basement, Khushnuma Complex, 7 Meerabai Marg (Behind Jawahar Bhawan), Lucknow-226001, UP, India
  Ph: +0522-4000032          e-mail: tiwari.lucknow@cbspd.com
- **Mumbai:** PWD Shed, Gala no 25/26, Ramchandra Bhatt Marg, Next to JJ Hospital Gate no. 2, Opp. Union Bank of India, Noorbaug, Mumbai-400009, Maharashtra, India
  Ph: 022-66661880/89          e-mail: mumbai@cbspd.com

### Representatives

| | | | | | | |
|---|---|---|---|---|---|---|
| • Hyderabad | 0-9885175004 | • Jharkhand | 0-9811541605 | • Nagpur | 0-8692091830 |
| • Patna | 0-9334159340 | • Pune | 0-9664372571 | • Uttarakhand | 0-9716462459 |

*Printed at* Neekunj Print Process, Haryana (India)

# FOREWORD

The poultry industry continues to be a major and cheapest source of animal protein. Scientists have increased and exploited birds' genetic potential to the fullest. But there has not been a corresponding improvement in the structure of vital organs. Increased stress on the body gives rise to conditions like ascites in broilers and fatty liver-haemorrhagic syndrome in layers. Moreover, the picture of poultry diseases keeps constantly changing. Therefore, an adequate knowledge of poultry diseases is vital. This is precisely what Dr. J.L. Vegad's book aims at.

By contributing such a useful book for farmers and poultry professionals, Dr. Vegad has rendered a great service to industry. I do hope the book proves valuable in controlling poultry losses - the basic objective for which it is written. This book provides scientific insights to the layman farmers and practical insight to the pure scientists.

V. N. Dubey
Chairman, Phoenix Group
and
Mayor, Nagar Nigam, Jabalpur

# PREFACE TO SECOND EDITION

The widespread popularity of the first edition among farmers and poultry professionals, feed and pharmaceutical personnel, poultry consultants, diagnostic laboratories, and veterinary students and teaching community has prompted me to bring out the Second Edition. I do hope this edition proves equally useful and is received with the same interest.

In the short period since the First Edition of the book was published in 2004, many things have happened. To begin with, the industry has been finally hit by avian influenza (bird flu), causing considerable disquiet and anxiety among poultry farmers. The industry at present has no potent weapon, such as an effective vaccine, to fight back. How then to contain the threat? Marek's disease has again raised its ugly head, inflicting up to 60% mortality in layers and ruining farmers' economy. Experts believe that useful life of Marek's disease vaccine is about 10 years. This is due to the evolution of more virulent strains. So, what next? The menace of diseases like Ranikhet and Gumboro, *E. coli* infection, mycoplasmosis, coccidiosis and others continues unabated. So much so that many antibiotics, that were once foolproof, are no longer that effective or reliable due to the phenomenon of drug resistance. Keeping these and several other points in view, the Second Edition is presented. It has been extensively revised and many chapters are completely rewritten. The changes in particular include:

- The section on avian influenza has been completely rewritten, covering all aspects of the disease with latest information. The disease is also illustrated with many coloured photographs showing changes in sick birds as well as the postmortem findings. **The pictures are from the recent Indian outbreak.** In addition, a summary of the Action Plan of the Government of India on the control and containment of avian influenza is given for general information.

- The section on Marek's disease has been revised and updated.

- A lot of new information has been added on necrotic enteritis, *E. coli* infection, Ranikhet disease, and almost on every aspect of poultry health.

- Chapter on **'The Avian Immune System'** has been revised and updated.

- In view of the problem of drug resistance and relative ineffectiveness of antibiotics, the major thrust in this Edition is on the prevention and control of diseases through biosecurity, hygiene, sanitation, and disinfection. For example, with avian influenza, the vaccinated flocks cannot be considered influenza-free. However, the use of vaccine reduces the amount of virus shed. Or, with Ranikhet disease, although vaccination protects the birds against the disease, virus growth and shedding still occur, though at a reduced level. For this reason, the chapter on disinfection has been revised and updated.

- Finally, a major effort has been made to update company's products. Those that were no longer marketed are deleted and new ones included. Also, attempts have been made to include products from as many companies as possible.

I am grateful to Mr. Suneel Gomber, Manager, International Distributing Co., Lucknow, for the publication of this book. I express my sincere appreciation to Dr. Priti Mishra, Nutritionist and Mr. Satish Shukla, Microbiologist, Phoenix Laboratory for their generous help in the compilation of tables on medicines and vaccines. I tender my thanks to them both. The coloured photographs on avian influenza were obtained through the courtesy of both Department of Animal Husbandry, Government of Madhya Pradesh, while lecturing on a Bird Flu Training Programme, and Prof. R.N. Sreenivas Gowda, Vice-Chancellor, Karnataka Veterinary, Animal and Fisheries Sciences University, Bidar. I am grateful to them both. Thanks are due to Dr. R. K. Tripathi, Dr. Vijay Makhija, Dr. Mrigen Dutta, Dr. Chand Bahar, Mr. Vijay Tripathi, Mr. Pritesh Gupta, Mr. Praveen S. Pathradkar, Mr. Ganga Ram Chaudhary and Mr. Gajendra Rajput who all helped me in procuring the literature on pharmaceutical products. My special thanks are due to Mr. Vijay Parmar of Jabalpur Graphics who was most generous in extending help relating to computer work. Finally, I am grateful to my wife Nita Vegad for her tolerance and faith in me and my work.

J.L. Vegad

## PREFACE TO FIRST EDITION

This book is written for poultry farmers and poultry professionals. The theme: effective disease diagnosis, treatment and control. The objective: prevention of losses, more profits and better economics.

The picture of poultry disease has changed over the years and the classical symptoms and postmortem findings, once so helpful in disease diagnosis, are no longer all that classical or helpful. Moreover, certain bacteria, like that of fowl cholera, have developed variations in their make-up through the years, giving rise to several different types of the same organism. Also, certain viruses, such as that of infectious bronchitis, have a natural tendency toward genetic mutation. This can lead to generation of new strains against which present vaccines may be totally ineffective. Such changes continually occurring in poultry health, and resultant disguised version of the disease, have not only confused the farmer but posed a serious challenge even for the professionals. In addition, several new diseases keep constantly knocking at the door. Therefore, unless diseases are properly diagnosed and effectively controlled, poultry farming can no longer remain a profitable proposition in the present competitiveness. It is with this objective that the book has been written, to acquaint the farmers with changing disease scenario and also with complexities of the problem. Change is the law of nature and poultry diseases are no exception. We must be well equipped for the challenges ahead. There will be no point in locking the stable door after the horse has run away!

The book has five sections, divided into 43 chapters. The first section deals with infectious, nutritional, and metabolic diseases as well as miscellaneous conditions. While the main emphasis is on diagnosis, treatment and control, other aspects have been dealt with for those interested to know more.

The second section is on disease diagnosis. The third relates to disease treatment/prevention. Apart from providing a comprehensive list of commercial medicines and vaccines, this section also covers important topics like antibiotic growth promoters, probiotics, mould inhibitors, toxin binders, enzymes, oligosaccharides, osmoregulators, methyl donors, acidifiers, and biosurfactants.

The fourth section discusses disease control. Disease-producing bacteria are abundant in the poultry world. This is because, like higher forms of life, they must also fight for their survival. Being small, they have been provided by nature with a survival potential and possess the ability to reproduce in extremely large numbers. These large numbers mean that their spread and presence will be extremely great. Therefore, to achieve the best results from any disease control programme, attention has to be given to the ways in which disease organisms can spread and examine management closely to find out where and how this spread can be minimized. All these aspects are dealt with in the first three chapters of this section, namely, biosecurity, disinfection, and sanitation.

ix

Another important aspect of disease control discussed in the fourth section is the subject of vaccines and vaccination. Already there are so many commercial vaccines in the market and new ones keep coming. Also, so much technical literature keeps pouring all the time on immunity and chicken's immune system that the farmer is often confused and even lost. Keeping this in view, the fundamentals and certain basic concepts of the chicken's immune system are discussed. This is followed by a discussion of the impact nutrients have in boosting immunity in the chicken and thereby prevent early chick mortality. The remaining two chapters of this section devote to properties of the vaccines and various vaccination schedules.

The fifth and final section, 'tips on rearing and management', has been added with the firm belief that origin of more than 80% of the poultry health problems lies in poor management, and that there can be no profitable poultry industry without proper management. In fact, management is the bedrock on which productive poultry farming rests.

I hope the comprehensive coverage of poultry diseases from various angles will prove valuable to farmers in their continuous struggle to minimize losses from sickness and death, and in improving growth and performance of the birds. This would make poultry farming a worthwhile enterprise.

The book contains the latest information in a simplified manner, so that it is readily understood. Also, it has photographs, line-diagrams, figures and tables to further increase understanding of the text.

Though the book is written to meet the requirements of poultry farmers, it will be equally useful to poultry consultants, diagnostic laboratories, and feed and pharmaceutical professionals. In addition, the book will acquaint veterinary students and teaching community with the practical aspects of poultry health management.

In conclusion, I shall greatly appreciate receiving any comments/suggestions to enable me to improve the future edition of this book.

J.L. Vegad

## ACKNOWLEDGEMENTS

The work of writing such a book inevitably involves many helping hands.

First, I would like to express my gratitude to Shri V.N. Dubey, Chairman, Phoenix Group and Mayor, Nagar Nigam, Jabalpur, for writing 'FOREWORD' of the book. I am especially grateful to Shri D.R. Dangi, Chief Executive, Phoenix Group, for his being most helpful. While preparing section, "Tips on rearing and management", suggestions given by Dr. P. S. Atkare were very useful. He also devoted a large amount of time. I am grateful to him.

Dr. P.K. Tiwari, Shri S.K. Gorasia and Shri S.G Atkare of Phoenix Group were generous in many ways. Shri J. Khare helped in the computer work, and Shri Nishit Tiwari willingly typed the lengthy Chapter of 'Medicines and Vaccines'. In fact, all the staff of Phoenix Group were most helpful. I tender my thanks to them all.

Dr. Priti Mishra, Nutritionist, Phoenix Lab, prepared chapter 19 on commercial medicines and vaccines. She was painstaking, meticulous and assiduously at it till the work was completed. Dr. Madhu Swamy, Associate Professor of Veterinary Pathology, took pains and gave enough time in going through the manuscript. I am grateful to them both. Thanks are also due to Miss Jyoti Tamsikar, Microbiologist, Phoenix Lab, for her help. I thank Shri Ganga Ram Choudhary of Phoenix Lab for discussions on practical aspects of poultry management, and Shri Gajendra Rajput for his assistance.

I am grateful to Shri Suneel Gomber, Manager, International Book Distributing Co., Lucknow, for publication of the book. Dr. Vijay Makhija gave useful suggestions and Shri Brajesh Shrivas of Sunrays Marketing was helpful. I am thankful to them both.

Shri Anand Parmar and Shri Vijay Parmar of Jabalpur Graphics; and Shri Sharad Vegad, Shri Dilip Vegad and Shri Amit Vegad were most generous in extending help related to scanning and computer work. Finally, it is indeed a great pleasure to express my appreciation to members of my joint family for their patience and understanding. I am especially grateful to my wife Nita and my eldest brother Amrit Lal Vegad for the moral support, and for their faith in me and my task.

J.L. Vegad

# ABBREVIATIONS

| | | |
|---|---|---|
| B.P. | = | British pharmacopoeia |
| BWD | = | Bacillary white diarrhoea |
| $^0$C | = | Degree Celsius |
| C.F.U. | = | Colony forming unit |
| CCRD | = | Complicated chronic respiratory disease |
| cm | = | Centimetre |
| CRD | = | Chronic respiratory disease |
| DNA | = | Deoxyribonucleic acid |
| e. g. | = | For example |
| EID | = | Egg infective dose |
| Exts | = | Extracts |
| $^0$F | = | Degree of Fahrenheit |
| FCR | = | Feed conversion ratio |
| Ft | = | Foot |
| g | = | Gram |
| G | = | Greek |
| Gal | = | Gallon |
| GI | = | Gastro-intestinal |
| h | = | Hour |
| hrs | = | Hours |
| HCl | = | Hydrochloric acid |
| i.e. | = | That is |
| I/M | = | Intramuscular |
| Inj | = | Injection |
| I.P. | = | Indian pharmacopoeia |
| I.U. | = | International unit |
| I/V | = | Intravenous |
| Kg | = | Kilogramme |
| L | = | Latin, also litre |
| Lb | = | Pound |
| LD50 | = | Minimal lethal dose |
| Liq | = | Liquid |
| M | = | Metre |

| | | |
|---|---|---|
| Mcg | = | Microgramme |
| ME | = | Metabolizable energy |
| mg | = | Milligram |
| M.I.U. | = | Million international unit |
| ml | = | Millilitre |
| mm | = | Millimetre |
| Pdrs | = | Powders |
| pH | = | Hydrogen ion concentration |
| pfu | = | Plaque-forming unit |
| ppb | = | Parts per billion |
| ppm | = | Parts per million |
| q.s. | = | Quantum sufficit |
| Qty | = | Quantity |
| % | = | Percent |
| S/C | = | Subcutaneous |
| Soln | = | Solution |
| SPF | = | Specific pathogen free |
| spp | = | Species |
| Vit | = | Vitamin |
| US | = | United States |
| USA | = | United States of America |
| USP | = | United States Pharmacopoeia |
| viz | = | Namely |
| v/v | = | Volume by volume |
| wt. | = | Weight |
| w/v | = | Weight by volume |
| w/w | = | Weight by weight |

# CONTENTS

## SECTION I: DISEASES

xvii

## SECTION II: DISEASE DIAGNOSIS

## SECTION III: DISEASE TREATMENT/PREVENTION

## SECTION IV: DISEASE CONTROL

xix

# Section I

# DISEASES

# Chapter 1

# Introduction

The word **'disease'** is of Latin origin. **'Dis'** in Latin means **'not'**. Disease (disease) then means **'not at ease'**. Thus, disease is that condition in which the individual suffers from discomfort.

## Causes

A wide variety of factors can cause disease in poultry. These include pathogenic (i.e. disease-producing) micro-organisms, parasites, nutritional deficiencies, metabolic disorders, fungal toxins, chemical agents and drugs, or even just lack of adequate oxygen. Pathogenic micro-organisms include viruses, bacteria, mycoplasma, fungi, and chlamydia; whereas parasites comprise helminths (i.e. worms), protozoa (such as coccidia), and insects. Each of these infectious agents, as well as the diseases produced by them, are discussed under the appropriate chapter.

## Cell Injury and Necrosis

In response to the injurious stimuli, cells within the body first try to adjust themselves, in an attempt to cope with the changed situation. But if the stimulus is powerful, the cell gets damaged and suffers from cell injury. If the stimulus is still more powerful, the cell gets irreversibly injured. That is, it reaches to a **'point of no return'** and cannot recover even if the harmful stimulus is gone. The cell then dies. This local death of cells or tissue (i.e. a group of cells) within the living body is called **'necrosis'**; an example in the poultry being **'necrotic enteritis'**.

## Inflammation

The living tissue with its blood vessels first tries to protect itself from injury. This reaction of the tissue against local injury is called **'inflammation'**. Its purpose is to destroy, dilute, or isolate the injurious agent and repair the damage caused. During inflammation, a lot of fluid and cells escape from the blood vessels into the tissue. The purpose is to dilute the irritant, to bring in protective cells into the area to destroy the disease-producing micro-organisms, and also to get antibodies that would help these cells in killing the pathogens. Thus, **inflammation is body's defensive response. Without inflammation, infections would go unchecked and wounds would never heal.** Inflammation is therefore fundamental to the survival of the bird. In fact, it is the most basic, the most important, and the most common response that occurs following an injury. Most diseases, at some time in their course, are inflammation. **In fact, more than 80% of the diseases in poultry are basically inflammatory in nature.**

The most common causes of inflammation in the chicken are the disease-producing micro-organisms, mainly viruses, bacteria, mycoplasma, and coccidia. Like higher forms of life, micro-organisms also fight for survival. Being small, they have been provided by nature with a large survival potential (capacity) through their ability to reproduce in extremely large numbers. These large numbers mean that their spread in the environment would be extensive. **Most micro-organisms are therefore abundant in the poultry world.**

Inflammation of an organ or tissue is described by adding suffix **'-itis'** after its name, which is mostly, is Latin or Greek. For example, **'enteritis'** is inflammation of intestine; **'hepatitis'** inflammation of liver; **'nephritis'** inflammation of kidneys; **'tracheitis'** inflammation of trachea; and **'dermatitis'** inflammation of the skin.

## Gangrene

When dead (necrosed) tissue is attacked by saprophytic bacteria, it undergoes putrefaction (decay). Saprophytes are those organisms which live on decaying or dead organic matter. This putrefaction of dead tissue in the living birds is called **'gangrene'**; the best example in poultry being **'gangrenous dermatitis'**.

## Tumour/Neoplasm/Cancer

In certain circumstances, following an injurious stimulus, tissue may not undergo necrosis or inflammation, but may proliferate (grow) without any control of the body, serve no useful function, and kill the bird. This growth of new cells is called a **'tumour'**, a **'neoplasm'**, or **'cancer'**; the best examples in poultry being lymphoid leukosis, **Marek's disease**, and reticuloendotheliosis.

## Lesion

Following disease, tissue undergoes abnormal changes in its structure and function. An abnormal structural alteration in the tissue, whether gross or microscopic, is called a **'lesion'**. Certain lesions are specific of a disease and indicate without doubt the cause of a particular disease. Such a typical lesion (or lesions) is called a **'pathognomonic lesion'**. Such lesions are most helpful in arriving at a diagnosis during the postmortem examination, particularly under field conditions. Examples include: swollen, inflamed, haemorrhagic bursa in Gumboro disease; pinpoint haemorrhages on the glands' of proventriculus in Ranikhet disease; and white chalky coating of urates on heart, liver, kidney and at other places in the body cavity in gout (see Chapter 17 for more information on characteristic (pathognomonic) lesions).

## Symptom

An abnormal change in the structure of an organ or tissue leads to its abnormal function. This abnormal function shows itself as a **'symptom'** of the disease. Thus, symptom is a manifestation of an abnormal function; examples in chicken include fever, difficult breathing, swelling, loss of appetite, diarrhoea, lameness, etc.

## Concluding Remarks

This section covers diseases caused by infectious agents, nutritional deficiencies, and also those brought about by metabolic disorders. One chapter also deals with miscellaneous conditions, such as heat stress, vices, effects of ammonia and several others. **All illnesses and ailments affecting poultry are covered.**

The sequence in which various diseases have been described includes: first, a brief introduction of the infectious agent or disease, followed by cause of that disease, its spread, development, symptoms, postmortem findings (i.e. gross lesions), diagnosis, treatment, and control. While the main emphasis is on diagnosis, treatment, and control, other aspects of the disease have also been dealt with fairly adequately for those interested to know more.

The descriptions of the diseases, though contain the latest information, all attempts have been made to present the complicated matter in a most simplified manner so that it is readily understood. Also, to the extent possible, technical terms have been used to a bare minimum so that the text is easily grasped. Only those terms that were essential or unavoidable, have been used. Although the technical terms, wherever they occur in the text, have been explained within brackets, they have also been given at one place in the next chapter as: **"Important Terms",** for easy reference.

# Chapter 2

# Important Terms

**Active Immunity:** Immunity produced by the bird against an infectious agent following natural exposure, or introduced by vaccination.

**Acute Disease:** A disease which has sudden onset, sharp rise, severe symptoms, and a short course. Not chronic (see 'chronic disease').

**Agglutination Test:** A test for the presence of antibodies. It is performed by mixing blood or serum with an antigen.

**Airsacculitis:** Inflammation of the airsac.

**Anaemia:** A condition in which the blood is deficient in red cells, in haemoglobin, or in total volume.

**Anthelmintic:** A drug capable of expelling, or destroying worms in the intestines.

**Antibiotic:** A substance that has the power to kill, or stop the growth of micro-organisms.

**Antibody:** A protective substance (a protein) formed in the body as a result of infection, or administration of vaccines.

**Antigen:** A substance that produces antibodies when introduced into the bird. In poultry, they are usually infectious agents.

**Antiserum:** A serum containing antibodies specific for a particular antigen.

**Ataxia:** Uncoordinated muscular movements.

**Attenuated organism:** A disease-causing organism which has been so altered that its disease-producing power (virulence) has been reduced.

**Avirulent:** An organism that is not capable of producing disease.

**Bacteraemia:** Presence of bacteria in the blood.

**Bactericide:** A substance that kills bacteria, but not necessarily their spores. Adjective is **'bactericidal'**.

**Bacteriostat:** A substance that stops the growth of bacteria without killing them. Adjective is **'bacteriostatic'**.

**B-Lymphocytes (B-Cells):** Cells of the immune system which are differentiated a developed in the bursa of Fabricius.

**Body cavity:** In birds, there is no diaphragm. In mammals, diaphragm separates thoracic and abdominal cavity. Therefore, cavity in the body of the birds is only one and is referred to as **'body cavity'**, and not as 'abdominal cavity'.

**Broad-Spectrum Antibiotic:** An antibiotic that stops the growth of many kinds of organisms. The more numerous the kinds of organisms, the wider is the spectrum.

**Bursa of Fabricius:** A sac-like organ touching the upper part of cloaca, involved in the processing and maturation of cells of the immune system.

**Cancer:** A mass of abnormal tissue that grows independently without any control of the body, serves no useful function, and kills the bird.

**Carrier:** A bird that shows no evidence of a disease, yet harbours (carries) the organism, and is capable of transmitting the disease to others.

**Caseous:** Cheesy (like cheese) in appearance.

**Catarrhal Inflammation:** Inflammation of the mucous membrane, usually of the respiratory tract.

**Cellulitis:** Inflammation of the deep tissues under the skin.

**Chronic Disease:** A disease which has a long duration, and is associated with sickness (morbidity) rather than death (mortality). Not acute (see 'acute disease').

**Coccidiostat:** A chemical compound added to the feed, or drinking water, to control coccidiosis by stopping growth of coccidia.

**Contagious Disease:** An infectious disease which is readily transmitted to other birds.

**Culture (noun):** Micro-organisms grown on artificial media in a laboratory.

**Cyanosis:** Bluish colour of an organ as a result of lack of oxygen.

**Dermatitis:** Inflammation of the skin.

**Disease:** Illness of the body, caused by infection or internal disorder.

**Disinfectant:** A compound used to kill disease-producing organisms. It is usually applied to inanimate (not living) objects.

**Endemic:** A disease which is regularly found in a particular area.

**Enteritis:** Inflammation of the intestine.

**Erythrocyte:** A red blood cell. It transports oxygen.

**Exudate:** Inflammatory fluid.

**Fomites:** Inanimate (not living) objects, such as clothes, equipment, etc. that mechanically carry and transmit disease-producing organisms.

**Gangrene:** Putrefaction of dead tissue in the living body.

**Gram-positive/negative:** This refers to the Gram's staining technique used for identification of bacteria.

**Haemorrhage:** Escape of blood from the blood vessels.

**Hepatitis:** Inflammation of the liver.

**Horizontal transmission:** Spread of infection from bird to bird by direct or indirect contact (Fig. 1).

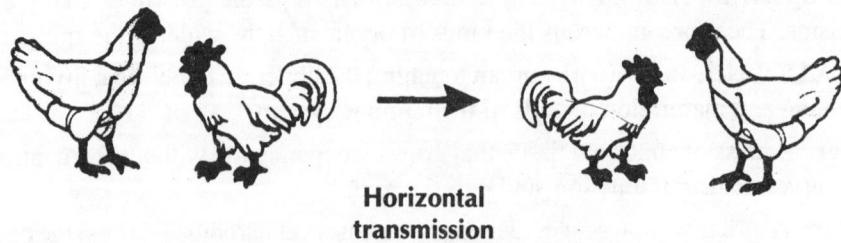

**Horizontal
transmission**

**Fig. 1.** Horizontal transmission.

**Host:** A bird that supports a parasite or a disease-producing organism.

**Host-specific:** An organism confined to a single host species.

**Immune:** Protected against a particular antigen (infectious agent).

**Immunity:** A condition of being able to resist a particular disease, by preventing the development of that disease-producing organism.

**Immunosuppression:** Immunosuppression means suppression of the natural immune responses. Certain diseases and other conditions affect the developing bursa of Fabricius and thymus in the young chick. These conditions cause destruction of the bursa and thymus in varying amounts. This results in suppression of the immune responses, known as **'immunosuppression'.**

**Inclusion Body:** An accumulation of virus particles found in the cells when the bird is infected with certain diseases.

**Incubation Period:** The period between exposure to infection and appearance of the first symptoms.

**Induced Immunity:** Immunity resulting from vaccination.

**Infection:** The entry of a disease-producing organism into a susceptible bird.

**Infectious Disease:** A disease produced by the entry of a disease-producing organism.

**Latent:** An infection that remains hidden or dormant (inactive), but may become visible at a later time.

**Lateral Transmission:** Spread of infection from bird to bird by direct or indirect contact.

**Lesion:** An abnormal structural alteration in the tissue, whether gross or microscopic, following disease.

**Lymphocyte:** A type of white blood cell. These are produced in increased numbers during an infection and are involved in controlling the disease.

**Lyophilization:** Stabilization of biological materials by rapid freeze-drying.

**Maternal Antibody:** Antibody passed from hen to the chick through the egg.

**Memory Cells:** Lymphocytes that 'remember' previous immune responses. They have the ability to produce an increased response against infectious agent as compared with lymphocytes that had not previously met the infectious agent.

**Micro-organism:** Living organisms that are too small to be seen without the help of a microscope.

**Morbidity:** Diseased birds in a flock.

**Mortality:** Birds that have died. It is usually expressed as a percentage.

**Mucosa:** Mucous membrane.

**Mucous Membrane:** A membrane rich in mucous glands. They line body passages and cavities, mainly respiratory and digestive tract.

**Mucus:** A sticky wet liquid secreted by mucous membranes and glands.

**Mycosis:** Any disease caused by a fungus.

**Necropsy:** Postmortem examination of an animal or bird.

**Necrosis:** Local death of cells or tissue within the living body. Adjective is 'necrotic'.

**Neoplasm:** A mass of abnormal tissue that grows independently without any control of the body, serves no useful function, and kills the bird.

**Oedema:** An excess of fluid in body tissues.

**Opisthotonus:** A sitting position in which neck is arched and the head rests on the back.

**Parasite:** An organism that lives in or on another organism, from which it derives its nourishment.

**Passive Immunity:** Immunity (antibodies) passed from the hen to the chick through the egg.

**Pathogen:** An organism capable of causing disease. Adjective is 'pathogenic'.

**Pathogenicity:** The capability of an organism to produce a disease.

**Peracute Disease:** A disease which is very acute or violent.

**Pericarditis:** Inflammation of the sac surrounding the heart.

**Peritonitis:** Inflammation of the peritoneum, a membrane in the body cavity.

**Perosis:** Deformity of the long bones.

**Plasma:** The clear liquid remaining after the cells have been removed from the blood.

**Polyvalent:** A vaccine containing several strains of an organism or organisms.

**Prebiotic:** A prebiotic is a non-digestible food ingredient. It is an indigestible carbohydrate that selectively stimulates the growth and/or activity of one or a limited number of bacterial species already present in the intestine of chickens. It thus improves bird's health. Examples: mannose, lactose, fructo-oligosaccharide (FOS), and mannan-oligosaccharide (MOS).

**Predispose (verb):** To make susceptible (prone) to disease.

**Predisposing Factor:** A factor that makes bird susceptible to a particular disease.

**Predisposition:** A tendency to develop a certain disease.

**Probiotic:** A probiotic is a live microbial feed supplement, which beneficially affects the chicken by improving its intestinal microbial balance.

**Rales:** Abnormal respiratory sounds.

**Renal:** Relating to the kidneys.

**Rodents:** A group of small animals with strong sharp front teeth, such as rats, mice, squirrels and beavers.

**Sanitizer:** A preparation capable of reducing the number of bacteria present. When added to water, it is called a 'water sanitizer'.

**Saprophyte:** An organism (bacteria) that grows on decomposing (decaying) organic matter. It is not a disease-producing organism.

**Septicaemia:** Invasion of the bloodstream by disease-producing micro-organisms.

**Serological Test:** A test performed on blood serum to determine the presence or absence of specific antibodies.

**Serotype:** A particular strain of a micro-organism.

**Serum:** The clear fluid remaining after the cells and clotting properties have been removed from the blood.

**Stress:** Anything that negatively affects the bird's well-being.

**Subclinical Disease:** A disease that produces so mild effects that they are not visible. That is, a very mild form of the disease.

**Synbiotic:** A synbiotic is a combination of probiotic and prebiotic. This combination improves the survival of the probiotic organism because its specific substrate is available. This is in the benefit of the chicken, both from micro-organisms and prebiotic. Examples: fructo-oligosaccharide (FOS) and bifidobacteria, and lactitol and lactobacilli.

**Syndrome:** A group of symptoms common to a specific disease.

**Tendon:** A tough dense tissue that unites a muscle to bone.

**Tendon Sheath:** Dense fibrous tissue covering of a tendon.

**Tenosynovitis:** Inflammation of a tendon sheath.

**Titre:** A value placed on the potency of a vaccine. It is the relative concentration of the specific antibody being measured in the blood/serum.

**T-Lymphocytes (T-cells):** Cells of the immune system that differentiate and develop in the thymus.

**Torticollis:** Twisting of the neck to one side.

**Tumour:** A mass of abnormal tissue that grows independently without any control of the body, serves no useful function, and kills the bird.

**Vaccine:** A preparation of micro-organisms (killed or living) which when given to the bird produces or increases immunity against specific disease.

**Variant:** One that shows variation. Regarding micro-organisms, one that is serologically, or physiologically different from the original form. It is usually the result of a mutation. Mutation is a basic change in form or structure. It results in a new type of micro-organism called 'variant'.

**Vector:** A living entity that carries and transmits a disease or parasite to poultry, such as the earthworm, which carries the chicken tapeworm eggs.

**Vermin:** Insects (such as lice, mites) and rodents (rats, mice) that spread disease, or cause damage.

**Vertical Transmission:** Spread of an organism (usually a virus) from hen to the chick through the egg (Fig. 2).

**Virulence:** The relative ability of a micro-organism to attack the bird and produce disease. That is, its disease-producing power/capacity.

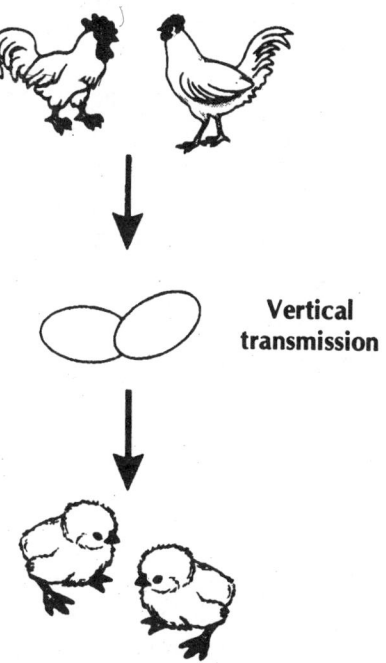

Vertical transmission

**Fig. 2.** Vertical transmission.

**Virus:** Infectious agents which are too small to be seen by a light microscope. They multiply only in living host cells. Some are capable of causing disease.

**Water Sanitizer:** A preparation capable of reducing number of bacteria in water to a safe level.

# Chapter 3

# Viral Diseases

**V**iruses are infectious agents that are too small to be seen by a light microscope. They are the smallest and simplest of all life forms. All other micro-organisms, such as bacteria, mycoplasma, chlamydia and protozoa occur in cell forms, **whereas viruses are not cells.** They contain mainly nucleic acid, RNA (ribonucleic acid) or DNA (deoxyribonucleic acid), **but not both. Thus, viruses are classified either as a RNA or DNA virus.**

Until a virus enters a cell, it is more dead than alive. It is as lifeless as a speck of dust. **Alone, that is, on its own, a virus cannot multiply. It can multiply only in living host cells.** This is because it depends on the host-cell machinery for its protein synthesis and multiplication. Virus uses cell's enzymes to complete these processes. Viruses are specific in their need for certain enzymes and find out a location in the body where such enzymes are produced. Thus, some viruses may affect liver, some the bursa of Fabricius, others the respiratory tract, and so forth.

Viruses vary in size, from about 20 nanometres (nm) to 300 nm. They attack the host cells, and it is this invasion that is thought to produce the disease, rather than any toxin formed. When a virus attacks the cells lining the respiratory tract and airsacs, the cell walls are ruptured and become a point of entry for other viruses and bacteria. In many cases the disease developed by the primary invader virus may produce little damage to the bird, but the secondary invader bacteria, such as *Escherichia coli*, may cause serious disease.

Since viruses live and multiply only within a cell, **antibiotics are of no value against diseases caused by viruses.** This is because antibiotics cannot penetrate into the cell and kill the virus. Bacteria, on the other hand, mostly multiply outside the cells. **Therefore, antibiotics can be successfully used to treat bacterial diseases in poultry.** However, antibiotics are sometimes given in viral disease outbreaks to prevent secondary infections with bacteria like *E. coli.*

**To conclude,** as viruses use the machinery of the host cell for reproduction, it becomes necessary to stop that machinery being used to prevent growth of the virus. Otherwise, it would damage those cells that are being targeted by that virus. This, in turn, would harm chicken. **As antibiotics are of no help in treating the viral infections, the most practical way to control the viral diseases in poultry and prevent losses is through timely vaccination.**

Viral diseases are among the most important of poultry diseases, and include dreadful infections like Ranikhet and Gumboro, which pose a real challenge to poultry farmers and each year, inflict heavy losses on poultry industry.

# RANIKHET DISEASE (NEWCASTLE DISEASE)

Also known as **'Newcastle disease (ND)'**, Ranikhet disease (RD) is a sudden and severe, rapidly spreading disease of poultry caused by a paramyxovirus. The disease is characterized by rapid onset, respiratory symptoms, also nervous manifestations, and varying mortality. It is worldwide in distribution. **In India, Ranikhet is the most dreaded viral disease of poultry and is, without doubt, number one in causing deaths every year.**

The first outbreaks of Newcastle disease were recorded in 1926, in Java, Indonesia, and in the same year, also in the town of Newcastle, in England. The name **'Newcastle disease'** was given because of its **first reporting from Newcastle.** In India, the disease was first reported from **Ranikhet**, a small town in Kumaon hills, District Nainital, Uttaranchal, in 1927, hence the name **'Ranikhet disease'.**

## Cause

Ranikhet disease is caused by a group of closely related viruses which form the avian paramyxovirus type 1 serotype. **There is only one serotype.** Paramyxoviruses are **enveloped**, single-stranded RNA viruses. Considerable antigenic variation exists between different strains of Ranikhet disease virus. Based on the nature of disease, **Ranikhet disease viruses have been divided into five groups.**

1.  Highly powerful disease-producing Ranikhet disease viruses **(viscerotropic velogenic viruses).** These viruses cause the most severe form of disease in which haemorrhagic changes are present in the intestines.

2.  Highly powerful disease-producing Ranikhet disease viruses which cause high mortality following respiratory and nervous symptoms **(neurotropic velogenic viruses).**

3.  Moderately powerful disease-producing Ranikhet disease viruses **(mesogenic viruses)** cause respiratory and sometimes nervous symptoms, with low mortality.

4.  Viruses which cause mild, or not clearly noticeable respiratory infection **(lentogenic respiratory viruses), and**

5.  Viruses that cause intestinal infection without showing any symptoms **(asymptomatic enteric viruses).**

## Disease

The severity of the disease depends mainly on the strain of virus, but dose, route of entry, age of the chicken, and environmental conditions all have an effect. With powerful viruses in the field young birds die suddenly without showing symptoms, while in older birds, the disease lasts longer and has characteristic symptoms. Infections through nose, mouth, or eye produce mainly respiratory form of the disease.

After infection it takes between 2 to 15 days (average 5-6 days) for the symptoms to appear. The speed with which symptoms appear depends on the infecting virus, age and immune status of the birds, infection with other organisms, environmental conditions, stress factors, route of infection, and dose of the virus.

## Spread

As Ranikhet disease virus is easily spread, **the disease is highly contagious. Methods of spread include:**

1. **Infection occurs through inhalation or ingestion,** and spread from one bird to another depends on the organs in which the virus grows, and also on the availability of the virus in an infectious form. Birds showing respiratory disease shed virus in fine particles of mucus (a respiratory tract secretion) suspended in air which may be inhaled by susceptible birds. **Coughing dislodges the virus, which then easily becomes airborne.** Viruses that are mainly limited to intestinal growth may be spread by ingestion of infected faeces, either directly or in contaminated food or water, or by inhalation of small infective particles produced from dried faeces.

2. Viruses transmitted by the respiratory route under crowded conditions, such as in an intensive broiler house, may spread extremely rapidly. On the other hand, viruses excreted in the faeces and spread mainly through the ingestion of contaminated feed or water by faeces, may spread very slowly, especially if birds are not in direct contact, such as layers in cages.

3. An important factor in the spread of Ranikhet disease is the **ability of the virus to survive in the dead bird or excretions** (waste products eliminated from the body). **In infected carcasses, virus may survive for several weeks at cool temperatures,** or several years if held frozen. **Faeces in which virus may be present in high concentrations is also an excellent medium for the survival of the virus, and even at $37^0$ C faeces remains infective for over a month.**

4. **Humans** play a very important role in the spread of Ranikhet disease virus. Spread usually is by the movement of live birds, substances capable of carrying infection (fomites), people, and poultry products (including dead birds and faeces for fertilizer) from affected premises to susceptible birds. Movement of people, contaminated vehicles, and fumigated eggs thus spread the virus.

5. Wild birds and other wildlife can also spread the disease, either by infection or by mechanical transfer, but their exact role has not been fully clarified.

6. Spread of virus from hen to progeny through the egg (vertical transmission) is

controversial.

7.  Cracked or broken infected eggs may serve as a source of virus for newly hatched chicks. In addition, the virus-rich faeces may contaminate the outside of eggs.

8.  Virus may also penetrate the shell after laying of an egg.

**The following methods of spread of Ranikhet disease virus have been involved in various outbreaks.**

1.  Spread through the air (airborne spread)

2.  Movement of people and equipment

3.  Contaminated poultry feed

4.  Contaminated water

5.  Contaminated vaccines

6.  Movement of poultry products

7.  Movement of live birds – wild birds, pet/exotic birds, game birds, racing pigeons and commercial poultry

8.  Movement of other animals

The importance of any of these factors depends on the situation in which the outbreak occurs. For example, in Great Britain, outbreaks of Newcastle disease were spread by feed that had been contaminated by infected wild pigeons.

Without doubt, the greatest possibility for spread of Ranikhet disease virus is by **humans and their equipment.** Humans may be infected in the conjunctival sac of the eye with the virus, and this then becomes a method of spread. However, a more common method is the mechanical transfer of the infectious material (usually faeces). Modern transport enables people to travel rapidly to any country in the world. **Therefore, spread by humans should not be treated as only a local or national threat.**

People carrying out vaccination (vaccinators), who move from farm to farm, have been involved in the spread of virus, as also the contamination of vaccines.

## Symptoms

As already mentioned, the disease which occurs following infection varies greatly with the type of virus. In addition, the immune status, and age and condition under which the chicks are reared, also influence the symptoms. Moreover, the presence of other organisms may make even the mildest of the disease more serious. Therefore, no symptoms can be considered as characteristic of the disease.

The **most harmful (highly virulent) viruses** may produce very severe (peracute) infections, the first indication of the disease being sudden death. Symptoms such as depression, weakness, lying down, increased respiration, diarrhoea, swelling of the face, and nervous signs may occur, ending in exhaustion and death. Green diarrhoea is usually seen in birds that do not die early in infection. Also, before death, muscular tremors, twisting of the neck to one side (torticollis), paralysis of legs and wings, and arched position of the body (opisthotonus) may be present. Mortality usually reaches 100% in flocks of fully susceptible chicks. In the adult chicken, the early symptom is the appearance of shell-less or soft-shelled eggs, followed by complete stoppage of egg laying.

The **moderately harmful (moderately virulent, mesogenic)** viruses usually cause severe respiratory disease and respiratory symptoms, with mortality up to 50% or more. In adult birds, there may be a marked drop in egg production that may last for several weeks. Nervous symptoms may occur but are not common. Mortality is usually low, except in very young birds.

The **viruses** which are **only mildly harmful** may cause no disease, or mild respiratory distress. However, the presence of other organisms or poor management may cause disease similar to that seen with more harmful virus. Other organisms include avian pneumovirus, infectious bronchitis and vaccine strains of Ranikhet disease. **Even symptomless infections may result in loss of weight gain in broiler chickens.** In young birds severe respiratory problems can be seen, usually resulting in mortality.

## Postmortem Findings

No postmortem findings are characteristic for any form of Ranikhet disease. **Viruses which cause symptomless infections produce no changes (lesions).**

The most harmful viruses usually cause haemorrhagic lesions of the intestinal tract. These are usually prominent in the proventriculus, caeca and small intestine. **The lesions include pinpoint haemorrhages** (i.e. small) **on the tips of the proventricular glands,** or bigger haemorrhages in the lining (mucosa) of the proventriculus; **enlarged and haemorrhagic caecal tonsils;** and **haemorrhagic lesions in the intestinal wall (in the lymphoid aggregates).** Spleen shows necrosis (white spots of dead tissue) on its outer surface, and also on the cut surface.

Viruses which cause respiratory disease may produce marked congestion of trachea, often with haemorrhages. The airsacs may be inflamed (airsacculitis) and appear cloudy and congested. Also, thickening of the airsacs with mucus (respiratory tract secretion) or cheesy inflammatory mass (caseous exudate) may be observed. However, gross changes are not always present in the respiratory tract.

Laying hens infected with powerful viruses usually show egg yolk in the abdominal cavity. The ovarian follicles are often soft, lack firmness and show haemorrhagic blood spots. Haemorrhage and discoloration of the other reproductive organs may occur.

## Immunity

### 1. Cell-Mediated Immunity

The initial immune response to infection is cell-mediated (i.e. protection through cells). (To understand the nature of cell-mediated and antibody-mediated immunity, refer to chapter 32: **"The avian immune system"**). This may be detected as early as 2-3 days after infection with live vaccine strains. This explains the early protection in vaccinated birds before a significant antibody response is seen. However, the importance of cell-mediated immunity in protection given by vaccines is not entirely clear.

### 2. Antibody-Mediated Immunity (Humoral Immunity)

Following vaccination, antibodies which protect the birds against Ranikhet disease, are produced. These antibodies are present in blood and can be measured by virus neutralization (VN) tests. Since the virus neutralization response is similar to the haemagglutination inhibition (HI) response, haemagglutination inhibition test is usually used to measure the protective response, especially after vaccination. These antibodies neutralize the Ranikhet disease viruses and thus protect the bird.

When chickens survive Ranikhet disease, antibodies can usually be detected in the serum within 6-10 days. The levels depend mainly on the strain of infecting virus, but generally peak response is at about 3-4 weeks. Decrease in antibody level is much slower than its development. Haemagglutination inhibition antibodies may remain detectable for up to one year in birds recovered from infection with moderately powerful disease-producing viruses (mesogenic viruses), or after a series of vaccinations. Re-infection, or vaccination some weeks after the level begins to decrease, produces a secondary response.

### 3. Local Immunity

Antibodies appear in the secretions of the upper respiratory tract and intestinal tract of chickens at about the same time when antibodies in the blood are first detected. In the upper respiratory tract, the antibodies (immunoglobulins) are mainly IgA, with some IgG. (For information on the nature of IgA, IgG and IgM antibodies, refer to chapter 32: **"The avian immune system"**). Similar antibodies can occur in Harderian gland following eye infection. (Harderian gland is a lymphoid organ located near the eye. It plays a role in the immune protection of the bird).

The exact function of local immunity in protection is not clear, although it is believed that it protects the respiratory tract independently of antibodies in the blood (humoral immunity). Vaccination in the eye with B1strain results in the growth of virus in the Harderian gland. This growth can be prevented by the presence of maternal IgG (i.e. IgG antibody obtained from hen) in tears (lachrymal fluid). Growth of virus in the Harderian gland results in the production of IgG, IgA and IgM in tears. In particular, the Harderian gland becomes the main site for IgA-antibody forming cells in the chicken. However, IgM may be the main antibody in the clearance of virus in eye infections.

## 4. Passive Immunity

Hens with antibodies to Ranikhet disease virus pass them to their progeny (i.e. newly hatched chicks) through the egg yolk. Levels of antibody in the day old chicks directly depend on levels in the hen. Maternal immunity (i.e. antibodies received from the hen) is protective, and thus must be taken into consideration when deciding the first vaccination of chicks.

## Immunosuppression

Immunosuppression means suppression of the immune response. This occurs due to infection with other viruses, such as Gumboro disease virus. The resulting inability of the bird to produce antibodies (immunoglobulins) has double effects. Firstly, it may result in a more severe Ranikhet disease, and secondly, such immunodeficient birds fail to respond adequately to vaccination (see **'Gumboro disease'** and **'vaccination failure'**). Immunosuppression from chicken infectious anaemia virus is also involved in the failure of birds to respond well to secondary killed Ranikhet disease virus vaccine.

## Diagnosis

1. None of the symptoms or postmortem findings may be considered as characteristic. At best, these can only indicate the presence of Ranikhet disease. However, the presence of pinpoint haemorrhages on the tips of glands in the proventriculus can be taken as highly suggestive of Ranikhet disease.

2. Confirmation of diagnosis depends on the isolation of virus and its characterization. Samples from live birds should consist of both cloacal (or faeces) and tracheal swabs, regardless of the symptoms. From dead birds, samples should be taken from intestines, intestinal contents and trachea.

3. A wide range of serological tests may be used to detect antibodies to Ranikhet disease virus in poultry blood (serum). The most widely used test is **'haemagglutination inhibition (HI) test'. Good correlation has been reported between ELISA and haemagglutination inhibition test.**

4. The value of any serological method in the diagnosis of disease depends on the immune status of the birds and is therefore complicated in the case of Ranikhet disease by the extensive use of vaccines.

5. Haemagglutination inhibition and other tests are used to measure the immune status of vaccinated birds.

6. At present, the early confirmatory method for Ranikhet disease diagnosis is isolation of virus and its characterization.

# Control

The basic objective of control is either to prevent susceptible birds from getting infected, or to protect the susceptible birds through vaccination.

# Vaccination

The best way to control Ranikhet disease is through vaccination. Vaccination would result in immunity against infection and growth of the virus. **Although vaccination usually protects the birds against the disease, but virus growth and shedding may still occur, though at a reduced level.** It must be remembered, however, that **vaccination cannot be considered as an alternative to good management practice, biosecurity, or good hygiene in rearing poultry.**

Vaccines against Ranikhet disease are usually made from the lentogenic or mesogenic form of the virus, and to some degree give protection to all forms of the disease. Thus, there are three types of commercially available vaccines for Ranikhet disease:

1. Live least harmful vaccines (live lentogenic),

2. Moderately powerful vaccines (live mesogenic), and

3. Killed (inactivated) vaccines

1. **Live least harmful vaccines (live lentogenic vaccines)** are derived from field viruses which have low disease-producing power, but produce an adequate immunity. These vaccine strains are LaSota, Hitchner B1, F strain and V4. **Of these, F strain vaccine has the lowest disease-producing power.** B1 strain is slightly more effective than the F strain, whereas LaSota strain vaccine is a bit more powerful than these two. LaSota and B1 are the most widely used vaccines. However, LaSota is usually not used for the first vaccination, but often as a booster after one or more B1 strain / F strain vaccines. After LaSota-based vaccines are given, there is mild bird-to-bird spread. It will not prevent the drop in egg production, when adult birds are challenged with a velogenic strain.

   These vaccines can be given by eye drop, in the drinking water, or by machines producing sprays. Although administration of vaccines through sprays enables rapid vaccination of large numbers of birds and the immune response is particularly fast, the small particle size can penetrate deeply into the respiratory tract and result in reactions that can be most severe in fully susceptible birds. Use of sprays of LaSota vaccine on such birds may result in heavy mortality.

2. **Moderately powerful vaccines (live mesogenic),** such as **Mukteswar (R2B),** Roakin, Komarow and H (Hartfordshire) are prepared in the laboratory from virulent (harmful) strains. Their use is restricted to areas where there is a problem of Ranikhet

disease from virulent viruses. The method of administration varies with the strain. Some are given in drinking water, while others require intradermal injection (i.e. in the skin) in the wing web. **Mesogenic vaccine viruses are capable of causing severe disease and must only be given after primary (earlier) vaccination with least harmful viruses (live lentogenic vaccines).** Mesogenic vaccines are capable of producing a high secondary immune response.

3.  **Killed (inactivated) vaccines** are usually prepared from virus grown on egg, which is killed by treatment with formalin. Both harmful (virulent) and harmless (avirulent) viruses have been used for the preparation of killed vaccines. Killed vaccines are given to birds by intramuscular (into a muscle) or subcutaneous (under the skin) injection. Thus, in addition to their high production costs, they are also much more expensive to administer than live vaccines.

4.  The **time of administration** and the type of vaccine are extremely important in the effectiveness of Ranikhet disease vaccination. Many different factors must be considered in planning vaccination programmes. These include disease situation, availability of vaccines, presence of other organisms, size of flock, expected life of the flock, available labour, climatic conditions, economics of vaccination or type of vaccine, and past performance of vaccination programmes.

5.  **Maternal immunity** poses a particular problem in the vaccination against Ranikhet disease. (Maternal immunity means immunity due to maternal antibodies. Chicks get these antibodies from the hen through eggs.) This is because maternal immunity may prevent the effectiveness of primary vaccination. To avoid this problem, birds are either not given primary vaccination until they are of 3-4 weeks of age, or vaccinated with live virus at one day old by eye drop or coarse spray. This establishes infection in some birds, which then spread it to others as they become susceptible. This is followed by re-vaccination at 3-4 weeks of age. Killed vaccines have also been successfully used in one day old, maternally immune chicks.

6.  Except during outbreaks of Ranikhet disease, vaccination after 3 weeks of age is usually practised only in egg-laying birds. To maintain adequate antibody levels, either slightly more powerful live vaccines than the primary vaccines are given at regular intervals, or killed vaccines are used. The killed vaccines may be followed by mild live vaccines at intervals to maintain the immune response.

## Hygiene and Biosecurity

1.  Under field conditions vaccination alone is not sufficient to control Ranikhet disease. It must therefore be accompanied by good hygiene.

2.  Under poorly managed, overcrowded, badly ventilated conditions with unavoidable underlying bacterial load, even the mildest live vaccines can produce disease severe

enough to resemble Ranikhet disease caused by a powerful disease-producing virus. **Good hygiene accompanied by good management is therefore of the greatest importance at all times and not only during an outbreak of disease.**

3.   Hygiene measures should involve both maintaining the birds in a healthy environment and exercising some degree of biosecurity (see 'biosecurity'). Some form of security should be imposed on all farms and houses to prevent the easy entry of humans and fomites (substances that can carry infection). Vehicles should be thoroughly disinfected while entering and leaving premises. Any movement directly between premises, such as food deliveries, egg collection, dead carcass collection, etc. should be particularly avoided. Even provision of facilities for change of clothes and taking a shower (bath) for staff entering and leaving the farm is highly desirable.

**Note:** For a list of various commercially available Ranikhet disease vaccines, see Chapter 19 under **'Ranikhet disease vaccines'.**

## INFECTIOUS BURSAL DISEASE (GUMBORO DISEASE)

Also known as **'infectious bursitis'**, infectious bursal or Gumboro disease is an acute (i.e. sudden and severe), highly contagious viral infection of young chickens. It is an extremely important disease of poultry throughout the world. **In India, it takes a heavy toll of bird life every year.** The disease was first described in 1962 and was called **'avian nephrosis'** because of the severe kidney damage it caused. The name **'Gumboro disease'** was given as it was first recognized in the Gumboro district of Delaware, a state in U. S. A.

**The disease is of great economic importance for two reasons:** 1. Due to the heavy mortality it causes in the chickens of three weeks of age and older, and 2. Because of the severe and prolonged suppression of the natural immune responses **(immunosuppression)** in chickens infected at an early age. Immunosuppression can lead to vaccination failures (see **'vaccination failures'**), *Escherichia coli* infection, gangrenous dermatitis, and inclusion body hepatitis-anaemia syndrome. The morbidity (sickness) and mortality (deaths) resulting from these other diseases in many cases is greater than that from Gumboro disease itself.

Gumboro disease affects young chickens, usually between 21 and 42 days of age. The acute form (i.e. severe form) is characterized by sudden onset, short course and extensive destruction of lymphocytes (one type of white blood cell), particularly in the bursa of Fabricius and also in other lymphoid tissue. Milder forms of the disease occur and also infections not clearly visible, but all forms damage the immune response of young birds.

**In fact, Gumboro is a disease of the immune system.** The bursa of Fabricius plays an important role in the disease. Bursa is the place where B-lymphocytes develop which later form antibodies (see chapter 32: 'The avian immune system'). Gumboro disease virus settles in the bursa and causes severe damage to the organ. If chicks are infected before 3 weeks of age, there can be permanent damage to the immune system. The antibody formation can be reduced or stopped altogether. Bursa may return to normal size once the disease subsides. But the tissues of the bursa are partially or permanently damaged. **Although clinical disease is not seen in chicks below 3 weeks of age, but subclinical infection** (i.e. mild infection not showing symptoms) **can have an extremely damaging effect on the immune system.**

## Cause

Gumboro disease is caused by a birnavirus, which is a **non-enveloped**, double-stranded RNA virus. The virus has **two main serotypes: serotype 1 and serotype 2.** Serotype 2 does not produce disease, **but serotype 1 does. Serotype 1 has several strains.** Some strains are so mild that they do not produce disease, whereas others are so harmful that they cause up to **50% mortality.** In contrast to serotype 2 viruses, these viruses have an attraction (tropism) for B-lymphocytes of the bursa and cause depletion of this organ. (For information on B and T-lymphocytes, refer to chapter 32: 'The avian immune system').

Serotype 1 virus causes an infectious and highly contagious disease. Following infection of growing susceptible chicks, the virus is excreted in faeces for 10-14 days. **It is very stable** and remains highly infectious in the poultry environment for many months. Thus, **the hardy nature of the virus is an important reason for its persistent survival in poultry houses, even when thorough cleaning and disinfection procedures are followed.**

## Spread

1.  **Gumboro disease is highly contagious** and the virus continues to remain in the environment of poultry house. The virus survives between outbreaks due to its resistance to heat and disinfectants. **Houses, from which infected birds are removed, remain infective for other birds up to 122 days. Water, feed and droppings taken from infected pens are infectious even after 52 days.**

2.  **The most common route of infection is by mouth,** but eye and respiratory tract may also be important.

3.  **There is no evidence that Gumboro virus is transmitted through the egg, or that a true carrier state exists in recovered birds.**

4.  Litter mites and mealworms (larvae of various beetles) are infective for up to 8 weeks, and mechanical vector (transmitter) such as wild birds, humans, and vermin (insects, such as lice, mosquitoes; rats, mice etc.) play a part in the spread of virus.

# Disease

The incubation period (i.e. period between the entry of a virus and appearance of symptoms) is very short, and **symptoms of the disease are seen within 2-3 days after infection.** In fully susceptible flocks, the disease appears suddenly and there is a high morbidity (number of birds affected), usually reaching 100%. Mortality (deaths) may be mild, but can be as high as 20-30%. **It usually begins on the 3$^{rd}$ day following infection, reaches its peak, and decreases in a period of 5-7 days.** Very virulent (harmful) strains of Gumboro virus can cause mortality of 90% to 100% in 4 weeks old susceptible birds.

**The first outbreaks on a farm are usually the most severe (acute).** Recurrent outbreaks in subsequent batches are less severe and usually go unnoticed. Many infections are silent either due to age of birds (less than 3 weeks old), or infections may be from non-disease-producing strains, or infections may be in the presence of maternal antibody.

# Development of the Disease

Four to five hours after infection by mouth, virus is present in macrophages (large tissue cells) and lymphoid cells in the caeca. An hour later, virus is present in the small intestine. The virus first reaches the liver. It then enters the blood and is distributed to other tissues, including the bursa. **The bursa is thus infected through the blood** and by 11 hours many cells in the organ contain the virus. A second massive blood infection (viraemia) occurs when the virus infects other organs, including spleen, Harderian gland and thymus. (**Harderian gland** is a lymphoid organ located near the eye. It plays a role in the immune protection of the bird). **B-lymphocytes and their earlier stages are the main target cells,** although virus may be found in macrophages. (To understand the nature of T and B-lymphocytes, refer to chapter 32: **'The avian immune system'**).

In some birds **kidneys are swollen and may contain urate deposits.** These deposits are due to blocking of the ureters by a markedly swollen bursa. The cause of haemorrhage in the muscles is unknown.

**Depletion (disappearance) of B-lymphocytes from bursa following infection in early life can result in extremely poor immune responses against micro-organisms.** The harmful effects of the suppression of natural immune responses (immunosuppression) are lowered resistance to diseases, and poor responses to vaccines given during this time.

The period of greatest susceptibility is between 3 and 6 weeks of age. Chickens younger than 3 weeks do not show symptoms. However, as already stated earlier, this subclinical form is economically important because it causes severe immunosuppression in the chicken.

## Role of Maternal Antibody

Young chicks with maternal antibody (i.e. antibody obtained from the hen through the egg) are resistant (immune) to infection when antibody levels are high. But they become susceptible when antibody levels (titres) drop. Some of the more recent extremely powerful and harmful strains (very virulent strains) are capable of breaking through the maternal antibody at an earlier stage. Older birds, in which the bursa is reduced in size and disappears, are more resistant to infection and do not develop the disease.

## Symptoms

The severity of disease depends upon age, breed and maternal antibody level of the chick as well as on the disease-producing power (virulence) of the virus.

The disease is limited to growing birds. The acute (severe) form is seen in chicks between 3 and 6 weeks of age (i.e. between 21 and 42 days) and occurs within 2-3 days after infection. One of the earliest symptoms of disease in a flock is the tendency for some birds to pick at their own vents. Other symptoms include depression, **white watery diarrhoea**, soiled vents, loss of appetite, ruffled feathers, unwillingness to move, trembling, closed eyes, lying down in exhaustion, and finally, death. Morbidity (number of birds affected) varies from 10% to 100%, and mortality 0% to 20%, sometimes reaching 50%. Strains of very virulent Gumboro virus (vvIBDV) cause 90% to 100% mortality.

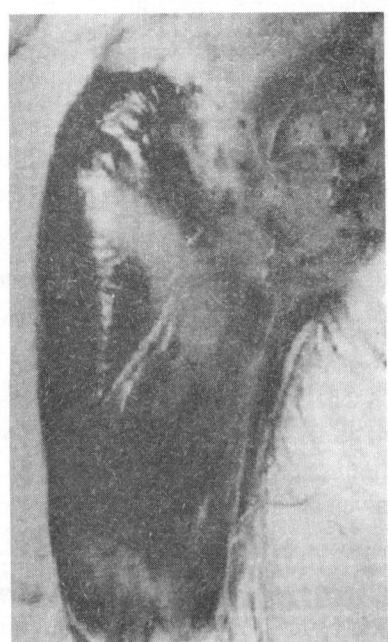

The mild form may not show any symptoms except poor growth, and sometimes an increase in the occurrence of other diseases. There is also a reduced response to vaccines.

The course of the disease in individual chicks is short, leading rapidly to death or recovery. However, in a flock where protective maternal antibody levels vary, the disease continues for a longer time with chicks dying when their antibody levels drop. **On the flock basis mortality reaches a peak 3-5 days after infection.**

## Postmortem Findings

Carcasses are dehydrated. Breast muscles are dark in colour. **Usually, haemorrhages are present in the thigh (Fig. 3)** and breast muscles, and sometimes on the lining (mucosa) of the proventriculus. There is increased mucus (a sticky fluid) on the intestine, and kidney changes are

**Fig. 3.** Haemorrhages in leg muscle typical of Gumboro disease.

prominent in birds that die, or are in the advanced stages of the disease. **Kidneys are swollen and white in appearance** due to dilatation of tubules with urates and fallen cells. Such changes are probably due to severe dehydration. In birds killed and examined during the course of disease, kidneys appear normal. The liver may be swollen and show areas of dead tissue near the margin.

As **bursa** is the primary target organ of the virus, it is important to understand the sequence of changes while examining birds at postmortem. On the 3rd day following infection, bursa begins to increase in size and weight because of accumulation of fluid (oedema) and more blood in the organ (hyperaemia). **By 4th day, bursa usually is double its normal weight and size**, and thereafter begins to decrease in size. By 5th day, the bursa returns to normal weight, but it continues to decrease in size. From the 8th day onward, it is about one-third its normal weight.

The **bursa** usually shows **necrotic foci** (areas of dead tissue), and **a cheesy mass** (caseous core) is found within its lumen from fallen cells of tissue. At times small and large **haemorrhages** on its inner surface (mucosal surface) are also seen. Sometimes widespread haemorrhages throughout the entire bursa are present **(Fig. 4)**. In such cases, birds may pass blood in their droppings.

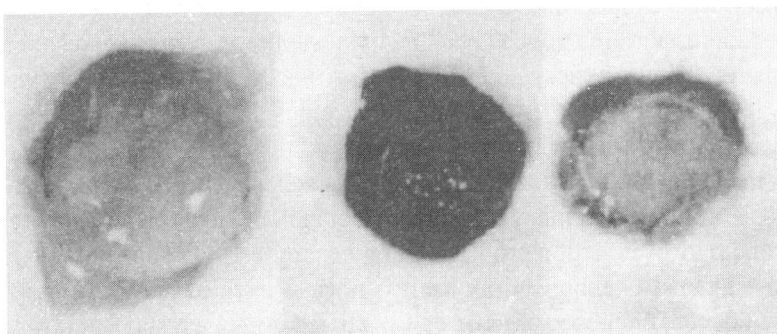

**Fig. 4.** Bursa of Fabricius from Gumboro disease. The swollen (oedematous) bursa on the left and haemorrhagic in the centre are typical of Gumboro disease. Bursa on the right is normal.

The spleen may be slightly enlarged and usually has small grey foci uniformly spread on the surface. Sometimes, haemorrhages are observed at the junction of the proventriculus and gizzard. Very virulent (harmful) strains of Gumboro virus also cause severe changes in the caecal tonsils, spleen, thymus and bone marrow, but changes in the bursa are similar.

# Immunity

## Active Immunity

Natural infection, or vaccination with either live or killed vaccines, stimulates active immunity. Antibody levels are normally very high after field exposure, or vaccination and virus neutralizing antibody titres greater than 1:1000 are common.

## Passive Immunity

Antibody transmitted from the hen, through the yolk of the egg, can protect chicks against early infection with Gumboro virus, and thus against the immunosuppression. The half life of maternal antibody is between 3 and 5 days. Therefore, if the antibody titre of the progeny is known, the time when chicks will become susceptible can be said. For example, it has been found that when antibody titres fall below1:100, chicks are 100% susceptible to infection. Titres from 1:100 to 1:600 give about 40% protection against infection. Titres must fall below 1:64 before chickens can be vaccinated effectively with a live vaccine. Use of killed vaccines to stimulate high levels of maternal immunity in parents is very common in the field. **Killed vaccines can stimulate adequate maternal immunity in parents to protect chicks for 4-5 weeks. Progeny from breeders vaccinated with live vaccines are protected for only 1-3 weeks.**

## Immunosuppression

Immunosuppression means suppression of the natural immune responses in the body. As a result, the bird fails to produce immunity and remains susceptible against infectious diseases. Gumboro virus produces profound immunosuppression. The effects of immunosuppression are in two ways. **Firstly**, it suppresses antibody response against vaccines, that is, following vaccination. This leads to vaccination failures (see **'vaccination failure'**). **Secondly**, not only is response to vaccines suppressed, but chicks infected early with Gumboro disease virus are more susceptible to *E. coli* infection, gangrenous dermatitis, infectious bronchitis, infectious laryngotracheitis, Marek's disease, coccidiosis, salmonellosis, chicken anaemia virus, and inclusion body hepatitis. It is interesting that while Gumboro virus infection produces immunosuppression against many organisms, the response against Gumboro virus itself is normal even in one day old susceptible chicks. The effect of Gumboro virus on cell-mediated immune responses is mild and less noticeable than that on antibody-mediated responses. (See chapter 32 for differences between cell-mediated and antibody-mediated immune responses).

## Diagnosis

1. The history, symptoms and postmortem findings are sufficient for the diagnosis of acute disease. In fact, **changes in the bursa are quite characteristic and confirm the diagnosis.**

2. In the case of disease without visible symptoms, or typical changes in the bursa at postmortem (subclinical cases), differential diagnosis from other diseases may be necessary. These include coccidiosis, Ranikhet disease, vitamin A deficiency, fatty liver and kidney syndrome, dehydration with swollen kidneys and excess renal urates, and haemorrhagic syndrome of muscles and other haemorrhages.

3.  Confirmation of the diagnosis can be made by enzyme-linked immunosorbent assay (ELISA), and isolation and identification of the causative agent. The bursa is the most commonly used tissue for isolation of the virus. **ELISA is the most commonly used serological test for the evaluation of Gumboro virus antibodies in poultry flocks.**

## Treatment

No curative or supportive treatment has been found to change the course of Gumboro disease.

## Control

1.  Due to the stable nature of the virus, and the large amounts excreted following infection, it is virtually impossible to remove all sources of infection once a rearing site has been contaminated.

2.  However, thorough cleaning and disinfection of houses between the flocks and the practice of **'all-in, all-out' management** reduces the virus. It may also delay infection. This would allow time for vaccines to produce immunity.

3.  It is known that contact with infected birds and substances that carry the infection (fomites) readily cause spread of the infection. Also, the relative stability of the virus to many physical and chemical agents increases the chances that it will be carried over from one flock to another. Therefore, the **hygiene and sanitary precautions** that are applied to prevent the spread of most poultry infections must also be strictly followed in the case of Gumboro disease.

4.  Formaldehyde and iodophors have been shown to be effective disinfectants. (See chapter 19 for a list of commercially available disinfectants).

5.  The possible involvement of other vectors, e.g. mealworms, mosquitoes and rats, has already been discussed. They could pose extra problems for the control of this infection.

6.  **Vaccination of chickens is the main method used for the control of Gumboro disease.** Especially important is the immunization of **breeder flocks** in order to provide **maternal antibodies to their progeny.** Such maternal antibodies protect the chicks from early infection. Maternal antibody will protect chicks for 1 to 3 weeks, but by boosting the immunity in breeder flocks with killed vaccines, passive immunity can be extended to 4 or 5 weeks.

7.  To obtain high levels of maternal antibody in progeny, parents are vaccinated between 4 and 10 weeks (some suggest between 10-14 weeks) of age with live vaccine, and again at about 16 weeks with killed vaccine. In the progeny, the maternal antibody levels decrease with time. These antibodies protect the bird against the disease up

to 2½ to 3½ weeks of age.

8.  **The main problem with vaccination of young passively immune chicks is in finding out the proper time of vaccination.** This varies with the level of maternal antibody, route of vaccination, and virulence (disease-producing power) of the vaccine virus. Monitoring of antibody levels in a breeder flock or its progeny (**antibody profiling**) can help in determining the proper time of vaccination.

9.  There are many choices for live vaccines. These are based on virulence and antigenic diversity. Generally vaccines prepared from strains of intermediate virulence and very mild virulence are used. Highly virulent, intermediate, and very mild strains overcome maternal antibody titres of 1:500, 1:250 and less than 1:100, respectively. Intermediate strains vary in their virulence and can cause bursal atrophy (reduction in the size of bursa) and immunosuppression in one day old chicks. If maternal antibody titres are less than 1:1000, chicks may be vaccinated by injection with very mild strains of virus.

10. Mild vaccine strains which cause no changes in bursa cannot be used in chicks with maternal antibodies until about 4 weeks of age as they are neutralized.

11. Moderately powerful vaccine strains (**intermediate strains**), that are less affected by maternal antibodies, can be given with some success as early as 2½-3 weeks depending on maternal antibody titres. As levels of maternal antibody vary within a flock and between flocks, repeated vaccination is practised by some in order to ensure that chicks are actively immunized as soon as the maternal antibody levels decrease to a level at which they do not neutralize the vaccine.

12. In countries where **antigenic variants** exist, chicks with maternal antibody to 'classical' strains become susceptible to infection at an early age with the variants. Live and killed vaccines for use in parent stock to provide maternal antibody therefore should contain both classical and variant strains to ensure broad-spectrum antibodies. Vaccines used for active immunization, however, need not contain variant strains as the antibody titres produced are sufficiently high to provide adequate cross-protection against current variants in the field.

13. **Killed vaccines are used to boost and prolong immunity in breeder flocks.** They are not used in young chickens. Killed vaccines are most effective in chickens that have been 'primed' with live virus in the form of vaccine. **Antibody profiling of breeder flocks should be done to assess effectiveness of vaccination and persistence of antibody.**

14. A common vaccination programme cannot be given because of the variability in maternal immunity, management and operational conditions that exist. Vaccination timing with mild and intermediate vaccines varies from as early as 7 days to 2 or 3 weeks.

**Note:** For a list of various commercially available Gumboro disease vaccines, see chapter 19 under **'Gumboro or infectious bursal disease vaccines'**.

# INFECTIOUS BRONCHITIS

Infectious bronchitis (IB) is a sudden, rapid, highly contagious respiratory disease of chickens characterized by abnormal respiratory sounds, coughing and sneezing. It affects chickens in every part of the world, and is a serious problem in India. It is **an important disease of young chicks,** causing high mortality. Besides causing disease of the respiratory tract, **the virus may also affect kidneys.** In fact, some strains specifically cause kidney changes which lead to higher than expected flock mortality. In laying birds, infectious bronchitis causes great economic loss through reduced egg production, watery albumen, and poor eggshell quality.

Infectious bronchitis is also of great economic importance because **it causes poor weight gain and feed efficiency.** The losses from production are usually more important than losses from mortality.

## Cause

The disease is caused by a coronavirus. It is an **enveloped**, single-stranded RNA virus. **There are 20 or more serotypes of the virus.** Some of the serotypes produce cross-immunity while others do not. **Coronaviruses have a natural tendency to undergo genetic mutation. This can lead to new field strains against which present vaccines may not give protection.** Therefore, it is best not to add new vaccine strains to any region when the specific serotype prevalent there has not been isolated. If this is not done, it may introduce new disease-producing strains, or induce mutations of field strains present.

**The best known serotypes include:**

1. Massachusetts
2. Connecticut
3. Holland
4. Arkansas-99
5. JMK, and
6. Florida

Of these, **Massachusetts** is the most common and also produces the most severe type of disease. It produces cross-immunity with the Connecticut strain. Both Massachusetts and Connecticut serotypes have a natural tendency for the respiratory tract. **Some serotypes cause kidney disease.** These serotypes are known as **'nephrotropic'** or **'nephropathogenic'.** Also, new serotypes appear from time to time.

Recently a serotype has been isolated which shows a tendency for the digestive tract. **Simultaneous infection of chickens with more than one serotype occurs.**

The **survival of the virus outside the bird** under farm conditions is believed to be from weeks to months. However, the virus is rapidly killed by common disinfectants.

## Disease

Birds of all ages are susceptible, but the disease is most severe in **young chicks**, causing some mortality. As age increases, chickens become more resistant to effects on the kidneys and oviduct, and mortality due to infection.

**The respiratory form** is more severe in young chicks, and the kidney form is mainly seen in birds less than 10 weeks of age. Infection at hatching causes developmental abnormality of the oviduct. However, infection of birds during laying can also cause damage to oviduct.

**The immune status of the bird** can influence protection. For example, both maternal immunity (immunity due to antibodies obtained from the hen) and active immunization (either from natural infection or vaccination), may prevent or reduce disease and limit virus excretion. **There is evidence that onset of laying can cause excretion of virus which has perhaps been latent in the hen for some months previously. Probably this is associated with hormonal changes.**

Infections with other disease-producing micro-organisms occurring during the course of infectious bronchitis produce more severe and prolonged respiratory disease. These include viruses of Ranikhet disease and infectious laryngotracheitis and bacteria such as *Haemophilus paragallinarum, Escherichia coli, Mycoplasma gallisepticum* and *M. synoviae*. In the **nephritic (kidney) form** of the disease, male birds are more severely affected, and high protein rations (particularly meat meal) are aggravating factors. Chilling in brooding chicks can also intensify any form of disease. Immunosuppressive diseases (i.e. diseases that suppress the natural immune responses), such as infections with Gumboro virus, may reduce the protective immune response to vaccination or natural infection with infectious bronchitis virus.

## Spread

1.  **By the air.** It takes just a few of the virus particles to infect a bird. **As the virus is easily spread by air, inhaling infected air is the most important means of spread.** The virus is known to travel over long distances by this route. However, spread through **infected faeces** may also be important.

2.  **Spread by people** and virus-contaminated substances (i.e. **fomites**) can occur. **The virus has not shown to be egg-transmitted.**

3.  **Carriers** (birds which carry infection without showing symptoms) also spread the disease. The great source of infection is those birds in which the virus is rapidly

growing and is being excreted. **Birds may shed the virus for as long as 4 weeks after recovery.** Such birds also include those in which virus growth has been stimulated by such factors as the **onset of laying.**

4.   The kidney and other non-respiratory organs are sites of persistence of infectious bronchitis virus, from where it is periodically shed in nasal secretions and faeces.

## Symptoms

Infection may be without symptoms, or may result in symptoms which point to disease of the respiratory or reproductive systems. In addition, there may be depression and reduced growth. All birds in the flock become infected, but mortality is variable. Mortality may be as high as 25% or more in chickens less than 6 weeks of age, and is usually very slight in chickens above this age.

**The respiratory form is the most common in birds of all ages.** The symptoms include abnormal respiratory sounds, gasping and sneezing, watery nasal discharge, sometimes accompanied by eye discharge, and facial swelling. Symptoms may be seen within 1-3 days following infection in almost all birds in a susceptible flock, because the infection spreads rapidly. Mortality is very slight in the uncomplicated disease, except in birds during early brooding when it can reach 30% of the flock, especially in the absence of maternal antibody. Mortality, sometimes up to 30%, may occur even in the **kidney form** in broilers. The uncomplicated disease may last 10-14 days, but other infections along the course of infectious bronchitis may increase severity and duration of disease and mortality, especially in intensively kept broilers.

**There are two forms of the disease involving the reproductive tract.** The **most common** damages the fully functional oviduct during laying and results in reduced egg production and quality. Thus, reduced egg production may occur in flocks which become infected at the time of laying, or when production is reaching to a peak, or after the peak production. **Drop in production may sometimes be more than 50%.** Return to full laying may take 4-6 weeks, but the expected production is never reached. Respiratory symptoms may or may not occur with the drop in egg production.

Egg production may become normal 3-4 weeks after the first signs of disease, but it may be accompanied by fall in egg quality. Eggs may be smaller than normal, they may be deformed, lack in symmetry or show folds on the surface. The shells may show loss of pigment, have calcareous deposits (i.e. containing calcium carbonate), be thinner than normal, or the shell may be absent entirely. Internally, the albumen loses its viscosity (**'watery whites'** - the quality of being sticky and glutinous) and the chalazae are usually broken so that the yolk floats free. (Chalazae are the two strings that hold the yolk in position). Small haemorrhages may be seen in the albumen or yolk. In other words, the albumen is **'thin'** and **'watery'** without definite demarcation between the thick and thin albumen of the normal fresh egg **(Fig. 5).**

The **less common form** of the disease **of the reproductive tract** is associated with abnormal development of the oviduct following infection of very young chicks. The oviduct may fail to develop completely or partially. At maturity affected birds ovulate normally but the ova are not taken up by the badly formed oviduct, and are shed into the body cavity. Such birds go through the process of egg laying but fail to lay and are known as **'blind layers'**. In some cases ova may pass through the open but abnormal oviduct to give eggs of reduced quality regarding shell and albumen.

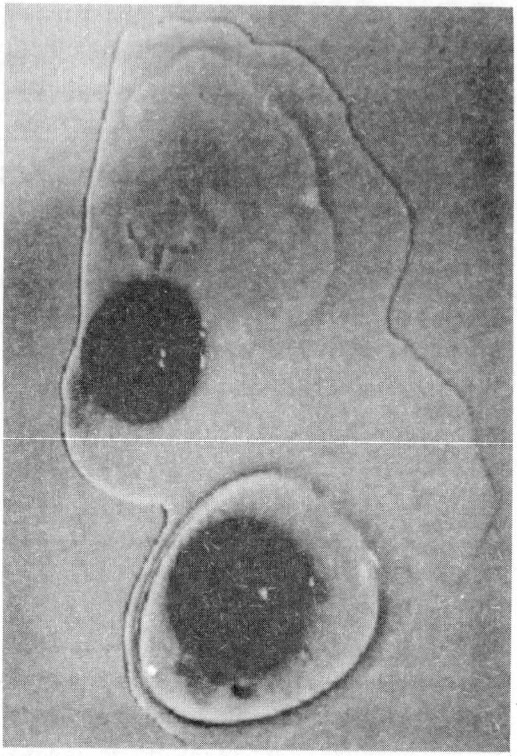

In the **kidney (nephritic) form** of the disease, there is marked depression, usually with respiratory symptoms and mortality as high as 30% of the flock in the **severe form**. This form usually affects young growing birds of 3-6 weeks of age. In the **milder form** there may be little or no mortality.

**Fig. 5.** Watery white. Contents of two eggs. The bottom egg is normal. The top egg is from a chicken with infectious bronchitis. Note that albumen is thin and watery without definite demarcation between thick and thin albumen of the normal fresh egg. The yolk is separated from the albumen and floats free.

During the last few years **another form of the disease** has been seen in which there are either very mild respiratory symptoms or no symptoms at all. There is a drop in egg production of 5-10% and reduction in the pigment of shells, some becoming completely white. In some cases production returns to normal in 2-3 weeks.

## Postmortem Findings

In the **mild respiratory form** there may be excess mucus in the respiratory tract. Lungs may be congested and airsac walls cloudy and thickened. **Airsacs** may contain a **yellow cheese-like mass (caseous exudate).** In the **more severe form, a caseous plug** may be found **in the lower trachea or bronchi** of chicks that die. In older chicks severe inflammation with reddening of the tracheal rings may be present.

Disease of the functional oviduct results in reduction in its size. Disease of the oviduct in the very young chick may result in varying degrees of abnormal development.

In the **kidney form**, the kidneys are swollen and pale, and the distended tubules are white with urates. The ureters are often distended with urates. In some birds there is **visceral gout**, in which case white granular material (urates) may coat the internal organs (see **'visceral gout'**).

## Diagnosis

1. The symptoms and postmortem findings may be suggestive, but are not diagnostic of infectious bronchitis.

2. The respiratory form may resemble the disease caused by other respiratory disease-producing micro-organisms, acting alone or in combination with others. Infectious bronchitis must be differentiated from other acute respiratory diseases, such as Ranikhet disease, infectious laryngotracheitis, and infectious coryza.

   Ranikhet disease is usually more severe than infectious bronchitis. Nervous symptoms may be seen with powerful strains of Ranikhet disease, and in the laying flocks drops in egg production may be more than with infectious bronchitis. Infectious laryngotracheitis spreads more slowly in a flock, but respiratory signs may be more severe than with infectious bronchitis. Infectious coryza can be differentiated on the basis of facial swelling which occurs only rarely in infectious bronchitis.

3. Decreased egg production and quality may be caused by a wide variety of factors, both infectious and non-infectious, including errors of management. Drop in production and shell quality problems in egg drop syndrome are similar to those seen with infectious bronchitis, except that internal egg quality is not affected in the case of egg drop syndrome.

4. Also there may be other causes of abnormal development of the oviduct, and kidney disease may be associated with nutritional deficiencies and unknown causes.

5. Confirmation of the disease depends on demonstration of the virus, or detection of specific antibodies in the sera. It is very easy to demonstrate the virus in the early stages of disease when it is growing most rapidly. **About 7-10 days after infection it is difficult to find the virus**. Serum samples can be tested by either ELISA or the haemagglutination inhibition (HI) test.

6. The most common method for the demonstration of virus is by inoculation of embryonated chicken eggs. Materials most likely to yield virus are trachea, lungs, airsacs, caecal tonsils, and kidneys in the kidney form.

## Treatment

There is no specific treatment for infectious bronchitis. In multiple infections, use of antibiotics may be recommended against *Escherichia coli* and mycoplasma. **In the kidney form** of disease, administration of electrolytes in the drinking water is useful.

## Control

1.  Management can be helpful if adequate attention is given to maintaining proper temperature and ventilation of young chicks.

2.  Treatment is of no value in the control of this virus. Also, because this virus is so commonly present everywhere and spreads rapidly, it is not practical to remove it by hygienic means in commercial operations. **Thus, control depends on increasing resistance of flocks by vaccination.**

3.  **Live and killed vaccines** are available and both have been shown to be of value. However, for killed vaccines to be effective, birds should have been **'primed'** with a live vaccine. To avoid interference, a period of at least 8 weeks should pass between the administration of live and killed vaccine.

4.  **It is important to note that outbreaks of infectious bronchitis often occur, even in vaccinated flocks. This is because the virus strains isolated from these outbreaks are usually, but not always, found to be a serotype different from the vaccine type.**

5.  Ideally, the live vaccine should contain serotypes of virus which will stimulate protection against those serotypes existing in a particular area. **The Massachusetts serotype of virus is the one most commonly included in commercial vaccines.** This is because it produces cross-immunity against many strains. However, depending on local circumstances it may be necessary to include other serotypes in order to obtain adequate protection.

6.  Live vaccines may be administered to day-old chicks by nasal route (through nose) or eye drop, and for older birds in the drinking water or even eye drop.

7.  The **schedule of vaccination** is usually planned for the type of flock involved, such as broilers, commercial layers and breeding birds. Whatever pattern is followed, **a very mild live virus vaccine is given first.** For broilers this may be given at hatching at the hatchery. It is given at this stage to prevent possible infections with such organisms as *E. coli* with which the disease appears at about 3 weeks of age. For other birds, the first vaccination is usually delayed until they are 3 weeks old and is given in the drinking water and may be followed at about 8 weeks by a second live vaccine. Several weeks before laying, a live, moderately strong vaccine may be given in the drinking water, or a killed vaccine is given intramuscularly.

8.  It is a common practice to give live vaccine against both infectious bronchitis and Ranikhet disease together at 3 weeks of age and at other times, and to give killed vaccines for infectious bronchitis, Ranikhet disease and Gumboro disease for breeding flocks a few weeks before laying.

**Important:** Broilers should be vaccinated only where the disease is a real problem. This is because the stress produced by bronchitis vaccination may cause greater flock morbidity (sickness) than the disease itself.

**Note:** For a list of various commercially available infectious bronchitis vaccines, see Chapter 19 under **"Infectious bronchitis vaccines".**

# INFECTIOUS LARYNGOTRACHEITIS

Also known as **'laryngotracheitis'**, infectious laryngotracheitis is an acute respiratory disease of chickens, caused by a herpesvirus. It may result in severe production losses due to mortality and decreased egg production. The disease is worldwide in distribution. Chickens of all ages are susceptible. Although the very young are the most susceptible, the disease is usually seen in birds between 3-9 months of age. In areas where the disease is prevalent, older birds are usually immune (resistant). In general males are more susceptible than females.

## Cause

The causal herpesvirus is an **enveloped**, double-stranded DNA virus. It affects only the respiratory tract and conjunctiva, and strains vary in their disease-producing power. The virus does not seem to be very highly invasive. **It does not enter the blood.** Multiplication of the virus is limited to respiratory tissues, and there is no viraemia (i.e. blood infection). It can survive away from the bird for several weeks under farm conditions, and longer when the environment is very cold. The disease becomes serious when other disease-producing agents, such as the viruses of Ranikhet disease, infectious bronchitis and fowl pox and also *Haemophilus paragallinarum* and *Mycoplasma gallisepticum,* occur at the same time. Deficiencies of vitamin A and excess of ammonia in the atmosphere also predispose to a more severe disease.

## Spread

1.  In affected birds, the virus is present in the discharges from nostrils, mouth, trachea and the conjunctiva. **The infection is spread by air. It enters into the body through the upper respiratory tract and conjunctiva.**

2.  Among recovered birds, and even in birds vaccinated with a live virus, **the virus can become latent.** That is, it is present but is not active and does not produce the disease. **Such birds become carriers of infection.** Thus, birds which appear healthy may excrete the virus from time to time for long periods, probably for several years. A number of factors, such as the movement of birds, handling, stress, and the onset of laying may bring about such excretion. The live affected bird is the most important source of infection and spread of disease, particularly in the early stages of infection. Movement of such birds, or even mildly affected birds or carriers, is an important method of spread.

3.  Because of the survival of the virus outside the body of the host, substances such as infected crates, receptacles, vehicles, equipment and buildings, and mechanical carriers such as people, wild birds, vermin (rodents, insects, etc.), and dogs and cats can be transmitters of the virus.

4.  **Spread through the egg is not known to occur,** and newly hatched chicks are free from infection.

## Symptoms

Infection may result in peracute (very severe), acute (severe), mild, or asymptomatic (without symptoms) disease. In the **peracute form**, the bird may be found dead without showing any symptoms, or they may show sudden severe respiratory distress with marked coughing and discharge of mucus and blood-stained material and blood clots from the mouth. This is followed by death in 1-3 days.

In the **acute form**, difficult breathing is a symptom but it is not as sudden in onset or as severe as in the peracute form. In some, obstruction of the trachea with exudates (inflammatory material) causes the bird to breathe with long gasps (i.e. quick deep breaths), with its head and neck upward and beak wide open. This is usually accompanied by a loud harsh cry. Abnormal respiratory sounds (rales) are always heard. In some birds there may be nasal discharge and conjunctivitis (inflammation of the conjunctiva of the eye). In birds with severe respiratory distress, there is cyanosis (bluish discoloration) of the face and wattles, and death usually occurs in 3-4 days. In other birds the respiratory distress first increases in severity and then subsides and recovery occurs in 2-3 weeks.

In the **mild form**, there may be respiratory sounds, slight coughing and head shaking, nasal discharge and conjunctivitis. Affected birds show depression and the more severely affected birds lie down on their hocks. Egg production is also affected and may stop completely for a time, but in uncomplicated cases it returns to normal.

The **asymptomatic form** occurs without symptoms and its presence may go undetected.

In some of the more severe outbreaks there is very high mortality and as many as 70% of the affected birds may die. In some outbreaks all forms of the disease may be seen, while in others only the milder form of the disease is present.

## Postmortem Findings

Postmortem findings vary with the severity of the disease, but in most cases are restricted to the upper respiratory tract. In the **peracute form**, there is haemorrhagic tracheitis. That is, the trachea is inflamed red and contains blood casts (blood moulded in the shape of trachea) throughout the entire or part of its length, or is filled with blood-stained mucus. The primary bronchi may also be affected.

In the **acute form** caseous exudate (i.e. cheesy inflammatory material), mucus and some haemorrhage occur in the trachea and usually produce obstructive plugs. Trachea itself is very congested and cyanotic (bluish). In the **mild form** there is excess of mucus in the trachea. The nares (nostrils) may show caseous exudate. Conjunctivitis is the most common eye lesion. Sometimes there may be caseous lesions in the larynx and this may be confused with the diphtheritic form of fowl pox, or with vitamin A deficiency. The lungs and airsacs are rarely affected, but there may be congestion of the lungs and some thickening of the airsacs.

## Diagnosis

1.  The history of disease, the region in which it occurs, and the symptoms and postmortem findings in the more severe forms in which there is gasping respiration and tracheal haemorrhage, are almost diagnostic of laryngotracheitis.

2.  However, the mild form cannot be differentiated on the basis of symptoms and postmortem findings from other mild respiratory diseases. In these cases, therefore, and for confirmation of infection, it is necessary to demonstrate the presence of virus, or antibodies to infectious laryngotracheitis virus. There are a number of ways by which the virus or the antibodies can be demonstrated, the most common being ELISA (enzyme linked immunosorbent assay).

3.  However, one of the diagnostic features is the presence of intranuclear inclusion bodies in the epithelial cells of trachea. These intranuclear inclusions can be demonstrated in tracheal sections following histological staining.

## Treatment

No drug has been shown to be effective in reducing the severity of disease. If a diagnosis of infectious laryngotracheitis is obtained early in an outbreak, vaccination of unaffected birds may produce adequate protection before they become exposed

## Control

1.  Use of **sound biosecurity measures** (see chapter 29: '**biosecurity**') will avoid exposure of susceptible chickens through contaminated material. The importance of **sanitation and hygiene** and prevention of movement of potentially contaminated people, feed, equipment, and birds is most important in the successful prevention and control of infectious laryngotracheitis. The virus is readily killed outside the body by disinfectants and warm temperatures. Thus, carry-over between successive flocks in a house can be prevented by adequate clean-up.

2.  Rodents (rats, mice, squirrels) and dog control measures should also be followed.

3.  In areas where the disease is prevalent, it is extremely difficult to prevent the entry of the virus into susceptible flocks, especially on continuous production sites. **In**

such circumstances vaccination is of value. For this purpose live vaccine is used. It produces very good immunity.

In high-risk areas it may be necessary to vaccinate at 1-3 days of age. In other areas vaccination may be delayed to any age between 3 and 18 weeks. Birds may be vaccinated more than once at an interval of 2-3 weeks. The methods of vaccination include eye drop, in the drinking water, or rarely cloacal scarification. The immunity produced varies but usually persists in a flock for several months. Because protection is rapid following vaccination, it is worthwhile considering vaccination in the face of an outbreak, especially in early stages. Vaccination during an outbreak will both limit virus spread and shorten duration of the disease.

4.  A disadvantage of the use of live vaccine is the possible spread of the virus within a week or 10 days of vaccination, and the production of carriers since the virus can become latent. This may lead to infection becoming established. For these reasons, in areas where the disease is not a serious problem, but where an outbreak has occurred, it would be economically better to dispose of all the chickens and thoroughly clean and disinfect the houses before re-stocking with birds free of the infection.

## FOWL POX

Fowl pox is a viral disease characterized by **skin lesions** (changes). Although there is another form of the disease (**diphtheritic form**), in which lesions appear in the mouth and upper respiratory tract, this form of the disease is also usually associated with skin lesions in some chickens. The disease was once widely prevalent worldwide, including India, but with the arrival of vaccination the incidence has been greatly reduced, although in some areas it still continues to be of considerable economic importance.

## Cause

Fowl pox is caused by an avipoxvirus. It is **enveloped** and has double-stranded DNA. **It is the largest virus known. Strain variations exist,** but there is a varying degree of cross protection. It now appears that some variant strains do exist that are not protected by vaccination. **Fowl pox virus infects birds of both sexes, and all ages and breeds.**

## Spread

1.  Fowl pox virus does not penetrate intact skin. **Some break in the skin is required for the virus to enter the cells, grow, and cause disease.**

2.  Infection occurs through mechanical spread of the virus to the injured skin. **Individuals handling birds at the time of vaccination may carry the virus on their hands and clothes, and may unknowingly deposit the virus in the eyes of susceptible birds.**

3. Spread of the virus from one chicken to another **by direct contact** is a major factor in the spread of disease. Most of the spread is the result of birds picking, fighting, or scratching one another. However, it has been shown that certain biting insects, such as **mosquitoes**, transmit the disease and produce eye infection. In warm climates this can result in a rapid spread of disease. **Mosquitoes have been shown to be capable of infecting a number of different birds after a single feeding on a bird infected with fowl pox virus.** In some cases, the virus may enter the body of the mosquito and mosquito will remain a carrier for several months.

4. In a contaminated environment, presence of virus in the air from feathers and dried scabs containing fowl pox virus, may lead to skin and respiratory infection. **The virus can survive in dried scabs for months or even years.** Lining of the upper respiratory tract and mouth appears to be highly susceptible to the virus, because infection may occur in the absence of trauma or injury.

5. Bad sanitary and hygienic conditions help in the spread of the disease. Therefore, measures to reduce this are important in control.

## Development of the Disease

Virus enters a skin cell, and then spreads from cell to cell locally. Some virus enters the blood to cause a blood infection (viraemia). Although there is spread to internal organs, no changes are seen. However, it is likely that there is some viral growth in certain organs, such as the liver and spleen, and a secondary viraemia occurs. Virus can enter again into the skin cells and a generalized disease can occur, although this is rare.

## Symptoms and Lesions

**Fowl pox can occur at any age.** Maternal immunity has no effect. There are **two forms of the disease: 1. Cutaneous or skin form (dry pox), and 2. Diphtheritic form (wet pox).**

In the **skin form**, lesions appear on the unfeathered skin of the head (**Fig. 6**), neck, legs and feet. A **diphtheritic form** also occurs in which lesions are present in the upper respiratory and digestive tracts. However, the skin form is usually the most common in disease outbreaks. Its beginning in the flock is usually gradual, and it is not noticed until the skin lesions become visible. The disease spreads slowly, and in some cases it may last several weeks. Fowl pox can cause a drop in egg production in layers.

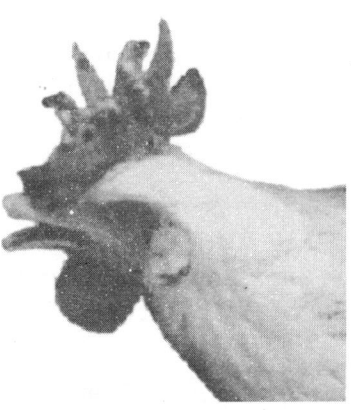

**Fig. 6.** Fowl pox lesions on the comb of an infected chicken.

**The skin lesions can vary in appearance.** First, there is **a papule** (a small raised red area) which rapidly progresses through the **vesicle** a small blister-like swelling containing fluid) to the **pustule** (small swelling containing pus), and finally to the **crust or scab stage.** In most outbreaks, this last reddish-brown to black scab stage is present on at least some of the chickens presented for diagnosis. After about two weeks the scab falls and a healed area is left which may or may not leave a scar.

In the **diphtheritic form (wet pox),** small white nodules are observed in the upper respiratory and digestive tracts. These nodules merge together to form raised yellow cheesy patches (plaques) on the mucous membranes (i.e. lining of the respiratory and digestive tracts). Most lesions are found in the mouth but others are present in the larynx, trachea, and oesophagus. These lesions may cause difficulty in breathing (dyspnoea) and/or loss of appetite. Lesions in the nares (nose) can give rise to nasal discharge, while those on the conjunctiva give rise to eye (ocular) discharge and in rare cases result in blindness. Mortality as high as 50% has been reported with the diphtheritic form, but is usually low.

Fowl pox in chickens usually causes weakness and poor weight gain. Egg production is temporarily stopped if layers are infected. The course of the disease is about 3-4 weeks, but if complications are present duration can be much longer.

## Diagnosis

1.  The presence of skin lesions is suggestive of fowl pox. No other poultry disease produces such lesions. In some outbreaks the diphtheritic form may be more common, but usually there are some birds with skin lesions.

2.  Bird transfer. A small amount of scab material from an infected bird is scratched on the surface of the comb of an uninfected bird. About 5 days later, typical pox lesions (scabs) appear when skin form is involved.

3.  Histological examination of the fowl pox lesions will show intracytoplasmic eosinophilic inclusions (**'Bollinger bodies'**). Material can be scraped from the lesions and smears made on the glass slides. Using the appropriate stain, Borrel bodies (virions) can be seen with the light microscope.

4.  The diphtheritic form is more difficult to diagnose on symptoms alone. The lesions are attached and if removed leave ulcers. This fact helps in differentiating fowl pox from infectious laryngotracheitis and vitamin A deficiency. However, in both forms of fowl pox, confirmation depends on the isolation of virus in material from the lesions.

5.  Infection may be diagnosed by serological means. Various tests have been used to detect fowl pox specific antibodies. The most sensitive test is the ELISA.

## Treatment

There is no satisfactory treatment.

## Control

1.  **Fowl pox can be prevented by vaccination**. Live vaccines are available. Various routes have been used for vaccination. **There are two main routes: the wing web and thigh.** In the former, vaccine is inoculated into the skin of the wing web, using a bifurcated needle, which has a grove that holds the vaccinal fluid. In the latter, feathers are removed from the thigh and vaccine brushed into the resulting follicles.

2.  Whichever method is used, the skin is examined 7-10 days later for the presence of pox lesions. A large number of birds should be examined in order to find whether the vaccine has been effective. If more than 10% of the birds do not have any lesions, then the vaccination has been unsuccessful.

    That is, about 10 days after vaccination, the birds should be examined for a **'take'**. If the vaccination has **'taken'**, a definite pox scab (lesion) will be seen on the wing-web where the puncture was made. If there is no scab, the birds should be re-vaccinated.

3.  **Vaccination is usually done in areas where fowl pox is prevalent, or there have been outbreaks in the past.** Most layers and breeders are vaccinated before they come into laying, that is. 3-5 weeks before egg production starts. It is best to vaccinate chickens when they are at least 6 weeks of age, but vaccination may be required earlier than this in some cases. In areas where fowl pox is prevalent, the first few affected birds should be culled (removed) and the remaining ones vaccinated. The vaccinated birds should be examined at regular intervals to check for any re-infection. Any affected birds are culled.

4.  Attenuated fowl pox vaccine is a mild form of pox vaccine. It gives good immunity without many of the side effects of fowl pox vaccine. However, it may not stand up to severe challenge. Pigeon pox vaccine is milder than fowl pox vaccine. Therefore, it can be used in cases where fowl pox vaccine produces a severe reaction, as in day-old or very young chicks, birds undergoing stress, or birds in egg production. In areas which have problems with the diphtheritic form, it has been found that pigeon pox vaccine may be helpful as a means of control.

5.  It is very important to follow the instructions given by the vaccine manufacturer. Do not vaccinate birds which are in poor condition, or under stress, or which are affected with any other condition. Because of the virulence (disease-producing power) of the vaccine virus, birds must be 5 weeks of age or older when vaccinated. **Precautions should be taken to minimize the spread of the vaccine virus,**

both on the birds and in the environment. **Being a live virus, it is capable of spreading the disease and therefore must be used carefully.** The entire flock should be vaccinated in a few days to prevent the vaccine from spreading to other areas in the house.

6.  Carcasses of dead or affected birds should be buried or burnt. After removal of the birds the house should be thoroughly disinfected, although the virus remains in the infected scabs and is difficult to clear from certain premises.

7.  A **mosquito-control programme** should also be made a part of the preventive procedure.

**Note:** For a list of various commercially available fowl pox vaccines, see Chapter 19 under **"Fowl pox vaccines"**.

# AVIAN INFLUENZA (BIRD FLU)

## Introduction

**Avian influenza**, commonly known as **'bird flu'**, has hit the country after all. After causing havoc in south-east Asian countries (Hong Kong, Vietnam, Laos, Cambodia, Indonesia, and Thailand) and the neighbouring Pakistan, avian influenza finally struck India in February 2006. Though brief, it inflicted heavy losses and jolted nation's economy. Poultry industry appeared paralyzed for a time, and fear of its spread to humans brought the industry to a virtual halt.

The disease had suddenly flared up in the Navapur area of Maharashtra and Gujarat, Jalgoan district of Maharashtra and Burhanpur district of Madhya Pradesh. Although a swift and rigorous action, jointly by the respective State Governments and Government of India, promptly brought the disease under control, poultry industry remains vulnerable nevertheless under the constant threat of bird flu, as the virus is not to go away that easily. On the contrary, it may stay, pose a threat to industry, and perhaps risk to humans. **It is on this account that the topic of 'bird flu' has been dealt with at some length, covering its all aspects, so that the latest information is readily available.** The basic theme is prevention of poultry losses, protection of the industry, and welfare of the people in view of its reportedly extremely rare human transmission.

## Definition

Avian influenza is a viral disease characterized by extremely high mortality. The virus affects the respiratory, digestive, and nervous system. Avian influenza viruses infect, besides chickens, a wide variety of wild and domestic birds, especially the free-living birds that live in or near water, such as ducks, geese, swans, shorebirds, gulls, terns (sea birds), doves, and others. **In fact, avian influenza (AI) viruses have been isolated from more than 90 species of free-living birds.** Migratory waterfowl, particularly ducks, have yielded more viruses than any other group. **However, most AI infections do not produce clinical disease in free-living birds.**

## History

Avian influenza is not a new disease. It was discovered 129 years ago in 1878 in Italy as **'fowl plague'**. It was so named because it dealt poultry a severe blow by causing heavy mortality. **'Plague'** is a Latin word and means **'blow'**. In 1901 its causative organism was shown to be a virus, but it was not until 1955 that its relationship to mammalian influenza A virus was demonstrated.

## Cause

Avian influenza virus is **an enveloped, single-stranded RNA virus.** Its surface is covered by two types of projections (Fig. 7). They are of glycoprotein. The **two projections** differ in shapes: (1) **Haemagglutinin (HA)** is a rod-shaped timer (i.e. made up of three subunits), and (2) **Neuraminidase (NA)** is a mushroom-shaped tetramer (made up of four subunits). AI viruses are classified on the basis of HA and NA surface antigens. At present there are **16 distinct (separate) HAs** and **9 distinct NAs.** Each virus contains one HA and NA subtype. Thus, there can be 144 subtypes. These are identified by haemagglutinin (H) and neuraminidase (N) typing. Each subtype differs in its disease-producing ability (pathogenicity), capability to infect different species, and transmissibility. Although AI viruses can occur in numerous subtypes, the subtype H5N1 has caused most outbreaks, followed by H7N7, H7N3, H5N2, and others (given under **'Myth about H5 and H7 subtypes'**).

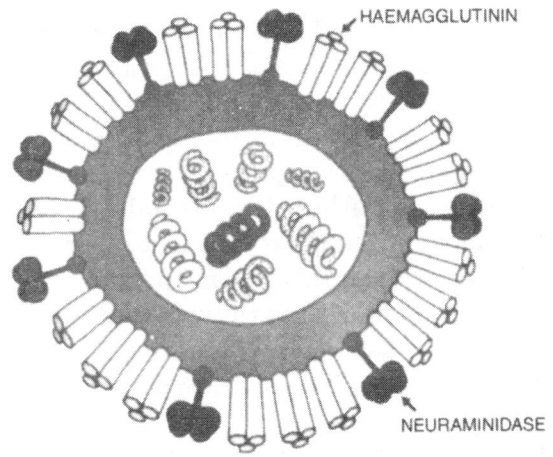

Fig. 7. Diagram of an **avian influenza virus.** Note **two projections** from its surface: (1) rod-shaped **haemagglutinin (HA),** and (ii) mushroom-shaped **neuraminidase (NA).** Its genome consists of **eight segments of single-stranded RNA** in the centre

Its genome (in the centre) consists of **eight segments of single-stranded RNA.**

The **haemagglutinin** is responsible for attachment of the virus to receptors present on the cell surface, and thus enables the virus to enter into the cell. On the other hand, **neuraminidase**, which is an enzyme, is responsible for release of the new virus from

43

the cell by its action on the neuraminic acid in the receptors. **Antibodies against HA and NA are important in protective immunity.** Antibodies against HA neutralize the virus and thus protect against infection. Antibodies against NA are also important in protection, by restricting the spread of the virus from infected cells.

The **viral genome** (genetic material) is composed of **eight segments of single-stranded RNA** that code for 10 proteins **(Fig. 7 )**.

## Chemical Composition

Avian influenza viruses are composed of 0.8-1.0% RNA, 5-8% carbohydrate, **20% lipid**, and 70% protein. **Lipids are present in the viral envelope** and are derived from the host cell.

## Growth of Virus within the Cell (Viral Replication)

**This process is very complex. Briefly,** the virus attaches to the host cell receptors containing sialic acid bound to glycoproteins. This initiates receptor-mediated endocytosis, that is, entry of virus into the cell. In the endosomes, that is, vesicles or sacs formed, envelope of the virus fuses with the endosome membrane. The cleavage (splitting) of the HA into HA1 and HA2 by proteolytic enzyme is essential for fusion and infectivity of the virus. The nucleocapsids of the virus (i.e. RNA and its surrounding protein) are transported to the nucleus where viral transcriptase complex synthesizes messenger RNA (mRNA). Transcription is initiated with 10 -13 nucleotide RNA fragments. (**Transcription** is the mechanism by which specific information encoded in a nucleic acid chain is transferred to the mRNA. This is brought about by the enzyme **transcriptase**.) Six mRNAs are produced in the nucleus and transported to the cytoplasm for **translation** into HA, NA and internal proteins of the virus. (**Translation** is the mechanism by which a particular base sequence in the mRNA results in production of a specific amino acid sequence in the protein.) The HA and NA proteins are glycosylated (i.e. contain glycosyl radicals, derived from glucose) in the rough endoplasmic reticulum, trimmed (cut) in the Golgi and transported to the surface. Here, they are embedded in the **plasma cell membrane** (i.e. cell membrane). The eight viral gene segments along with internal viral proteins assemble and migrate to certain areas of the plasma membrane.

## Susceptibility to Chemical and Physical Agents

Avian influenza viruses are **relatively unstable** in the environment. Heat, extremes of pH, and dryness can inactivate AI viruses. Because AI viruses have **lipid envelopes**, they are inactivated by organic solvents and **detergents**.

**In the presence of organic matter,** AI virus can be destroyed by chemical inactivants such as **aldehydes** (formaldehyde and **gluteraldehyde**) and **beta-propiolactone. After removal of organic matter,** chemical disinfectants such as phenolics, ammonium ions (including quaternary ammonium disinfectants), oxidizing agents (such as **sodium hypochlorite**), dilute acids, and hydroxylamine can destroy AI viruses.

## Laboratory versus Field Conditions

**In the laboratory conditions,** commonly used detergents and disinfectants (such as phenolics, quaternary ammonium surfactant compounds and sodium hypochlorite) inactivate AI viruses.

**However, under field conditions, influenza viruses are protected by organic material such as nasal secretions or faeces. These increase their resistance to physical and chemical inactivation.** Cool and moist conditions favour long survival of AI viruses in the environment. AI viruses have remained viable (alive) in liquid manure **for 105 days in the winter** and in faeces for 30-35 days at 4° C and for 7 days at 10° C.

**To control field infection, it is essential to destroy the virus. This requires an integrated approach. First,** heat the buildings to 90-100° F for one week. Then, remove and properly dispose of manure and litter. This is followed by cleaning and disinfection of buildings and equipment, and allowing a 2-3 weeks vacancy period before re-stocking. **Virus in manure and litter must be inactivated or disposed of by burial, composting, or incineration.** Effective disinfectants against AI viruses on clean surfaces include **5.25% sodium hypochlorite,** 2% sodium hydroxide (lye), phenolic compounds, acidified ionophor compounds, chlorine dioxide disinfectants, strong oxidizing agents, and 4% sodium carbonate/0.1% sodium silicate. **However, organic material must be removed before disinfectants can work properly. '**

## Nature of the Disease

**Avian influenza viruses produce diseases that range from: (1) asymptomatic infection** to (2) **respiratory disease and drops in egg production** to (3) **severe, systemic disease with 100% mortality.** This last form of the disease results from infection by highly powerful (highly pathogenic, HP) AI viruses. Thus, based on their disease-producing power, **avian influenza viruses are of two types:** (1) those that are mildly harmful (of low virulence). These have been termed as '**low pathogenic or mildly pathogenic (MPAI) viruses,** and (2) those that are extremely harmful (of high virulence), capable of causing a severe disease in poultry and inflicting up to 100% mortality. These are called **'highly pathogenic or HPAI' viruses.**

Although in the laboratory only two pathotypes of AI viruses have been demonstrated, namely, one of low disease-producing power (**MPAI**) and the other of high disease-producing power (**HPAI**), **in the field, natural infection by AI viruses results in a wide range of clinical diseases.** This depends on virus strain, host species, and environmental factors. **From the mortality patterns, symptoms and lesions, avian influenza in the field occurs in four different forms: (1) Extremely harmful, that is, highly virulent form.** It results from infection by highly pathogenic H5 or H7 AI viruses in chickens (discussed later). It occurs as a severe, systemic disease that affects most organs, including brain and heart. **Morbidity (sickness in birds) and mortality (deaths) reach 100%.** (2) **Moderately harmful (moderately virulent) form.** This form results from infection by mildly pathogenic viruses, of any HA or NA subtype (discussed later), but associated with (co-infection) by secondary pathogens (i.e. disease-producing bacteria). The mortality rates may vary but range from 5-97%, and occurs mainly in young birds, reproductively active hens, or birds under severe stress. Lesions occur in the respiratory tract, reproductive organs, kidney, or pancreas. (3) **Mildly harmful (mildly virulent) form.** This form results from infection by mildly pathogenic AI virus with low mortality and mild respiratory disease or drop in egg production. Mortality is usually less than 5%, typically in older birds. (4) **Asymptomatic (avirulent) form.** This form results from infections by mildly pathogenic AI viruses. There is no mortality or symptoms of the disease. **This form is the most common in wild birds with infection by mildly pathogenic AI viruses. In fact, disease is usually absent with AI virus infection in most wild bird species.**

## Incidence and Distribution

Avian influenza viruses have a worldwide distribution. **The most common source of AI viruses has been free-flying aquatic birds, that is, those living in or near water, especially ducks and geese,** and also shorebirds, gulls, and terns (sea birds). These are considered as reservoirs of all AI viruses. **In these species, AI viruses usually cause no disease (MPAI viruses),** exception being high mortality in common terns of South Africa during 1961 outbreak of bird flu. Most combinations of the 16 HA and 9 NA subtypes have been reported in free-flying birds. **Chickens and turkeys are not natural reservoirs of AI viruses. Most influenza infections in domestic poultry are from avian-origin influenza viruses.**

## Myth about H5 and H7 subtypes

The outbreaks of highly pathogenic avian influenza between 1901 and mid-1950s involved isolates that today have been classified as **H7N1** and **H7N7** subtypes. However, an outbreak during 1959 in chickens of Scotland and during 1961 in common terns (sea birds) of South Africa involved subtypes H5N9 and H5N3, respectively. **This led to the wrong conclusion (myth) that all H5 and H7 AI viruses are highly pathogenic.** However, since 1971 numerous **H5** and **H7** mildly pathogenic AI viruses have been isolated and characterized. **This has clarified the situation that subtypes H5 and H7 do not always mean high pathogenicity.**

**Following is the list of 20 documented outbreaks of highly pathogenic avian influenza (HPAI) virus since the discovery of AI virus as the cause of fowl plague in 1955:**

| S.No. | Country | Year | Subtype | Species Affected |
|-------|---------|------|---------|------------------|
| 1. | Scotland | 1959 | H5N1 | Chickens |
| 2. | South Africa | 1961 | H5N3 | Common terns |
| 3. | England | 1963 | H7N3 | Breeder turkeys |
| 4. | Canada | 1966 | H5N9 | Breeder turkeys |
| 5. | Australia | 1976 | H7N7 | Laying chickens, broilers and ducks |
| 6. | Germany | 1979 | H7N7 | Unknown |
| 7. | England | 1979 | H7N7 | Commercial turkeys |
| 8. | USA | 1983 | H5N2 | Chickens and turkeys |
| 9. | Ireland | 1983 | H5N8 | Meat turkeys |
| 10. | Australia | 1985 | H7N7 | Broiler breeders, laying chicks, and broilers |
| 11. | England | 1991 | H5N1 | Turkeys |
| 12. | Australia | 1992 | H7N3 | Broiler breeders |
| 13. | Mexico | 1994 | H5N2 | Chickens |
| 14. | Australia | 1995 | H7N3 | Laying chickens |
| 15. | Pakistan | 1995 | H7N3 | Broilers and broiler breeder chickens |
| 16. | Hong Kong | 1997 | H5N1 | Chickens and other domestic birds in contact with the chickens |
| 17. | Australia | 1997 | H7N4 | Broiler breeders and broilers |
| 18. | Italy | 1997 | H5N2 | Chickens, turkeys, ducks, pigeons, geese |
| 19. | Italy | 1999 | H7N1 | Laying chickens, meat and breeder turkeys, broiler breeders and broilers |
| 20. | Hong Kong | 2001 | H5N1 | Birds |

## Antigenic Variation of Strains – Drift and Shift

**Human influenza viruses** have a high frequency of antigenic variation in the surface glycoproteins (HA and NA) because of two phenomena, **drift** and **shift**. This explained the antigenic change that occurred in human influenza viruses within human population. However, it is at present doubtful if such a phenomenon occurs in avian influenza virus.

**Antigenic drift** in mammalian influenza virus arises from point mutations in the HA and/or NA genes that result in **minor antigenic changes in the coding proteins.**

**Antigenic shift** arises from genetic re-assortment between the gene segments of two influenza viruses that infect the same cell. **This results in the production of new HA and /or NA antigens.**

## Protective Characteristics of the Virus

**HA** is the major antigen that produces antibodies which protect birds against death and clinical signs. **Such antibodies are HA type specific. That is, protection of the bird is HA subtype specific and lasts for more than 35 weeks.** Antibodies produced against the NA provide protection against NA subtypes in birds.

Antibodies against internal proteins (of the virus), mainly nucleoprotein, do not protect from death or clinical signs.

## How to determine whether avian influenza virus is highly pathogenic?

To categorize it as a highly pathogenic AI virus, it must fulfil the **following requirements:**

1. It must kill 6, 7, or 8 of eight 4 to six-week-old susceptible chickens within 10 days following intravenous inoculation with 0.2 ml of a 1:10 dilution of a bacteria-free infectious allantoic fluid.

2. Any H5 or N7 virus that does not meet the requirement in item 1, but has an amino acid sequence at the end of the haemagglutinin cleavage site that is compatible with HPAI viruses.

3. Any influenza virus that is not an H5 or H7 subtype, which kills 1-5 chickens and grows in cell culture in the absence of trypsin.

These criteria emphasize the importance of *in vivo* testing (i.e. in the living body) in deciding high pathogenicity of the virus, but recognize the importance of *in vitro* tests (i.e. laboratory tests) for identifying AI viruses that have the potential to become highly pathogenic.

**Recently, these tests have revealed that antigenic sub-typing is not an indicator of high pathogenicity. <u>Only a small percentage of H5 N7 AI viruses are highly pathogenic.</u> By contrast, all H1 to H4, H6, and H8-15 AI viruses are of low virulence, that is, mildly pathogenic for birds.**

## Spread

**AI virus is excreted from the nares (nose), mouth, conjunctiva, and cloaca of infected birds into the environment.** This is because virus grows in the respiratory, intestinal, renal (kidney), and/or reproductive organs.

1. The virus is spread by **direct contact** between infected and susceptible birds, or **indirect contact through fine droplets suspended in air**, or exposure to virus-contaminated **fomites** (inanimate objects).

2. **Air spread** is important because of high virus concentrations in the respiratory tract. However, the large volume of lower concentration of AI virus in infected faeces makes **fomites a major means of transport.** Thus, AI viruses are readily transported to other premises **by people (contaminated shoes and clothing) and equipment.**

3. **Sources of infection** for the first introduction of the virus into poultry include: (1) other domestic and confined poultry, (2) migratory birds (waterfowls), (3) domestic pigs, and (4) pet birds. **It has been found that spread through air has a limited role as compared to mechanical movement of fomites on equipment, clothing, and shoes.**

4. Introduction of AI viruses, **especially mildly pathogenic,** from **wild birds,** especially migratory waterfowl, has been documented. **The source is contaminated faeces from ducks** either through direct contact with poultry, or indirectly through contamination of feed or water.

5. **Spread of AI virus during an outbreak** is by mechanical transmission of virus on fomites, by air, or movement of infected poultry.

6. Whereas horizontal spread of AI virus commonly occurs, **it does not spread vertically.** However, AI virus infection of hens results in virus recovery from the **eggshell surface** and the **internal contents of the eggs. Cleaning of faecal material and disinfection of egg shells may be necessary to prevent the hatchery-associated spread of AI viruses.**

7. **Once a flock is infected, it should be considered a potential source of virus for life.**

8. Some infections of free-living perching birds, such as **sparrows,** have been associated with outbreaks on poultry farms where they may have acquired infections from close contact with poultry.

## Role of Migratory Birds in the Spread of AI Virus

It is widely believed that migratory birds spread the AI infection to poultry. On the contrary, **migratory birds are natural reservoirs for low pathogenicity virus.** In **wild ducks,** the viruses grow mainly in the intestinal tract, cause no signs of the disease, and are excreted in high concentrations in the faeces. This can lead to heavily contaminated pond water that could be a source of infection for other wild birds, **or for poultry. Ducks occupy a very important position in the spread of AI virus.**

**Mildly pathogenic AI viruses** are maintained in wild birds living in or near water. At times, they cross over to poultry and cause outbreaks of **mild disease. Highly pathogenic AI viruses do not have a recognized wild bird reservoir. Highly pathogenic AI viruses arise from mildly pathogenic AI viruses through mutations**

**in the haemagglutinin (HA) surface protein.** Virulence shifts in **H5** and **H7** subtypes occur that facilitate the spread from wild birds to domestic poultry, resulting in highly pathogenic situations.

**Migratory birds maintain mildly pathogenic AI viruses and do not appear to play a significant role in the spread of highly pathogenic AI viruses. For example, in Australia,** despite the occurrence of five outbreaks of avian influenza in poultry caused by H7 subtypes, there has not been a single isolate of this subtype from wild birds. The non-pathogenic subtypes isolated from wild aquatic birds included H1, H3, H4, H5, H6, H11, H12, and H15.

However, in the Asian avian influenza outbreaks, the presence of H5N1 viruses in dead migratory birds suggests that **wild populations may be involved.** While it is not known whether the **H5N1** virus has become established in wild bird populations, **its potential role must be considered. To conclude, the extent of infection in the wild birds, their involvement in virus spread, and the range of species involved are, at present, not known.**

## Incubation Period

Incubation period is the interval between exposure to an infection and the appearance of the first symptoms. The incubation period in avian influenza is **3 days** in naturally-infected **individual birds** and up to **14 days in a flock.** It depends on the dose of the virus, the route of exposure, the species exposed, and the ability to produce symptoms.

## Symptoms

The symptoms are extremely variable and depend on factors such as species of the bird, sex, concurrent infections, acquired immunity, and environmental factors. However, **the pathotype of the AI virus,** whether it is mildly pathogenic **(MPAI)** or highly pathogenic **(HPAI), has the greatest impact on the clinical manifestations of the disease**

## Symptoms in Mildly Pathogenic Avian influenza Viruses (MPAI)

**In wild birds**, MPAI viruses produce no symptoms.

**In chickens,** the most common symptoms include mild to severe respiratory symptoms. These include coughing, sneezing, abnormal respiratory sounds (rales), and excessive discharges from the eyes (lacrimation). **In layers and breeders,** hens may show increased broodiness and **decreased egg production.** In addition, they show huddling, ruffled feathers, depression, decreased activity, **reduced feed and water consumption**, and sometimes diarrhoea. Emaciation (thinning) is uncommon because AI is an acute and not a chronic disease.

## Symptoms of Highly Pathogenic Avian Influenza Virus (HPAI)

**In wild birds and ducks,** HPAI viruses grow poorly and therefore produce almost no symptoms. The one exception is common terns (sea birds) in the South African outbreak of AI in 1961 which produced sudden deaths without showing any other symptoms.

**In chickens,** symptoms vary depending on the extent of damage to specific organs and tissues. **That is, not all symptoms are present in every bird.** In most cases, **the disease attacks suddenly and is extremely severe.** Some birds are found dead before any symptoms are seen. If the disease is **less severe** and birds survive for 3-7 days, individual birds may show nervous disorders, such as tremors of head and neck, inability to stand, twisting of the neck, and unusual positions of head and legs. The poultry houses are usually quiet because of decreased activity and reduction in normal vocal sounds of the birds. Depression and decrease in feed and water consumption are common. **Sudden drops in egg production occur in breeders and layers. The drops go on increasing, and within six days there is total stoppage of egg production.**

**Respiratory symptoms are less common than with MPAI viruses,** but can include abnormal respiratory sounds (rales), sneezing, and coughing.

## Morbidity and Mortality

**In chickens,** morbidity (sickness in birds) and mortality rates are as variable as the symptoms. These depend on disease-producing power of the virus and the host as well as age, environment, and concurrent infections. **For MPAI viruses,** high morbidity and low mortality rates are typical. Mortality is usually **less than 5%,** unless accompanied by secondary pathogens (i.e. bacteria), **or if the disease is in young birds. With the HPAI viruses** morbidity and mortality rates are very high (50 – 90%) and can reach 100% in certain flocks.

**In wild birds,** MPAI viruses usually produce no disease or deaths. However, high mortality was reported in the outbreak in South African terns (sea birds) during 1961.

## Postmortem Findings

**Postmortem findings are extremely variable,** depending on the pathogenicity of the infecting virus, and presence of secondary pathogens.

## In Mildly Pathogenic Avian Influenza Viruses (MPAI)

**In poultry, the most common lesions (changes) are in the respiratory tract,** especially sinuses, and are characterized by different types of inflammation. **The tracheal mucosa** (i.e. internal lining of trachea) **can be swollen** (oedematous) **with congestion and sometimes haemorrhages. Tracheal exudates** (inflammatory fluids) may vary from serous (resembling serum) to caseous (cheese-like) with, at times, **blockage of airways** resulting in **asphyxiation** (suffocation). **Airsacculitis** (inflammation of airsacs) may be present. The inflammation is usually associated with secondary bacterial infections. The infraorbital sinuses (i.e. present below the eyes) may be swollen and mucus to mucopurulent nasal discharge occurs. **Bronchopneumonia** can result when secondary pathogens such as *E. coli* and *Pasteurella multocida*.

**In the body cavity,** there may be catarrhal to fibrinous **peritonitis** (i.e. inflammation of peritoneum, a membrane in the body cavity), and even **egg yolk peritonitis** may be observed. **Enteritis** (inflammation of the intestines) may be observed in the caeca and/ or intestine. **Inflammatory exudates** may be found **in the oviduct** of laying birds, and the last few eggs laid have reduced calcium deposition within the eggshells. Rarely eggs are misshapen and fragile with loss of pigmentation. **Ovaries undergo regression, beginning with haemorrhage in the large follicles and progressing to colliquation. That is, the ovary becomes softened and liquefied. The oviduct may be swollen (oedematous) and contain exudates (inflammatory fluids) before undergoing involution (shrinkage).** In a few cases in laying hens, kidneys may be swollen, and accompanied by visceral gout.

## In Highly Pathogenic Avian Influenza Viruses (HPAI)

**In poultry,** HPAI viruses produce a variety of oedematous, haemorrhagic, and necrotic lesions in internal organs and the skin. However, if the death is sudden, no gross lesions may be seen. **In chickens, swelling of the head, face, upper neck (see Plate 1)** and feet are common as a result of subcutaneous oedema (i.e. accumulation of fluid under the skin). **The eyes may show excessive discharge,** and swelling surrounding the eye is common (see **Plate 2**). These changes are accompanied by **small to large haemorrhages below the skin in the feet** (see **Plate 3**). Necrotic foci (areas of dead tissues), haemorrhage, and **cyanosis** (bluish to purplish discoloration of the skin due to deficiency of oxygen in blood) of the non-feathered skin is common, **especially wattles, combs, and legs** (see **Plate 4, 5 and 6**).

**Lesions (changes) in the internal organs** vary with virus strain, but are **mostly haemorrhages** on serosal or mucosal surfaces and **foci of necrosis** inside the internal organs. Most common are prominent haemorrhages on the surface of the heart (epicardium) (see **Plate 7 and 8**), in the breast and leg muscles (see **Plate 9**, and in mucosa (lining) of the proventriculus (see **Plate 10**) and gizzard and, at times, in small intestine. Necrotic foci are common in pancreas, spleen (see **Plate 11**), and heart, and sometimes in liver and kidney. **Trachea** may be highly congested and in severe cases may exhibit severe haemorrhages (see **Plate 12**). **This was particularly seen in the Indian outbreak.** Lungs show pneumonia with oedema. The lungs can be congested or haemorrhagic.

**NOTE: The postmortem lesions** described, at best, only suggest that the disease may be avian influenza. **They are by no means specific for AI,** since such findings can also be seen in certain other diseases of poultry. Definitive diagnosis is established

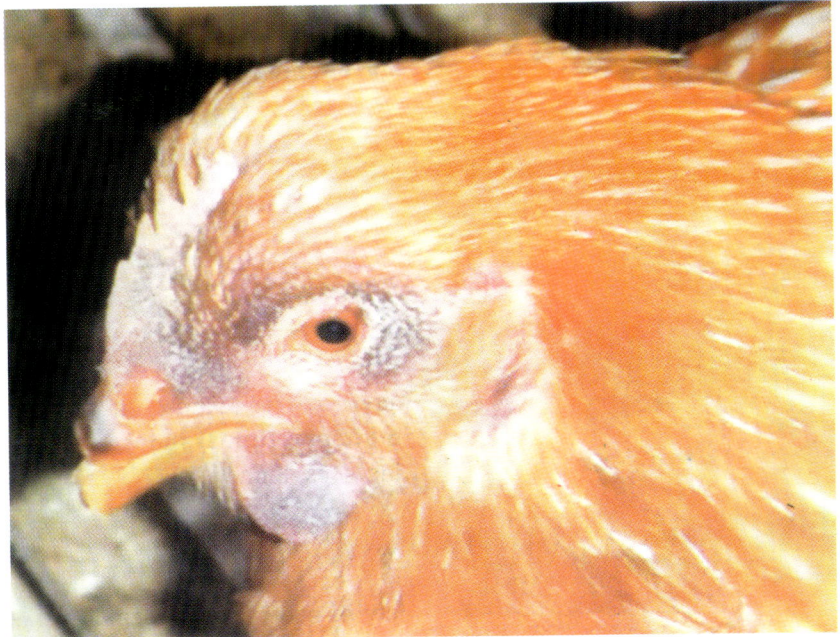

**Plate 1. Avian Influenza (Bird Flu).** Note swelling of the head, face and upper neck of a chicken.

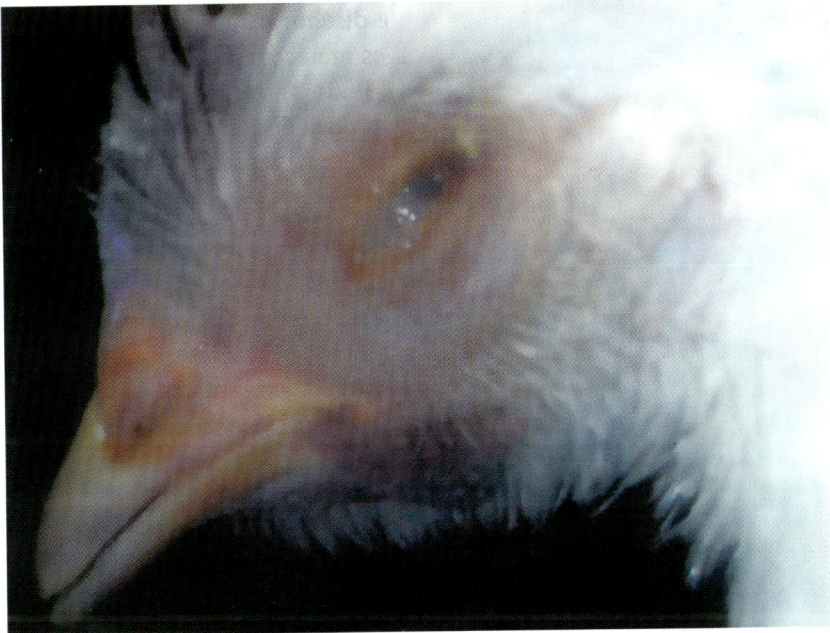

**Plate 2. Avian Influenza (Bird Flu).** Note excessive discharge from the left eye of a chicken. Note also the swelling surrounding the eye.

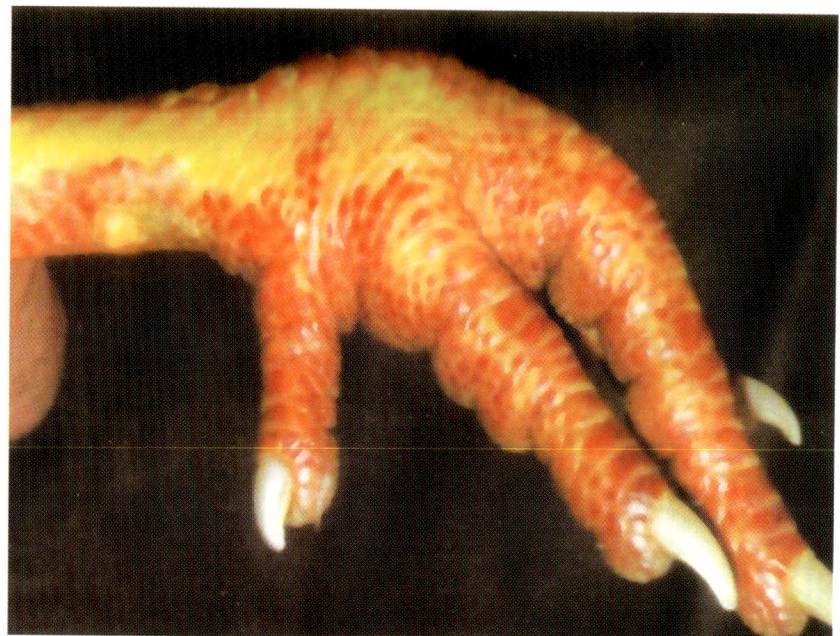

**Plate 3. Avian Influenza (Bird Flu).** Note haemorrhages under the skin (subcutaneous) in the feet of a chicken.

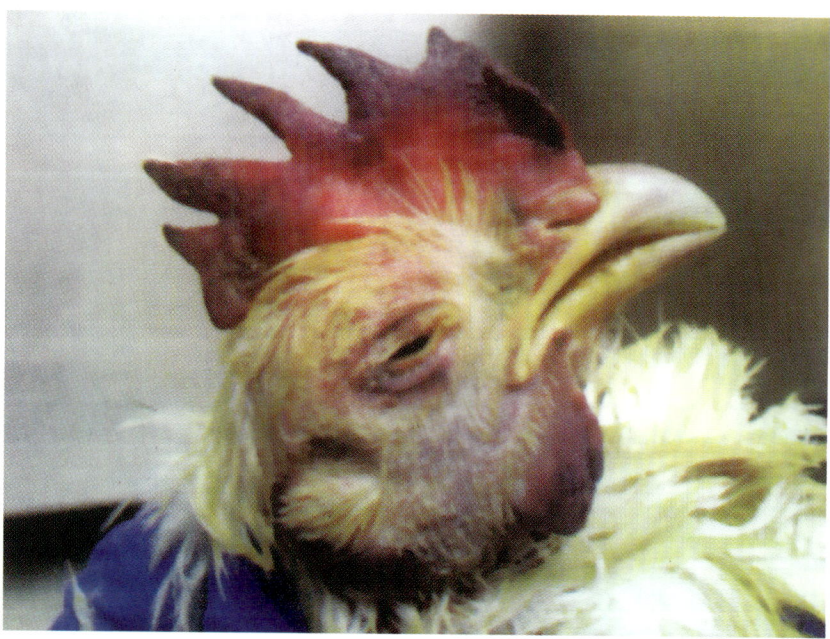

**Plate 4. Avian Influenza (Bird Flu).** Note cyanosis (bluish to purplish discoloration) on the comb and wattles of a chicken.

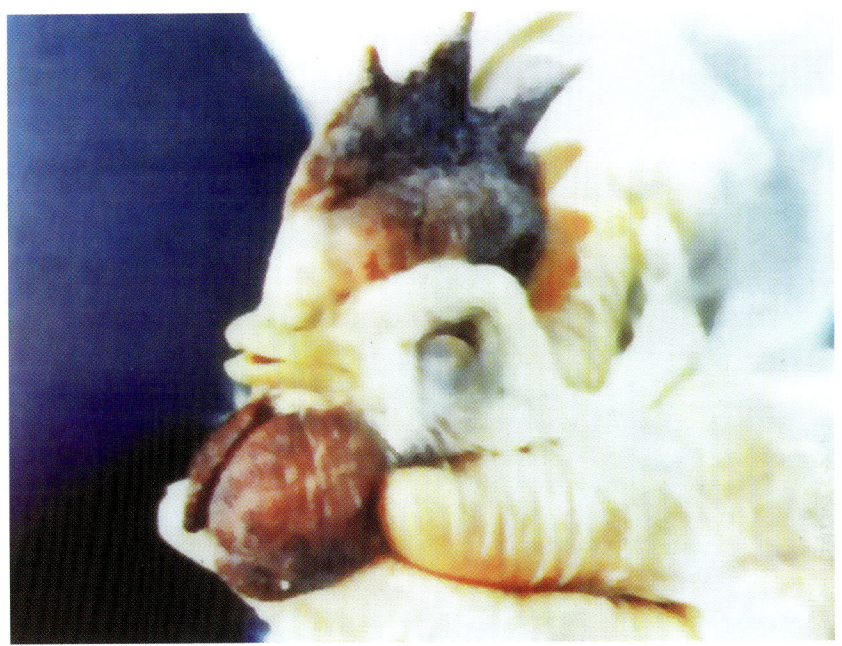

**Plate 5. Avian Influenza (Bird Flu).** Cyanosis (bluish to purplish discoloration) of comb and wattles from another bird. Note both comb and wattles are extremely swollen, haemorrhagic, and necrotic (i.e. dead).

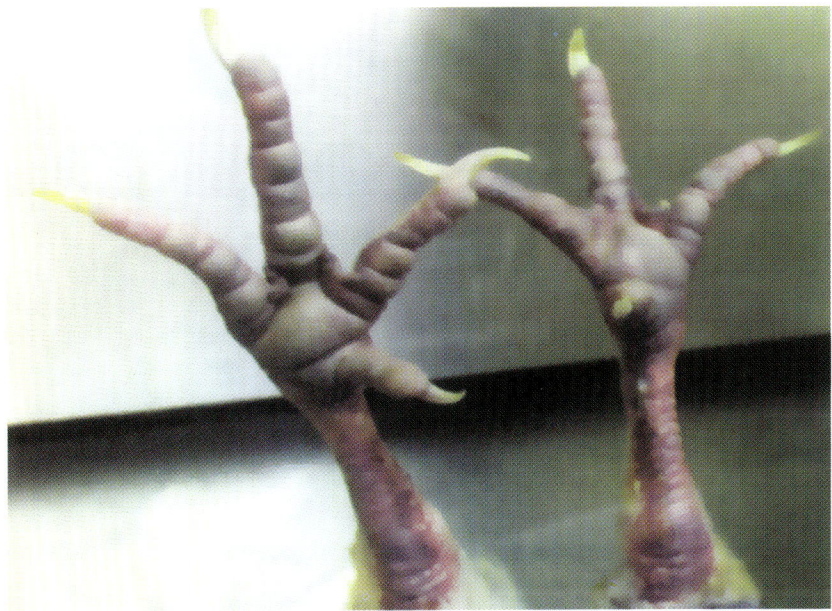

**Plate 6. Avian Influenza (Bird Flu).** Note cyanosis (bluish to purplish discoloration) on the feet and toes of a chicken.

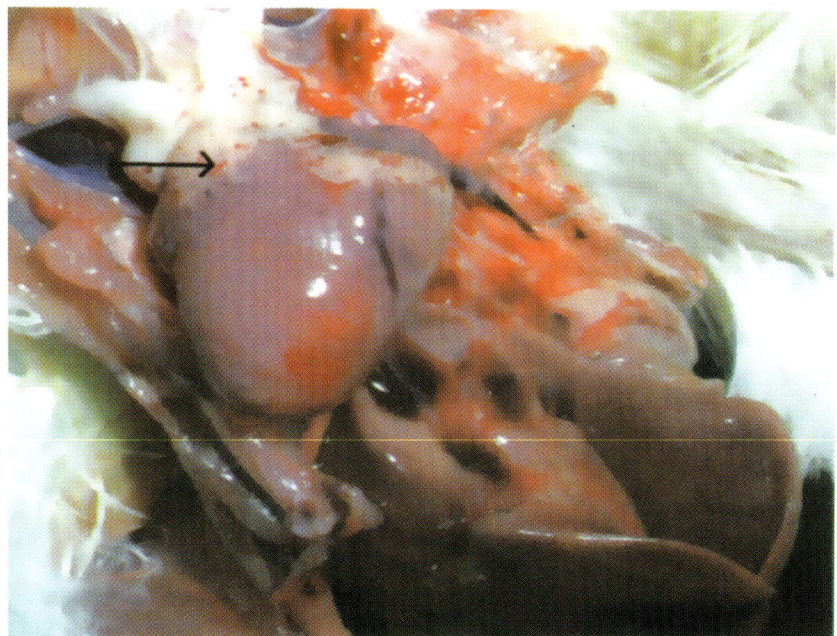

**Plate 7. Avian Influenza (Bird Flu).** Note small but prominent haemorrhages (arrow) on the upper portion of the heart (in the yellow fat) of a chicken.

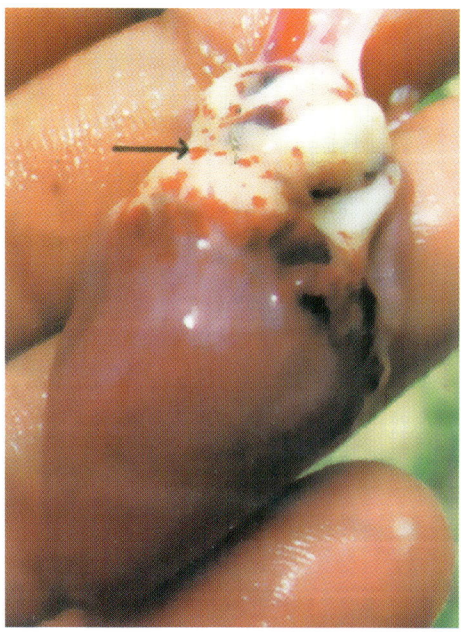

**Plate 8. Avian Influenza (Bird Flu).** Note prominent haemorrhages (arrow) on the upper portion of the heart of another chicken.

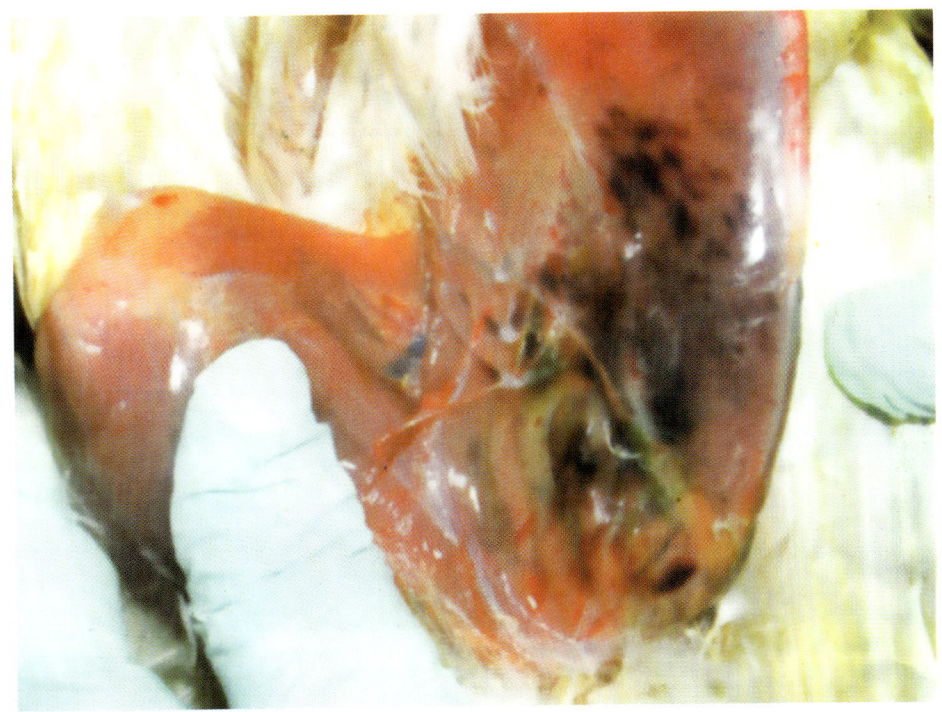

**Plate 9. Avian Influenza (Bird Flu).** Note big haemorrhages in the leg muscles of a chicken.

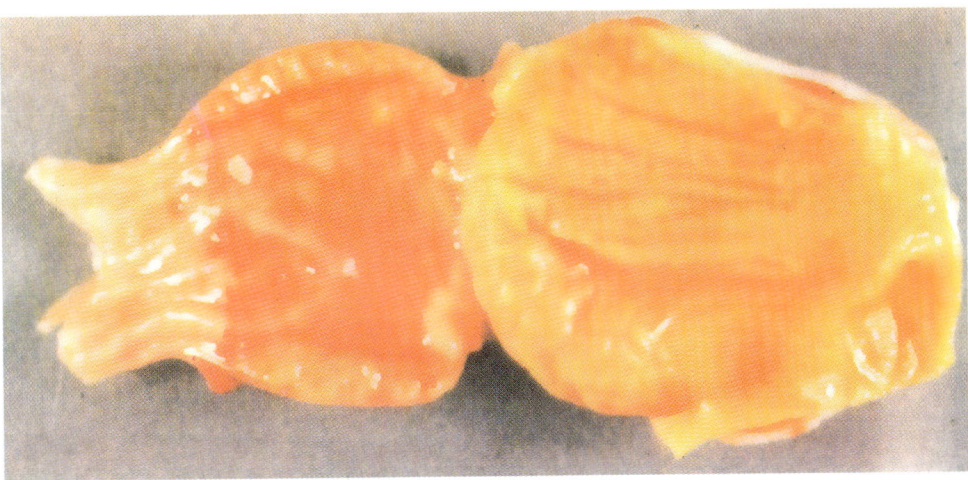

**Plate 10. Avian Influenza (Bird Flu).** Note prominent haemorrhages in the mucosa (internal lining) of the proventriculus of a chicken.

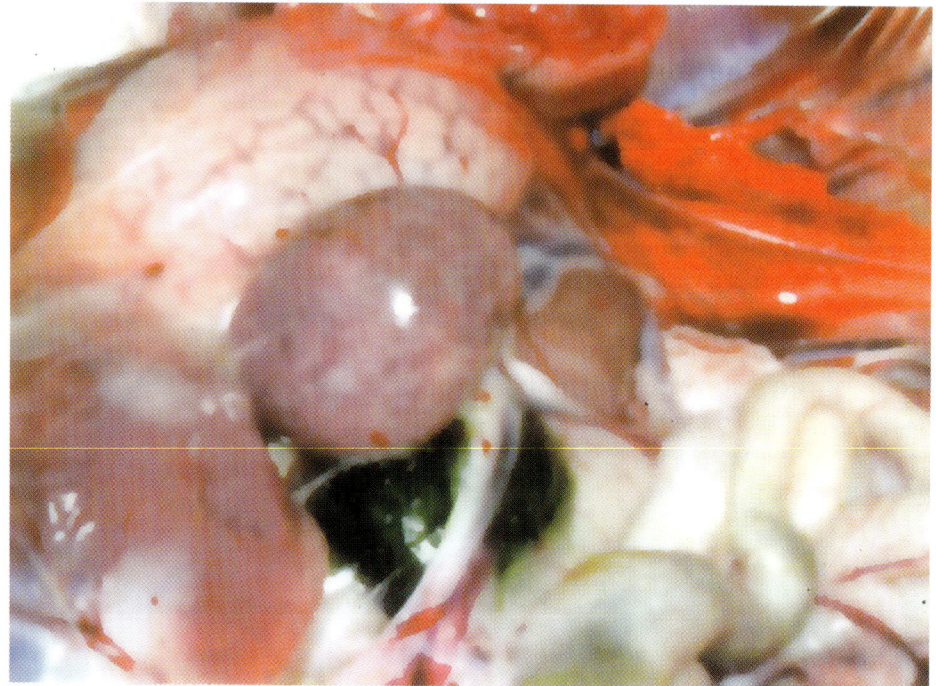

**Plate 11. Avian Influenza (Bird Flu).** Note that spleen of a chicken is enlarged and shows haemorrhagic/necrotic foci on its surface.

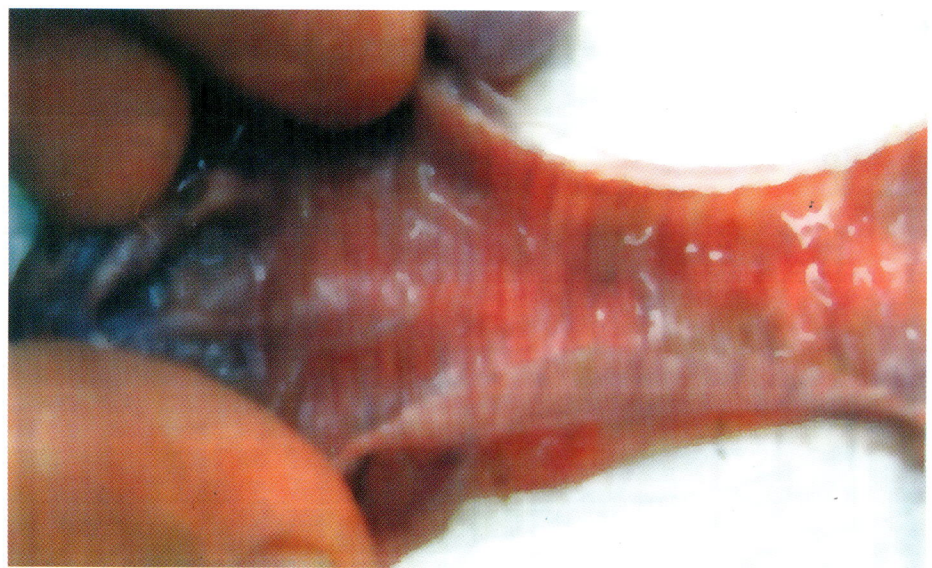

**Plate 12. Avian Influenza (Bird Flu).** Note trachea is not only severely congested but also shows diffuse haemorrhages on its left.

only by isolation and identification of the avian influenza virus (see Diagnosis).

## Development of the Disease

The disease begins by **inhalation** or **ingestion** of MPAI or HPAI viruses. **In poultry**, the nasal cavity is a major site of initial growth (replication).

**With HPAI viruses**, the virions invade the submucosa of the respiratory or intestinal tract, and enter into minute blood vessels (capillaries). The virus replicates (grows) within endothelial cells of these vessels and spreads through the vascular or lymphatic systems to infect and grow in a variety of different cells in internal organs, brain, and skin. It may also happen that it may spread to different organs, before its extensive growth in the endothelial cells of the vessels. **Symptoms and death are due to multiple organ failure.** Damage caused by AI viruses is the result of any one of these three processes: (1) **direct virus growth in cells,** tissues, and organs. (2) **indirect effects** from production of cellular mediators such as **cytokines**, and (3) ischaemia (inadequate flow of blood) from **vascular thrombosis** (i.e. blood clotting in vessels)

**With MPAI viruses, replication (growth) is usually limited to the respiratory or intestinal tract. Like HPAI viruses, it does not spread to internal organs. Illness or death is usually from respiratory damage**, especially if accompanied by secondary bacterial infections. Sometimes, the MPAI viruses spread systemically, replicating and causing damage in kidney, pancreas, and other organs.

## Immunity

### Active

Infection with AI viruses as well as immunization with vaccines produces a **humoral antibody response at both systemic and mucosal levels.** This includes systemic **IgM response** 5 days after infection, followed soon by an **IgG response**. The **mucosal immune response** is poorly characterized.

**Antibodies against the surface proteins of the virus (HA and NA) are neutralizing and protective.** Protection is mainly associated with antibodies directed against the HA protein. However, either HA, NA, or both prevent clinical signs and death. **Duration of protection is unknown,** but in layers, protection against symptoms and death has been shown to be at least for **30 weeks following a single immunization.** Birds that have recovered from field exposure are protected from the same HA and NA subtypes.

**Immune response against internal proteins does not prevent symptoms and death, but may shorten the period of virus replication and shedding.** However, the mechanism of this limited protection is unknown, but may be the result of **cell-mediated immunity.**

## Passive

Not much is known on the protective role of **maternal antibodies**. But based on evidence available for other diseases, protection against symptoms and death from the avian influenza virus is likely for the first two weeks after hatching.

## Diagnosis

A **definitive diagnosis** is established by: (1) Direct detection of AI viral proteins or genes in specimens such as tissues, swabs, cell cultures, or embryonating eggs, or (2) Isolation and identification of AI virus. **A presumptive diagnosis can be made by detecting antibodies to AI virus.**

## Sample Selection and Storage

1. Avian influenza viruses are usually recovered from **tracheal or cloacal swabs** of either live or dead birds. This is because most HP and MPAI viruses replicate in the respiratory and intestinal tracts.

2. The swabs should be placed in sterile transport medium containing high levels of antibiotics to reduce bacterial growth.

3. Tissues, secretions, or excretions from these tracts are appropriate for virus isolation.

4. **Tissues** can be collected and placed into sterile plastic tubes or bags.

5. In the examination of organs for virus, collect and store internal organs separately from the respiratory and intestinal tract tissues **because isolation of virus from internal organs may be an indication of systemic spread and is usually associated with HPAI viruses.** In case of systemic infections produced by HPAI viruses, almost every organ can yield virus because of the high levels of viraemia or replication in parenchymal cells.

6. If the samples can be tested within 48 hours, they may be kept at 4°C. However, if the sample has to be held for a longer time, storage at -70° C is recommended.

7. Before testing for virus, tissues should be ground as a 5-10% suspension in the transport medium and clarified by low-speed centrifugation.

## Direct Detection of AI Viral Proteins or Nucleic Acids

The direct demonstration of influenza virus RNA or viral proteins in samples from animals is not routinely used for diagnosis at this time.

## Virus Isolation

**Chicken embryos,** 10-11 days-old, are inoculated through the allantoic cavity with about 0.2 ml of sample.

The death of inoculated embryos within 24 hours after inoculation usually results from bacterial contamination or inoculation injury. **These eggs should be discarded.** A few viruses may grow rapidly and kill the embryos by 48 hours. However, in most cases the embryos will not die before this time. **After 72 hours,** or at death, the eggs should be removed from the incubator, chilled, and allantoic fluids should be collected. **The presence of virus is demonstrated by chicken erythrocyte haemagglutinating activity in the allantoic fluid.**

Generally, if virus is present in a sample, there will be enough growth in the first passage to result in **haemagglutination**, and repeated passage is unnecessary. Repeated passage of samples increases the risk of cross-contamination in the laboratory.

Long-term storage of virus should be done at -70° C.

# Virus Identification

1.  Standard methods for testing the egg fluids for the presence of haemagglutinating activity (antibodies) are through the use of chicken erythrocytes by macro- or micro-techniques. **Allantoic fluid positive for haemagglutination is used for virus identification.**

2.  It is important to find out whether the haemagglutinating activity detected in the allantoic fluid is due to influenza virus, or other viruses such as Ranikhet disease virus (Newcastle disease virus). **Therefore, the isolate is tested in HI assays against Ranikhet disease and other antiserum.**

3.  If negative, the virus is then tested for the presence of the type A specific antigen to confirm **that an influenza A virus is present.**

4.  The next step in the identification is to **determine the antigenic subtype of the surface antigens, HA and NA.** The NA subtype is identified by a **micro-NI assay** with antisera prepared against the 9 known NAs. This NI assay is usually the first assay that is done on an isolate.

5.  **The HA is identified in the HI test using a panel of antisera prepared against the 16 distinct HAs.**

6.  The final identification is done by the **Government of India's High Security Laboratory** located at Bhopal, Madhya Pradesh, India.

# Serology

1.  Serological tests are used to detect the presence of AI-specific antibodies **as early as 7 days after infection.**

2.  Several techniques are used for serological surveillance and diagnosis. For surveillance, **a double immunodiffusion test for the detection of anti-NP antibody is generally used.** This is because it detects antibodies to type A specific

antigens shared by all influenza A viruses.

3. **ELISA assays (tests)** have been developed to detect antibody to influenza. Once influenza is detected by immunodiffusion **or ELISA, HI tests can be used to determine HA subtype.**

## Differential Diagnosis

1. Infections that must be considered in the differential diagnosis include **Ranikhet disease, infectious bronchitis, infectious laryngotracheitis, and mycoplasmosis.**

2. Concurrent infections with other viruses or other bacteria are commonly observed.

## Treatment

There is no satisfactory treatment. Supportive care and treatment with broad-spectrum antibiotics may reduce the effects of concurrent bacterial infections.

## Prevention and Control

The basic approach in the control of avian influenza is **preventing the first introduction of the virus and controlling the spread if it is introduced.** One critical aspect in the prevention and control is the education of the poultry industry regarding **how the viruses are introduced, how they spread, and how such events can be prevented.**

## Prevention

1. The most important source of virus for poultry is **other infected birds.** Therefore, the first step towards prevention of infection is the **separation of susceptible birds from infected birds and their secretions and excretions** (see Biosecurity). **Biosecurity is the first line of defence.**

2 **Spread** can occur when susceptible and infected birds are in close contact, or when infectious materials from infected birds are introduced into the environment of susceptible birds. Such introductions occur with the movement of equipment, footwear (shoes, etc.) and clothing, vehicles, insemination equipment, feed, water, etc. **The presence of virus in faecal material is the source for its movement through equipment and people.**

3. There should be **no contact with recovered flocks**, because the length of time birds within a population shed virus is not clearly known.

4. **Wild birds** are the reservoir of influenza viruses. **They should be considered a major source of infection for poultry.** Therefore, it is important to reduce the contact between these two groups.

## Control

1.  **Influenza virus is excreted from both respiratory and digestive systems.** Therefore, within a poultry house, bird-to-bird transmission is **by air and ingestion. Contaminated poultry manure (faeces) is the most important source of spread between flocks.**

2.  After the avian influenza has been introduced into commercial flocks, certain things must be identified that contribute to its spread. These include **unclean equipment and people, marketing an actively infected flock, and inadequate cleaning and disinfection.**

3.  **All methods for controlling the spread of influenza are based on preventing contamination and controlling the movements of people and equipment. Persons** who have direct contact with birds or their faeces have been the cause of most disease spread between houses or premises. **Equipment** that comes in direct contact with birds or their faeces should not be moved from farm to farm **without adequate cleaning and disinfection.** Also, it is important to monitor that the **traffic area** near the poultry house does not get contaminated with faeces/manure.

4.  Even before the occurrence of avian influenza, vigorous control measures must already be in operation. If a virus turns out be highly pathogenic, it could take a few weeks from initial sickness until a government emergency can be declared. **Therefore, voluntary industry efforts to control the initial outbreak are most important.**

5.  The farm-to-farm spread of influenza virus must first be brought under control before the disease can be eradicated.

6.  **Most of the influenza virus shed from an infected flock occurs during the first two weeks of infection. Serologically positive (sero-positive) flocks are not associated with a high risk of spread. Usually by four weeks after the infection, virus cannot be detected.**

7.  Orderly and well-timed marketing of birds or eggs is appropriate after an MPAI outbreak.

8.  **In the case of MPAI outbreaks, efforts must focus on preventing spread of the disease beyond the first cases.** In the past, outbreaks in USA, Mexico, and Italy have shown that **HPAI can emerge from MPAI outbreaks.** In these cases, HPAI emerged after MPAI H5 or H7 viruses circulated widely in susceptible poultry flocks for several months. In contrast, 20 outbreaks of H5 or H7 MPAI eliminated within 3 months in USA did not result in the emergence of HPAI. **This illustrates the need for prompt responses against MPAI outbreaks. Prevention and control of mild influenza outbreaks are the most important steps to prevent**

outbreaks of HPAI.

9.   **With HPAI virus eradication procedures (quarantine, slaughter, disposal, and clean-up) must be employed. Area quarantines are essential to prevent spread and to achieve eradication.** It is important to detect new outbreaks and contain them.

## Vaccination

1.   **Inactivated influenza virus vaccines have been used.** Their effectiveness in preventing symptoms and mortality is well documented. **However, protection is virus subtype specific.** Birds are susceptible to infection with influenza viruses belonging to any of the 16 HA subtypes. Moreover, there is no way to predict their exposure to any particular one. It is not practical to use preventive vaccination against all possible subtypes. **However, after an outbreak occurs and the subtype of the virus is identified, vaccination may be a useful tool.**

2.   Inactivated monovalent and polyvalent virus vaccines, with adjuvants, are capable of producing antibody and providing protection against mortality, morbidity, and egg production drops.

3.   Carefully controlled use of vaccines in a MPAI H5 or H7 outbreak may delay and reduce the chance of the emergence of HPAI viruses. **However, their use is still debated.**

4.   **Vaccinated flocks cannot be considered influenza virus-free.** However, use of vaccine reduces the amount of virus shed in experimentally vaccinated and challenged birds. **This reduces shedding and potential spread of the virus to other birds.**

5.   **Controlled, effective vaccine use will reduce the population of susceptible poultry and reduce the quantity of virus shed if infection occurs.**

6.   **To conclude,** because of the large number of influenza A viruses in migratory and wild bird populations, the viruses will continue to cause serious disease problems in the commercial poultry industry. **Judicious use of vaccines may therefore be appropriate to reduce spread and decrease susceptibility of poultry to the viruses. This would enable implementation of eradication methods before the disease spreads and becomes endemic (i.e. prevalent in the area).**

## Summary of the Guidelines (Action Plan) Given by the Government of India on the Control and Containment of Avian Influenza (AI):

The strategy of the Government of India is to contain the disease at the source, that is, at the level of the affected bird itself. This will reduce its spread and possible human infection.

1    Surveillance (close watch) on AI must include poultry and migratory birds.

2.   Poultry owner must report unusual mortality and sickness in birds to State Veterinary Hospital.

3.   **Routine Surveillance**: The State Governments must periodically collect random samples (cloacal and tracheal swabs, serum) of poultry from different parts of the State and get them tested as part of the routine surveillance against bird flu. This should also include migratory and wild birds.

4.   **Sample Collection, Packing, and Transportation**

   - For routine surveillance, collect 4-5 samples (cloacal and tracheal swabs, serum) from a particular poultry farm. The sampling should be representative.

   - **Ensure quality of the samples. The samples should be packed in isotonic phosphate buffered saline (PBS), pH 7.0-7.4, containing antibiotics, and dispatched on ice.**

   - **It is most important that cold chain is maintained while despatching the samples,** otherwise samples would get contaminated or putrefied and will have to be discarded.

   - The samples must accompany the proforma prescribed by the Government.

5.   **Types of samples to be sent to laboratory:**

   The following samples must be collected and sent to **High Security Animal Disease Laboratory (HSADL), Bhopal.**

   - At least five diseased birds (either dead, or sick birds after killing them) for postmortem examination.

   - Pooled tracheal and lung samples from at least five dead birds.

   - Pooled intestine samples from at least five diseased birds

   - Cloacal and tracheal swabs from at least 10 healthy birds. **Swabs must contain at least one gram of faecal material.** Then, immerse them in **phosphate buffered saline (PBS).**

   - At least 10 blood samples.

6.   Pack the samples in leak-proof containers, and wrap them in at least two plastic bags.

7.   Transport them in a cold chain to the laboratory inside a polystyrene box (ice box) containing ice packs. The samples must be accompanied by the appropriate form.

8.   Samples should be sent to the laboratory immediately through a special messenger.

9.   **Following an outbreak of avian influenza, following steps must be taken**

**immediately:**

- Restrict movement of people from the infected premises.

- Restrict movement of vehicles from the infected premises.

- Restrict movement of equipment from the infected premises.

- Eliminate (destroy) the entire stock of diseased and in-contact birds.

10. **Disposal of Dead Birds, Eggs, and other Materials:**

- The dead birds must be disposed of by **burning** or **burial**. They must not be moved out of the infected site.

- **For burning** about 5 quintals of wood per 100 Kg of dead birds would be required.

- **For burial,** a pit must be prepared. It must be at least two meters long, two meters wide, and two meters deep. This size pit enables disposal of about 1800 birds. If it is made one meter deeper, its capacity increases to 3000 birds.

- The carcasses must be covered with a layer of **calcium hydroxide**, and then with a layer of earth (at least 40 cm deep). Then, alternate one layer with the other till the pit is covered up to the ground level.

- The burial pit should be marked and must not be opened for at least five years.

- All the infected materials must be destroyed. Litter, feed and feathers be either buried in the pit with carcasses or burnt. Eggs and egg products may be buried in the pit.

11. **Clean-Up and Disinfection:**

- The infected premises must be disinfected after birds and infected materials have been destroyed and disposed of.

- **Wash and disinfect** walls, floors and ceilings of the infected poultry premises, after removing all the organic matter. Wash floor and walls with **3% calcium hydroxide solution**, sprinkle **beaching powder** and **lime** on the floors of sheds. Then spray the areas with **4% formalin.**

- **Fumigate** closed chambers and sheds with potassium permanganate and formalin

- Treat all equipment with **2% sodium hypochlorite solution** for 48 hours.

12. **List of Active Disinfectants:**

- **Rectified spirit**, or **Savlon**, or **Dettol (1% solution)** can be used for cleaning of hands and feet of farm workers.

- **2% solution** of **sodium hydroxide** (NaOH) should be used at the entrance on foot mats to clean the shoes. This solution can also be used to scrub and clean gumboots and other items.

- **Sodium hypochlorite:** 2% active chlorine solution for disinfection of equipment.

- **Quarternary ammonium salts:** 4% solution for treatment of walls, floors, ceilings, and equipment.

- **Calcium hydroxide:** 3% solution for treatment of walls and floors.

- **Synthetic phenols:** 2% solution for treatment of floors.

- **Formalin** and **potassium permanganate** for fumigation.

13. **Vaccination:**

- Vaccination is not to be taken as routine prophylaxis. It is to be undertaken only during hours of crisis.

- **Vaccination alone is not sufficient to bring the outbreaks in poultry under control. Vaccinated birds may get protected against the disease, but continue to spread the infection. Therefore, vaccination must be used together with the comprehensive strategy already discussed, that is, culling of affected birds, strict biosecurity, quarantine, and other measures to prevent further spread of the disease.**

- **Monitoring and surveillance in the event of vaccination:** The flock must be under constant clinical surveillance. Serum samples should be collected after 21 days to determine the immunity level. The samples must be drawn from at least 1% of the total poultry population and sent to HSADL, Bhopal. The second vaccination, if required, may be carried out after 4-6 weeks. Again, there should be testing of the samples.

- **A strategy that is capable of differentiating infected from vaccinated birds has been recommended.**

14. **Biosecurity Measures:**

    The best way to control avian influenza is to prevent exposure by imposing **strict biosecurity measures**. The poultry owners must therefore adopt the following measures:

- **Keep distance:** Only those people who take care of the poultry farm should be allowed to go close to the birds. Unnecessary people should be restricted from entering the sheds.

- **Keep cleanliness:** Cleanliness inside the sheds and around the farms is a must. It prevents germs and bacteria from multiplying.

- **Don't let the disease enter the farm.** The new birds should be kept away from healthy flock for at least 30 days. Disinfect and wash shoes, clothes and hands before and after contact with poultry to prevent spread of the disease.

- **Don't borrow the disease:** If equipment, tools or poultry supplies are borrowed from other farms, always clean and disinfect them before bringing in contact with healthy birds.

- **Know the signs:** A check must be kept on birds. An increase in deaths must be recorded. Swelling around the eyes, neck, head, nasal discharge, discoloration of the wattles, combs, legs, drop in egg production, are warning signs.

- **Report sick birds:** Every unusual sickness or death of birds should be immediately reported to the nearest veterinary centre.

- **Follow uniform age group policy.** This is best done by adopting **'all-in-all-out' production system.**

- **Guidelines for farm personnel:** Inter-sectional movements of farm personnel should be restricted. While leaving the farm premises, farm personnel should clean themselves thoroughly with disinfectants and change their clothing and shoes.

## AVIAN INFLUENZA: IT'S PUBLIC HEALTH SIGNIFICANCE

Since the discovery of avian influenza virus in 1955, the world has experienced more than 25 documented outbreaks in poultry caused mostly by **H5N1** subtype, or even by H7N3 or H7N7 and others. **The H5N1 subtype had never produced a disease in humans until the outbreak of avian influenza in Hong Kong in 1997.** The AI virus appeared to have crossed the species barrier from poultry to humans for the first time. This raised the alarm.

During 1997, the **'highly pathogenic avian influenza (HPAI)'** virus (H5N1) resulted in the **hospitalization of 18 people** and **six deaths** in Hong Kong. The patients had fever and symptoms of upper respiratory and gastrointestinal disease, including vomiting, diarrhoea, and pain. **Patients that died had severe bilateral pneumonia.**

Despite this, since 2003 only about 164 people have died from H5N1 strain of the virus worldwide. This is because, in general, influenza viruses exhibit host species adaptation, and **transmission usually occurs between individuals of the same species,** or occasionally inter-species transmission to closely related species. Only on very rare occasions avian influenza viruses have shown inter-species transmissibility to humans. **Therefore, compared to the hundreds of millions of human infections by human-adapted influenza viruses that occur each year, transmission of avian influenza viruses to humans are rare.** Recently it has been shown that AI viruses have a preferential binding for **alpha 2, 3-galactose linkage receptors** present on the avian respiratory epithelium. On the other hand, human influenza viruses preferentially bind to **alpha 2, 6-galactose linkage receptors.** Avian respiratory epithelium has predominantly 2, 3-linkage; human respiratory epithelium has 2, 6-linkage; and swine respiratory epithelium has a mixture of alpha 2, 3-linkage and alpha 2, 6-linkage. This accounts for the slightly greater number of reports of swine influenza viruses than avian influenza virus transmission to humans.

These findings explain why avian influenza viruses are not easily transmitted to humans. However, the fact that 164 people have died worldwide from avian influenza (H5N1) does indicate **that, though extremely rare, the virus can infect humans.** More recently it has been found that humans do have some alpha 2, 3-galactose linkages in the alveoli, but these are located deep into the lung. **This is the reason why avian influenza virus is not easily transmitted to humans, unless humans come in very close contact with poultry over a prolonged period.**

However, **the major threat** posed by avian influenza viruses to humans may come **from the genetic reassortment of gene segments between avian and human influenza viruses.** Waterfowl, mainly **ducks**, and other aquatic birds are the primary reservoir of all influenza viral genes. The appearance of avian influenza viral genes in human influenza viruses have been rare events, covering a large span of time and resulting from the reassortment of RNA gene segments between avian and human influenza viruses. Although the probability of an AI virus entering the human population, reassorting, and establishing a new form of human influenza virus is extremely **rare, this is consistent with the long association between these two viruses and the emergence of new human pandemic influenza viruses in the past.**

For example, analysis of nucleotide sequence data has established that the **1957 (H2N2) human pandemic influenza viruses** resulted from the assortment of three avian influenza viral genes with five human influenza viral genes (**'Asian' flu**). This resulted in the development of a **'new'** strain (genetic reassortment) having the ability to produce human pandemic. Similarly, in **1968 (H3N2) human pandemic influenza virus** resulted from the assortment of two avian influenza viral genes with six human influenza viral genes (**'Hong Kong' flu**). This resulted in the development of another **'new'** strain having the ability to produce human pandemic. **Birds appear to be the source. Both, the H2 that appeared in 1957 and the H3 that appeared in 1968, came from influenza viruses circulating in birds.** Recent sequencing of genes of the influenza virus from a US soldier and a US lady who had died in 1918 in the human pandemic (**'Spanish' flu**), and whose tissues were either preserved or had remained frozen, **has revealed that its genome resembled bird flu genome more closely than those of human strains. Ducks** and **pigs** have been proposed as the **'mixing vessel'** for co-infection by influenza viruses from birds and mammals.

The concern among public health experts is that H5 influenza virus could be the cause of the next worldwide pandemic of human influenza. When a different 'H' subtype emerges as the cause of human influenza, severe disease and death losses can occur, because no one then has residual immunity to the 'new H' strain from vaccination, or past infection. Humans have had long experience with infections and vaccines by both H1 and H3 flu viruses (strains used in human vaccines). But the human population has absolutely no immunity against any H5 viruses.

## MAREK'S DISEASE

Over the past four years, Marek's disease has emerged as a big threat to poultry industry. So much so that, despite proper vaccination, it has inflicted up to 60% mortality among layer birds and virtually ruined farmers' economy. Causes for such vaccination failures are difficult to ascertain, although early exposure and the emergence of new strains of the virus, are important. Regardless of the reasons, Marek's disease has undoubtedly emerged as a serious threat.

Marek's disease (MD) is a tumour-causing viral disease of chickens. It is characterized by marked enlargement of the nerves, or marked enlargement of the liver, spleen and kidneys due to diffuse growth of certain cells (lymphoid cells).

The disease was first described by the Hungarian veterinarian Jozsef Marek in 1907, after whom it was named as Marek's disease. Involvement of nerves leads to paralysis which is a prominent symptom of the disease, and has given it names such as 'fowl paralysis', 'range paralysis', and 'polyneuritis'. Marek's disease is an economically important disease of worldwide distribution, including India. However, it was effectively controlled by vaccine. But now it has reappeared. It usually occurs between 2 and 8 months of age. Sometimes it also occurs after the birds have come into egg production. This form is referred to as 'late Marek's'. In a rare case, on postmortem examination, author observed Marek's disease in an 18-month-old layer.

## Cause

Marek's disease is caused by an enveloped, alphaherpesvirus which contains double-stranded DNA molecule (ds DNA). It is highly cell-associated, but readily transmitted, and its virulence varies and evolves. Marek's disease virus (MDV) occurs in three serotypes: 1, 2, and 3. Serotype 1 contains disease-producing strains of the virus; serotype 2 contains a group of non-disease-producing strains of the virus; and serotype 3 which is also a non-disease-producing strain but is related to herpesvirus of turkeys. It is commonly called the herpesvirus of turkeys (HVT).

Thus, it can be seen that disease-producing power is associated only with serotype 1 viruses. Serotype 2 and 3 have no disease-producing power and do not produce the disease. However, serotype 1 strains differ markedly in their disease-producing power. Based on their disease-producing ability, serotype 1 strains have been classified into four types: **(1) mildly harmful** (mMDV), **(2) harmful** (vMDV), **(3) very harmful** (vvMDV, and **(4) very very harmful** (vv+MDV). **Birds may become infected early in life, and remain infected until death.**

Another important feature of Marek's disease virus is that it is strictly cell-associated, except in the feather follicles, where cell-free virus is produced. Because of its cell association, it escapes action of antibodies after it gains entry into the body.

## Spread

1.  The virus spreads rapidly from infected to uninfected birds. It grows readily in the cells lining the feather follicles. The feather dander is a rich source of virus. The virus is present in cells shed from the feather follicles and in secretions from the mouth, nose, and trachea. **Cells from the feather follicles are the most important source of infection,** and are responsible for the infectivity of dander (minute scales from feathers or skin), poultry dust, and litter.

2.  **Virus spreads through the air (airborne spread), and infection by the respiratory tract is considered to be the most important route.** Marek's disease is highly contagious. Infected dander can transmit the disease over great distances. Material from the feather follicles is shed off as fine particles which are inhaled by the birds. Dander and feathers from infected chickens are infectious because they contain cell-free virus from the feather follicle epithelium **bound to cellular debris. Such materials remain infectious for 4-8 months at room temperature, and at times even up to one year.**

3.  Direct or indirect contact between birds spreads the virus. When feather dust and dander settle on clothes, equipment, etc., the virus is easily transmitted to other poultry houses and to poultry-producing areas.

4.  Many seemingly normal birds are carriers (i.e. carry the infection without showing symptoms) which can transmit the disease. Infection probably persists indefinitely.

5.  Beetles can carry the virus for several weeks, but insects are not considered to be an important means of infection.

6.  **The virus is not transmitted through the egg,** and thus chicks are hatched free of infection. The age at which birds become infected varies according to management and hygiene conditions. Commercial flocks are usually infected within a few weeks of hatching.

7.  **Once contracted, the infection persists throughout the life of the chicken and infected birds continue to contaminate the environment by shedding the virus.** Continued shedding of the virus by infected birds and hardiness of the virus are responsible for the prevalence of infection.

## Factors Influencing the Disease

There are a number of factors which affect the symptoms and severity of Marek's disease in individual bird and the severity of an outbreak of disease in a flock. These are:

1.  The genetic constitution of the chicken greatly influences the incidence and severity of Marek's disease. Genetically controlled resistance is not resistance to infection, but resistance to the development of disease after infection.

2.  The sex of the chicken also influences the incidence of disease: **females are more susceptible than males.**

3.  The age at infection and immune status of the chicken are also important. Resistance to the development of disease increases with the age. Chickens with passive immunity (due to maternal antibodies obtained from the hen) or active immunity (antibodies acquired following vaccination) are more resistant.

4.  The strain of virus is also important. Strains that have greater disease-producing power have more chances of producing the disease.

5.  Apart from all above, stress is the main environmental factor associated with increased incidence of Marek' disease. Transport, vaccinations, handling, debeaking, and changes of feed are the stresses that are of great importance.

## Development of the Disease

**The virus enters through the respiratory tract, by inhalation**, and then it grows within certain cells of the lungs. A quickly developing and severe phase of the disease occurs within 3-4 days, characterized by destruction of lymphocytes (one type of blood cell) mainly in the bursa of Fabricius, thymus, and also spleen. The primary target cells in all these organs are **B-lymphocytes.** (For information on B-lymphocytes, see Chapter 32: **'The avian immune system''**). Infected birds usually recover from this acute phase of the disease.

**After 6-7 days, the infection becomes latent (i.e. it exists but is not active).** This coincides with the development of immune responses. **Cell-mediated immunity** has been shown to be important. Most latently infected cells are CD4+ T-cells, although CD8+ T-cells and B-cells may also be involved. (To understand cell-mediated immunity and the role of T-lymphocytes, refer to Chapter 32). The virus is spread throughout the body by infected lymphocytes, and is present in the blood in a cell-associated form. The latent infection persists, and can last for the life of the bird.

**A secondary destructive infection** occurs in the feather follicles two weeks after the primary infection, and cell-free virus capable of producing infection is produced and shed into the environment in feather debris and dander. This is because feather follicle is the only known site of complete virus growth. Here, infection results in the development of large numbers of **enveloped, fully infectious virus particles.** At other places, most of the virus particles are **non-enveloped,** and therefore **non-infectious. To be infectious, virus particles must be enveloped, and this occurs only in the feather follicle epithelium.**

**Proliferation (multiplication) of the lymphocytes is the final response** and progresses to tumour (an abnormal mass of new tissue) formation. T-lymphocytes transform into tumour cells and proliferate in nerves and other tissues and organs. This results in infiltration of these cells in the nerves and lymphoma (tumour of lymphocytes) formation. Lymphomas consist mainly of T-lymphocytes, although some B-lymphocytes are also present. **Death of the birds from lymphomas may occur at any time from 3 weeks onward.**

**Vaccination changes development of the disease.** It severely reduces or eliminates the early destructive phase. Also, the level of latent infection is greatly reduced and immunosuppression (suppression of the immune responses) does not occur. Immunity following vaccination suppresses the active viral infection and thereby reduces the incidence of tumours.

## Symptoms

Marek's disease affects chickens from about 6 weeks of age. It occurs usually between 12 and 24 weeks of age, but older birds may also be affected. The incubation period (the interval between exposure to infection and appearance of symptoms) may be as short as 3-4 weeks in some, and several months in others. Clinical disease occurs in several forms.

## Classical Marek's Disease

**This form is now rarely seen.** Mortality varies, but is rarely more than 10-15%. In some outbreaks, mortality is confined to a few weeks, while in others a low incidence continues over many months. The symptoms depend on which nerve is affected. Involvement of brachial and sciatic nerves is common, and **leads to paralysis of the wings and legs (Fig. 8).** A particularly characteristic posture is that in which the bird has one leg stretched forward and the other backward as

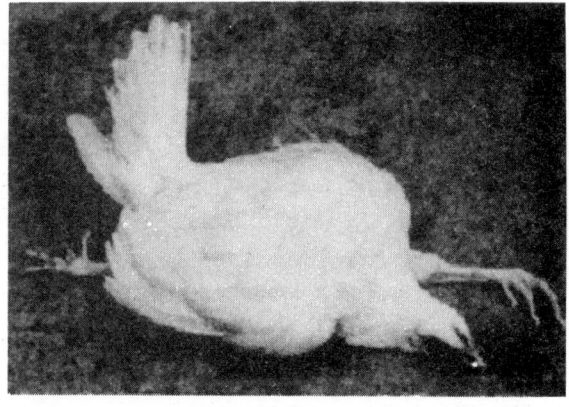

Fig. 8.   Paralysis of the legs of a chicken affected with Marek's disease.

a result of one sided paresis (partial paralysis) or paralysis of the leg. Sometimes, when the cervical nerves (i.e. of the neck) are involved, there may be torticollis (twisting of the neck to one side); and if the vagus and intercostal (i.e. between the ribs) nerves are affected, respiratory symptoms may develop. The interval between onset of symptoms and death varies from a few days to several weeks. Rarely, birds may recover.

## Acute Marek's Disease

**This form is the most common in our country.** Mortality in this form is usually much higher than in the classical form. Mortality of 10-30% of the flock is common, and outbreaks involving up to 80% of the flock are recorded. Many birds die suddenly without any preceding symptoms. Others appear depressed before death, and some show paralytic symptoms similar to those seen in the classical form.

## Postmortem Findings

**Classical Marek's disease:** The characteristic finding is marked enlargement of one or more nerves. Nerves commonly affected are the sciatic and brachial plexus (network), coeliac plexus, abdominal vagus, and intercostal nerves. **Affected nerves are up to 2-3 times the normal thickness (Fig. 9).** The normal striated and white glistening appearance is lost, and the nerve may appear greyish and sometimes oedematous (i.e. swollen from fluid accumulation). Some paralyzed birds show no visible enlargement at postmortem, but characteristic nerve changes are found microscopically. Sometimes, tumours (lymphomas) are present in addition to nerve changes. These tumours usually occur in the ovary, and are often small, soft, and grey in appearance, or rarely large, yellowish, and lobulated. Lungs, kidney, heart, and liver are sometimes affected by lymphomas.

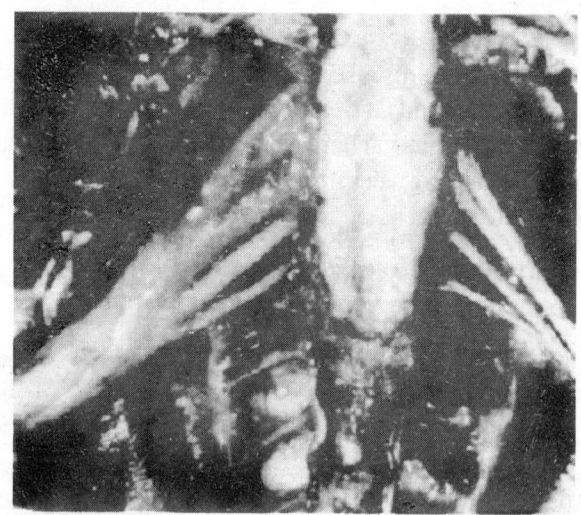

**Fig. 9.** Enlarged left sciatic nerve network in a chicken with Marek's disease. The right sciatic network is normal.

**Acute Marek's Disease:** A characteristic postmortem finding of Marek's disease in our country is **marked enlargement of the liver and spleen,** several times their normal size, showing white spots of cancerous tissue on the surface. Other typical finding is significant **enlargement of the proventriculus.** When opened, its wall is greatly thickened and the internal lining shows irregular, somewhat diffuse, blotchy haemorrhages, quite different from those seen in Ranikhet disease. There may also be enlargement of the kidneys, lungs, gonads (ovary, testes), and heart. In younger birds, liver enlargement is moderate, but in adult birds the liver is greatly enlarged, which is similar to that in lymphoid leukosis.

## Immunity

The vaccine-induced immunity is an anti-tumour immune response because vaccination does not prevent super-infection with a very virulent plus (vv+MDV) virus, **but does prevent tumour development.** However, vaccination reduces the early destructive phase of infection, and thus prevents extensive damage to the immune system. **Inactivated (killed) vaccines produce only antibody responses and not cell-mediated responses.**

Chickens infected with Marek's disease virus develop precipitating and virus neutralizing antibodies (humoral immunity) within 1-2 weeks. A transient Ig M response is replaced by IgG. However, **most of the antibodies have no role in protection of the bird.** This is because due to the cell-associated nature of the virus, antibodies are of not much importance in Marek's disease immunity. **It is the cell-mediated immunity that protects the bird.**

## Vaccinal Immunity

The sequence of events which occur following vaccination are: (1) **Natural killer cells** are activated as early as 3 days after vaccination. They produce **gamma-interferon** and kill a limited number of virus infected B-cells. Gamma-interferon also reduces virus replication. In addition, it stimulates macrophages. (2) **Activated macrophages,** in turn, produce enzyme nitric oxide synthase. This enzyme produces **nitric oxide (NO)** between 3 and 7 days post vaccination. NO limits the replication of field virus. (3) The antigen-specific **cytotoxic lymphocytes** start developing from 7 days and kill cells infected with field virus. The combination of these mechanisms pushes the field virus into latency. Memory cytotoxic T-lymphocytes quickly eliminate re-activated virus infected cells. **Thus, cell-mediated immunity prevents tumour formation.**

## Immunosuppression

Marek's disease affects the bursa of Fabricius, a gland necessary in the production of antibodies (see Chapter 32). **Damage to the immune response in Marek's disease results directly from destruction of lymphocytes in the bursa of Fabricius and thymus.** Both antibody-mediated and cell-mediated immunity are depressed. Thus, Marek's disease virus can increase susceptibility of birds to infection with coccidia. It must be remembered that while there is suppression of the immune responses, there is not a total loss of function. In fact, both antibody-mediated and cell-mediated immunity develop in competent birds after infection with Marek's disease virus. Antibody-mediated immunity is due to the development of antibodies. Antibodies remain throughout the life of the bird. A protective role for passively acquired maternal antibody has been observed in chicken. However, as antibodies are not required in immune resistance of Marek's disease, **it is the cell-mediated immunity that is important.** Thus, functional T-lymphocytes are required for resistance as well as for the development of immunity following vaccination (vaccinal immunity). (To understand the relative importance of antibody-mediated and cell-mediated immunity, see Chapter 32.) Permanent immunosuppression correlates with eventual tumour development and is seen only in birds that have already developed tumours. Thus, it is difficult to distinguish between cause and effect.

## Diagnosis

1.  Diagnosis is made on the basis of symptoms, **postmortem findings,** and microscopic changes. Classical Marek's can be tentatively diagnosed from symptoms of lameness or paralysis, and **acute Marek's disease by the presence of tumours in internal organs, on postmortem.** The tumours in birds under 18 weeks of age are usually caused by Marek's disease, but **'late Marek's'** may continue for another 10 weeks.

    Classical disease can often be diagnosed by the presence of peripheral nerves that may be yellowish and have lost their typical cross striations. However, diagnosis of Marek's disease is difficult under field conditions. This is because there is no truly characteristic postmortem finding, and also because changes in Marek's disease can closely resemble those of lymphoid leukosis, which is also a common disease. However, Marek's disease and lymphoid leukosis can be differentiated microscopically by the type of cells present in various organs.

2.  Infections not accompanied by symptoms are detected by virus isolation, or by demonstration of viral antigen in feather tips by agar-gel precipitation tests, or antibody in blood. However, it must be remembered that diagnosis of Marek's disease cannot be made by virological and serological tests alone. Other tests are required.

3.  Differentiation of Marek's disease from lymphoid leukosis is important. The main differentiating features are presented in Table 1.

## Differential Diagnosis

In lymphoid leukosis, chickens usually have gross tumours in the bursa of Fabricius. Tumours are absent in bursa in Marek's disease.

## Treatment

There is no treatment for Marek's disease.

## Control

Control is based on management methods, which include: (1) Isolation of growing chickens from sources of infection, (2) use of genetically resistant stock, and (3) vaccination.

**Table 1.** **Features useful in differentiating Marek's disease from lymphoid leukosis**

| Feature | Marek's disease | Lymphoid leukosis |
|---|---|---|
| Age | Six weeks or older | Not less than 16 weeks |
| Symptoms | Usually paralysis | Non-specific |
| Incidence | Usually above 5% in unvaccinated flocks | Rarely above 5% |
| **Postmortem findings:** | | |
| Enlargement of nerves | Common | Absent |
| Bursa of Fabricius | Diffuse enlargement or reduction | Nodular tumours |
| Tumours (lymphoid) in liver, heart, ovary, testes, skin, muscle, and proventriculus | May be present | Usually absent |
| Type of lymphocyte involved | T-lymphocyte | B-lymphocyte |

## Management and Hygiene

1. Because transmission of infection through eggs (vertical transmission) does not occur, chicks hatched and reared in isolation will be free of Marek's disease virus. However, this is difficult because of the highly infectious nature of the disease and widespread presence of the virus. Virus associated with **feathers** and **dander** is infectious, and contaminated poultry house dust remains infectious for several months. Chicks are mostly exposed to Marek's disease virus by contact with residual dust and dander, or by the introduction of these materials by aerosols (suspended fine particles in the air) from the nearby chicken houses, fomites, or personnel. **Once infected, chickens appear to shed virus indefinitely.**

2. Although it is very difficult to keep the flocks at farms free of Marek's disease virus, **management measures** can be used to reduce or delay infection and thus minimize the chance of serious disease. Young chicks should be reared in isolation from older stock for the first 2-3 months of life. This is the period when infection has serious effects. **An all-in, all-out policy should be adopted.** In this way it should be possible to break the infection cycle through disinfection when the houses are empty. Houses should be so constructed to allow thorough disinfection. **The failure to prevent early exposure is the most important single cause of vaccination failure.** Improved hygiene has played a key and cost-effective role in the control of excessive Marek's disease losses in vaccinated flocks.

3.  Because insects may act as reservoirs of infection, treatment of premises with insecticides is desirable.

4.  Vaccines should not be used as an alternative to good hygienic measures, but be taken as an additional step.

## Genetic Resistance

Poultry breeders can select for increased genetic resistance to Marek's disease and thus reduce susceptibility to the disease.

## Vaccination

Development of successful vaccines for control of Marek's disease is an important achievement, both in poultry science and basic cancer research. This is because Marek's disease, before vaccination, had become the most costly poultry disease, and also because this was the first time an important cancer had been controlled through vaccination in any species. Vaccination remains for now and also future the central strategy for the control of Marek's disease. Genetic resistance and biosecurity are also important additional measures to vaccination and may come to have greater significance in future as we come to know more about the limitations of vaccination.

**Marek's disease vaccinations are very effective, usually achieving more than 90% protection under commercial conditions.** However, at times, there are increasing numbers of flocks in which Marek's disease losses are excessive. The causes for such **'vaccination failures'** are difficult to determine. However, early exposure and **emergence of 'new' strains of the virus** with increased disease-producing power may be important.

**Commercially available vaccines are derived from all three serotypes (see under 'causes'), for use either alone or in combination.**

**All vaccines are used mostly as a single dose in day-old chicks, usually administered at the hatchery.** The vaccine is injected subcutaneously (i.e. under the skin) in the nape of the neck. The recommended dose is 1000 plaque-forming units per chick. A significant level of protection is developed within about a week and **protection lasts throughout the life of the chicken. However, the vaccines do not prevent re-infection, or a second infection with disease-producing field viruses.**

## Serotype 1 Vaccines

1.  Vaccines are produced from serotype 1 whose disease-producing power has been completely removed. The first commercial vaccine was of this type. It is available only in a **cell-associated form.** Commercially its widespread use was soon replaced by the HVT (herpesvirus of turkey-serotype 3).

2.  The next category includes vaccines produced from serotype 1 whose disease-

producing power has been markedly reduced. Example of this type of serotype 1 is the **CVI-988 (Rispens) strain of Marek's disease virus** which retains very slight disease-producing ability. It is a **cell-associated vaccine.** More recently it has been used in combination with HVT vaccine.

## Serotype 2 Vaccines

Serotype 2 viruses are naturally occurring non-disease-producing strains of Marek's disease virus. They are widespread among poultry flocks and may provide natural immunization (vaccination) against Marek's disease. An example of this serotype is the **SB-1 strain** which is protective, in a **cell-associated form**, against most strains of harmful Marek's disease virus, but is less protective against very harmful Marek's disease virus. In combination with the HVT, however, SB-1 provides good protection against very harmful Marek's disease virus. SB-1 vaccine is available commercially in India.

## Serotype 3 Vaccines

The turkey herpesvirus falls in serotype 3. An example of this serotype is the **FC-126 strain.** It is widely used commercially in either a **cell-associated form** or a **cell-free form**, and is highly effective against harmful Marek's disease virus. **A cell-associated form requires storage in liquid nitrogen,** which is difficult, but even then it has been most widely used because it is more effective than cell-free virus in the presence of maternal antibodies.

HVT vaccine has been most extensively used because it is economical to produce, and the cell-free virus extracted from infected cells can be lyophilized (freeze-dried) for more convenient storage and handling. To lyophilize or freeze-dry is to dry in a frozen state under high vacuum for preservation.

## Combination of Two or Three Vaccines

It was observed that when serotype 1, 2 or 3 vaccines were used alone, they did not provide adequate protection against very harmful Marek's disease virus. **However, when used in combination of two or three vaccines they show a synergistic effect and provide good protection.** (Synergistic effect means that the combined effect of two or more vaccines is greater than the sum of their individual effects.) **A combination of two consisting of the SB-1 strain of serotype 2 and FC-126 strain of serotype 3 (HVT), that is, a bivalent vaccine, has been found to be particularly effective and is now in commercial use in India in a cell-associated form.** Other bivalent vaccines used are CV1- 988 Marek's disease virus and HVT; and attenuated HPRS-16 Marek's disease virus and HVT (serotype 1 and 3).

## Factors Affecting Effectiveness of Vaccine/Vaccination

1.  **Vaccine is usually given at hatching.** Both cell-associated and cell-free vaccines are given by subcutaneous injection. The amount of the vaccine administered is

very important. The quantitative measure is in plaque-forming units (PFUs). **Proper and adequate immunization in the layer chicks requires at least 5000 PFUs.** When the dosage is 0.2 ml, each dose should contain 5000 PFUs, or more. In broilers, the vaccine is usually diluted to one-half or one-third strength.

2.  The intramuscular (within the muscle) route is slightly more effective than the subcutaneous (below the skin) route.

3.  The shorter the interval between vaccination and exposure to the disease-producing field virus, the poorer the level of protection. **Early exposure is one of the most important causes of excessive Marek's disease in vaccinated flocks. This is because at least seven days are required for a solid immunity to be produced and also because field exposure usually occurs very soon after placement of chickens.**

4.  Keeping the chicks under **strict biosecurity in the first week** also allows vaccines to stimulate immunity in the chicks before Marek's disease virus infects them.

5.  The strain of chicken is also an important factor (see **'genetic resistance'.**) For example, HVT vaccine in a genetically resistant chicken produces better immunity than a combination of HVT + SB-1 vaccine in a susceptible chicken.

6.  In an attempt to improve the effectiveness of vaccination, **increased vaccine doses or revaccination at 7-12 days were tried without any success.** However, keeping in view the need for more effective immunity, vaccine manufacturers have increased recommended doses. **Many layer and breeder chickens now receive up to 10,000 PFU of HVT at hatchery. Revaccination** has been used in Europe and sometimes also in the United States, **but there is no convincing evidence of its effectiveness.**

7.  Stress interferes with the maintenance of vaccinal immunity. It is believed that immunosuppressive stress may play an important role in Marek's disease losses, especially in those that occur after the onset of egg production.

8.  Marek's disease vaccines as a class are usually effective, often achieving greater than 90% protection under commercial conditions. However, even then at times some flocks show excessive losses despite proper vaccination. Causes for such vaccine failures are difficult to ascertain, although **early exposure and the emergence of new Marek's disease virus strains with increased virulence may be important. The failure to prevent early exposure is perhaps the most important single cause of vaccine failures.**

9.  The tendency of Marek's disease virus to evolve to greater virulence is critical in the overall planning and use of vaccines for Marek's disease. **Experts believe that the useful life of a Marek's disease vaccine is about 10 years under present management conditions.**

10. There is no direct evidence that late losses in Marek's disease are due to recent or late exposure to a 'new' viral strain. In fact, this is unlikely due to the natural resistance of older chickens to Marek's disease infection, and also because this resistance is increased by earlier vaccination and exposure to other field strains.

11. Various other infections, such as Gumboro disease, chicken infectious anaemia, reovirus, and reticuloendotheliosis have been reported to interfere with the production of immunity following vaccination.

12. Naturally occurring infection with non-disease-producing serotype 2, or with serotype 1 having low disease-producing power, may provide protection against subsequent exposure to disease-producing viruses. They may also help vaccination in producing effective immunity.

13. Proper handling of vaccine during thawing (i.e. making liquid from a frozen state) is very important. Also, **vaccination of breeders with a serotype 1 or 2 virus, rather than HVT, would make progeny respond better to vaccination with HVT.**

14. Outbreaks associated with very harmful strains of Marek's disease virus in flocks vaccinated with HVT can usually be controlled by vaccination with vaccines composed of all three serotypes, or of serotype 2 and 3. **The combination of serotype 2 and 3 is much more effective against infection with very harmful strains of Marek's disease virus.**

15. As already mentioned under combination of vaccines, **synergism is best seen with viruses of serotypes 2 and 3. Vaccines composed of the FC-126 strain of HTV combined with either the SB-1** or 301B/1 strains of serotype 2 Marek's disease virus **give excellent protection and are widely used.** A variety of other combinations are also used, such as serotype 1 and 3, or vaccines having all three serotypes. Although the advantage of three combinations (polyvalent vaccine) compared to simpler combinations has not been shown, there are also no negative effects of their use.

16. As already mentioned in the beginning, Marek's disease in recent years has become a serious economic threat to the poultry industry causing heavy losses. **This is because vaccines are not 100% effective.** The main reason being the emergence of 'new' strains of the virus with increased virulence (disease-producing power). **In fact, poultry industry worldwide remains concerned about the possibility that vaccines may ultimately fail due to the evolution of more virulent strains of Marek's disease virus, resulting in serious losses.**

## Conclusion

The emergence of increasingly powerful and harmful viral strains of Marek's disease, associated with a reduction in the effectiveness of vaccines during the past 20 years, has caused anxiety. This indicates that vaccination by itself does not provide a complete control programme, and certainly it is not the final solution for Marek's disease. Strict biosecurity procedures (see **'biosecurity'**) to reduce early exposure, and the presence of genetic resistance, are essential additional requirements for a successful vaccination programme.

**Note:** For a list of commercially available Marek's disease vaccine, refer to Chapter 19 under **"Marek's disease vaccines"**.

## LEUKOSIS/SARCOMA GROUP OF DISEASES

There is a group of viruses called **'avian leukosis/sarcoma viruses'**. These viruses produce a number of conditions in poultry known as **'leukosis/sarcoma group of diseases'**. The main characteristic of these diseases is that they are **neoplastic or cancerous in nature**. That is, they are characterized by an abnormal and unlimited growth of cells in the body which usually causes bird's death. These diseases include lymphoid leukosis, erythroid leukosis (erythroblastosis), and myeloid leukosis (myeloblastosis and myelocytomatosis). **Of these, only lymphoid leukosis is sufficiently common to be of economic importance.** It is a significant cause of loss to the poultry industry in India. The other conditions are rare and unimportant. Therefore, only lymphoid leukosis will be discussed.

More recently, **a subclinical infection by avian leukosis virus,** without producing a cancerous condition, has been found to reduce egg production. This has made prevention of infection by avian leukosis viruses all the more important.

## LYMPHOID LEUKOSIS

**Lymphoid leukosis is the commonest disease caused by avian leukosis/ sarcoma viruses.** It is a tumour-producing viral disease, and is **characterized by marked enlargement of the liver.** Other organs are also enlarged. Nodular growths can be found in the bursa of Fabricius in almost all cases. Lymphoid leukosis occurs any time after 14 weeks of age. **However, incidence is usually highest at about sexual maturity. Lymphoid leukosis is usually a problem of breeders and laying hens.** However, some new strains are known to affect young broiler chicks.

### Cause

Avian leukosis/sarcoma are **enveloped**, single-stranded RNA viruses (alpharetroviruses), and widely prevalent in commercial chickens. Infection occurs in all chicken flocks. By sexual maturity, most birds are exposed. **However, the incidence of clinical disease is usually low.**

### Spread

1.  **Lymphoid leukosis virus is transmitted both vertically from hen to progeny**

through the egg, and also horizontally from bird to bird by direct or indirect contact.

2. Usually only a small number of chicks are infected vertically, and the majority becomes infected by contact with vertically infected chicks during rearing. Although only a small number of chicks are infected vertically, this route of spread is important because it provides a means of maintaining the infection from one generation to the next. Most birds become infected by close contact with vertically infected birds. Although vertical spread is important in maintaining the infection, horizontal infection is also necessary to maintain a rate of vertical spread sufficient to prevent the infection from dying out. The infection does not spread readily from infected birds to birds not in direct contact, such as in separate pens or cages, **because of the relatively short life of the virus outside the birds.**

3. Vertical infection occurs from hens which shed virus from the oviduct into the **egg albumen,** from where it passes into the chick embryo. Vertical infection of the embryo is associated with shedding by the hen of lymphoid leukosis virus into egg albumen and with presence of virus in the vagina of hens.

   **Shedding of virus into egg albumen and spread to the embryo is a result of virus production by albumen-secreting glands of the oviduct.** Recent studies have revealed a high degree of virus growth in the magnum. Magnum is that portion of the oviduct which comes after the infundibulum. Egg stays in the magnum for nearly 3 hours, and 3 layers of albumen are added here. Virus growth also occurs in various cells of the ovary, but not in the follicular cells or ovum, and trans-ovarian infection (i.e. through the ovary) is not important. Not all eggs that have virus in the albumen give rise to infected embryos or chicks. Only about one-half to one-eighth of embryos are reported to be infected from eggs with virus in the albumen. This intermittent vertical spread may be a result of neutralization of virus by antibody in the yolk, and also from loss because of heat inactivation.

4. Chick embryos do not become infected from the male. The virus does not multiply in germ cells. The cock therefore acts only as a virus carrier and source of contact of venereal infection (through sex) to other birds.

5. Vertically infected chicks develop immunological tolerance to lymphoid leukosis virus. Because of this tolerance, they fail to develop antibodies but continue to have virus in the blood. When such chicks become hens, hens of this class have much virus in the oviduct and shed it into most of their eggs and embryos.

6. Chicks infected horizontally have virus in their blood for only a short time, and then develop virus-neutralizing antibodies without virus in the blood. Such birds are usually virus carriers. That is, they carry the virus/infection without suffering the disease. A small number of hens of this type have an oviduct infection, and shed the virus to their progeny periodically.

7.  The incidence of lymphoid leukosis decreases if horizontal infection occurs after the first few weeks of life. Virus is present in the saliva, faeces, and feather debris of infected birds, **but its survival outside the body is relatively short (a few hours only). Therefore, lymphoid leukosis virus is not very contagious.**

8.  Older hens (2-3 years of age) spread virus in their eggs less regularly and at a lower level than birds under 18 months.

9.  Virus particles are present in the pancreas (an abdominal gland) and many other organs of infected chicken embryos. These particles, which are highly infectious, are shed in droppings of newly hatched chicks. Infectious virus is also present in saliva and faeces of older birds that provide a source of horizontal infection to other birds.

10. Avian retroviruses have high lipid content in the envelope (30-35%), **and therefore their infectivity is destroyed by lipid solvents and detergents.**

## Certain Features of Lymphoid Leukosis

1.  Usually only a small number of infected birds develop lymphoid leukosis. The others remain **carriers** and **shedders**.

2.  Incidence of lymphoid leukosis decreases rapidly if infection by natural routes occurs after the first few weeks of age.

3.  Immunosuppression (suppression of the immune responses) caused by Gumboro disease virus increases the rate of shedding of lymphoid leukosis virus.

4.  Resistance of birds to lymphoid leukosis increases with age.

5.  The genetic constitution of the bird has a strong influence on the response to lymphoid leukosis virus.

6.  **Females are more susceptible to lymphoid leukosis than males.**

## Development of the Disease

The incubation period, that is, the interval between exposure to infection and appearance of the first symptoms is 4 months or more. The basic cell that transforms itself into a cancerous cell in lymphoid leukosis and then spreads into different organs of the body comes from bursa of Fabricius. These transformed cells are **lymphoblasts**. These cells proliferate and give rise to **nodular growths (tumours) into the bursa** which are visible from about 14 weeks of age. **It is now established that lymphoid leukosis is a cancer of the bursa-dependent lymphoid system.** In fact, lymphoid leukosis always begins as a tumour in the bursa of Fabricius and remains localized until the bursa atrophies (i.e. is reduced in size) at sexual maturity. **Therefore, the incubation period is 4 months or more.** (To get an idea of the bursa-dependent lymphoid system, see Chapter 32: "The avian immune system").

Sometimes losses up to 30% can occur from mortality occurring between 5 to 9 months of age in egg-laying and breeding stock. Subclinical infections by lymphoid leukosis virus have adverse effects on egg production, egg size, fertility, hatchability and growth rate, and they also increase non-specific mortality.

## Symptoms

. The symptoms are non-specific. The bird may be weak and emaciated, and show loss of appetite. The comb may be pale, shrivelled, and sometimes cyanotic (i.e. of bluish discoloration). Diarrhoea may occur and the wattles may be pale. The abdomen is usually enlarged because of the massive liver. Enlargement of liver, bursa of Fabricius and/or kidneys can often be detected on palpation. Once symptoms begin to develop, the course is usually rapid.

## Postmortem Findings

**The liver is greatly enlarged (Fig. 10).** The spleen, bursa of Fabricius, kidneys and ovary are also usually enlarged. Bone marrow is often tumourous.

Grossly visible **tumours** almost always involve liver, spleen, and bursa of Fabricius. Size of tumour is highly variable as are number of organs affected. In addition to the liver and spleen, these may include kidney, lung, gonad (ovary, testes), heart, bone marrow and mesentery.

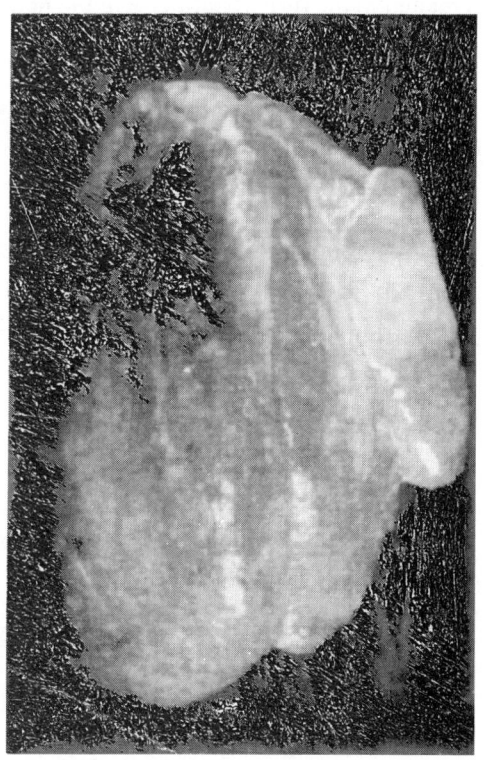

**Fig. 10.** Lymphoid leukosis (diffuse form). Note marked enlargement of the liver.

Tumours are soft, smooth, and glistening. A cut surface appears slightly greyish to creamy white. Growth may be nodular, granular, or diffuse, or a combination of these forms. In the **nodular form,** lymphoid tumours vary from 0.5 mm to 5 cm in diameter, are usually spherical and may occur singly or in large numbers. The **granular form** consists of numerous small nodules less than 2 mm in diameter and uniformly distributed throughout the liver. In the **diffuse form,** the liver is uniformly enlarged, slightly greyish in colour, and usually very friable. Sometimes, the liver is firm, hard, and almost gritty.

## Immunity

Antibodies from infected hens are passed through the yolk to progeny chicks. This provides them passive immunity (maternal antibodies) against contact infection, which lasts for 3-4 weeks. This passively acquired antibody delays infection by lymphoid leukosis virus, reduces incidence of tumours, and also the incidence of viraemia (presence of virus in blood) and shedding of the virus. Level and persistence of antibody in the chick is related to the titre of antibody in the hen's blood.

## Genetic Resistance

Two types of genetic resistance to lymphoid leukosis virus are recognized: (1) Resistance to virus infection, and (2) resistance to tumour/cancer development.

## Diagnosis

1.  Postmortem findings may suggest lymphoid leukosis. However, correct diagnosis requires pathological and virological examinations.

2.  **Pathological diagnosis:** Diagnosis of lymphoid leukosis is made by gross and microscopic examination of freshly killed or recently died birds. Microscopic examination of the impression smears of fresh tumour tissue, stained with May-Grunwald-Giemsa stain, is very helpful in arriving at a diagnosis. If possible, several birds should be examined. The tissues to be examined include liver, spleen, bursa of Fabricius and bone marrow, and any other tumour tissue. **Differentiation of lymphoid leukosis from Marek's disease is important and is described under differential diagnosis.**

3.  **Virological Diagnosis:** This involves isolation and identification of the causative agent. Blood (plasma, serum) and tumour tissue are the best materials for isolation of lymphoid leukosis virus. The presence of infection can be demonstrated easily by detection of neutralizing antibodies in serum. Virus can also be detected from tumour tissue such as liver, vaginal and cloacal swabs, egg albumen, and embryos. Because the virus is easily destroyed at room temperature, samples should be collected from live or freshly killed birds, or from newly laid eggs, and stored at -70$^0$ C.

## Differential Diagnosis

1.  **Lymphoid leukosis and Marek's disease can be differentiated only with difficulty.** This is because similar lymphoid tumours may occur in both diseases in the same organs during the same age period. Lesions in the organs in these two diseases cannot be differentiated by gross examination alone. **Diagnosis is possible in most cases on careful microscopic examination.** However, considerable experience is necessary.

2. In coming to a decision, history, symptoms, gross and microscopic changes, and cytology (cell picture) should all be considered. For example, lymphoid leukosis usually does not occur before 14 weeks of age and most of the mortality occurs between 24 and 40 weeks. On the other hand, Marek's disease may occur as early as 4 weeks, and the mortality peak varies from 10 to 20 weeks. Sometimes, losses continue and may reach a peak after 20 weeks.

3. **Nodular tumours of the bursa** can usually be palpated through the cloaca **in birds infected with lymphoid leukosis.** Paralysis associated with gross lesions in nerves is specific for Marek's disease.

4. As stated, the bursa of Fabricius plays a central role in the development of lymphoid leukosis. **When distinct lymphoid tumours are present in the bursa, a diagnosis of lymphoid leukosis can be made.** Such tumours are sometimes quite small and may be overlooked. Marek's disease, on the other hand, usually causes a premature reduction in the size of the bursa.

5. Cytologically (cell picture-wise), lymphoid leukosis tumours are usually composed of a homogeneous population of lymphoblasts. In contrast, tumours of Marek's disease usually contain lymphoid cells varying in size and maturity from lymphoblasts to small lymphocytes. Plasma cells may also be present.

6. **Lymphoid leukosis tumours are composed almost entirely of B-lymphocytes** and have surface IgM markers, whereas 60-90% of **Marek's disease tumour cells are T-lymphocytes that** lack IgM markers and only about 3-25% are B-lymphocytes.

## Treatment

No treatment or vaccines are available.

## Control

1. Control must be based on high standards of hygiene and flock management to reduce infection from the environment.

2. Also, birds used should be from a disease-free source of genetically resistant stock.

3. Because the infection is egg transmitted, it cannot be prevented by rearing in isolation.

Taking these facts into consideration, control is discussed under three heads: (1) Eradication, (2) Selection for genetic resistance, and (3) Immunization.

## Eradication

1. **Eradication of infected breeding hens is the best method of controlling lymphoid leukosis.** Since egg transmission is the number one method of spreading the disease, removal of carrier birds from the breeding flock has been highly

successful in reducing the infection in their progeny. In such cases, mortality due to tumours has been reduced and egg production has increased. **Breeder hens are tested by various methods for the presence of lymphoid leukosis virus, and those that test positive are discarded.**

2.  Lymphoid leukosis virus can be eradicated (removed) from flocks. Eradication of infection depends on breaking the vertical spread of virus from hen to progeny. To establish a leukosis-free flock it is necessary to hatch, rear, and maintain in isolation a group of chickens free from vertical infection. To achieve this, eggs must be obtained from hens that are not transmitting virus to their progeny.

3.  An approach for eradication of lymphoid leukosis virus involves:

    (i)   Selection of fertile eggs from hens negative in the egg albumen or vaginal swab test,

    (ii)  Hatching of chicks in isolation in small groups (25-50) in wire-floored cages, avoiding manual vent sexing, and also avoiding vaccination with a common needle to prevent mechanical spread of any residual infection.

    (iii) Testing of chicks for the virus, discarding reactors and contact chickens, and

    (iv)  Rearing lymphoid leukosis virus-free groups in isolation.

4.  Chicks are most susceptible to contract infection by lymphoid leukosis virus during the period immediately after hatching. **Vertically infected chicks are the main source of such infection.** However, there are several methods that can reduce or eliminate infection remaining from previous flocks. Incubators, hatchers, brooding houses, and all equipment should be thoroughly cleaned and disinfected between each use. Chick boxes should not be reused, and each farm should have only one age group of chickens. The danger of introducing strains of virus not already present in the flock can be prevented if eggs or chicks from different sources are not mixed, or if chicks are reared under isolation conditions that will prevent cross-contamination of flocks.

## Selection for Genetic Resistance

Resistance to infection is controlled by recessive genes that are present in varying frequency in commercial strains. Commercial breeding companies can increase the frequency of the resistance genes and develop stocks resistant to lymphoid leukosis.

## Immunization

Possible use of activated vaccines to increase bird's resistance can be extremely helpful in controlling lymphoid leukosis. However, attempts to produce attenuated strains of virus that do not cause the disease have so far failed.

# AVIAN ENCEPHALOMYELITIS

Avian encephalomyelitis (AE) is a viral disease of young chickens. It is characterized by muscular incoordination and rapid tremors, especially of the head and neck. Because of the tremor (trembling or shaking), it is often called **'epidemic tremor'**. The disease is worldwide in distribution, including India. Its economic importance is due to the infection it causes in **chicks**, reduced egg production in laying hens, and a lowered hatchability of fertile eggs. It is a disease of the intestinal tract and central nervous system.

Avian encephalomyelitis is caused by an enterovirus, which is a **non-enveloped**, single-stranded RNA virus. The virus is relatively resistant to physical and chemical agents. However, the virus is susceptible to a single exposure to formaldehyde fumigation. Beta-propiolactone inactivates the virus.

## Factors Influencing the Disease

1. The **immune status of the bird** influences the outcome of infection. Maternal antibodies protect young chicks against infection. It is usually difficult to produce the disease in chicks as they become older. This is due to increasing ability to produce antibodies with age and development of a protective antibody response.

2. In adult birds, the immune response to natural infection or vaccination, prevents egg transmission of the virus. It also provides protective maternal immunity which lasts through the highly susceptible period in the life of the young bird.

## Spread

1. **Transmission through egg (vertical transmission) is a very important means of virus spread.** Transmission of the virus occurs through the egg, from infected to susceptible birds housed together. Egg transmission occurs between the period of infection of laying hens and the development of immunity, a period of 3-4 weeks. Spread of infection from chicks, who acquired infection while inside the eggs (**congenital infection**), to susceptible chicks can occur in the hatchery and during breeding and also in older flock.

2. Under natural conditions, avian encephalomyelitis is basically an intestinal infection. As the virus multiplies in the intestinal tract, it is shed in the faeces. Since the **virus is very resistant to environmental factors,** contaminated water and feed are sources of spread from bird to bird and house to house. Similarly, transfer of faecal material to uninfected houses or premises will cause an outbreak. Disease can be transmitted by people and equipment contaminated with virus-containing faeces. **Ingestion is the usual route of entry. Exposure through the respiratory tract is unimportant,** apart from the simultaneous exposure of the digestive tract.

3. Spread also occurs through fomites (i. e. substances capable of mechanically carrying infection) and mechanical carriers. Infected litter is a source of virus that is easily

transmitted horizontally (laterally) by fomites. Infection spreads rapidly from bird to bird within a pen or house once introduced, and from pen to pen on farms where no special precautions are taken to prevent spread.

4. Some birds carry the infection in their intestine without showing the symptoms (**enteric carriers**). Such birds excrete the virus in their droppings for a period of several days. **Because it is quite resistant to environmental conditions, it remains infectious for long periods of time.** The period during which the virus is excreted in faeces depends on the age of the bird when infected. Very young chicks may excrete virus for more than 2 weeks, whereas those infected after 3 weeks of age may shed virus for only 5 days. Survival of the virus outside the body promotes indirect spread through fomites.    '

## Development of the Disease

The virus enters the tissues from the infected egg, when the infection is already present in the eggs laid. **After hatching, the virus enters through the mouth (oral route).** In young chicks the virus may be spread in a variety of tissues, including brain, organs, and muscles. A number of infected embryos may be killed during the last few days of incubation. **In chicks** which hatch, the period of incubation (period between the entry of virus and appearance of first symptoms) is 1-7 days. In those chicks which are infected after hatching, the period of incubation is at least 11 days. Thus, the disease pattern varies. There may be a reduction in hatchability and symptoms appear during the first 10 days of life in those chicks which acquire infection while still inside the eggs, whereas symptoms appear between 2-5 weeks in those infected after hatching. Although infection may be generalized following entry of the virus at any age, disease of the nervous system is seen only in the first few weeks of life.

## Symptoms

Avian encephalomyelitis **usually makes its appearance when chicks are 1-2 weeks of age.** Symptoms include depression, muscular incoordination (ataxia), and tremors. **In layers,** there is some drop of egg production, with reduced hatchability. The nervous symptoms may be seen at or soon after hatching, but are usually seen at one week of age. The ataxia varies from slight incoordination to sitting on the hocks, or lying down on one side. In such a condition death occurs from not reaching to the feed (starvation), or getting crushed by other members of the flock. **Birds over 4 weeks of age rarely show evidence of avian encephalomyelitis.**

**Very mildly affected birds recover completely.** Tremors may be absent in some outbreaks, or may occur in only a few birds. They usually occur after the early stages of incoordination and may be confined to the head and neck, or may be observed over the entire body. Morbidity (number of birds affected) may be as high as 60%, but is usually 15% of the flock. Mortality, however, is high and could be more than 50%. Fresh cases rarely occur after 5-6 weeks of age.

**In layers,** the drop in egg production is about 5-10% and lasts for 5-14 days, after that it returns to full production. The fall in hatchability accompanies the drop in production and is about 5% of fertile eggs.

## Postmortem Findings

There are no gross lesions (changes) in the young or older birds.

## Diagnosis

1.  The symptoms in young birds, absence of gross changes at postmortem, together with the absence of other virus infections and nutritional deficiencies affecting the nervous system, are strongly suggestive of avian encephalomyelitis.

2.  However, a definitive diagnosis requires demonstration of the virus by isolation or other means. Laboratory tests include histopathological examination of the brain, fluorescent antibody test, and enzyme-linked immunosorbent assay (ELISA).

3.  In differential diagnosis it is necessary to consider other diseases affecting the nervous system, including virus infections such as Ranikhet and Marek's disease and nutritional encephalomalacia (see under 'vitamin E deficiency'.)

## Treatment

Treatment is of no value.

## Control

1.  Under commercial conditions it is not possible to eliminate infection by high standards of hygiene alone. Thus, control depends on the vaccination of birds, and using hatching eggs from breeder flocks that are free from avian encephalomyelitis.

2.  **Live and killed vaccines** are available. **Live vaccines** can be given in the drinking water, and produce a lasting and adequate degree of protection (see Chapter 19, under 'avian encephalomyelitis vaccines'). However, the live vaccine usually causes a drop in egg production if it is given in laying birds. A **killed-virus** vaccine may be used for flocks in production. There is less effect on egg production.

3.  Vaccination is carried out to protect mainly against the spread of virus through the egg and development of disease in the progeny, and also against a fall in egg production and hatchability. **Commercial layers are usually not vaccinated because the total fall in egg production is small.**

4.  The age at which the birds are vaccinated with the live vaccine should be selected such that the virus does not produce harmful effects, or fail to produce immunity. During the first 6 weeks of life live vaccine might produce disease, and during the

first 8 weeks maternal antibody may interfere with the immune response. **Live vaccine given to birds while in laying may cause egg transmission and disease in the progeny.** Thus, such vaccines are usually given between 8 and 16 weeks of age. A period of at least 2 weeks, on either side of vaccination, is to be given between this and the administration of other vaccines. Vaccination can be done through drinking water. **Immunity against avian encephalomyelitis is long lasting.**

About 4 weeks after vaccination, serum should be submitted to diagnostic laboratory for an evaluation of the presence of antibodies. The enzyme-linked immunosorbent assay (ELISA) test is most frequently used.

5.　In an outbreak in chicks, affected birds are best destroyed since most will die.

6.　**Killed vaccines** may be used for protecting laying flocks without causing a drop in egg production, as might occur with live vaccines.

7.　Although certain aspects of the spread of this disease are not understood, **hygienic precautions** such as cleaning and disinfection between flocks and disposal of carcasses and litter must be followed. **This will, at least, limit the concentration of virus.**

**Note:** For a list of commercial vaccines available against avian encephalomyelitis, refer to Chapter 19 under **"Avian encephalomyelitis vaccines"**.

# AVIAN NEPHRITIS

Avian nephritis is an acute, highly contagious, typically subclinical disease of young chickens that produces **changes in the kidneys.** Avian nephritis virus was first described in Japan in 1976. It was isolated from the rectal contents of a normal 1-week-old broiler chicken. Chickens of all ages are infected, but 1-day-old chicks are the most susceptible. Avian nephritis virus is a RNA virus. It has been shown to be an astrovirus.

## Spread

Avian nephritis virus is distributed worldwide in chickens. Spread readily occurs by direct or indirect contact, through ingestion of faecally contaminated material. Egg transmission has been suggested on the basis of field observations.

## Disease

Chickens of all ages may be infected, but it has been observed that **1-day-old chicks are most susceptible.** The virus is widely distributed and is present in kidney, small intestine, rectum, bursa of Fabricius, spleen, and liver, but not in brain or trachea.

## Symptoms

Symptom in 1-day-old chicks is only mild diarrhoea, but not all chicks show the symptom. The affected chicks reveal significantly lowered body weight. In broiler chickens, clinical symptoms vary from none (subclinical) to outbreaks of the so-called runting syndrome and baby chick nephropathy.

## Postmortem Findings

There is mild to severe discoloration and swelling of the kidneys. Even visceral urate deposits may be observed. Chalk-like urate crystals are deposited on the surface of the peritoneum (a membrane in the body cavity) and liver. The heart is white due to heavy urate deposits on its surface.

## Diagnosis

Antibodies to avian nephritis virus can be detected by indirect immunofluorescence, virus neutralization tests, and ELISA. Of these, serum neutralization test is the most sensitive, but is costly and laborious.

## Control

Until the role of avian nephritis virus becomes known, it is difficult to suggest control measures.

## EGG DROP SYNDROME (EDS 76)

**Egg drop syndrome is a disease of laying hens.** Since its first description in 1976 in The Netherlands (Holland), egg drop syndrome has become a major cause of loss in egg production throughout the world. There is a sudden drop in egg production around the peak. The syndrome is characterized by otherwise healthy birds producing thin-shelled or shell-less eggs. The disease is caused by a group III adenovirus. It is **non-enveloped** and contains DNA. **Only one serotype is recognized. Once common, the disease is now relatively rare.**

Although disease outbreaks have been recorded only in laying hens, the **natural hosts** for egg drop syndrome are **ducks** and **geese**. The virus got introduced into the chicken, probably through a contaminated vaccine grown in duck cells. In the laying hens, the virus usually remains latent until birds come to peak production.

## Spread

The disease occurs in **three patterns.**

1. In the **classical form**, the **breeders** are infected, and the **main method** of spread is **vertical transmission**. That is, the virus is passed from parents to progeny. However, infected chicks excrete no virus and usually show no serological evidence of the disease **until egg production reaches 50%.** At this stage, virus is reactivated and excreted, resulting in rapid lateral spread.

2. The **second pattern (endemic form)** results from **lateral (horizontal) spread** between flocks. This is mainly due to the contaminated eggs or trays, and is usually seen in commercial egg layers. In India, once 32.6% of poultry flocks were found to be infected. Laying flock of any age may be affected. **Lateral spread** of virus is slow and occurs at intervals. It may take up to eleven weeks to spread through a cage house. Spread of virus between birds on litter is usually faster, but is slow in cages.

3. The **third (sporadic) form** occurs in **occasional isolated cases**, and is also seen in any age or breed of bird. It results from introduction of infection from ducks, geese or any infected wild bird, either through direct contact or indirectly through contaminated water.

Although faeces do not contain virus, droppings are contaminated because of the exudate (inflammatory fluid) from the oviduct. Lateral spread between flocks through contaminated people or substances can occur, but does not appear to be a major risk. Other methods of spread could be contaminated needles and, possibly, biting insects.

## Symptoms

The first symptoms are loss of shell strength and colour in pigmented eggs. This is soon followed by **thin-shelled, soft-shelled and shell-less eggs.** Eggshells may show mineral deposits. However, deformed eggs and eggs with ridges are not a feature. It is not clear whether there is an actual drop in egg numbers, or whether the drop in production is due to affected eggs being eaten or lost in the litter. The birds are normally healthy, but sometimes they appear slightly depressed. Diarrhoea has been described, but there is probably an excess of oviduct secretion in the droppings.

**Classical form** is characterized either by a drop in egg production (by 40 to 50%) around peak, or by a failure to achieve or hold expected production. In the first case the flock has no detectable antibody before the drop in production. In the second case, a small percentage of the flock develops antibody during the growing period. The birds with antibody reduce the spread of virus, so that there is a prolonged period of some birds having egg drop syndrome. A similar situation is observed when the virus is spread laterally in a cage unit.

## Postmortem Findings

Inactive ovaries and a decrease in the size of oviducts (atrophy) are usually the only postmortem findings. But these are not always present.

## Diagnosis

1. **A sudden fall in egg production, associated with thin-shelled, soft-shelled and shell-less eggs in a flock of healthy birds, is almost diagnostic.** Shell-less eggs are usually a feature, but are often missed because birds eat them.

Therefore, an inspection should be made early in the morning before eggs can be eaten. If birds are on litter, a careful search will show egg membranes. While shell-less, soft-shelled and thin-shelled eggs are characteristic, deformed eggs and eggs with ridges are not a feature. In an infected flock in which vertical transmission has occurred, most if not all cases occur around peak production, but flock of any age can be infected by lateral spread.

2.  Detection of antibodies against egg drop syndrome virus by the haemagglutination inhibition (HI) and serum neutralization tests. ELISA is also useful.

3.  Virus isolation is difficult because it is often not easy to identify the correct bird for taking the sample.

## Treatment

There is no successful treatment. Various treatments have been tried, such as vitamins, increasing calcium or protein in the ration, but no effect could be observed.

## Control

1.  **The classical form has been eliminated from all primary breeders and therefore the problem of vertically transmitted infection has decreased.**

2.  Disease prevalent in a particular area can be controlled by vaccination. **Efficient killed vaccines are available.** These are given intramuscularly between 14 and 18 weeks of age and are usually combined with other viruses, such as Ranikhet disease virus or infectious bronchitis virus.

3.  Since the main method of horizontal spread is through the infected egg and tray, wherever possible plastic trays should be washed and sterilized before returning to the farm. Other methods of spread, such as contaminated transport, people and needles, are much less important. Spread by air is not important.

4.  **Strong biosecurity should be practised.** Visitors should not be permitted to enter poultry houses.

**Note:** For a list of commercially available vaccines, see Chapter 19 under **"Egg drop syndrome vaccines"**

## AVIAN REOVIRUSES

Reovirus infections are present worldwide. Reoviruses have been isolated from a variety of disease conditions in chickens. They are commonly found in the digestive and respiratory tracts of apparently healthy chickens. But more than 80% of reoviruses isolated from chickens are non-disease-producing. The nature of the disease that occurs following reovirus infection depends on the age of the bird, type of virus, and route of exposure.

Reoviruses are **non-enveloped,** double-stranded RNA viruses. The virus is resistant to pH 3 and is also heat resistant. They are also resistant to 3% formalin, but are inactivated by a 5% solution of hydrogen peroxide. Economic losses caused by reovirus infections are usually the result of **lameness** and a **general lack of performance**, which include reduced weight gains, poor feed conversion, and a reduced marketability of affected birds.

## Spread

**Spread occurs from bird to bird, mainly through the faeces. Horizontal spread is the primary means of spread of the disease. Transmission through egg also occurs, but is low.** The virus is widely spread in intensive poultry flocks. **It can persist in birds for nearly a year.**

## Development of the Disease

Soon after infection the virus is present in the blood (viraemia). Virus grows in almost all organs. It is present in highest concentration in the digestive tract, spleen, tendons, and respiratory tract.

## Diseases

Reoviruses are associated with intestinal conditions, such as cloacal pasting (vent pasting) and ulcerative enteritis (inflammation of the intestine); respiratory disease; pericarditis (inflammation of the covering of heart), hydropericardium (accumulation of fluid under the covering of the heart); anaemia, inclusion body hepatitis (inflammation of the liver), and death. Reoviruses are also involved in the syndrome in broilers characterized by runting (stunting syndrome), abnormal feather development, proventriculitis, and skeletal changes.

Reoviruses have been associated with **viral arthritis** (inflammation of a joint) or tenosynovitis (inflammation of a tendon and its sheath). This condition is found mainly in **meat-type chickens** between 4 and 8 weeks, but has also been diagnosed in egg-type birds. In broilers, in some birds the hock joint is immobilized. **It produces lameness and the birds are reluctant to move.** Also, it affects their growth, increases mortality, and decreases feed efficiency. While morbidity (number of birds affected) varies, mortality (deaths) is usually under 1% but can reach 10%.

In addition, reoviruses can aggravate conditions caused by other disease-producing organisms, such as chicken anaemia virus, *Escherichia coli,* and Ranikhet disease virus. The increased susceptibility to other infectious agents, following or concurrent with reovirus infection, may result from damage to immune system.

Apart from the above, to be familiar with the full impact of reoviruses on poultry, it is important to know the following.

1.  Certain strains of reoviruses are **immunosuppressive** (i.e. they suppress the immune response) in chickens. This may explain the increased disease-producing ability of the chicken infectious anaemia virus in the presence of reovirus.

2.  Also immunossuppression caused by chicken infectious anaemia virus infection increases disease-producing ability of reovirus.

3.  **Infection with reoviruses can predispose to gangrenous dermatitis.**

4.  There are interactions between reoviruses and *Mycoplasma gallisepticum* (cause of CRD).

5.  Numerous avian reoviruses have been isolated from chickens affected with blue-wing disease.

6.  *Ascaridia galli* (roundworm of chickens) has been shown to contain and transmit avian reoviruses.

7.  Reovirus infection interferes with the production of immunity in Marek's disease following vaccination.

8.  Reovirus has been found to be associated with enlargement of the proventriculus and proventriculitis (inflammation of proventriculus).

9.  Reovirus infection damages vitamin A status of the bird by decreasing absorption and increasing endogenous (internal) losses.

## Diagnosis

Since there are no specific symptoms or postmortem findings, it is difficult to diagnose infections of reoviruses. Their association can be confirmed only by isolation of the virus and immunological tests. Faeces and spleen are the best source of virus. If arthritis is present, synovial fluid and synoviae from the tendon sheaths should also be included. Fluorescent antibody tests can identify the viral antigens in the tissues. The ELISA test can show an increase in antibody titre, further indicating reovirus infection.

## Treatment

No known treatment for an infected flock is available.

## Control

Avian reoviruses are present everywhere, are stable, and associated with modern, high-density rearing practices. **This makes their control very difficult.**

1.  However, thorough cleaning of poultry houses appears to prevent infection in the subsequent groups after removal of an infected flock.

2.  **Killed vaccines** have been used in the parent birds to reduce egg transmission of the virus, and to stimulate good levels of maternal antibody in the chickens.

3.  **Live vaccines,** using attenuated reoviruses, have also been used. However, it is not clear how much cross-protection there is, if any, between the reovirus serotypes. It is also not clear which serotypes are most important in causing viral arthritis. Therefore, reports on the effectiveness of the vaccines have differed.

**Note:** For a list of various commercially available reovirus vaccines, see Chapter 19 under **"Reovirus vaccines".**

## AVIAN ROTAVIRUSES

Rotavirus infection occurs worldwide in poultry, and is usually associated with **outbreaks of diarrhoea.** Rotaviruses are **non-enveloped,** double-stranded RNA viruses.

### Spread

Rotaviruses are **stable viruses** which are excreted in very large numbers in the faeces. This leads to heavy and persistent environmental contamination. As a result, infection accumulates and persists in houses where litter is re-used.

Lateral spread occurs readily between birds in direct and indirect contact. **Egg transmission of rotaviruses has not been demonstrated.** There is no evidence for a carrier state in birds, or biological vectors.

### Development of the Disease

**Rotavirus infection is confined to the intestinal tract.** Rotaviruses grow mainly in the mature epithelial cells, which line the small intestine. Some rotaviruses also grow in the large intestine. **Infected epithelial cells are destroyed.** The destroyed mature epithelial cells are replaced by immature cells. But immature cells are deficient in digestive enzymes, and also in their ability to transport water and electrolytes. It is believed that the frothy fluids found in the caeca of infected birds may result from defective digestion and absorption of carbohydrates and sugars. This, in turn, may lead to their fermentation by caecal bacteria, producing metabolites that draw water into the caeca by osmosis. **This leads to diarrhoea.**

### Disease

**Rotaviruses cause intestinal disease in chickens.** There are watery droppings, lasting 2-5 days. This may be accompanied by litter eating, vent pecking, abnormal thirst, and retardation of growth. Due to the excess fluid, litter deteriorates in quality. This can lead to lesions (changes) on the breast **(breast burns),** legs **(hock burns),** and sole of the feet. **However, rotavirus infections in chickens are mostly subclinical** (i.e. not producing any visible effects).

Most of the rotavirus infections have been reported in young birds in the first five weeks of life. However, there is no age resistance to infection, and rotavirus-associated diarrhoea has been recorded in 92-week-old birds.

## Symptoms

In broilers, symptoms vary from subclinical infections to **outbreaks of diarrhoea** associated with dehydration, poor weight gains, and increased mortality. Morbidity is high. Most faecal specimens taken from birds in affected flocks contain rotaviruses.

## Postmortem Findings

The most common finding at postmortem is the presence of abnormal amounts of fluid and gas in the intestinal tract and caeca. Secondary findings include dehydration, inflamed vents, and litter in the gizzard.

## Diagnosis

Since the symptoms and postmortem findings of rotavirus infection are not characteristic, laboratory diagnosis is necessary. Rotavirus infection must be differentiated from other conditions causing diarrhoea. **It is important to remember, however, that rotavirus infection does not necessarily result in disease.**

Serological diagnosis of rotavirus infections is difficult and not recommended. In developed countries, the classical way to diagnose rotavirus infections in the laboratory is to identify the virus in faeces or intestinal contents by **direct electron microscopic examination**.

## Treatment

At present, no specific treatment or means of control exists.

## Control

Because of the widespread occurrence of rotavirus infections in chickens, it is not possible to keep commercial flocks free from infection.

1.  If serious problems arise, it is recommended that litter be removed and the house and equipment be thoroughly cleaned and fumigated with formaldehyde before re-stocking with a new flock.

2.  Litter should not be re-used, as it results in a build-up of infection. Use fresh litter for each batch of birds.

3.  The effect of diarrhoea on the litter can be minimized by increasing ventilation and temperature, and by adding fresh litter.

4.  Vaccines have not yet been developed.

# CHICKEN INFECTIOUS ANAEMIA

Chicken infectious anaemia is a disease of **young chicks (less than 3 weeks of age),** the day-old birds being most susceptible. It causes **anaemia**. It may also cause haemorrhages under the skin and in the muscles. The disease is **immunosuppressive** (i.e. suppresses the immune responses).

Chicken infectious anaemia is caused by a **non-enveloped** virus known as 'circovirus', more recently 'gyrovirus'. The virus is extremely small and contains circular single-stranded DNA. The virus was first reported in Japan in 1979. **Chicken anaemia virus is remarkably resistant**. Its infectivity resists heating at $80^0$ C for 15 minutes and exposure to pH 3. **It is therefore difficult to eradicate this virus from the environment.** All viruses isolated so far belong to a single serotype. The disease has recently been reported to be widely prevalent in India, using polymerase chain reaction (PCR) technique.

## Spread

**The virus can be transmitted vertically from the hen through the hatching egg to the chick, and horizontally from chicken to chicken.** If the breeder flock is undergoing chicken infectious anaemia, infected eggs are produced. **Vertical transmission through the egg is the most important means of spread and results in clinical infection.** Chicks that hatch without maternal antibodies are most susceptible. These chicks then spread the virus rapidly through the flock. **Horizontal infection usually occurs through the mouth by ingesting infected material,** but infection through the respiratory route is also possible. **Horizontal transmission results in only subclinical infection** (i.e. infection without symptoms).

**Vertical transmission** occurs when breeder flocks with no previous exposure to the virus become infected as they come into egg production. In the newly hatched chicks, the virus causes an acute disease (i.e. sudden and severe) with clinical symptoms appearing between 10-14 days of age. Mortality is highest in the 3rd week and varies between 5% and 10%, but up to 60% has been recorded. Usually chicks hatched from eggs laid over a period of 3-6 weeks are affected. After this time the breeder flocks develop sufficient antibody to stop transmitting the virus through the egg.

**Horizontally** acquired infections, in older chickens lacking maternal antibody, usually originate from virus surviving in poultry houses between flocks. Infection can also come from virus excreted by a small number of vertically infected hatch-mates (i.e. birds of the same hatch), or from an outside introduced virus. Clinical symptoms do not normally develop, but the growth and health of the birds are affected.

**Embryo infection** can also be caused by semen of infected cocks. The virus is present in high concentration in the faeces of chickens 5-7 weeks after infection.

## Development of the Disease

**The disease occurs in those chicks which have no maternal antibodies.** Maternal antibody is protective. Chicks with maternal antibody usually show no disease or anaemia, but may shed the virus. Maternally derived immunity persists for about three weeks.

Double infection of chicken anaemia virus and other viruses which suppress the immunity, such as Marek's disease virus, Gumboro virus, and reticuloendotheliosis virus, increases the harmful effects of chicken anaemia virus. This results in a very severe disease and greater mortality. In such double infections, the protective effect of maternal antibody is overcome. **Chicken anaemia virus is also immunosuppressive.** That is, it suppresses the natural immune responses of the bird. The main sites of its growth are **lymphoblasts** in the thymus and **haemocytoblasts** in the bone marrow (i.e. soft tissue in the cavity of bones). Destruction of these cells causes **immunosuppression** and **anaemia**. Anaemia is a condition in which the blood is deficient in red blood cells, in haemoglobin, or in total volume. **Age resistance** develops rapidly during the first week of life and is complete by three weeks, or even earlier in immunologically competent chickens.

## Symptoms

No symptoms are seen in the parents.

Infected chicks are depressed and pale, experience slow weight gain, and are very susceptible to infections from other agents due to **immunosuppression**. Mortality can be as high as 60%, but usually is in the 5 to 10% range. The most important changes are **anaemia** and **atrophy (reduction in size) of the thymus, bursa of Fabricius and spleen.** Anaemia may be so severe that haematocrit values as low as 10% (usually 27% and below) have been recorded. The normal haematocrit in healthy chicks is 32-37.5%. Haematocrit is the volume of red blood cells packed by centrifugation. Anaemia is easily seen on comb, wattles, eyelids, and legs.

The disease is also characterized by **skin lesions**, usually appearing on wings, which are prone to secondary bacterial infections. Haemorrhages may occur under the skin and throughout the skeletal muscles (mainly thigh, leg and breast muscles). Enlarged liver and gangrenous dermatitis may also be present. Other names for this condition are: **'chicken anaemia virus syndrome', 'blue-wing disease', 'anaemia dermatitis syndrome', and 'haemorrhagic syndrome'.**

Surviving chicks recover from anaemia by 20-28 days after infection. However, recovery may be associated with secondary viral and bacterial infections. Secondary infections cause more severe clinical symptoms. Subclinical infection (i.e. infection without any symptoms) of the progeny of immune breeder flocks is common. This occurs soon after maternally acquired antibodies have disappeared at about 3 weeks of age.

## Postmortem Findings

The most important finding is a marked **reduction in the size of thymus, bursa of Fabricius,** and to a lesser extent, the **spleen**. The bone marrow changes from a red colour to a yellow or white colour. Bone marrow in femur is fatty and yellowish. Atrophy of thymus may result in complete disappearance of the organ. The liver is often swollen. Haemorrhages in the proventriculus, under the skin, and in the muscles are sometimes associated with severe anaemia.

## Diagnosis

This is based on the characteristic symptoms and gross changes. Laboratory diagnosis is based on a number of complicated tests, including polymerase chain reaction (PCR). The virus is very difficult to isolate. An ELISA test is available to check breeder flocks and chicks for the presence of antibodies.

## Treatment

No effective treatment is known. Treatment of secondary infections with appropriate antibiotics is helpful. The addition of vitamins to the drinking water is a general supportive therapy.

## Control

1. As chicken anaemia virus infection is very common, it is virtually impossible to maintain breeder flocks free of infection throughout their lifetime. This is mainly because of the **high resistance of the virus to disinfection.**

2. Immunization of parent flocks several weeks before egg production prevents outbreaks of chicken infectious anaemia in their progeny. A live vaccine administered through drinking water is now available in several countries. Vaccination should be performed at about 13-15 weeks of age, but never later than 3-4 weeks before the first collection of hatching eggs to avoid the risk of vaccine virus being spread through the eggs.

3. **Monitoring of breeder flocks for the presence of chicken infectious anaemia virus antibody should be done to avoid vertically transmitted chicken anaemia virus infections,** or to test the efficacy of vaccinations.

4. At present there are no means of controlling the losses among chicks by vaccination. Therefore, attention should be paid to **management and hygiene** to prevent immunosuppression by environmental factors, or other infectious diseases, and to prevent early exposure to chicken infectious anaemia virus.

**Note:** For a list of various commercially available vaccines against chicken infectious anaemia, see Chapter 19 under **"chicken infectious anaemia vaccines".**

# RETICULOENDOTHELIOSIS

Reticuloendotheliosis includes **three disease conditions,** caused by retroviruses of the reticuloendotheliosis group. They contain single-stranded RNA. The three disease conditions are: (1) Acute neoplasia, (2) Runting disease syndrome, and (3) Chronic neoplasia. These are different from those caused by the leukosis/sarcoma group of viruses, such as lymphoid leukosis. **These diseases are not common, although infection appears to be widespread.**

**Natural infections by reticuloendotheliosis viruses cause neoplastic disease.** A neoplastic disease is characterized by the formation of a new growth (neoplasm). This new growth serves no useful function but grows at the cost of bird and has characteristics of **cancer.** Regarding the occurrence of reticuloendotheliosis in India, the exact position is at present not known. On the basis of reported clinical disease elsewhere, the economic importance of reticuloendotheliosis is not much.

## Spread

The infection can spread by direct contact with infected chickens (**horizontal transmission**). The reticuloendotheliosis virus is present in faeces. Infected hens **transmit the virus vertically (vertical transmission)** to some of their progeny, although usually at low frequency compared to avian leukosis virus. Spread has also occurred through the use of **contaminated vaccines.**

## Disease

As mentioned, the disease occurs in **three forms:**

## 1. Acute Neoplasia

Infection of newly hatched chicks results in high morbidity (number of birds affected) from acute neoplastic diseases. The latent period can be as short as 3 days, but death occurs usually 6-12 days after infection. Due to the rapid onset of the disease, there are few symptoms in newly hatched chicks, and mortality rates often reach 100%. Affected birds have enlarged livers and spleens. Ovary, testes, heart, kidney and pancreas may also be slightly enlarged. This form of the disease is not common in the field.

## 2. Runting Disease Syndrome

The runting disease syndrome is characterized by poor growth, and has occurred in chicken accidentally vaccinated with reticuloendotheliosis virus-contaminated vaccines. It may also occur naturally in association with necrotic dermatitis in chickens. Affected birds are stunted and pale. Reduction in weight in infected chicks can be detected as early as 6 days of age. Some chickens may have abnormal feather development, particularly of wing. A few birds may show paralysis. Reticuloendotheliosis virus infection can cause immunosuppression (i.e. suppression of the natural immune responses).

The postmortem findings indicate runting, reduction in the size of bursa of Fabricius, enlargement of nerves, abnormal feather development, inflammation of the proventriculus (proventriculitis), enteritis (inflammation of the intestine), and the presence of small patches of dead tissue (necrotic foci) in the liver and spleen.

## 3. Chronic Neoplasia

These neoplasms take a much longer time for their formation, and are of two types: (1) Non-bursal lymphomas, and (2) Bursal lymphomas. ('Lymphoma' is a tumour of lymphoid tissue/lymphocytes).

## Non-Bursal Lymphoma

These lymphomas have latent periods as short as 6 weeks and involve thymus, heart, liver, spleen, and nerves, but not the bursa of Fabricius. These neoplasms superficially resemble those of Marek's disease. The cell type has been defined as **a T-cell** on the basis of cell surface markers. (For information on T-cell and B-cell, see Chapter 32: **"The avian immune system"**).

## Bursal Lymphomas

These lymphomas involve mainly liver and bursa of Fabricius. The neoplastic cells are B-cells. Bursal lymphomas cannot be differentiated from lymphoid leukosis, and occur in chickens after a long latent period (4-10 months).

No characteristic symptoms are seen during the development of chronic neoplasia.

## Diagnosis

1.  Diagnosis of reticuloendotheliosis requires not only the presence of typical postmortem findings (gross lesions), but also the demonstration of reticuloendotheliosis virus. Birds with lesions (changes) are the best source of virus for isolation and identification.

2.  The presence of infection in a flock can be detected by examining blood (serum) for the presence of antibodies, using the ELISA test. A number of other serological tests are also used.

3.  Viral antigen (i.e. virus) can be detected in blood (serum) from affected birds using the agar precipitin test.

4.  Reticuloendotheliosis virus-induced neoplasms (tumours) can be confused with those of Marek's disease and lymphoid leukosis. Therefore, serological diagnosis of the presence of reticuloendotheliosis virus is required to support a pathological diagnosis.

## Treatment

No treatment for reticuloendotheliosis is known.

## Control

No control procedures have been developed. This is mainly because the disease is not common, occurs singly, or in scattered instances, and is self-limiting; and also because the necessary techniques and knowledge are not available. However, methods similar to those used for the control of avian leukosis viruses can be applied.

## ADENOVIRUS INFECTIONS

Adenoviruses are widely distributed throughout the world. **They are also widely distributed in healthy birds.** Adenoviruses are very common in chickens. Therefore, isolation of adenoviruses from diseased birds forms no basis for assuming that they are the cause of the disease.

**Adenoviruses have been isolated from almost every condition.** They are usually associated with inclusion body hepatitis, respiratory disease, falls in egg production, diarrhoea, tenosynovitis (inflammation of a tendon sheath), poor growth, and reduced feed conversion. Chickens of all ages are susceptible. In contrast to the clear association of group III adenoviruses with disease (egg drop syndrome), the role of group I avian adenoviruses being discussed, is not well defined. Group I adenoviruses contain double-stranded DNA. They are **non-enveloped.**

## Spread

1.  **Adenoviruses are transmitted through the egg. Vertical transmission is very important** because this is the main method of spread from one generation to next. Afterwards, **horizontal (lateral) spread** by contact with infected faeces occurs. In natural infections adenovirus is excreted in the faeces for about 3 weeks, with the peak excretion between 4 and 7 days. Other observation records that adenoviruses are excreted from week 3 onward, and in broilers peak excretion occurs between 4 and 6 weeks of age. In layers, virus excretion is maximum from 5 to 9 week, but is still at 70% after 14 week. **Chickens infected with adenovirus are potential carriers for life.** Carriers probably excrete the virus at intervals throughout their life.

2.  There is a second period, around peak production, when adenoviruses are usually present. The stress of egg production (i.e. during laying), or high levels of sex hormones, **cause re-activation of the latent virus,** and the virus is excreted through the egg. This ensures maximum egg transmission to the next generation.

3.  **Horizontal (lateral) spread** is also important. Virus is present in faeces and nasal (of nose) lining (i.e. mucosa), and kidneys. Therefore, virus can be transmitted in all excretions, but highest levels are found in the **faeces.** Horizontal spread appears to be mainly by direct faecal contact.

4.  Spread by the air is not important unless the birds are infected with disease-producing organisms that cause respiratory distress, such as infectious bronchitis virus. It is only then that spread by the air becomes effective.

5.  Spread by virus-contaminated substances (fomites), or people and transport is possible because **adenoviruses are relatively resistant to inactivation (destruction) outside the body of the bird.**

6.  When the maternal antibody (i.e. antibody obtained by the newly hatched chick from the hen through the egg) is lost, virus excretion begins. Chicks in contact will be infected.

# INCLUSION BODY HEPATITIS

Inclusion body hepatitis is a disease of **young chickens** characterized by the sudden onset of mortality, anaemia, and hepatitis (inflammation of the liver).

This condition is **usually seen in broilers** between 4-9 weeks of age. However, it has been recorded in older birds and in growers. Outbreaks of inclusion body hepatitis in chickens under 3 weeks of age with mortality up to 30% have occurred in Australia. Immunosuppression (suppression of the immune responses) produced by Gumboro disease (infectious bursal disease) helps adenoviruses in causing inclusion body hepatitis. This disease is similar to **'leechi disease'**. The only difference between inclusion body hepatitis and leechi disease is that the mortality rate and occurrence of hydropericardium (accumulation of fluid under the covering of heart) are more in leechi disease (see **'leechi disease'**).

## Cause

Inclusion body hepatitis is caused by a group I adenovirus. It is **non-enveloped**. A number of different serotypes of adenovirus may be involved. The disease is much more severe when there is underlying immunosuppression caused by infections such as Gumboro disease or chicken infectious anaemia virus.

## Symptoms

Inclusion body hepatitis is characterized by a sudden onset of mortality, which is maximum after 3-4 days and usually drops on 5th day, but sometimes continues for 2-3 weeks. Mortality may reach 10% and sometimes as high as 30%. It is usually seen in **broilers 3-7 weeks of age,** but it has also been reported in birds as young as 7 days and as old as 20 weeks. Morbidity (number of birds affected) is low. Sick birds adopt a crouching position with ruffled feathers and also die within 48 hours, or recover. The other birds in the flock usually look normal, or they may be depressed for a few days. Overall feed conversion and weight gain are usually decreased.

## Postmortem Findings

The main finding is pale, friable (easily broken) swollen liver. Small and large haemorrhages may be present in the liver and skeletal muscles. The kidneys are also swollen. Anaemia and jaundice of the skin over the legs, breast, and the subcutaneous fat (i.e. fat under the skin), characterized by paleness and haemorrhages of various organs, especially the muscles and bone marrow, are usually present. In some outbreaks the bone marrow lesions are the most noticeable. Bone marrow is thin and watery.

## Respiratory Disease

Adenoviruses are usually isolated from airsacs, lungs and trachea of birds with respiratory disease. However, they are not believed to be the primary disease-producing organisms of the respiratory tract. But they do appear important as secondary disease-producing organisms. Mild to moderate inflammation of trachea with excess mucus are the only postmortem findings.

## Falls in Egg Production

Adenovirus infection has been reported to cause a 10% fall in egg production, or to affect eggshell quality. However, adenoviruses can be isolated from commercial flocks, even when there are very high levels of production and fertility.

It is possible that exposure of layers to an adenovirus may result in a fall in egg production. However, under most management systems it is unlikely that birds will reach sexual maturity without being infected by a large number of adenoviruses. Falls in egg production due to adenovirus infection appears to be relatively unimportant in chickens.

## Effect on Feed Conversion and Growth

Adenovirus infection has been reported to cause decreased food consumption. However, there is little evidence to indicate that naturally occurring infection causes either reduced food utilization or growth. But, slowing of growth does not occur in naturally infected birds.

## Viral Arthritis / Tenosynovitis

**Arthritis** is inflammation of a joint. **Tenosynovitis** is inflammation of a tendon sheath. (A tendon sheath is the tissue by which muscle is attached to the bone.) Adenoviruses are usually isolated from the joints or tendons of birds with these conditions. However, their exact role in producing arthritis / tenosynovitis is not known.

## Diagnosis

1. Diagnosis depends on isolation and identification of the virus. Virus may be isolated from the affected organ or faeces. **However, as adenoviruses are widely**

distributed in healthy birds, their isolation from birds with disease is not necessarily diagnostic.

2.  Antibody against adenovirus can be detected by indirect immunofluorescent test, agar-gel precipitin test, and enzyme-linked immunosorbent assay (ELISA). ELISA is both inexpensive and sensitive. However, the main problem with any serological test for adenoviruses is in the interpretation of the results. Antibodies are common in both healthy and diseased birds, and birds are usually infected with a number of serotypes. **That is, adenoviruses are so widespread that it is difficult to interpret the results.**

## Treatment

No treatment for the disease is available.

## Control

1.  The first step is to control or eliminate Gumboro disease virus and chicken anaemia virus. This is because both of these viruses increase the harmful effects of adenoviruses.

2.  **Adenoviruses are resistant, and it is almost impossible to eradicate (remove) them from commercial flocks.** This is because the virus is so effectively spread vertically through the eggs that viruses are easily introduced into the next flock. **Therefore, control would have to be started at primary breeder level.** Also, breeding birds with inclusion body hepatitis should not be used for producing hatching eggs.

3.  Normal sanitation procedures should be followed.

4.  Wild birds should be prevented from entering into the poultry house.

## LEECHI DISEASE

Also known as **'hydropericardium-hepatitis syndrome', 'hydropericardium syndrome',** and **'Angara disease',** leechi disease is a sudden and severe infectious disease of chickens. It is characterized by high morbidity (number of birds affected) and mortality (deaths caused), excess accumulation of fluid under the covering of the heart (pericardium), and by the presence of many areas of dead tissue (necrotic foci) in the liver.

Hydropericardium-hepatitis syndrome (leechi disease) was first recognized in flocks at a place called Angara Goth, near Karachi, Pakistan, in late 1987. Because the disease was recorded first at this place, it was named **'Angara disease'.** Within 12 months, the disease spread rapidly, affecting flocks in most of the intensive broiler growing areas in Pakistan. It caused between 20 and 80% mortality, ruining the national broiler industry. Typically, mortality began at 3 weeks, peaked in 4th and 5th week, and then decreased.

During 1994, hydropericardium syndrome appeared in the high density poultry areas in the neighbourhood of Delhi, in India. **The disease in India has been called as 'Leechi Disease', because following excessive accumulation of fluid under the covering of the heart, the heart looked like a peeled leechi fruit.** The condition has since been reported from the northern states of Jammu and Kashmir, Punjab, Uttar Pradesh, and also from several other states of India. Although 3-5 week old broilers are usually affected, the condition has been also recorded in immature broiler breeders and commercial layers.

This disease is similar to inclusion body hepatitis. The only difference between leechi disease and inclusion body hepatitis, as pointed out earlier, is that the mortality rate and occurrence of hydropericardium are more in leech disease (see **'inclusion body hepatitis'**).

## Cause

Leechi disease appears to be caused by a disease-producing group I adenovirus (serotype 4). It is **non-enveloped.** Other agents may increase the severity of the disease. These include immunosuppressive diseases (i.e. those which suppress the immune responses), such as Gumboro disease (infectious bursal disease), Marek's disease, and chicken infectious anaemia. Prevalence and severity of leechi disease outbreaks are linked to the density of the poultry population in an area.

Leechi disease **occurs usually in 3 to 5 week-old healthy broilers** and immature broiler breeder replacements.

## Spread

1.  Because it is believed that group I adenovirus are involved in producing leechi disease, it is presumed that leechi disease can be transmitted **both vertically** (egg transmission) **and horizontally** (laterally).

2.  Adenoviruses may remain latent in breeding stock until the onset of maturity, and then are shed following immunosuppression or stress.

3.  After 3 weeks of age, progeny of infected parent stock may excrete virus for up to 14 weeks. Horizontal spread of virus by carriers (birds carrying infection without showing symptoms) may be an important method of spread among flocks on multi-age farms, or in operations without adequate biosecurity (see **"biosecurity"**).

4.  Growth of virus in the intestinal tract indicates that faecal contamination of clothes, footwear and equipment, including transport crates and vehicles, may spread infection under commercial conditions. Lack of biosecurity, closeness of multi-age farms, and live-bird trading increase spread of viral agents.

5.  Contaminated vaccine prepared in embryonated eggs derived from infected flocks

could also be a source of infection. In Pakistan, it was found that visits to farms by persons carrying out vaccinations usually caused outbreaks of hydropericardium-hepatitis syndrome.

## Symptoms

Non-vaccinated broilers and immature breeder flocks can have mortality as high as 80% if they are exposed to a very powerful form of Ranikhet disease, very powerful form of Gumboro disease, and infections such as mycoplasmosis. Duration of the disease usually varies from 9-14 days with morbidity (number of birds affected) of 10-30% and daily mortality of 3-5%.

Flocks with leechi disease show no specific symptoms. The birds remain active until just before death. However, sudden onset of high mortality, dullness, crowding (huddling together) with ruffled feathers, and yellow, mucoid (resembling mucus) droppings are characteristic, but there is no morbidity (sick birds). Mortality starts at about 3 weeks of age and reaches its peak at 4 to 5 weeks, without showing any symptoms. Decreased albumin (a blood protein) because of liver damage is thought to be responsible for the hypoproteinaemia (low protein level in blood) in affected birds. This low protein level in the blood contributes to accumulation of fluid under covering of the heart, the condition being known as '**hydropericardium**'.

## Postmortem Findings

**The most striking postmortem finding is the presence of up to 20 ml of clear, straw-coloured, jelly-like fluid in the pericardial sac (i.e. under the covering of the heart).** That is, hydropericardium. General congestion and accumulation of fluid in the lungs (pulmonary oedema) are seen. Liver and kidneys are usually enlarged, pale and friable (easily broken). Very small haemorrhages may be present on the pericardium and beneath the capsule of the liver.

## Diagnosis

1.  Presence of large quantity of fluid in the pericardial sac (hydropericardium) and microscopic demonstration of basophilic intranuclear inclusion bodies in liver cells are considered highly suggestive of leechi disease.

2.  To confirm diagnosis, adenovirus has to be isolated by infecting embryonic chick liver cells. The presence of adenovirus in tissue culture is indicated by characteristic changes within the cells.

3.  Certain serological tests, such as agar gel diffusion, counter immunoelectrophoresis and ELISA are specific and reliable.

## Treatment

There is no specific treatment for leechi disease. However, use of an iodophor in the drinking water of affected flocks (0.07-0.1% of a 2.5% solution) reduces mortality and severity of the disease.

## Control

1.  Under Indian conditions, it is neither possible nor economically practical to maintain strict levels of biosecurity to ensure that adenovirus is prevented from entering broiler units and is kept out.

2.  Breeder flocks must be protected from infection by applying **a good biosecurity programme**. Measures include locating farms at least 2 kilometres away from the commercial units, and operating an all-in, all-out placement programme with thorough decontamination of houses between successive flocks.

3.  Feed should be delivered in bulk and all people should be decontaminated before entering a breeding farm.

4.  Live vaccines given to breeders and their progeny should be free from disease-producing organisms including adenoviruses and chicken infectious anaemia virus.

In areas where leechi disease is prevalent, it is necessary to protect the flocks against the adenovirus responsible for the condition through vaccination. It is believed that killed (inactivated) vaccines provide even up to 80% protection against infection. (Refer to Chapter 19 for a list of commercially available vaccines against leechi disease, under **"Leechi disease vaccines"**).

## INFECTIOUS STUNTING SYNDROME

There are many causes of poor growth in broiler chickens. However, in 1976 a new disease was recognized in USA and Europe. It was characterized by a small percentage of the flock (1-5%) becoming stunted, and about 10 to 50% of the remaining growing poorly. The affected birds were not ill. They were active with huge appetites. Financial loss was great due to excessive culling (removal), poor feed conversion, and reduced weight for age. Within a few years, this disease was reported from most broiler-producing countries of the world. More recent reports indicate that high mortality (**spiking mortality**) can occur in this disease. In India, infectious stunting syndrome is a serious problem in broilers, and every year inflicts great financial losses.

Infectious stunting syndrome is also known by several other names. These include **'malabsorption syndrome', 'runting and stunting syndrome', 'broiler runting syndrome', 'pale bird syndrome', 'infectious runting',** and **'helicopter disease'.** The term **'stunting'** pointed to the poor growth of affected chickens, whereas severely stunted birds which did not grow when given plenty of good feed are usually described as **'runted'**. Other names have been applied based on symptoms (**'helicopter feathering'**), or lesions (changes) thought important by those studying the disease (**'osteoporosis'**). **However, none of these names are specific and their use has** created confusion.

## Cause

**Infectious stunting syndrome is caused by a group of viruses.** The viruses may include calicivirus, enterovirus, parvovirus, reovirus, or togavirus. Recent studies indicate that picornavirus may also be involved. The rapid worldwide spread of this disease indicates that the causative agent is very strong and highly infectious, and a picornavirus fulfils these requirements.

## Predisposing Factors

These are those factors which make the bird easily prone to disease.

1.  All breeds and strains of chickens are susceptible to infectious stunting syndrome. However, **suppression of growth is most noticeable in broilers due to their rapid growth.**

2.  Cockerels are more severely affected than growers, again due to the greater growth rate of cockerels.

3.  Harmful management factors, such as overcrowding, cold stress during the first week and draughty conditions (i.e. allowing cold air in), and poor disinfection of poultry houses before housing chickens, have been associated with severe outbreaks of infectious stunting syndrome.

4.  Some farms are more often and more severely affected than others, and some broiler houses are more often affected than neighbouring houses. This indicates an important role for environmental and/or management factors.

5.  Many cases of infectious stunting syndrome are seen in chicks obtained from young breeder flocks. However, it is not known if this is due to vertical transmission (egg transmission), or a more general phenomenon of increased susceptibility of chicks from young breeders to infection.

6.  Suppression of growth in infectious stunting syndrome is increased by a slight decrease in vitamin concentrations in the feed, or by the presence of slightly more mycotoxins and/or subclinical infections (i.e. infections not showing symptoms) with various agents.

7.  Age at infection is important in the later development of this disease. Infection of chickens of 1 day old is associated with greater suppression of growth than infection at a later date.

## Development of the Disease

**The changes (lesions) are most marked in the middle of the small intestine.** Picornavirus-like particles are seen in the cells lining the villi. These viruses are associated with death of individual villus cells. At this stage, there is significant villus atrophy (reduction in size), but within 2 weeks the villi restore their normal height. However, they are populated by biochemically immature cells. Therefore, the activity of many enzymes involved in digestion and absorption of nutrients is greatly reduced. In addition, the arrangement of villi is altered. Therefore, ingesta transit times are decreased. This results in defective digestive ability and leads to **poor growth**, the characteristic feature of infectious stunting syndrome.

Some manifestations of the disease originate from secondary metabolic problems. For example, poor carcass pigmentation is due to reduced absorption of vitamin A and other carotenoids, osteodystrophy due to reduced vitamin D3 absorption, and encephalomalacia (brain softening) due to reduced vitamin E absorption. Slow feathering is probably due to reduced digestion and absorption of sulphur-containing amino acids.

## Symptoms

**Typically, birds are affected within the first two weeks of life and usually show diarrhoea, nervousness, slowing of growth (stunting), litter eating, and excessive drinking.**

The presence of stunted (small) chickens in an affected flock varies from 1% to 75%. However, it is difficult to estimate this exactly because birds tend to crowd together towards the outer side of the house and around feeders. **At 4-8 days,** the stunted chickens are 20-40 gram lighter than normal birds in the same flock. Sometimes symptoms, such as ruffled feathers, unwillingness to move, eating of faeces, and diarrhoea with pasting of faeces around the cloaca are seen after a short period in the first week, but none of these are specific nor are they restricted to stunted chickens.

**After one week,** the stunted chickens are characterized by slow feathering on their heads and necks, and pendulous (enlarged and hanging down) abdomens. At this stage they eat well and are very active. Mortality is not normally a feature, although in some affected flocks there is a slight increase in non-specific causes of death.

**At about 2 weeks of age**, affected chickens are usually called **'yellow heads'**. This is because of the easily visible retained down feathers (a covering of soft feathers) on the head and neck. Broken and displaced primary wing feathers (**'helicopter feathering'**) are sometimes seen in a small proportion of stunted chicks at 3-4 weeks, but it also occurs in well-grown birds. Lameness due to secondary (non-specific) bone defect (osteodystrophy) is seen in stunted chickens at 2-4 weeks and this further intensifies their poor weight gain. Pale shanks (i.e. portion of legs between the hock joint and foot) are seen in stunted chickens given high carotenoid (yellow pigment) diets. Stunted chickens without complications grow to a fairly good weight when given adequate feed, but feed conversion rates are poor

One of the features of infectious stunting syndrome is the occurrence of **severely stunted (runted) chickens,** which remain small despite their huge appetites. Their incidence is low, usually 1-5%, and if allowed to live 6 weeks they weigh only 100-200 gram. **These small chickens become more noticeable after 2 weeks,** whereas the unaffected birds grow rapidly. Their feathering is slow, but they are extremely active and difficult to catch. **It is better to remove (cull) these chickens as they eat excess food and tend to die from mishap, starvation, and/or dehydration.**

## Postmortem Findings

Affected birds are not in good bodily condition. In chickens fed carotenoids in high concentrations (yellow pigments), fat below the skin is pale compared to the normal. Therefore, the name was given as **'pale bird syndrome'**. The intestine may contain poorly digested contents and are distended and pale. The condition has been called as **'malabsorption syndrome'.** In chickens which do not get a chance to reach the food, the intestines usually contain clear watery fluid. This condition is sometimes called as **'mucoid'** or **'catarrhal enteritis'**. The caeca are sometimes distended. During the normal postmortem procedure the hips are separated (disjointed), but in chickens with infectious stunting syndrome separation of head of the femur from the underlying bone occurs on its own (traumatic separation). This is seen in birds with osteodystrophy (a bone defect). The exposed bone is red, but this is not **'femoral head necrosis'**. Osteodystrophy is usually found in infectious stunting syndrome-affected broiler chickens more than 2 weeks of age.

## Diagnosis

The causative agent of infectious stunting syndrome has not been characterized (identified) and serological tests are not available. Therefore, diagnosis depends on identifying the characteristic features of this disease. These include severely stunted (runted) but active chickens with retained down feathers on the head and neck at 2-3 weeks of age, and poor growth in a varying percentage of the remaining flock of 2-4 weeks. Other infections, management and metabolic diseases in which poor growth occurs should be ruled out.

## Control

1. **It is believed that this disease is due to infection of chickens at a young age with a very strong virus**. Control of infection requires attention to basic disease control principles. Farms should be operated on all-in, all-out basis. Thorough disinfection of a broiler house after an outbreak of infectious stunting syndrome, including fumigation with formaldehyde, usually reduces the incidence of severe stunting in the subsequent flock.

2. **Small chicks from young breeder flocks appear to be more susceptible to infectious stunting syndrome.** They are more likely to be vertically infected **(egg transmission)** than chicks derived from older breeder flocks. Therefore,

such chicks should be reared separately. Vertical transmission appears to involve faecal contamination of eggshells. Therefore, only clean eggs should be set.

3.  Young chicks are usually given starter feed on papers or cardboard. But the faeces which accumulate on the papers can be a source of infection for other birds. **Therefore, the papers should be removed as soon as possible.**

4.  Cold, as a stress factor, appears to increase the severity of stunting in infectious stunting syndrome. Therefore, adequate and constant temperatures should be maintained for young chicks.

5.  Supplementation with vitamin A, D3 and E may reduce the severity of the secondary effects of infectious stunting syndrome, such as poor carotenoid pigmentation, osteodystrophy and encephalomalacia. However, the dosage required will have to be greater than for normal chickens because of the poor nutrient absorption of affected chickens.

Economic loss from infectious stunting syndrome can be reduced by strict culling (removal) of severely stunted chicks (up to 10% of the flock). These birds are very active and have huge appetites, but do not grow well. Therefore, there is poor feed conversion in affected flocks. These stunted chicks can be caught easily between 10 and 28 days of age. After this age, catching them creates undue disturbance to the rest of the flock.

# Chapter 4

# Bacterial Diseases

**B**acteria are microscopic organisms composed of a single cell. Disease-producing bacteria are abundant in the poultry environment. These organisms are capable of attacking the chicken, in which they multiply rapidly through cell division and produce abnormal changes in the bird, which it cannot withstand. Sickness follows, and if the reaction is severe, death may occur.

Bacteria multiply by division, each cell separating into two equal parts. Once the disease-producing bacteria enter into the chicken, multiplication of the cells is rapid in susceptible birds. One cell divides into 2, 2 into 4, 4 into 8, 8 into 16, and so forth. Soon the numbers are so large that they produce disease in the bird.

In most cases, a disease is the result of the entry of the disease-producing bacteria into the bird, and the multiplication that follows. The organisms also produce **toxins**, which harm the bird. The greater the amount of toxin, either because of increased production by the bacteria or because the number of bacteria is large, the greater is the effect of the disease.

On the basis of Gram's staining, bacteria can be divided into two groups: **Gram-positive** and **Gram-negative**. The cell wall of Gram-positive bacteria is mainly composed of peptidoglycan (a substance composed of polysaccharide and peptide chains). The cell wall in Gram-negative bacteria is a polysaccharide-lipid-protein structure. The cell wall lipopolysaccharides of Gram-negative bacteria are toxic and are called **endotoxins.**

Most bacteria are primary pathogens (i.e. disease-producing organisms), and produce disease. Other bacteria are secondary pathogens, and produce disease only when birds are stressed by other micro-organisms, or by a disturbance in their environment or nutrition.

Most bacteria multiply outside the cells. They do not require host-cell machinery for multiplication, like viruses. As they live and multiply outside the cells, antibiotics are effective against diseases caused by bacteria. **Therefore, bacterial diseases can be successfully treated by antibiotics.**

## COLIBACILLOSIS (*E. coli* Infection)

*E. coli* **infection or colibacillosis is the most common, the most troublesome, and economically the most important bacterial disease of poultry.** It occurs throughout the year, and is difficult to deal with.

Bacteria of the species *Escherichia coli* normally live in the digestive tract of birds, and most strains do not produce disease. Certain strains, however, can cause disease in poultry. These diseases include colisepticaemia (blood infection) and yolk sac infection in **young chickens**; and egg peritonitis (inflammation of the peritoneum, a membrane in the body cavity) and coligranuloma in **adult chickens.** *E. coli* is also involved in a number of other conditions. These include synovitis (inflammation of the synovial membrane), arthritis (inflammation of a joint), osteomyelitis (inflammation of the bone and marrow), salpingitis (inflammation of oviduct), panophthalmitis (inflammation of the eye), and localized abscesses. All these conditions are collectively referred to as **"colibacillosis"**.

*E. coli* causes disease only when there is a serious managemental fault, or some other underlying disease-producing organism is present. In other words, colibacillosis occurs when bird's defences have been damaged or overpowered. **Collectively, infections caused by *E. coli* are responsible for huge economic losses to the poultry industry.**

# Cause

*Escherichia coli* is a Gram-negative, motile organism. In addition to **endotoxin**, a structural component of the organism's cell wall, disease-causing *E. coli* produces **several toxins** important in disease. These include **enterotoxins, cytotoxins, haemolysins, and haemagglutinins**, and several disease-producing **virulence factors**, such as **adhesins.**

# Development of the Disease

After *E. coli* enters into the bird, there is an acute inflammatory reaction in the tissues. Vascular permeability increases and fluid and protein accumulate in the tissues. Even after 12 hours, the inflammatory fluid (exudate) continues to accumulate and finally undergoes caseation to form a firm, dry, yellow, irregular, cheese-like mass. The fluid is rich in **fibrin.**

**E. coli infection in poultry occurs in two forms:** (1) **Systemic infection.** This infection is caused by the presence of *E. coli* in the blood circulation, technically called 'colisepticaemia'. (2) **Localized infection**. In this the infection is restricted to a specific or limited area. Both, systemic and localized forms of *E. coli* infections (**colibacillosis**), will now be discussed.

# SYSTEMIC FORMS OF *E. coli* INFECTIONS

# 1. COLISEPTICAEMIA

Colisepticaemia means the presence of *E. coli* in the blood circulation. It is most common in young chickens, and is also the most serious form of colibacillosis. The disease rose to prominence with the development of broiler industry. When the broiler industry expanded, large numbers of birds were kept under extremely crowded conditions and in poorly ventilated houses. Many broiler flocks were infected with **Mycoplasma gallisepticum**, which predisposed to or aggravated colisepticaemia. Coccidiosis, viral infections, Ranikhet disease or infectious bronchitis (even in live vaccine form), Gumboro disease, and nutritional deficiencies all predispose the bird to this disease. That is, make them more prone to colisepticaemia.

## Sources of Infection

1.  ***E. coli* is a common inhabitant of the intestinal tract of poultry and is present at concentrations up to $10^6$ g.** That is, one gram of intestinal content contains up to ten lakh (one million) organisms. Higher numbers are found in young birds, particularly in the lower intestinal tract and caeca. *E. coli* from the intestinal tract are continually being shed through faecal material. **These bacteria then dry and float in the air and gain entry into uninfected individuals through the respiratory tract.** Their presence in the drinking water indicates faecal contamination. Among normal chickens 10-15% of the intestinal *E. coli* are of the types that can produce disease under suitable conditions/environment. For example, poor incubation resulting in weak chicks is an important cause of their increased susceptibility to infection. In hens, *E. coli* may leave the intestines, acquire disease-causing ability, then enter into circulation and produce blood infection, when their resistance is weakened by hunger, thirst, cold, or lack of good ventilation. *E. coli* infection following vaccination is also documented.

2.  The egg lies in the cloaca prior to being laid. **The most important source of infection is the faecal contamination of eggs during laying and afterward penetration of *E. coli* through the shell.** There may be as many as 8000-10,000 pores (small openings) per egg on the eggshell. Through these pores, air passes into the egg to supply oxygen to the developing embryo and carbon dioxide and moisture are removed. In the freshly laid egg, the pores are almost completely closed, but as the egg ages, or is washed, the number of open pores is greatly increased. *E. coli* being a motile organism penetrates the shell through these tiny pores. A sudden difference in the temperature between that within the body and the external environment, when the egg is laid, creates a negative pressure or suction inside the gg. **This helps in the penetration of *E. coli*. As a result, in some cases, 0.5-6% of the eggs laid may contain the organism.** More bacteria are added to the shell when the egg remains in the nest. *E. coli* may then spread to other chicks during hatching and this is usually associated with high mortality rates, and may give rise to yolk sac infection.

3.  Egg transmission of disease-producing (pathogenic) *E. coli* through faecal contamination is common and can be responsible for high chick mortality. Pathogenic

*E. coli* are more common in the intestine of newly hatched chicks than in eggs from which they are hatched. **This indicates their rapid spread after hatching.**

4.  Transmission through the ovary is possible when the birds are shedding *E. coli* through the oviduct (uterine) infection. Infected breeder hens thus transmit the disease to the newly hatched chicks. Hens with infected oviducts continue to lay eggs of which 2.7% contain *E. coli.*

5.  *E. coli* can be found in litter and faecal matter. **Dust in poultry houses may contain between one lakh (1, 00000) to ten lakhs (one million) *E. coli* per gram ($10^5$ - $10^6$ *E. coli*/g).** These bacteria persist for long periods, particularly when dust is dry. After wetting of dust with water, they get reduced up to 84-97% within 7 days.

6.  **Feed is usually contaminated with pathogenic *E. coli*,** but these can be destroyed by hot pelleting processes.

7.  Rodents (rats, mice) droppings usually contain pathogenic *E. coli.*

8.  Pathogenic *E. coli* can also be introduced into the poultry flocks **through contaminated well water.**

## Predisposing Factors

Predisposing factors are those factors which make the bird easily prone to infection. They greatly influence the occurrence of colibacillosis. Young birds are most susceptible and the infection is also very severe in them.

Normal healthy birds with intact defences are remarkably resistant to *E. coli*. Infection occurs when skin or lining of the respiratory or digestive tracts (mucosal barriers) are damaged. Examples include: unhealed navel wounds; mucosal damage from viral, bacterial, or parasitic infections; and lack of normal flora.

Certain factors cause immunosuppression. That is, they suppress the natural immune responses. The bird is therefore unable to fight *E. coli* and succumbs to infection. For example, viral infections and toxins, such as mycotoxins, cause immunosuppression and predispose the birds to colibacillosis.

**However, the factors which act directly on birds in producing *E. coli* infection are:**

1.  Contaminated water

2.  Dry, dusty conditions. *E. coli* persist for long periods outside the bird's body in dry, dusty conditions

3.  Poor ventilation

4.  Overcrowding

5.  Poor litter condition

6.  Exposure to ammonia

7.  Faecal/water restriction

8.  Temperature extremes (too hot or too cold)

9.  Abnormal stress (too little or too much)

10. Infection with infectious bronchitis virus. This is due to the interaction between infectious bronchitis virus and *E. coli.*

It is interesting that moderate stress has been reported to increase resistance. This may be due to the development of immunity after contact of organisms with the immune system, or as a result of developing and exercising the defence mechanisms and keeping them in a state of readiness.

Because majority of the cases of colibacillosis occur secondarily to one or more of the factors stated above, these predisposing causes must be identified and corrected before the disease can be effectively controlled.

## Postmortem Findings

A layer of white fibrin covers heart (pericarditis) and liver (perihepatitis). **This is typical of blood infection by *E. coli.*** Infected airsacs are thickened and usually contain cheese-like material.

## 2. Respiratory Tract Infection

Inhalation of *E. coli*-contaminated dust is the most important source of infection for airsacs, and produces the most common type of colisepticaemia (blood infection). Exposure to chicken-house dust and ammonia destroy cilia (minute hair-like processes) of the upper respiratory tract. Cilia by their continuous beating action throw the disease-producing micro-organisms out of the respiratory tract. Their destruction by dust and ammonia (see '**Effects of ammonia**') permits inhaled *E. coli* to establish, grow and cause respiratory infection.

*E. coli* usually infects the respiratory tract of birds already infected with infectious bronchitis virus and Ranikhet disease virus, including vaccine strains, and mycoplasmas. The damaged respiratory tract becomes very much prone to invasion by *E. coli*. The resulting disease is called '**airsac disease**' or '**chronic respiratory disease (CRD)**'. In addition to inflammation of airsacs (airsacculitis), pneumonia (inflammation of lungs), pleuropneumonia (inflammation of both lungs and pleura, i.e. covering of the lungs), pericarditis (inflammation of the pericardium, covering of the heart), and perihepatitis (inflammation of the liver surface) are also usually present. Airsac disease occurs mainly between 4 to 9 week old broiler chickens. Heavy economic losses occur from morbidity (number of birds affected) and mortality (deaths caused).

## Postmortem Findings

Infected airsacs are thickened and usually contain cheese-like inflammatory material (exudate).

## 3. Pericarditis

Most *E. coli* cause pericarditis following septicaemia (blood infection). The pericardium becomes cloudy and is covered with a light-yellow inflammatory material (exudate).

## 4. Osteoarthritis and Synovitis

Inflammation of the joint (**arthritis**) associated with degeneration of the cartilage and bone of joints (**osteoarthritis**), or inflammation of the synovial tissues in a joint (**synovitis**), are usually the result of blood infection. Localization of the *E. coli* in bones and synovial tissues is a common occurrence in colisepticaemia. **Symptoms** include mild to severe lameness and poor growth. Affected birds are more likely to be victims of cannibalism. Hock, stifle, hip, and wing joints are sites where arthritis usually occurs.

## 5. Coligranuloma

Also known as '**Hjarre's disease**', this condition occurs in adult hens, usually as a cause of occasional death. It is caused by *E. coli.* Although Hjarre's disease is an uncommon form of systemic infection caused by *E. coli*, it can cause mortality up to 75% when a flock is affected. The **symptoms** are non-specific. Affected birds are usually found dead, or die after depression and loss of condition. **Postmortem examination** shows characteristic hard, yellow nodular growths in the wall of the intestine, particularly the caeca. Sometimes the liver is similarly affected, and is hard, discoloured and swollen, but spleen is not affected. There is no effective treatment or method of control.

## Localized Forms of *E. coli* Infections

## 1. Omphalitis and Yolk Sac Infection

**Omphalitis**, also known as '**mushy chick disease**' is inflammation of the navel (umbilicus). In birds, the yolk sac is usually involved because of its closeness with navel. **Yolk sac infection is the commonest cause of mortality in chicks during the first week after hatching, that is, early chick mortality.** *E. coli* is present in the yolk of about 70% of chicks with yolk sac infection. Other bacteria include staphylococci, **Proteus** species, **Bacillus** species, enterococci, **Pseudomonas**, and clostridia.

Low brooding temperature, or **fasting after hatching**, increases the incidence of infection and mortality. Egg dipping at 18 days of incubation increases infection than dipping at one day.

## Routes of Infection and Spread

1.  Infection occurs after **contamination of the unhealed navel** with powerful strains of *E. coli. E. coli* enters through the unhealed navel. **Faecal contamination of eggs is the most important source of infection.**

2.  Bacteria may enter into the egg if the hen has oophoritis (inflammation of ovary) or salpingitis (inflammation of oviduct), or through contamination following artificial insemination.

3.  Yolk sac infections can also result from transfer of bacteria from the chick's intestine, or from the bloodstream. In these cases, the navel is not affected. It is common to recover low numbers of *E. coli* from normal yolk sacs. Between 0.5 and 6% of eggs from normal hens contain *E. coli.*

    *E. coli* grows rapidly in the intestines of newly hatched chicks and infection **spreads** quickly from chick to chick in the hatchery and brooders. A hatchery environment that is not sufficiently humid is usually associated with a high incidence of yolk sac infection.

## Losses

Some embryos may die before hatching, particularly late in incubation. Others die at, or soon after hatching. The numbers of cases increase after hatching and decrease after about 6 days. However, occasional losses continue up to 3 weeks. **As few as 10 organisms of the powerful type can cause 100% mortality in day-old chicks following yolk sac infection.** With less powerful strains, there is no embryo or chick mortality, the only symptoms of infected yolk sacs being retained cheese-like yolk and reduced weight gain.

## Symptoms

**The navel of the affected birds is swollen, red and may even show small abscesses.** The abdomen is distended and blood vessels on the abdominal surface are prominent and full of blood. In severe cases, the wall of the navel and overlying skin undergo lysis (destruction) and are wet and dirty. Chicks having such soft and pulpy skin are known as **'mushy chicks'** and the condition as **'mushy chick disease'.** ('Mush' means a 'soft pulpy mass'. The disease is so called because the skin after lysis becomes a soft pulpy mass.)

## Postmortem Findings

The blood vessels below the skin and in the yolk sac are dilated and filled with blood. **The most important finding is an inflamed, unabsorbed yolk.** The yolk appears increased in amount because it has not been absorbed. **It is abnormal in colour, consistency, and smell.** Yolk may be yellow and thickened, or brown-green and watery, and is usually very foul-smelling. Peritonitis and haemorrhages on the surface of intestines are common. A profuse growth of *E. coli* may be obtained from the abdominal organs, particularly from the yolk on direct culture. **The blood vessels of the yolk are usually prominent.** Chicks which live more than 4 days may have **pericarditis** as well as **infected yolks**. This indicates spread of the organism from the yolk sac. The wall of the yolk sac is oedematous (swollen) with mild inflammation. There may also be non-specific changes, such as dehydration, visceral gout, emaciation, vent pasting, and enlarged gallbladder.

## Harmful Effects of Yolk Sac Infection

1. Deprivation of nutrients and maternal antibodies to newly hatched chicks.

2. Absorption of toxins in the body of the chicks.

3. Spread of *E. coli* by extension into the body cavity, or systemically through bloodstream may produce colisepticaemia.

4. The survivors are usually stunted and perform poorly. Afterwards, the yolk sac contracts, but an abscess remains for a long period. *E. coli* **usually persists in the inflamed yolk sac for weeks or months.**

## 2. Salpingitis and Peritonitis in Layers

Inflammation of the oviduct (**salpingitis**) caused by *E. coli* results in decreased egg production and occasional deaths in laying hens and breeders. **It is one of the most common causes of mortality in laying hens.** Infection occurs when *E. coli* enters into the oviduct from the cloaca. Spread to the oviduct from infected airsacs is also possible, but this occurs usually in young birds as part of a systemic infection. **Heavy egg production and associated oestrogenic activity predispose to salpingitis by relaxing the sphincter between the vagina and cloaca.** The oviduct is distended markedly with single or multiple masses of caseous material (exudate). The mass of caseous material may expand to the point that it fills much of the body cavity. The caseous material often contains a central egg, shells, and/or membranes. **It is very foul-smelling.**

Extension of infection into the body cavity through the oviduct wall leads to concurrent **peritonitis** (inflammation of the peritoneum, a membrane that lines the body cavity). Peritonitis in the absence of salpingitis can also occur due to free yolk in the body cavity (see 'egg peritonitis'). If *E. coli* is also present because of an ascending infection from cloaca, peritonitis may be severe. **Affected birds cannot produce and lay eggs.** Peritonitis is characterized by sudden deaths and free yolk in the body cavity.

## 3. Diarrhoeal Disease (Enteritis)

Primary enteritis (inflammation of the intestine) in poultry caused by *E. coli* is rare.

## 4. Coliform Cellulitis (Inflammatory Process)

**Cellulitis** is inflammation of the loose connective tissue situated under the skin, that is, subcutaneous tissue. It is rare in mammals, but relatively common in birds. It has many causes, but *E. coli* infection is the most common cause in chickens. For this reason, cellulitis is usually called **'coliform cellulitis'**. Because this form of *E. coli* infection has emerged as a significant disease problem in **broiler chickens**, it is covered separately at some length at other place (see 'avian cellulitis).

## 5. Swollen Head Syndrome

This is an acute (severe) form of **cellulitis** and involves areas surrounding the eye and nearby subcutaneous tissue of the head. It is important in **broilers** and is usually caused by *E. coli*. Because of its importance, this condition is also covered separately (see 'swollen head syndrome').

## Diagnosis (for all *E. coli* Infections)

Diagnosis based on characteristic postmortem findings is usually adequate to recommend treatment so that economic losses can be prevented. Bacteriological examination should be carried out to confirm the presumptive diagnosis and determine antibiotic sensitivity. *E. coli* are isolated and identified on artificial media in the bacteriology laboratory.

## Treatment and Control

These are discussed collectively at the end.

## Egg Peritonitis

Egg peritonitis is inflammation of the peritoneum caused by the presence of a broken egg in the abdominal cavity. Egg peritonitis also includes a number of reproductive disorders of poultry, such as salpingitis (inflammation of oviduct) and impaction (tight packing) of the oviduct. Almost always egg peritonitis is caused by *E. coli*.

## Incidence

In any flock of laying birds there will be a small number of deaths, usually about 1% a month. This is considered as unavoidable. However, when this 'acceptable' mortality is increased, it may be due to various types of egg peritonitis. Apart from this, however, egg peritonitis can occur as a greater flock problem. When this happens it is usually associated with inadequate management. Flock peritonitis outbreaks are usually linked with cannibalism and vent pecking. Overcrowding and huddling (crowding together in a small space) lead to vent pecking and egg peritonitis.

## Postmortem Findings

Postmortem examination reveals the presence of scattered pieces of yolk, thickened yolk, cheese-like material, or milky fluid in the abdominal cavity. There is also inflammation and distortion of the ovaries and salpingitis. In some cases the oviduct may be obstructed by thickened inflammatory material which may sometimes result in the rupture of oviduct wall. A complete, or partially formed, egg may be found impacted in the oviduct. Almost always a profuse pure growth of *E. coli* can be isolated from the oviduct and cheese-like thickened material in such cases. Unless the carcass is examined immediately after death, the importance of *E. coli* may be difficult to determine because the organism is a common and rapid contaminant.

## Treatment and Control

These are discussed collectively, next.

## Treatment (for all *E. coli* Infections)

Any treatment must begin with a complete sanitation programme as most *E. coli* infections start with dirty surroundings and various environmental stresses. Broad-spectrum antibiotics may be helpful in treating the conditions. However, **many *E. coli* are resistant to the commonly used poultry antibiotics.** An antibiotic sensitivity test is essential in identifying the best drug to use in a treatment programme.

1.  Antibiotics reduce mortality. *E. coli* may be sensitive to many drugs, such as ampicillin, chloramphenicol, chlortetracycline, neomycin, nitrofurans, gentamicin, ormethiprim-sulphadimethoxine, nalidixic acid, oxytetracycline, polymyxin B, streptomycin and sulpha drugs. Recently, fluoroquinolones (enrofloxacin, sarafloxacin) have generally proved to be highly efficacious.

    Antibiotics should be given for not less than 4-5 days. Best results are obtained if the medication is commenced early in the course of disease. **Once peritonitis and perihepatitis etc. are present, no treatment is effective.**

2.  Yolk sac infection and early chick mortality can also be reduced through medication during the first few days of life. Severely affected birds do not respond to medication because of their inability to eat and drink.

3.  *E. coli* from poultry is usually resistant to one or more drugs, especially if they have been used widely over a long period, for example, tetracyclines and now also enrofloxacin. The best approach is to isolate *E. coli* from the diseased birds and carry out a sensitivity test to select the most suitable antibiotic for the treatment. However, in the face of disease, it is necessary to start treatment before the sensitivity test result is available.

4.  Furazolidone at a level of 0.04% in the feed for 10 days, or chlortetracycline in the water at the rate of 600 mg/5 litres for 5 days, is usually effective in reducing morbidity (number of birds affected) and mortality (number of deaths).

5. Even a highly effective drug may not show improvement of the flock if too little is used, or it is incapable of reaching the site of infection. **Under-dosing stimulates development of resistance.**

# Control

1. The best method of controlling colisepticaemia is to maintain the highest standards of management and to obtain chicks only from disease-free, well-managed breeding flocks and hatcheries.

2. Avoid overcrowding.

3. Avoid dry, dusty conditions. Wetting the litter can reduce the cases of colisepticaemia.

4. Provide adequate ventilation in the poultry house.

5. Avoid build-up of ammonia. Maintain proper litter conditions. Good litter management and properly ventilated houses are very important factors in the control of colisepticaemia. The litter should be dry but not dusty (see **'litter management'**). The air flow through the houses should be controlled to avoid pockets of stagnant air, or build-up of ammonia fumes.

6. Protect the birds against extremes of temperature, heat or cold.

7. Ensure supply of clean water. Chlorination of drinking water is recommended. Also use water sanitizers (see **'sanitization'** and **'water sanitizers'**). Remember contaminated water can contain organisms in high numbers.

8. To prevent yolk sac infection and early chick mortality, provide the best possible brooding conditions (see **'brooding management'**).

9. The birds should be fed a well-balanced diet to avoid mineral deficiencies and malnutrition. Ensure a supply of high protein, vitamin A, vitamin E, and vitamin C and zinc (see Chapter 33).

10. Provide probiotic in the very first drinking water given to chicks, and continue to use it for at least a week, and thereafter in the feed. This way *E. coli* can be competitively excluded from the intestines of chicks (see **'competitive exclusion'** under **'probiotics'**).

11. Remember pelleted feed has fewer *E. coli* than mash.

12. Also remember that rodent (rats, mice) droppings are a source of pathogenic *E. coli.*

13. Use of nipple watering systems decreases the occurrence of colibacillosis.

14. The most important source for transmission of pathogenic *E. coli* between flocks is **faecal contamination of hatching eggs**. Transmission can be reduced by collecting

eggs frequently, keeping nest material clean, not using floor eggs, discarding cracked eggs or those with faecal contamination, and fumigating or disinfecting eggs within 2 hours after they are laid. If infected eggs are broken during incubation or hatching, the contents are a serious source of infection to others, especially when people and egg-handling equipment are contaminated. Eggs are particularly susceptible just before hatching. Contaminated chicks survive better if kept warm and not starved.

15. *E. coli* infection of the respiratory tract can be reduced by **raising mycoplasma-free birds** and reducing exposure of birds to viruses causing respiratory diseases. Also, they should have been vaccinated against Gumboro disease, Ranikhet disease, infectious bronchitis, and any other disease that is a local threat.

16. There have been encouraging reports of killed vaccines. These protected birds against mortality and respiratory disease following infection with pathogenic *E. coli*. Use of a killed vaccine in breeder produces passive protection in progeny. Protection is complete for 2 weeks and partial for several additional weeks after hatching.

17. Broiler breeder hens are to be vaccinated at 6-12 weeks of age. Vaccination is repeated 14-18 weeks of age. The interval between vaccinations has to be at least 6 weeks. The antibodies against *E. coli* are transferred to the progeny through the eggs. These antibodies help to protect the newly hatched broiler chicks against the effects of colibacillosis.

**Note:** For a list of commercially available vaccines against colibacillosis, refer to Chapter 19 under **"Avian colibacillosis vaccines"**.

## INFECTIOUS CORYZA

Also known as **'fowl coryza'**, infectious coryza is an acute respiratory disease of chickens caused by the bacterium, *Haemophilus paragallinarum*. The disease is characterized by swelling of the face, and discharges from the eyes and nostrils. The greatest economic losses occur from poor growth in growing birds and marked reduction in egg production (10-40%) in layers. Infectious coryza can turn into a chronic respiratory disease.

Infectious coryza occurs worldwide and is extremely common in India, both in broilers and layers. Chickens of all ages are susceptible, but older birds suffer more severely. It causes economic losses due to an increased number of culls (worthless birds) in growing chickens and reduced production in layers.

### Cause

*Haemophilus paragallinarum* is a Gram-negative organism. It is a delicate bacterium which dies quickly outside the bird. Survival outside the body under farm conditions is not more than 48 hours. *H. paragallinarum* occurs in **three serotypes** (serogroups): **A, B, and C.** It is believed that in India only type A and C are prevalent. **Presence of serotype B has not been confirmed so far.**

## Spread

1.  Clinically affected and carrier birds (birds which carry the infection without showing symptoms) are the main source of infection.

2.  As only a few organisms are required for infection, **the infection can be spread by drinking water contaminated by nasal (from the nose) discharge, as well as by the air (airborne) over a short distance.**

3.  Lateral spread occurs readily by direct contact.

4.  Spread between cages with nipple drinkers occurs more slowly.

5.  **Infectious coryza is not an egg-transmitted disease.**

## Development of the Disease

After entry, the organism first attaches itself to minute, short, hair-like processes (cilia) present on cells lining the upper respiratory tract. It then grows here. The toxic substances released from the organism during growth produce changes in the lining mucosa, and also the symptoms of the disease.

**The organism is non-invasive.** That is, it does not penetrate deeper into the tissues, because it has a strong affinity (attraction, liking) for the lining cells. It migrates into the lower respiratory tract (lungs and airsacs) only after combined (synergistic) interaction with other infectious agents, or when encouraged by immunosuppression (i.e. suppression of the natural immune responses). Other infections occurring during the course of this disease, such as with infectious bronchitis virus, laryngotracheitis virus, *Mycoplasma gallisepticum*, or *Escherichia coli,* and also unfavourable environmental conditions, make infectious coryza more severe and also a prolonged disease (**chronic respiratory disease**).

## Symptoms

The disease in flocks on deep litter is characterized by rapid spread, high morbidity (birds affected) and low mortality. The incubation period is 1-3 days after contact infection and all susceptible birds in the flock show symptoms within 7-10 days. If not complicated by other infections, the course of the disease is not more than 10 days in the mild form and about 3 weeks in the more severe form.

The first typical symptoms include sneezing, mucus-like discharge from the openings of the nose and eyes, and **swelling on the face (facial oedema) (Fig. 11).** In severe cases, marked conjunctivitis (inflammation of conjunctiva) with closed eyes, swollen wattles, and difficulty in breathing can be seen. Feed and water consumption is usually decreased. This results in a drop in egg production, or an increase in the culling of inferior, weaker, and worthless birds. A drop in egg production of more than 20% indicates involvement of other diseases/factors. If complicated with other infectious agents a more severe and prolonged disease may develop with the symptoms of a chronic respiratory disease.

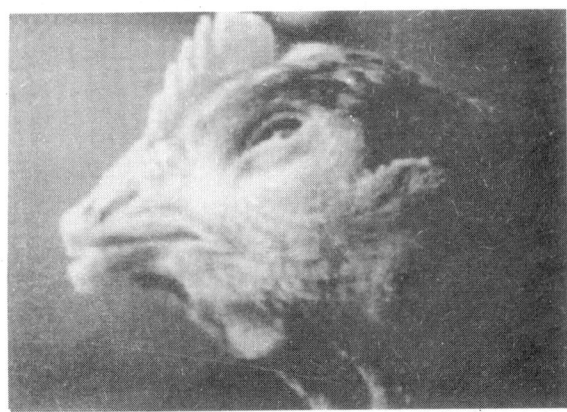

Fig. 11. Infectious coryza. Note typical swelling on the face.

## Postmortem Findings

There is inflammation of the nasal passages and infraorbital sinus (i.e. space present below the eye) and conjunctivitis characterized by the presence of mucus, or pus with fibrin. Swelling of face and wattle due to the accumulation of fluid under the skin (subcutaneous oedema) is prominent. The upper trachea may be involved, but the lungs and airsacs are only affected in chronic, complicated cases.

## Diagnosis

The history of a rapidly spreading disease and its symptoms and postmortem findings help in making a tentative diagnosis. This has to be confirmed by isolation and identification of the causal organism. Isolation should be attempted by taking swabs from the infraorbital sinus of 2 or 3 diseased birds on blood agar plates. The nasal exudate is usually contaminated. Swabs from the trachea and airsacs may be taken, although *H. paragallinarum* is less frequently isolated from these areas.

## Treatment

Various sulphonamides and antibiotics are useful in treating the disease. The combination of sulphonamide trimethoprim, tetracyclines, as well as the new second generation quinolone derivatives, such as enrofloxacin, esafloxacin and norfloxacin may be used. Erythromycin and oxytetracycline are the two commonly used antibiotics. After 5-7 days treatment the symptoms usually disappear, but relapse may occur after the treatment is discontinued. This is not because the drug is inefficient, but because it is not capable of eliminating the organism in all birds in a large population as well as from the environment. Therefore, the symptoms do not disappear completely before a specific immunity has been developed in most of the affected birds of the flock.

## Control

1. To eliminate the agent from the farm it is necessary to dispose of the infected or

recovered birds because such birds remain as a reservoir of the bacterial agent. After cleaning and disinfection of the houses and equipment, the premises should be allowed to remain vacant for 2-3 weeks before re-stocking with clean birds. Only day-old chicks, or older birds which are known to be free from *H. paragallinarum,* should be used for re-stocking. This is not possible in multi-age farm conditions.

2.  Improved management practices, such as culling of birds, good sanitation, traffic control and avoiding birds of multiple ages would help in breaking the disease cycle. Keep only birds of the same age on the farm. **Practise all-in, all-out management.**

3.  Because of the difficulty of controlling infectious coryza by sanitary measures, drug therapy and/or vaccination are used.

4.  Vaccination with an inactivated (killed) vaccine can protect chickens against the disease (see Chapter 19, under **'infectious coryza vaccines'**). Such a vaccine can provide serotype-specific immunity, but does not protect against all serotypes. All the same, appropriate vaccination is economically worthwhile because it usually protects against the more severe drops of egg production. Two doses of vaccine, each of which must consist of at least $10^8$ colony-forming units / ml, are recommended. Vaccine should be injected preferably subcutaneously (below the skin) 3-6 weeks apart, the first injection being given at about 16 weeks of age. Another approach is to give injection between 10 and 20 weeks of age. They give best results when given 3-4 weeks before an expected outbreak. Two injections given about 4 weeks apart, before 20 weeks of age, result in better performance of layers than a single injection.

Vaccines involving live *H. paragallinarum* organisms stimulate a more protective response, but they give rise to carriers and may cause disease. However, controlled exposure is practised in some areas where the disease is regularly found after vaccination with a killed vaccine.

Vaccines containing thimerosal as the killing agent for the organisms are more efficient than formalin. One study indicates that both subcutaneous and intramuscular routes are effective. Injection into the leg muscle gives better protection than when injected into the breast muscle.

Serotype B must be included in killed vaccine in areas where serotype B is prevalent, since it has been confirmed as a true serotype with full disease-producing power. **It may be necessary to prepare an autogenous killed vaccine (i.e. vaccine derived from the affected flock) for use in areas where the B serotype is prevalent.**

**Note:** For a list of commercially available infectious coryza vaccines, refer to Chapter 19 under **"Infectious coryza vaccines"**.

# NECROTIC ENTERITIS

Necrotic enteritis is a disease of the intestinal tract. It is an important disease of chickens, particularly in birds of 4 weeks of age. Sometimes it is also seen in adult birds. There are sudden deaths, and mortality in untreated flocks can reach 10% or more, and is **most common in broilers. The disease is most often established after an outbreak of coccidiosis.**

## Cause

Necrotic enteritis is caused by the proliferation of bacterium, *Clostridium perfringens* **(type A or C)** in the caeca and large intestine. Afterwards it migrates to the small intestine where it produces **toxins (alpha** and **beta).** These toxic substances are responsible for the death of intestinal lining (mucosal lining) and characteristic lesions (changes) of necrotic enteritis. *C. perfringens* is a Gram-positive organism.

Apart from *C. perfringens*, various predisposing factors are also involved in the development of the disease. These include environmental, health, and dietary factors. These factors modify the intestinal environment, and promote development of *C. perfringens*. **Necrotic enteritis is therefore a multi-factorial disease and its development is quite complex.**

## Occurrence

*C. perfringens* can be found in faeces, soil, dust, water, contaminated feed and litter, worker's clothing, shoes etc., and also in the intestinal contents. It is the main obligate anaerobe bacterium in the intestinal tract of **normal chickens.** That is, it thrives only in the absence of oxygen. It therefore lives in the caeca, where conditions for the absence of oxygen (anaerobiosis) are best.

Normally, *C. perfringens* is found in small numbers in the intestinal tract of healthy chickens. It is found in the crop, gizzard, the small intestine and caeca. **However, the presence of *C. perfringens* by itself does not produce the disease.** For example, between 75% and 95% of birds contain the organism at low levels, but only a few of these ever show symptoms of the disease. However, if the conditions, particularly in the small intestine alter due to a change in the type of feed or presence of some disease, then the circumstances go in favour of *C. perfringens*. The organisms then begin to proliferate and increase in number. At some critical number, they begin to produce **toxins** and destroy the cells lining the small intestine. The intestinal lining then usually gets covered by a layer of fibrino-necrotic material, i.e., dead cells containing fibrin.

Necrotic enteritis is an **enterotoxaemia** caused by *C. perfringens* types **A** and C. That is, a condition characterized by the presence in blood of toxins produced in the intestines by the organisms. Necrotic enteritis is therefore associated with high numbers of *C. perfringens* in the intestinal tract of poultry. *C. perfringens* strains **types A and C** produce **alpha** and **beta-toxin. Usually, the damage of the intestinal tract is associated** with **coccidiosis.**

*C. perfringens* is a spore-forming anaerobe. **Its ability to form endospores makes it extremely resistant to external environmental influences** and increases its ability to spread. An **endospore** is the resting stage of certain bacteria. Under unfavourable conditions the nucleus and cytoplasm of the bacteria get enclosed within a tough protective coat, **allowing the bacteria to survive.** On return of favourable conditions, the spore changes back to the normal form of bacteria.

Outbreaks of necrotic enteritis occur in chickens from 2 weeks to 6 months of age. Majority of reports have been in 2-5-week-old broiler chickens raised on litter. However, outbreaks in 3-6- month-old layers raised in floor pens have also been reported. Outbreaks of necrotic enteritis and coccidiosis have been reported in 12-16-week-old cage-reared growers. **Sub-clinical necrotic enteritis in broilers** causes decreased growth rate and feed utilization, that is, feed conversion efficiency.

## Sources of Infection

**Contaminated feed and contaminated litter** act as sources of infection.

## Predisposing Factors

These are those factors which make the bird easily prone to infection. In case of necrotic enteritis, these include:

1. **Outbreaks of coccidiosis, especially mild and subclinical.** Necrotic enteritis can be reproduced by dosing (administering) chickens with sporulated oocysts of **Eimeria** species (*E. maxima*). Oral administration of *C. perfringens* alone has not been successful in producing necrotic enteritis.

2. Partial impaction of the lower intestine due to litter and/or grain ingested without the provision of insoluble grit.

3. **Changes in feed.** Change of feed can affect the number of *C. perfringens* in the intestinal tract. **Their numbers are greatly influenced by the nature of the ration.** For example, high levels of fish meal, or high levels of wheat, barley, or rye in the feed can precipitate outbreaks of necrotic enteritis.

4. Removal of antibiotic growth promoters from the feed results in a significant increase in the incidence of necrotic enteritis. This is because of their direct effect on control of the causative organism *C. perfringens.*

5. **Damage to the intestinal mucosa** (lining) is another predisposing factor. Factors such as high-fibre litter or various strains of coccidia combined with higher than normal numbers of *C. perfringens,* can result in necrotic enteritis.

6. **Changes in the microflora of the intestine** may also result in the disease. This may be brought about by rapid changes in feed components. The changes upset the intestinal microflora and **allow *C. perfringens* to grow.**

7. **Immunosuppression** from Gumboro disease may precede necrotic enteritis.

8. Inadequate cleaning of houses, utensils, and equipment between batches of chickens.

## Factors Influencing Development of the Disease

**These factors are discussed at some length for two reasons. Firstly,** because of the great economic importance of necrotic enteritis due to its increased occurrence, and **secondly,** in view of the scientific advances made recently, particularly on this aspect of the disease.

The factors that allow *C. perfringens* to proliferate and produce **alpha-toxin** and cause necrotic enteritis are not known. However, when the disease does occur, it is characterized by an increased and localized population of *C. perfringens* associated with **increased levels of alpha-toxin.** Other factors that change the intestinal tract environment and allow excessive growth of *C. perfringens* are also required to produce the disease. **Several of these risk factors now have been identified.** The development of necrotic enteritis in a poultry flock depends on the interactions between these various factors. **These factors are:**

## 1. Dietary Factors (dietary ingredients)

There is a strong relationship between certain feed ingredients and the occurrence of necrotic enteritis. Some feeds containing cereals such as wheat, barley, and rye (**but not maize**) that contain indigestible water-soluble **non-starch polysaccharides (NSP),** for example, beta-glucans and arabinoxylans, encourage the development of necrotic enteritis. Also, feeds containing increased levels of protein, such as **fish meal,** predispose birds to overgrowth of *C. perfringens* and thus to necrotic enteritis.

Feeds that are imbalanced in their nutrient content can cause **nutritional stress in poultry.** For example, if the energy-to-protein ratio is low, the birds will consume more feed and exceed their requirements for protein. **This will increase the nitrogen content of the digesta (intestinal content) and excreta (faeces, urine).** Feeds that contain high concentration of protein, and also those with imbalanced profiles of amino acids, have reduced digestibility in the upper intestinal tract and therefore increased concentrations of these compounds and their metabolites are found in the lower intestinal tract. Similarly, poorly digested proteins concentrate in the lower intestinal tract and thus act as substrates for microflora. A substrate is a specific substance(s) on which a given enzymes acts.

**In the lower intestinal tract, proteins are degraded to ammonia and amines. This encourages the proliferation of *C. perfringens*.** An amine is an organic compound containing nitrogen and is derived from ammonia. The presence of these nitrogenous degradation products **raises the pH of the lower intestinal tract (makes it more alkaline),** because of their high pKa values and also because they counteract the pH changes that normally occur from the production of acetic and lactic acids by bacteria. (The pKa value is the pH in which half of the acid molecules are ionized). **The alkaline pH increases proliferation of** *C. perfringens.*

**Another result of higher dietary nitrogen**, an imbalance of amino acids, and reduced digestibility of proteins is that **the amount of nitrogen that is excreted is increased.** For efficient excretion to occur, more quantities of water are required. As a result **litter becomes wet and has higher nitrogen content.** This, in turn, leads to litter having more amounts of ammonia, and thus **higher pH (alkaline),** since ammonia is an **alkaline** compound of nitrogen. **The alkaline pH of litter favours proliferation of** *C. perfringens* **in the litter, which aggravates the problem.**

**Non-starch polysaccharides (NSP)** and **starch** can provide a ready source of energy for bacteria to utilize and proliferate. It has been found that the presence of NSP in the feed does not only encourage the growth of *C. perfringens* but also suppresses the growth of other useful bacteria such as **Lactobacillus** species. In contrast to starches, **NSP** present in cereals, legumes and other feedstuffs, are not utilized by poultry and cause a variety of effects in the intestinal tract of birds. They cannot be broken down by the enzymes present in the chicken. On the other hand, these compounds act as substrates for microflora within the intestinal tract **and thus allow the proliferation of pathogenic (disease-producing) bacteria.**

Moreover, NSP being hydrophilic increase the water content of the digesta. This has a number of effects. The increased association of water with NSP makes birds to consume more water to maintain body balance (homeostasis). However, the increased water intake also increases water excretion, affecting litter quality and **providing an opportunity for pathogenic bacteria to proliferate within litter**. These bacteria worsen the situation and perpetuate bacterial proliferation within the intestinal tract of the bird. The increased water content of digesta also encourages pathogenic bacterial proliferation. Moreover, the viscosity (glutinous consistency) of digesta increases in the presence of NSP. Viscosity decreases digestibility of nutrients and their absorption is reduced because of the increased time required for nutrients to migrate to villi, where nutrients are absorbed. Some NSP interact with the proteins and glycoproteins of the epithelial cells of the intestine, cause their damage, or stimulate them to secrete mucin. **This allows disease-producing microorganisms in the intestinal tract to adhere to the mucin or epithelial cells, and proliferate.**

In addition to the importance of the type of cereal used in the poultry feeds, the type of **animal protein**, like **fish meal** also increases the occurrence of necrotic enteritis. *C. perfringens* **lacks the ability to produce 13 out of 20 essential amino acids.**

Therefore, its growth is increased in an environment rich in protein, particularly **fish meal**. When fish meal is included in the diet, population of *C. perfringens* can increase to disease-producing levels. **The combination of NSP and protein in the diet can greatly complicate the problem.** The unfavourable effect of cereal combinations (high wheat or barley, low maize) on necrotic enteritis worsened when **animal proteins** were included in the feed.

## 2. Antinutrients, Antinutritive Factors and Toxins

**Antinutrients**, such as **lectins** (a group of proteins and glycoproteins) from **soybeans** and wheat interact very strongly with intestinal epithelial cells. They damage the cells, cause changes in the microbial population, and affect the immune response in birds. **Since soybean meal is the major ingredient in the feeds of poultry in India, these effects are highly important.** Protease inhibitors, found in heated soybean meals, reduce digestibility of proteins in the intestinal tract. Thus, they help in increasing the concentration of nitrogen in the lower intestinal tract, **thereby increasing the proliferation of *C. perfringens.***

**Mycotoxins are free radical generators.** Thus, they challenge the antioxidant responses within the poultry. When the birds are under some **nutritional stress** they become more susceptible to disease-producing bacteria, such as *C. perfringens.* Then an extra supply of the relevant protective nutrient, for example, an antioxidant such as vitamin E, is necessary.

**The size of the feed particles can influence necrotic enteritis.** Small feed particles move more rapidly through the intestinal tract. This denies *C. perfringens* the chance of adhering to the intestinal cells. For development of necrotic enteritis, increased numbers of *C. perfringens* are required to adhere to the intestinal cells. The particle size of the feed also influences the presence of **Eimeria** species, cause of coccidiosis, a disease closely associated with the development of necrotic enteritis.

## 3. Feed Additives with Protective Effects against Necrotic Enteritis

Enzymes, such as xylanases and beta-glucanases, break down the NSP components of the feed and increase the availability of nutrients. In general, addition of these enzymes **reduces the viscosity of the digesta** and may offer some protection against adhesion of *C. perfingens* and thus disease outbreaks.

Supplementation of poultry feeds or the drinking water with **organic acids (acidifiers)** can influence the numbers of *C. perfringens* and thus the occurrence of necrotic enteritis by **two mechanisms**: (1) Acids with high pKa values reduce the pH of the intestine and thus increase the growth of non-disease-producing bacteria, and (2) Acids with low pKa values are absorbed by the bacteria through the cell wall, they then disrupt the biochemical pathways within the bacteria, and thus prevent their proliferation. **The provision of organic acids indirectly to chickens, for example in litter, also**

**reduces the exposure of the birds to disease-producing organisms.**

Addition of **lactose** in the feeds reduces significantly the number of *C. perfringens* present in the caeca. **Lactose is not absorbed in the small intestine of chickens** and is therefore available to organisms such as **Lactobacillus** species in the caeca. The availability of lactose can alter the microbial population in favour of non-disease-producing bacteria and away from *C. perfringens*. Dietary lactose also reduces the pH of caeca (makes acidic), a condition that is unfavourable for *C. perfringens*. Addition of lactose in chicken feeds also reduces the level of *Salmonella typhimurium*.

## Interactions with other Disease-Producing Organisms

**There is an interaction between coccidiosis and necrotic enteritis.** Coccidiosis usually occurs just before or along with outbreaks of necrotic enteritis in the field, both in broilers and layers. **It is believed that coccidiosis usually occurs before necrotic enteritis.** This is because coccidia damage cells lining the intestinal tract which allows *C. perfringens* to take hold. Moreover, the sloughed cells from the damaged villi provide nitrogen. Certain coccidiostats control necrotic enteritis. Recently it has been reported that use of an anticoccidial vaccine also protects against necrotic enteritis.

## Management Factors that Influence the Development of Necrotic Enteritis

1. Any factor that causes **stress in broiler chickens** can change the environment in the intestines in such a way that the chances for necrotic enteritis are increased. For example, change from starter to grower feeds, causes such stress in the intestinal tract of young birds that *C. perfringens* can take advantage of the charged environment and proliferate. This may be due to changes in pH, feed composition (e.g. NSP content), enzyme supplementation, or to changes in host resistance through effects on the immune system.

2. **Contamination of feed by** *C. perfringens* is also involved in necrotic enteritis outbreaks. *C. perfringens* **spores** may be present in the raw ingredients used to produce poultry feeds, and the heat treatment of feed ingredients may activate the clostridial spores. Heat treatment may also inactivate enzyme supplements that would have otherwise reduced the level of NSP in the feed, thus increasing the risk of necrotic enteritis.

3. *C. perfringens* may be transmitted **vertically** or **horizontally**. The hatchery has been identified as a source of *C. perfringens* in a number of studies. Organisms have been recovered from 20% of eggshells, hatching paper, and feather dust. *C. perfringens* was recovered from faecal samples in 94% of flocks tested and also in materials transported from the hatcheries when chicks are delivered. Colonization of chicken intestinal tract with *C. perfringens* may therefore occur in the eggs

before hatching, or at a very early age after hatching.

Increasing stocking density (**overcrowding**) can also increase the incidence of necrotic enteritis. This is due to an increased **build-up of** *C. perfringens* **spores in the litter,** poor litter quality (wet, with high levels of nitrogenous compounds) and the increased risk of spread by contact or by air. **High fibre litter** increases the risk of necrotic enteritis through increased damage to the intestinal tract.

## Author's Observations

During rainy season, at two layer farms, investigation into the cause of mortality in caged growers revealed simultaneous occurrence of necrotic enteritis, intestinal coccidiosis, and Ranikhet disease (RD). LaSota vaccination had failed to control RD. Microscopic examination of the intestinal scrapings revealed presence of *Eimeria maxima* oocysts in large numbers. Necrotic enteritis was treated by oral administration of neomycin sulphate, but it occurred again. It was brought under control only after coccidiosis was treated. RD could be controlled only after both necrotic enteritis and coccidiosis were successfully treated. This observation has since been confirmed in several other outbreaks, including those in broilers.

**Interpretation**: Intestinal coccidiosis caused by *E. maxima* facilitated the occurrence of necrotic enteritis. Since, both necrotic enteritis and coccidiosis severely damaged the intestinal tract, LaSota vaccination remained ineffective, because its proper absorption in adequate amounts may have been interfered with.

**Conclusion: The most important predisposing cause of necrotic enteritis, both in broilers and layers, appears coccidiosis. Therefore, in every outbreak of necrotic enteritis coccidiosis must be ruled out, and if present, must also be treated. Likewise, every outbreak of coccidiosis must also be examined for the presence of necrotic enteritis, and if present, must be treated.**

## Symptoms

There may be no symptoms, and birds are suddenly found dead. Or, the appearance may resemble that of coccidiosis. The birds show depression, loss of appetite, unwillingness to move, reduced growth rate, diarrhoea, ruffled feathers, and increasing mortality.

**Outbreaks of 'coccidiosis' that do not respond to treatment should be looked with suspicion.** On a flock basis the disease lasts for 7-10 days.

## Postmortem Findings

Postmortem changes are usually confined to the middle part of the small intestine. The intestine is distended with gas and filled with a foul-smelling brown fluid. However, changes in the caeca may also occur. **The small intestine is greatly thickened due to extensive velvet-like necrosis (death) of the mucosal lining (Fig. 12). The** mucosa is lined by a loose to tightly attached yellow or green layer (a false membrane), and is deeply cracked. Spots or small patches of blood may occur, but haemorrhage is not a feature.

## Diagnosis

1. Diagnosis can be made from typical postmortem findings.

2. Stained smears of intestinal scrapings show large numbers of Gram-positive rods. For confirmation causal agent may be isolated from intestinal

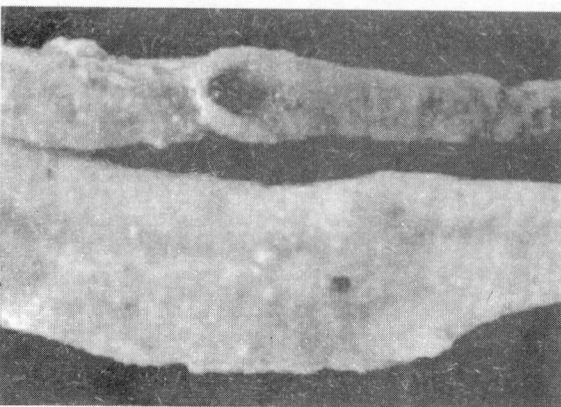

**Fig. 12.** Necrotic enteritis in a broiler chicken with concurrent coccidiosis. Note the congestion and diffuse necrosis of the mucosa with ulceration.

contents or scrapings of intestinal wall. Identification of the causative agent will confirm the diagnosis.

3. Diseases that must be differentiated from necrotic enteritis are ulcerative enteritis (see 'ulcerative enteritis') and coccidiosis.

4. In necrotic enteritis changes are usually confined to small intestine, and there is no involvement of caeca or liver, whereas in ulcerative enteritis, there are areas of necrosis (tissue death) in caeca and liver. For coccidiosis, microscopic examination of faecal smears or intestinal scrapings should demonstrate the presence or absence of coccidia (oocysts or schizonts).

5. Usually, necrotic enteritis and coccidiosis occur together in a flock, and demonstration of one or both agents is necessary.

## Treatment

1. A number of antibiotics in the feed reduce the number of *C. perfringens* shed in the faeces. These include virginiamycin, tylosin, penicillin, ampicillin, lincomycin, bacitracin, and furazolidone.

2. **Betaine**, through its function as an osmolyte (see Chapter 25), can increase the ability of an anticoccidial to minimize the intestinal damage caused in coccidiosis. As a result, both intestinal and digestive integrity are better maintained, and less nitrogen can enter the caeca. This will help in reducing losses from subclinical and clinical necrotic enteritis. For a list of commercial osmolyte preparations available in the market, see Chapter 19 under **'Osmoregulators and methyl donors'**.

# Control

1. Drugs which have an effect on Gram-positive organisms, such as lincomycin, penicillins, virginiamycin, may be included in the feed.

2. Probiotics, such as *Lactobacillus acidophilus* and *Streptococcus faecium* reduce the severity of necrotic enteritis.

3. Anticoccidial drugs, e.g. the ionophores, can also play a role.

4. Removal of fish meal from the ration can help in the prevention of necrotic enteritis and clostridial infection in general, in poultry.

5. **Good management and sanitation practices should be employed.** Improved biosecurity and management strategies are most important. Where a high bacterial load exists (high soil spore counts) and repeat breaks are common, addition of sodium chloride (NaCl) to chicken house dirt floors after a thorough clean out may prevent recurrence of the disease. **Due attention should be given to house maintenance, dietary ingredients, and nutrition.**

# GANGRENOUS DERMATITIS

Gangrenous dermatitis is characterized by areas of death (necrosis) of the skin and underlying tissues, including muscle. Also known by a variety of other names, such as **'wing rot', 'necrotic dermatitis', 'gangrenous cellulitis', 'gangrenous dematomyositis', 'avian malignant oedema', 'gas oedema disease'**, and in some cases, as a part of **'blue-wing disease'**, gangrenous dermatitis is a serious disease **and usually results in death.** It is also quite common. Gangrenous dermatitis is primarily a disease of the broilers over 4 weeks of age, but also occurs in growers up to 18 weeks, and in layers between 6 and 20 weeks. Occurrence is more common in warm, humid conditions. **Mortality ranges from 1 to 60%.**

# Causes

1. Bacteria, known as *Clostridium septicum, Clostridium perfringens* type A, *Staphylococcus aureus*, and *Escherichia coli*, either singly of in combination, are involved. **Combined infections are usually more severe.** When birds receive small injuries to the skin, they may then become infected by the bacteria.

   *Staphylococcus aureus* **is an extremely hardy organism and remains viable for long periods of time in exudates** (inflammatory fluids). It is also a very powerful disease-producing organism and produces a total of **10 enzymes and toxins.** These include **hyaluronidase (spreading factor), deoxyribonuclease, fibrinolysin, lipase, protease, haemolysins, leukocidin, dermonecrotic toxin (causes death of skin), exfoliative toxin, and enterotoxins.** These are responsible for the disease-producing power of the organism.

2.    Gangrenous dermatitis also has a link with those diseases which produce an immunosuppressive effect, such as Gumboro disease, chicken infectious anaemia, and inclusion body hepatitis.

3.    Other predisposing factors are unhygienic management (poor sanitation), overcrowding, **mycotoxins**, nutritional deficiencies, and also chicken infectious anaemia virus and reovirus.

## Development of the Disease

Most cases in broiler chickens occur between 4 and 6 weeks, in commercial layers between 6 and 20 weeks, and in broiler breeders during the 20th week.

Clostridial organisms are present in soil, faeces, dust, contaminated litter or feed, and in the **intestinal contents (mainly caeca).** Staphylococci exist everywhere and are common inhabitant of skin and mucous membranes of poultry. Mucous membranes are the linings of the digestive, respiratory and urinary tracts. **For infection to occur, a breakdown in natural defence mechanisms of the bird must occur.** In most cases, this involves damage to the natural barriers like skin and mucous membranes. That is, **infection occurs through injuries in the skin.** The open navels of newly hatched chicks, debeaking, or even vaccinations provide additional means of entry for staphylococci.

In many cases, gangrenous dermatitis follows diseases caused by other infectious agents, such as Gumboro virus, chicken infectious anaemia virus, reticuloendotheliosis virus, Marek's disease virus and avian adenovirus infections, including inclusion body hepatitis. In these diseases the bursa of Fabricius or thymus is damaged and the immune system is compromised (damaged). Another condition predisposing chickens to gangrenous dermatitis is **'blue-wing disease'.** Characteristic changes in blue wing disease are haemorrhages in the skin, underlying tissue and muscle. Gangrenous dermatitis usually occurs secondarily to the skin haemorrhages. This is because all these infectious agents produce immunosuppression, and a damaged immune system is the underlying predisposing factor allowing gangrenous dermatitis to develop.

## Symptoms

**There is increased mortality in the flock.** Affected birds are usually very depressed, show loss of appetite, leg weakness, drooping of one or both wings, incoordination of movement, **and die within a few hours.** The period of illness is very short, **usually less than 24 hours.** Mortality ranges from 1 to 60%.

## Postmortem Findings

Carcasses rapidly decompose (putrefy) with a foul smell. The skin and underlying tissues under the wings, between the thighs and over the ribs and flanks (i.e. sides between the ribs and the hip) of the birds are very dark, moist, usually devoid of feathers, and show extensive sloughing (falling off). Deep red and swollen areas are found on the feet, legs and sometimes around the feather follicles of the wings. There is blood tinged watery fluid under the skin. The surrounding muscle is usually coloured and oedematous (i.e. contains fluid). If clostridial organisms are involved, gas is produced in the muscle. The kidneys, heart and liver are often congested. In some birds, the lungs are markedly congested and oedematous, and resemble a mass of dark red jelly. The bursa of Fabricius may be very small and lacks firmness. This may be due to Gumboro virus infection.

## Diagnosis

**The postmortem picture is almost diagnostic**. However, gangrenous dermatitis should not be confused with **'blue-wing disease'** (chicken anaemia virus) which occurs in younger birds. Bacterial culture can be misleading, since both staphylococci and clostridial organisms are present on the skin of normal chickens.

## Treatment

No treatment has proved completely successful. This is because of the nature of the lesions (**dead tissues cannot be treated**), and also because many kinds of causes are involved in production of the disease. The underlying viral causes are not controlled. However, penicillins, tetracyclines, chlortetracycline, oxytetracycline, erythromycin, or bacitracin may be given in the drinking water. Follow up should be done by the addition of antibiotics in the feed.

## Control

1.  Avoid overcrowding to prevent injuries in the skin. High stocking densities (overcrowding) result in feather breakage and entry of bacteria into the skin.

2.  Maintain good standards of hygiene in management. Improve litter condition, reduce moisture and bacterial levels in the environment, and minimize trauma (injury) to the bird. Excess moisture in the litter promotes bacterial growth (see **'litter management'**).

3.  Control of the disease has also been achieved to a great extent with the use of **water acidifiers** and **acidification of litter.**

4.  Protect the birds against immunosuppressive diseases like Gumboro disease and others by carrying out proper and timely vaccinations.

5.  **Remove daily dead birds as quickly and as often as possible.**

6.  House sanitation should be carefully controlled. Feeder, water and litter management are very important.

7.  Good nutrition and prevention of stress are also helpful.

8.  Vaccination against Gumboro disease helps in removing the immunosuppressive factor in   this disease.

# ULCERATIVE ENTERITIS (QUAIL DISEASE)

Ulcerative enteritis is an acute bacterial infection of young chickens characterized by sudden onset and rapidly increasing mortality. The disease was first noticed in quail (a small game bird), and was therefore named **'quail disease'.** Since then it became known that many other species of birds, other than quail, are susceptible and therefore the earlier name was replaced by **'ulcerative enteritis' because of ulcer formation in the intestine.** Ulcerative enteritis is worldwide in distribution, and is widely prevalent in India.

Ulcerative enteritis is caused by a Gram-positive bacterium called *Clostridium colinum.* **The organism is extremely resistant to chemical agents and physical changes due to spore formation.** Ulcerative enteritis is more commonly seen in young birds. It occurs in chickens 4-12 weeks old. Outbreaks usually accompany or follow coccidiosis, chicken infectious anaemia, Gumboro disease, or stress conditions, including poor hygiene.

## Spread

Ulcerative enteritis is spread through droppings. Birds become infected by ingesting contaminated feed, water or litter. **The organism produces spores** (a resistant form of the bacterium), **which results in permanent contamination of premises** after an outbreak has occurred. Chronic carriers have been considered to be one of the most important factors in the continuance of ulcerative enteritis.

## Symptoms

**Birds may die suddenly without showing any preceding symptoms.** They are usually well muscled and fat, and have feed in the crop. As the disease progresses, infected birds become depressed, show loss of appetite, are huddled with eyes partly closed and feathers dull and ruffled. Extreme emaciation with reduction of breast muscles is seen in birds affected one week or longer. Mortality in chicken varies from 2% to as high as 12%.

## Postmortem Findings

There is severe haemorrhagic enteritis (inflammation of the intestine with blood), mainly in the duodenum. In birds which survive the infection for several days, there is necrosis (death of tissue) and ulceration (ulcer formation) in any portion of the intestine and caeca. Early lesions (changes) are small yellow foci with haemorrhagic borders. As ulcers increase in size they may merge to form a large necrotic patch. Perforation of ulcers occurs, resulting in peritonitis (inflammation of peritoneum, a membrane in the body cavity).

Liver may show large irregular yellow areas along the edges. Other lesions are yellow circular foci, sometimes surrounded by a pale yellow rim. Spleen may be congested, enlarged, and haemorrhagic. Gross changes are absent in other organs.

## Diagnosis

The postmortem findings are usually sufficient, but diagnosis should be confirmed by demonstration of the organism in the intestine, liver or spleen, by culture or by immunofluorescence. Dead liver tissue can be crushed between two slides, fixed by heat, and stained by Gram's technique. Large Gram-positive rods, with sub-terminal and free spores, can be seen. If necessary, *C. colinum* can be isolated from liver or spleen.

Ulcerative enteritis should be differentiated from coccidiosis and necrotic enteritis. Frequently, coccidiosis in chickens precedes or occurs together with ulcerative enteritis. Both diseases may be present in the same flock. It is therefore very important that a differential diagnosis between the two is made because treatment of each disease is separate.

## Treatment

Drugs that affect Gram-positive organisms are very useful and are administered in the water or feed. The most effective drugs are bacitracin or streptomycin. Bacitracin is used in the feed at a concentration of 0.005-0.01%, and streptomycin at 0.006%. Each drug can be given in the drinking water both for prevention and treatment.

## Control

1. Since the infectious **organism** is in the droppings and **remains alive indefinitely in litter,** contaminated litter on problem farms must be removed and clean litter should be used for each batch. Avoid all the predisposing causes and maintain a high standard of hygiene in management.

2. Avoid stresses caused by overcrowding, keep coccidiosis under control, and use preventive measures against those viral diseases which may act as stress factors and/or cause immunosuppression (i.e. suppression of natural immune responses).

3. Survivors of an outbreak may be carriers and should not be mixed with unexposed birds. A carrier bird is one which harbours the disease-producing organism without showing any symptoms, and is potentially capable of spreading that organism to others.

## PULLORUM DISEASE

Pullorum disease is a highly contagious, **egg-transmitted disease.** It is mainly a septicaemic disease (blood infection) of chickens. The disease is characterized by **white diarrhoea in young chicks.** It was previously known as **'bacillary white diarrhoea or BWD'**, but as white diarrhoea is not always a symptom, it became known as **'pullorum disease'**.

The disease is worldwide in distribution. It is caused by a Gram-negative, **non-motile** bacterium called ***Salmonella pullorum***. The organism can survive outside the body for many months, and for **several years** in a favourable environment. Mortality from pullorum disease is usually confined to the first 2-3 weeks of age.

## Spread

1. **The most important method of spread is from an infected hen through the eggs to the newly hatched chicks.** A significant number of birds become **adult carriers** (i.e. they carry the infection without showing any symptoms), with *S. pullorum* persisting in the ovary and being excreted in the ova **(egg transmission) (Fig. 13).** Such infected hens do not lay many eggs and only a small percentage of eggs are likely to be infected. The fertility and hatchability of infected eggs is also below average. The number of eggs infected with *S. pullorum* can be as high as 33% of the total laid by an infected hen.

2. However, viable chicks (i.e. chicks that survive) do hatch from such infected eggs and become a source of infection. Fluff (soft feathers) from such chicks is heavily contaminated with *S. pullorum*, and as it dries, the bacteria are rapidly spread through the incubator or brooder. Thus, pullorum disease is passed from hen to chick by **vertical transmission** (i.e. through ovary), and then there is lateral spread **(horizontal transmission)** from chick to chick in hatcheries and rearing units **(Fig. 13).**

3. Young chicks with the disease shed *S. pullorum* organisms through faeces. This is the major method of spread. However, in adult birds the faecal material contains few *S. pullorum* and is not a major means of spread.

4. Contaminated feed, water and litter can also be sources of *S. pullorum* infection.

5. Attendants, visitors, feed dealers and chicken buyers who move from house to house, and from farm to farm, may carry infection unless precautions are taken to disinfect footwear, hands, and clothing. Similarly, trucks, crates, and feed sacks may also be contaminated. Contaminated equipment may also be the source of infection.

6. Wild birds, animals, and flies may mechanically spread the organism.

7. Spread may also occur within a flock as a result of cannibalism (see **'cannibalism'**) of infected birds, egg eating, and through wounds on the skin. **Because of the septicaemia (blood infection), cannibalism is an important means of spread, as blood is transferred from bird to bird.**

8. Beak-trimming (debeaking) machines can be a means of transferring the bacteria from bird to bird.

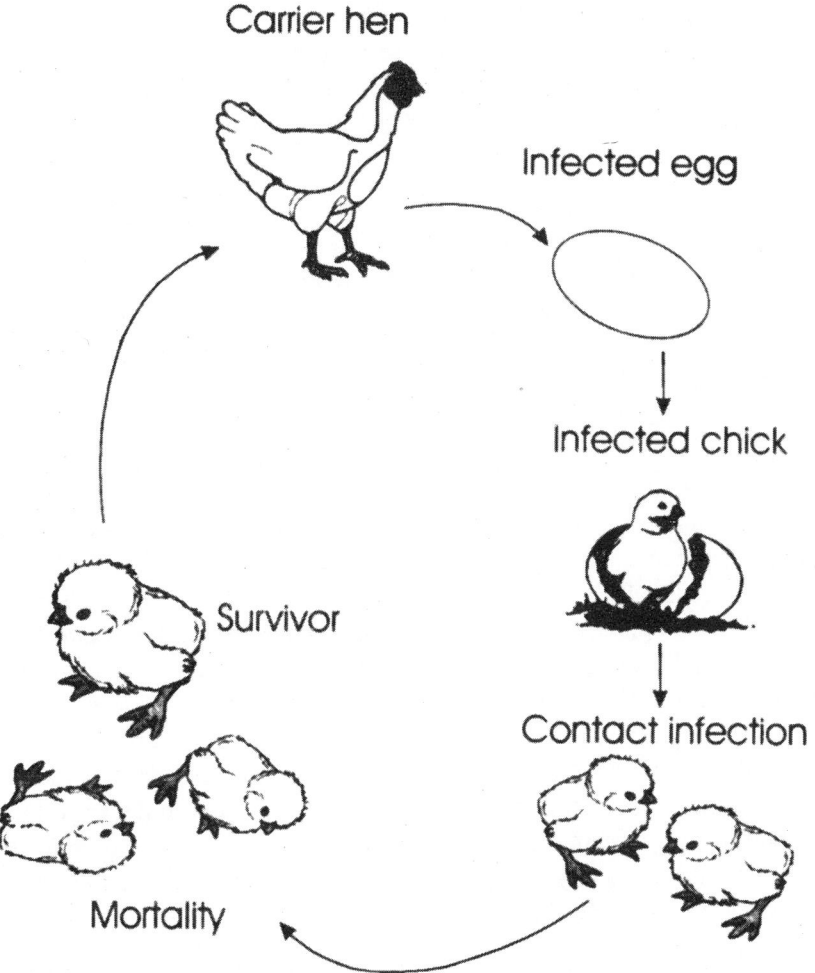

**Fig. 13. Pullorum disease.** A carrier hen (infected hen) spreads infection through the infected egg to the newly hatched chick. Some of the infected chicks may die. A proportion of those that survive become adult carriers with ***S. pullorum*** persisting in the ovaries and being excreted in the ova. Chicks which hatch from such infected eggs become a source of infection as **carriers** when they become adult, **and the cycle is repeated.**

9. Spread through shell penetration and feed contamination by *S. pullorum* has been reported, but appears to be of minor importance.

## Symptoms

**Pullorum disease is considered mainly a disease of chicks. It is seen in chicks below 3 weeks of age.** The first indication is usually a large number of dead-in-shell chicks, and deaths soon after hatching. Affected birds show different and non-specific symptoms which include depression with tendency to huddle (crowd together in a small space), respiratory distress, loss of appetite and **white viscous** (thick and sticky) **droppings** that stick to the feathers around the vent. Death may soon follow. The peak mortality usually occurs during the 2nd or 3rd week. **The mortality varies greatly and in extreme cases can be 100%.**

**In young birds,** a subacute form (less severe form) with lameness and swollen hock joints may be seen and result in poor growth rates. **Older birds** may appear depressed and have pale and shrunken combs with ruffled feathers. Low egg production may be the only symptom of the disease when adult birds are affected. Both growing and older birds may show **greenish-brown diarrhoea.** The condition is rare, however, in adult birds.

## Postmortem Findings

**Chicks** that die soon after hatching usually have peritonitis (inflammation of the peritoneum, a membrane in the body cavity) with an inflamed, unabsorbed yolk sac. The lungs may be congested and the **liver** dark and swollen with haemorrhages visible on the surface. Sometimes, in chicks that die in the acute (severe) phase of the disease, there are no specific lesions (changes) or only those of a septicaemia (blood infection) with liver congested and the blood vessels under the skin dilated and prominent. Chicks that die after showing signs of disease for 1 or 2 days may have typhlitis (inflammation of the caecum). The caeca are enlarged and distended with hard, dry, necrotic (dead) material. **Distinct, small, white, necrotic foci (area of dead tissue) are also usually found in the liver, lungs, heart and gizzard wall.** Sometimes, white nodules in lungs and heart may be most prominent. In growers affected with arthritis (inflammation of a joint), the hock joints are usually enlarged due to the excess of gelatinous material around the joints. **In general, the lesions are neither characteristic nor constant.**

**In adult birds,** the characteristic lesion is an **abnormal ovary, the ova being irregular, cystic, deformed, discoloured and pedunculated (attached) with prominent, thickened stalks.** There may also be peritonitis, arthritis and pericarditis (inflammation of the covering of heart). In some infected adult hens the ovary is inactive, the ova being small, pale and undeveloped.

## Diagnosis

1.  The symptoms and postmortem findings may vary and are not sufficiently characteristic to make a firm diagnosis. The disease is diagnosed in the chick by isolating *S. pullorum* from liver or lungs.

2.  Infection in the older birds can be detected by demonstrating *S. pullorum* antibodies in blood samples by agglutination tests. Positive serological findings are of great help in detecting infection, **but negative results are not enough for final diagnosis.** This is because antibodies take several days to appear and maximum

antibody production may not occur until 100 days **after initial infection**. Antibodies therefore may not be detected until the bird has reached immunological maturity at 16 weeks of age. Similarly, positive results should be interpreted with caution because of cross reactions with other serogroup D salmonellae such as *S. enteritidis.*

Once a bird has been infected with *S. pullorum,* antibodies specific for *S. pullorum* are present in the bloodstream. These antibodies clump with killed *S. pullorum* organisms in the test antigen. A number of tests are available to detect antibodies, but the two most commonly used are:

1. Rapid slide agglutination test performed on whole blood using a stained antigen, and

2. Tube agglutination test carried out on serum

## Rapid plate agglutination test (whole blood test, WBT)

This is a rapid test which can be used on the farm for the detection of *S. pullorum.* It is a cheap test to perform and requires little equipment. A measured drop (0.5 ml) of antigen is placed on a testing plate. Next a blood vessel (a vein) on the underside of the wing is punctured and a drop of blood is picked up by a loop of wire. The blood is then mixed with the antigen. The plate is rotated in a circular motion to facilitate mixing and clumping. If the blood contains *S. pullorum* antibodies, it will clump with the bacterial cells of the antigen creating a positive reaction. Such birds are known as **reactors**. If no antibodies are present in the blood, the mixture remains clear, and the bird is known as a **non-reactor**, i.e. is negative to the test. The simplicity of this test makes it easy to run in the field, thus getting immediate results. The reactors can then be immediately separated for further testing.

Reaction in most cases occurs immediately on mixing the blood and antigen, **and reaction is almost always completed within 30 seconds.** A doubtful reaction occurs if fine, pinpoint blue granules appear, either throughout the mixture or only at the margin. **Any reaction which occurs between 1 and 2 minutes must be considered doubtful, and all reactions which occur after 2 minutes must be taken as negative.**

**This test is excellent for flock testing.** It is quick and easy to perform. The reactor birds can be identified at one handling and do not have to be leg or wing banded. Labour is thus reduced to a minimum. **Two successive clear tests, one month apart, are necessary before a flock can be considered free of pullorum disease.** All doubtful and positive reactors should be culled from the flock.

Sometimes **non-pullorum reactors** cause problem in interpretation. A variety of bacteria possessing antigen in common with, or closely related to those of *S. pullorum* may infect birds and produce an agglutinin response. Non-pullorum reactors vary from a few birds in a flock to as high as 30-40%.

## Rapid Slide Agglutination Test

In the laboratory, the rapid slide agglutination test may be done using serum. 0.02 ml serum is mixed with 0.02 ml polyvalent crystal violet-stained antigen. The interpretation of the results is the same as for the whole blood test.

## Tube Agglutination Test

This test can be used as a confirmatory test to rapid plate agglutination test. It is also run on serum, and is carried out in the laboratory. Tube agglutination test has the advantage of being quantitative. The result is expressed as a specific dilution, and the test is a useful back-up check for the plate test.

More recently, enzyme-linked immunosorbent assay (ELISA) has been used for screening large numbers of blood samples.

## Treatment

A number of antibiotics reduce the morbidity (birds affected) and mortality. **However, no treatment is effective in the complete removal of carriers from an infected flock.**

Various sulphonamides followed by nitrofurans and several other antibiotics have been found to be effective in reducing mortality. **Furazolidone** at the concentration of 0.04% in the feed for 10 to 14 days is highly effective in preventing mortality in carriers among chicks. Furazolidone water medication has also been shown to be effective in reducing mortality in chicks infected with *S. pullorum*. Various antibiotics such as **chloramphenicol** at a concentration of 0.5% in feed for 10 days and **chlortetracycline** at 200 mg/kg level in the feed are effective in reducing mortality. None of these antibiotics, however, is totally effective in eliminating *S. pullorum*. Spraying eggs with neomycin sulphate before incubation has also been helpful in controlling pullorum disease in chicks.

## Control

1. **Control the disease by removal of carriers.** The basis of this programme is to test repeatedly the blood of breeding flocks (parents) and **remove reactors.** This must be combined with high management standards and hatching discipline. **Birds are tested between 16 weeks and time of laying.** Two successive clear tests one month apart followed by an annual clear test can be taken as evidence that a flock is pullorum free.

2. Replacement birds must be purchased only from flocks known to be free of the disease, or kept isolated until they have been tested and found to be pullorum free.

3. Eggs from pullorum-free flocks should be incubated and hatched only in hatcheries receiving eggs exclusively from clean flocks.

**To conclude,** the only requirement to control pullorum disease is to **make breeding flocks free of** *S. pullorum* and to hatch and rear their progeny under conditions that prevent direct or indirect contact with infected chickens.

# FOWL TYPHOID

Fowl typhoid is a septicaemic disease (blood infection) like pullorum disease, affecting chickens. **Although fowl typhoid is usually referred to as a disease of adult birds, it can also cause high mortality in young chicks.** Fowl typhoid can cause mortality as high as 26% in chicks during the first month. The disease is a serious poultry health problem. It is caused by a Gram-negative, **non-motile** bacterium, *Salmonella gallinarum*. Like *Salmonella pullorum* this organism can survive outside the bird's body for many months, and **for several years** in a favourable environment.

## Spread

1.  *S. gallinarum* is passed out by infected birds in the droppings. Lateral spread occurs by the ingestion of such material in contaminated food or water. *S. gallinarum* continues to exist in faeces for at least a **month** and in the infected carcasses for much longer periods.

2.  Recovered birds usually remain carriers (i.e. carry infection without showing symptoms) for long periods. Movement of such birds readily spreads the disease.

3.  **Egg transmission also occurs.** Chicks hatched from infected eggs become a source of infection. **The disease is thus passed from hen to chick through egg,** and then there is lateral spread from chick to chick in hatcheries and rearing units. The number of eggs infected with *S. gallinarum* can be as high as 33% of the total laid by an infected hen.

4.  Attendants, visitors, etc. may carry infection from one farm to another, unless proper disinfection practices are followed.

## Symptoms

Fowl typhoid **occurs usually in growing and adult chickens. In acute (severe) outbreaks,** the first symptom is an increase in mortality followed by a drop in food consumption. In the untreated flocks, mortality may run as high as 50%. If the birds are in laying, there is drop in egg production. Affected birds are depressed, stand still with ruffled feathers and their eyes closed. This is a common feature. Respiratory distress with rapid breathing can occur, but the most characteristic symptom is **a watery to mucoid (resembling mucus) yellow diarrhoea.**

In birds which do not die within 2 or 3 days of developing the above symptoms, **a chronic phase occurs.** There is a loss of condition and a severe anaemia (deficiency in blood of red cells, haemoglobin, or in total volume) which produces shrunken pale combs and wattles. If untreated, the disease spreads rapidly through the flock and can cause losses up to 50% or more.

**Subacute (less severe) outbreaks** may cause occasional mortality over a long period. **Egg transmission can occur,** and leads to an increase in dead-in-shell embryos and small, weak or dead chicks on the hatching trays.

When **young chicks** are affected, the symptoms are non-specific and similar to those seen in pullorum disease or salmonellosis. There may be weakness, unwillingness to move, a tendency to huddle (crowd together) and a drop in food consumption. Yellow, pasty droppings, which stick to the feathers around the vent, are also seen. Sometimes there is respiratory distress with rapid breathing and gasping.

## Postmortem Findings

If the birds have died in the acute phase of the disease, the carcasses have a septicaemic, jaundiced appearance. Blood vessels under the skin are congested and prominent. An important and consistent finding is that the **liver is swollen, friable (breaking easily) and has a dark red or almost black colour.** Its surface has a **characteristic coppery bronze sheen** (i.e. has a reddish-brown shine). The spleen may also be enlarged. There is enteritis (inflammation of the intestine), and intestines contain thick sticky, bile-stained material. If birds have died in the chronic phase, the carcasses are emaciated and severely anaemic with focal necrosis (areas of dead tissue) in the heart, intestines, pancreas, and liver. Pericarditis (inflammation of pericardium, a covering of the heart) with turbid yellow fluid in the pericardial sac and fibrin attached to the surface of the heart is a feature of chronic fowl typhoid.

In young chicks, additional findings may be distinct necrotic foci in the lungs and gizzard. The egg yolk is usually unabsorbed. In laying birds there may be retained yolks which may later rupture.

## Diagnosis

**The symptoms and postmortem findings are not specific to make a firm diagnosis.** The disease is diagnosed by isolating *S. gallinarum* from liver or spleen. The organism grows readily on most laboratory media and may be identified both bacteriologically and serologically. Agglutination tests may be used to determine if adult birds are carriers.

## Treatment

Treatment with antibiotics will reduce symptoms and mortality. **Furazolidone** continuously in the feed for 10 days, at a level of 0.04%, is usually considered to be the best treatment. Recently enrofloxacin has been used. Such treatment, however, does not remove *S. gallinarum* infection completely, **and infected carrier birds** (i.e. birds that carry infection without showing symptoms) **remain even after treatment.** Re-infection of susceptible birds with the development of disease may also occur, and the disease may recycle in the flock. Therefore, treatment should be accompanied by culling (removal) of chronically affected birds and reactors to a blood test. Moreover, all the affected birds should be properly removed and burnt.

## Control

1.  Systematic blood testing of breeding flocks for *S. pullorum* infection with removal of reactors is the main reason why fowl typhoid has been virtually eradicated. *S. gallinarum* has the same antigenic structure as *S. pullorum*. **Therefore, the whole blood or rapid plate agglutination test using standard *S. pullorum* antigen can be used to detect carriers of *S. gallinarum*.** Positive birds can then be removed from the flock. The blood test thus supports treatment and vaccination programme.

2.  If an early diagnosis of fowl typhoid is made, treatment with furazolidone or other suitable antibiotic, followed by vaccination after the effect of the drug is gone, is a useful control procedure.

3.  **Vaccination with fowl typhoid vaccine usually gives solid, long-lasting immunity.** Vaccine reduces mortality in infected flocks. It does not reduce egg production when used in flocks free of the disease. However, vaccine must be used with caution since vaccinated birds can carry and excrete the rough strain of *S. gallinarum* for long periods, **and it can also be transmitted through the eggs laid by vaccinated birds.**

4.  The only requirement to control fowl typhoid is to **create breeding flocks free of *S. gallinarum*,** and to hatch and rear their progeny under conditions that prevent direct or indirect contact with infected chickens.

**Note:** For a list of commercially available vaccines against fowl typhoid, refer to Chapter 19 under **"Fowl typhoid vaccines".**

## Paratyphoid Infections

Besides *S. pullorum* and *S. gallinarum,* there are many other salmonellae that affect poultry. These have been called as **'paratyphoids'.** Important ones are *S. enteritidis* and *S. typhimurium.* Most paratyphoid bacteria do not cause much disease in chicken, **except for young chicks.** Many can infect humans, particularly the young and old, or those weakened by chronic or immunosuppressive disease. **It is the human infection that is of greatest significance. Some food-borne illnesses in humans have been traced to Salmonella infection.** Therefore, poultry industry must take extreme measures of sanitation in poultry and egg processing plants.

**'Paratyphoid infections'** or **'salmonellosis'** in poultry are bacterial infections caused by motile salmonellae ('salmonellae' is plural of 'salmonella' organisms), the most common species being **S. enteritidis** and **S. typhimurium. S. pullorum** which causes pullorum disease and **S. gallinarum** which causes fowl typhoid (already discussed earlier) are also salmonella organisms, but both of them are **non-motile.**

Salmonella organisms are found virtually in every part of the world, and salmonellosis in chickens is a serious problem in India. Salmonella organisms are Gram-negative. **They are quite stable in the environment, and most can live in water and feed for weeks.**

## Sources of Infection

Once salmonella becomes established in a primary **breeding flock**, it can infect poultry in other units through hatcheries by both **vertical (egg transmission) and lateral spread.** It is therefore important to know how infection can be introduced into a salmonella-free breeding flock.

If a **breeding flock** is infected with salmonella, **a cycle is established.** The organism passes through the egg to the progeny, and even to chicks hatched from eggs laid by infected progeny. This cycle can occur by transmission through ovaries, as is the case in pullorum disease and **S. enteritidis.**

However, **spread through faecal contamination of the surface of the egg is more common.** As the egg passes through the cloaca, salmonella in faeces attach themselves to the warm wet surface of the shell and are drawn inside as it cools. **Being motile salmonella, S. enteritidis penetrates easily.** Penetration of the shell occurs more quickly if the eggs are stored above room temperature. When the chicks from infected eggs hatch, there is lateral spread to contact chicks in hatcheries and brooding and rearing units. Salmonellae are thus commonly introduced into a unit with purchased poultry, and can also be introduced into a country with importation of live poultry, or hatching eggs.

## Disease

Paratyphoid salmonellae infections have very different effects on newly hatched chicks and on more mature birds. In very susceptible **young chicks,** paratyphoid infection can sometimes cause **serious illness and death.** Older birds are much less susceptible to the harmful effects. They may have growth in the intestine, and even systemic spread, without significant morbidity (number of birds affected) and mortality (deaths caused).

Environmental and management factors influence the susceptibility of poultry to paratyphoid salmonellae. **Exposure to stressful conditions facilitates salmonella infection.** For example, lowering the brooding temperature of chicks by $5^0$ to $8^0$C increases significantly mortality among newly hatched chicks.

## Spread

1. **Paratyphoid salmonellae can be introduced into poultry flocks from many**

**different sources.** Humans, rodents (rats, mice), insects, water and feed can all introduce infection into a poultry unit. The most common sources are **contaminated feed** and various animal and insect vectors (i.e. transmitters).

**Staff on a poultry farm can carry salmonellae mechanically from one unit to another on contaminated footwear (shoes, 'chappals' etc.), clothing, and hands.** Humans may also be salmonella excreters and infect poultry in their charge. For these reasons visitors to poultry farms should be restricted to those on very important business. Moreover, adequate protective clothing should be provided to them and hygienic procedures strictly followed.

2.  Salmonellae can be **transmitted vertically (egg transmission)** from infected breeder flocks to the progeny and **horizontally (lateral spread)** within and between flocks. Salmonellae can spread from unit to unit from movement of vehicles, equipment and utensils, including hatchery egg trays and trolleys contaminated with the organism.

3.  **Vertical spread (egg transmission)** of paratyphoid salmonellae to progeny of infected breeder flocks can occur from the production of eggs contaminated by salmonellae in the contents, or on the surface.

**Eggshells are usually contaminated with paratyphoid salmonellae by faecal contamination during egg laying.** The paratyphoid organisms are found in great numbers in the intestinal tract. When the egg is laid, these organisms are drawn in through the shell pores (i.e. small openings on the eggshell). **Contaminated litter or nesting material is a major source of the organism on the eggshell.** The penetration of salmonellae into the shell can result in direct spread of infection to the developing chick. Also, it can lead to exposure of the chick to organisms when the shell is broken during hatching. Some salmonellae, particularly *S. enteritidis,* can be deposited in the contents of eggs before laying. The resulting **transovarian transmission (i.e. spread through the ovary)** of infection to progeny is an important aspect in the occurrence of *S. enteritidis* in chickens.

**Regardless of the mechanism,** any salmonella carried in or on eggs can be spread extensively in the hatchery. As chicks pip through (i.e. break through) the eggshells, salmonellae are released into the air and circulated around hatching cabinets on contaminated soft feathers (fluff) and other hatching material. **Newly hatched chicks lacking protective bacteria in the intestine, are highly susceptible to infection.** After introduction into poultry, salmonellae can **spread horizontally (laterally)** within and between flocks. Organisms can spread rapidly from infected day-old chicks to others reared on litters. Contaminated poultry house environments are the main sources of salmonellae. Lateral spread occurs by direct bird-to-bird contact, contaminated water, people and equipment, and a variety of other mechanisms.

4.  **Contaminated feedstuffs** are a common and important source by which a poultry flock becomes infected with salmonellae. Animal proteins included in the ration in the form of **fish meal,** meat meal and bone meal, and poultry offal (wastes) have been found to be frequently contaminated with salmonellae. Similarly, vegetable protein may become contaminated either before or during processing.

5.  **Domestic flies and beetles** are both capable of transmitting salmonellae, and infection can persist through the contamination of their eggs and larvae. Insects, including cockroaches and mealworms (larvae of various beetles), can carry salmonellae and spread them throughout poultry houses.

6.  **Rats and mice** are an important source of salmonella. Also, they are attracted to the poultry houses by the plenty of easily available food. Mice have been shown to be vectors (transmitters) of *S. enteritidis*. They become infected during the life of a flock, move outside the house after disposal of the flock, then re-enter and infect the next crop of chickens.

7.  **Water** can also be source of salmonella. Care should be taken to ensure that storage and header tanks do not become contaminated by wild birds, rats, and mice. Chlorination may be desirable.

8.  **Wild birds** are not only infected with salmonella, but can also mechanically carry material contaminated with bacteria on their feet. Although environmentally-controlled houses are bird-proof, poultry kept on free range could come into direct contact with wild birds and contaminated equipment.

9.  **Heat treatment of poultry feed in the pelleting process may remove the organism,** but in many cases insufficient temperatures and conditioning times only reduce the number of organisms. Treatment of feed with chemicals, such as formic or propionic acid, or fumigating with formaldehyde or methyl bromide has been shown to reduce the level of salmonellae in feed.

## Symptoms

**Disease caused by salmonella is usually seen in chicks below 2 weeks of age, and rarely in birds over 4 weeks of age.** The morbidity and mortality vary greatly, and deaths are usually less than 20% of the affected group, but in exceptional cases can reach 100%. The symptoms are not specific, and are similar whichever type of salmonella is involved.

Affected birds are depressed and unwilling to move. They stand with their eyes closed and with ruffled feathers and drooping (falling) wings. Profuse watery diarrhoea is usually seen, often resulting in dehydration and pasting of the feathers around vent area. Loss of appetite and emaciation are common. Affected birds are usually seen to shiver (tremble) and huddle (crowd together) near heat sources. Blindness and lameness have sometimes been associated with paratyphoid infections.

## Postmortem Findings

These vary greatly, from the complete absence of any visible changes to that of lungs, liver, spleen and kidneys being swollen and congested. When baby chicks are affected an inflamed, unabsorbed yolk sac is a common finding. Distinct necrotic lesions (i.e. white areas of dead tissue) in the lungs, liver and heart; peritonitis (inflammation of peritoneum, a membrane in the body cavity); and haemorrhagic enteritis (inflammation of the intestine with blood) may be seen in birds that do not die suddenly in the acute phase of the disease.

The most characteristic postmortem finding, seen in about one-third of birds dying of salmonellosis, is **typhlitis** (inflammation of the caecum). **The caeca are distended by hard white masses of dead tissues.** In broilers with salmonellosis due to *S. enteritidis,* there are usually gross postmortem findings of septicaemia (blood infection), pericarditis (inflammation of pericardium covering the heart) and perihepatitis (inflammation of the liver surface). The pericardial sac is distended with a great quantity of turbid fluid containing large masses of salmonellae.

## Diagnosis

1.  Confirmation of the diagnosis requires isolation and identification of the causative organism. Salmonellae are readily isolated from infected tissues by direct culture. Thus, in chicks dying of septicaemia (blood infection), direct isolation can be made from the liver, gallbladder, or yolk sac. In older chicks salmonellae are usually confined to the intestine, with the **caeca being the best site for isolation.**

2.  While identifying infection in large populations, it must be kept in mind that the frequency of infection may be very low. Therefore, methods have been developed to collect samples from the environment as an indirect indication of flock infection. These methods include samples from the floor litter, accumulated dust, and nest. It is also important to take samples for bacteriological culture after cleaning and disinfection following disposal of birds, and to confirm that mice are not acting as a reservoir of infection on the site.

3.  The value of serological tests for diagnosis depends to some extent on the salmonella serotype involved. *Salmonella pullorum* and *S. gallinarum* do not grow in (colonize) the digestive tract, but infect the rest of the bird's body. This stimulates the production of antibodies which can be detected by serological tests. Other salmonella serotypes grow in the digestive tract, but do not enter into the tissues, and therefore may not stimulate the production of antibodies.

## Serological Diagnosis

1.  A number of serological tests have been developed for the diagnosis of salmonella infections in poultry. The **whole blood test (WBT)** and the **serum agglutination**

test (SAT) have been used successfully for more than 50 years for the identification of flocks infected with *S. pullorum* and *S. gallinarum* (see '**pullorum disease**' and '**fowl typhoid**'). Because *S. enteritidis* possesses the same group antigen as *S. pullorum*, the whole blood test and related tests can be used for the diagnosis of infection. In recent years other tests, such as the enzyme-linked immunosorbent assay (ELISA) have been developed for the identification of *S. enteritidis*-infected flocks and are now in use.

2.    Serological methods should be used to identify infected flocks rather than to identify the infected individual birds, and bacteriological confirmation should always be obtained. This is because some poultry with a positive serological reaction may not be infected with salmonella organisms. Similarly, poultry which are actively excreting salmonellae in the early stages of infection may be serologically negative.

3.    If immunization is used to control salmonella infections in the flock, it is necessary to differentiate the vaccine response from that of actual infection.

4.    Newly hatched chicks are immunologically immature and do not respond serologically to salmonella (antigen) until 2-3 weeks of age. Chicks may, however, acquire salmonella antibodies passively from their parents through the yolk, which may indicate an infected parent flock. Egg yolk may also be tested for antibodies to salmonella, and eggs may provide a method to screen laying flocks.

## Treatment

A number of antibiotics are useful in reducing morbidity and mortality within a flock. The more commonly used drugs include furazolidone, spectinomycin, ampicillin, tetracyclines, and more recently enrofloxacin. None, however, is capable of removing infection in a flock. Chicks are sometimes treated with antibiotics for prevention of infection after hatching. They are given an antibiotic in their feed and water for one to two weeks to minimize possible morbidity and mortality.

If it is decided to treat an outbreak of salmonellosis, it is better to check the sensitivity of the organism involved by laboratory tests.

Although treatment may appear to be effective, a number of birds may become carriers and antibiotic-resistant strains of salmonella might appear.

## Monitoring for Salmonella

1.    Monitoring, either by culture or serology, should be carried out at all stages of the production cycle.

2.    **At the hatchery**, the inner surfaces of the hatchers and broken eggshells from the hatcher trays should be cultured every two weeks. Other samples such as meconium (first faeces of a newly hatched chick) and surface swabs from different parts of

the hatchery and dead-in-shells are also helpful in checking for the presence of salmonellae as well as the effectiveness of routine hygiene measures.

3. **At the rearing site** the presence of salmonellae can be checked by culture of chick box liners (i.e. material that lines boxes) or swabs from the bottom of the boxes, and chicks dead on arrival and those culled or dying within a few days of arrival. During the rearing period litter samples and dust from various sites, for example, exhaust fans, provide the most convenient method of monitoring. When the breeders are in laying, the most reliable samples are nest box floor swabs, nest box litter, and dust from egg sorting tables and carriers. **For grandparents, more frequent sampling is desirable.**

4. **After disposal of the birds,** and when cleaning and disinfection have been completed, buildings should be checked for the persistence of salmonellae. Samples should include drag swabs of earth floor surfaces or floor sweepings from concrete floors, nest box floors, feed hoppers, beams and pipes, and electric fittings. In laying flocks, additional samples include sweepings or swabs of the egg store area, egg sorting table, egg handling room floor and, if rodents (rats, mice) are numerous, these should be trapped and examined.

## Cycle of Infection

When poultry over 4 weeks of age are infected with salmonella the organisms may grow in the intestine, but almost all such chickens become free of infection within 60 days. However, a small percentage of infected birds excrete salmonellae either continuously or intermittently for long periods. Stress, such as onset of laying, may also reactivate infection and excretion. Although most of the infected birds carry salmonellae for only short periods, the conditions in intensive poultry units allow infection to recycle from bird to bird. The period of salmonella excretion by an infected bird may also be extended by antibiotic treatment.

## Control

**Effective control requires that breeding stock is free of salmonella infection to prevent vertical transmission through the egg to progeny.** Exposure must be prevented in the hatchery and throughout the life of the flock by **high standards of management and flock security.**

## 1. Hatching Egg Hygiene

Preventing spread of salmonella from infected parents in the hatchery to chicks, following contamination of the outside of the eggshell, is an important factor in control. Eggs from flocks infected with the paratyphoid salmonellae are usually sterile (free from organisms) when laid. **Contamination occurs in the nest box from contact with faeces.** Therefore, strict attention should be given to management of nest boxes.

151

Adequate clean, dry litter should always be available and regularly changed. Use of an appropriate disinfectant is very helpful.

**Eggs should be collected as frequently as possible and never less than three times each day.** Cracked, dirty, and floor eggs should not be used for hatching and should be kept separate from clean eggs. Lightly soiled eggs can be washed in bactericidal (i.e. solution that will kill bacteria) used at the concentration and temperature recommended by the manufacturer. **All eggs used for hatching should be disinfected on the farm as soon as possible after collection and cleaning.** Dipping the eggs in 0.5% glutaraldehyde solution at $40^0$ C for 3 minutes, or fumigation with formaldehyde gas for 20 minutes, are both effective methods of egg disinfection. The eggs should then be stored and transported correctly. They should be kept in a clean, dry vermin-proof (i.e. proof against rats, mice, insects, etc.) area at a temperature of between $13^0$ C and 75% relative humidity. They should be packed firmly and correctly in suitable containers to prevent damage during transit to the hatchery.

## 2. The Hatchery

Salmonellae are introduced into a hatchery by incubation of unidentified infected eggs. However, it is difficult to prevent this because infection of supply flocks is not normally identified before infected eggs are produced. **Control of salmonella spread within, and from the hatchery, is of the utmost importance.** A code of effective hatching hygiene practice should be designed for each premise. A good programme of general hygiene control within a hatchery has a beneficial effect on chick quality and salmonella control, although visible clean surfaces may still harbour salmonella.

## 3. Biosecurity

As already stated, salmonella organisms can spread from unit to unit through movement of vehicles, equipment and utensils, including hatchery egg trays and trolleys contaminated with organisms. Control of salmonella from such sources can be achieved only by maintaining a **high standard of management** and implementing a **good biosecurity programme** (see 'biosecurity'). Houses should be thoroughly cleaned and disinfected between flocks, and fresh clean litter used. The disinfectant should be product which has a high activity against salmonella and applied thoroughly at an effective application rate.

## 4. Cleaning and Disinfection

Complete and effective cleaning and disinfection are very important to prevent any carrying over of salmonella organisms to the new flock. After a poultry building falls vacant following disposal of birds, all manure should be removed and the building must be cleaned and disinfected with an approved disinfectant. If the flock being disposed of is suspected or known to be salmonella positive, it is important to carry out an effective terminal disinfection.

5.    Strict attention should be given to control and, if possible, removal of **rats and mice** (which **are known sources of salmonella**) from poultry houses.

## 6. Competitive Exclusion

Competitive exclusion is the term used for the activity of normal intestinal bacteria. These normal bacteria restrict the growth (colonization) of disease-producing bacteria that cause infection of the intestine; including salmonella (see **'competitive exclusion'** under **'probiotics'**). In poultry farming, birds are usually reared in an environment which prevents the entry of those bacteria that are necessary for protection. **If chicks are provided with these useful bacteria, good protection occurs within 32 hours which effectively restricts the prevalence of salmonella infection within a flock.** Competitive exclusion works against heavy continuous environmental exposure and usually prevents infection when low levels of salmonella are present. This is because the protective bacteria either compete with salmonella for intestinal receptor sites, or produce substances that inhibit salmonella growth (see **'probiotics'**).

## 7. Vaccination

A variety of vaccines are being developed and some are now commercially available abroad for the control of *S. enteritidis* infection.

## FOWL CHOLERA

Fowl cholera is a septicaemic disease (blood infection) of chickens. It is caused by a Gram-negative bacterium, *Pasteurella multocida*. In its severest form (peracute form) fowl cholera is one of the most harmful (virulent) and highly contagious diseases, inflicting high morbidity (birds affected) and mortality (deaths caused), but chronic (less severe) and harmless conditions also commonly occur. The disease is worldwide in distribution.

Strains of *P. multocida* vary in their disease-producing power (virulence). Some are most harmful, others moderately so, and a certain number harmless. Outside the body of the bird the organisms are very susceptible to drying and disinfectants. *P. multocida* is easily destroyed by ordinary disinfectants, such as 1% solution of formaldehyde, phenol, or sodium hydroxide. Sunlight, drying, or heat, kill the organism within 15 minutes at $56^0$ C and 10 minutes at $60^0$ C.

Losses from fowl cholera usually occur in laying flocks, because bird at this age is more susceptible than younger chickens. **Chickens less than 16 weeks of age are usually quite resistant.** Mortality often ranges from 0 to 2%, but greater losses have been reported. Reduced egg production and persistent localized infection usually occur. Chickens are more susceptible to fowl cholera after withdrawal of feed and water, or after sudden change of diet.

The immune status of the bird may give protection against the strain of the organism with which they have previously had contact, **but they are often susceptible to other**

153

**strains.** Therefore, it is advisable to use an **autogenous** vaccine (i.e. a vaccine derived from the affected flock), if possible.

## Spread

1.  Sources of infection include carrier birds (i.e. survivors of a natural outbreak), clinically diseased chickens and their excretions, and carcasses of birds which have died from the infection. Many healthy birds harbour the organism in their nasal or upper respiratory passage. It is believed that survivors of an outbreak become the reservoir of infection as healthy nasal carriers. That is, **recovered birds become chronic carriers.** Carrier birds among the older flocks, kept for more than two years, provide a reservoir of infection for young susceptible growers housed with them. **The organism enters the body through the respiratory or digestive tract.**

2.  Spread of *P. multocida* within a flock is mainly by excretions by the mouth, nose, and conjunctiva of diseased birds. These excretions contaminate their environment, **particularly feed and water.** Thus, spread can be through contaminated feed and water. Faeces very rarely contain viable (live) *P. multocida.*

3.  Airborne spread of infection does occur between pens, but **spread through water and feed troughs is more important.**

4.  The disease is **not known to be egg-transmitted.**

5.  Contaminated crates, feed bags, or any equipment used previously for poultry, introduce fowl cholera into a flock. Spread can also be by people, their clothing and footwear. Ulcerated wattles are a source of infection. Organisms are spread by the carcasses of birds that die of acute fowl cholera. They serve as a source of infection, especially because chickens tend to consume such carcasses.

6.  **Free-flying birds** having contact with poultry may be a source of fowl cholera organisms. Sparrow and pigeons carry organisms without showing symptoms. A healthy bird pecking at a contaminated bird may be a means of spreading the disease through blood or nasal exudate (discharge).

7.  **Rats** are also reservoir for *P. multocida,* and may also transmit fowl cholera.

Disease tends to recur on the same site. **Poultry may be infected through oral (mouth), nasal (respiratory) and conjunctival (eye) routes and through wounds.** *P. multocida* usually enters tissues of birds through mucous membranes of the pharynx or upper air passages, but it may also enter through the conjunctiva or skin wounds.

## Symptoms

**The disease occurs in several forms.** These include peracute (severest), acute (severe), chronic (less severe), and localized. In the **peracute form**, there may be no preceding symptoms and a large number of birds in the flock are found dead, in good bodily condition. 50% or more of the birds may die. **Birds between 12 and 18 weeks of age seem very susceptible.** In the **acute form,** marked depression, loss of appetite, mucus discharges from the orifices (openings), ruffled feathers, cyanosis (bluish discoloration) in comb and wattles, and foul-smelling diarrhoea may be seen. Droppings in **diarrhoea** are first watery and whitish in colour, but later become **greenish** and contain mucus. Birds that survive the initial acute septicaemic stage may later die from weakness and dehydration, may become chronically infected, or may recover.

The **chronic form** is seen in birds which survive the more acute disease. Or, it may occur from infection with an organism having low disease-producing power. Symptoms are usually related to localized infection. The symptoms include depression, difficult breathing, and sometimes later in the infection, lameness, torticollis (twisting of the neck to one side), and **swelling of the wattles, particularly in male birds.** Chronically infected birds may die, remain infected for long periods, or recover.

## Postmortem Findings

Postmortem findings in the peracute and acute forms include marked congestion of the carcass, numerous pinpoint haemorrhages throughout the internal organs and multiple pinpoint necrotic foci (areas of dead tissue) in the liver. The **liver** may be enlarged, and may also show **very small haemorrhages** on the surface. In laying hens free yolk may be present in the abdominal cavity. In the less severe disease, oedema of the lungs (i.e. accumulation of fluid), pneumonia (inflammation of lungs), and perihepatitis (inflammation of liver on its surface) are seen. Chronic lesions include caseous (cheesy) arthritis (inflammation) of the hock and foot joints, and swelling with hardening of one or both wattles.

## Diagnosis

The history of the disease, symptoms and postmortem findings are helpful, but all forms of the disease can be confused with other infections. Demonstration of *P. multocida* confirms the diagnosis. In the peracute form impression smears of the liver or smears of the heart blood will show **bipolar organisms** when stained with methylene blue. In the pneumonic form smears from the lungs may be helpful.

*P. multocida* can be isolated readily from internal organs of birds that die of acute fowl cholera, and usually from lesions of chronic cases. Bone marrow, heart blood, liver, or localized lesions are preferred for culturing, isolation, and identification.

## Treatment

Peracute cholera is so rapid that treatment is rarely of value. In the less acute form a number of drugs have proved to be effective. They include sulphonamides and antibiotics. Sulphonamides used are sulphamethazine, sodium sulphamethazine, sulphadimethoxine, sulphaquinoxaline, and sulphaethoxypyridazine. The main disadvantage of the sulphanomides is that they only inhibit the growth of bacteria (are bacteriostatic) and do not kill them (are not bactericidal). Moreover, they are unable to cure localized abscesses and have a toxic effect on birds. **Extreme care should be taken when treating with sulphonamides as birds may be forced out of egg production, and under certain conditions mortality may occur from kidney damage.**

In antibiotics, penicillin, streptomycin, oxytetracycline, chlortetracycline, and erythromycin have been used successfully. Tetracyclines may be given in feed, in water, or by injection. In some outbreaks treatment for 7-10 days may be followed by a longer period during which drugs are given at a lower dosage. Along with the medication, the use of sodium salicylate in the drinking water for 3 days appears to help in recovery.

Although the treatment may bring the disease under control and reduce mortality, relapses are frequent once the drug is withdrawn.

## Control

1.  To control infection at farms, it is necessary to dispose of all birds and clean and disinfect the buildings thoroughly. Also, control vermin (rodents, insects, wild birds, etc.). **Good management practices** with emphasis on **sanitation** are the best means of preventing fowl cholera. **Dead birds should be picked up frequently to reduce spread.**

2.  Fowl cholera is not a disease of hatchery. Infection occurs after birds are in the hands of the farmers, and care must be taken of the many ways by which infection is introduced into a flock.

3.  The main source of infection is the sick bird, or those that have recovered and still carry the organism. Only young birds should be introduced as new stock. They should be raised in a clean environment completely isolated from other birds. Isolation should also be practised in housing. Separate houses should be provided for first year and second year flocks.

4.  If an outbreak of fowl cholera occurs, the flock should be disposed of as soon as economically suitable. All houses and equipment should be cleaned and disinfected before bringing other batch.

5.  Housing chickens in cages appears to reduce the chances of infection with *P. multocida.*

6.  **Vaccination** should be considered in areas where fowl cholera is prevalent, but it **should not be substituted for good sanitary practice.** Vaccination using a variety of strains of live or killed organisms is used. Commonly produced bacterins (killed vaccines) and live vaccines are available. **But better protection is obtained with autogenous vaccines** (i.e. vaccines prepared from bacteria obtained from

the affected flock) **of killed organisms.**

**Note:** For a list of commercial vaccines available in the market against fowl cholera, see Chapter 19 under **"Fowl cholera vaccines".**

# STAPHYLOCOCCOSIS

Staphylococcosis is caused by the bacterium, *Staphylococcus aureus. S. aureus* infections are common in poultry, the most common sites being bones, tendon sheaths and joints of the legs. **A wide variety of conditions** are associated with disease-producing strains of *S. aureus.* These include arthritis (inflammation of a joint) and tenosynovitis (inflammation of a tendon and its sheath), gangrenous dermatitis, yolk sac infection, subdermal abscesses (bumble foot), spondylitis (inflammation of a vertebra), osteomyelitis (inflammation of the bone and marrow), staphylococcal septicaemia (i.e. blood infection) usually with endocarditis (inflammation of the internal lining of the heart), and granuloma (small nodules) on the liver, spleen and other organs.

Although there are about 20 different species of staphylococci, *S. aureus* **is the only species which produces disease in poultry.** *S. aureus* is a Gram-positive, and is usually found on the skin, in the nares (the pair of openings on the nose), on the beak and on the feet of **normal chickens,** as well as in the air of poultry houses. *S. aureus* produces a number of toxins and enzymes which influence its disease-producing power. These include **hyaluronidase (spreading factor), deoxyribonuclease, fibrinolysin, protease, haemolysins, lipase, leukocidin, dermonecrotic toxin** (causes death of skin), **exfoliative toxin,** and **enterotoxins.**

Most staphylococci are considered as normal flora. They help in suppressing the disease-producing organisms through interference or **competitive exclusion** (see **'competitive exclusion').** Some have the ability to cause damage and produce disease if allowed entry through the skin or mucous membranes (i.e. linings of the respiratory, digestive and urinary tracts).

**Staphylococci are extremely tough.** The organism can survive away from the bird **for many months,** particularly under dry conditions and in pus. Some strains are heat and disinfectant resistant.

## Spread

1. **For infection to occur, injury to the skin or mucous membranes is essential.** In most cases, this involves a skin wound or inflamed mucous membrane, as in pecking and in fowl pox. *S. aureus* enters through the broken barrier and travels to internal locations where a focus of infection (e.g. osteomyelitis, i.e. inflammation of bone marrow) is established. In newly hatched chicks, the open navel provides a route of entry leading to omphalitis (inflammation of navel) and other types of infection. Minor surgical procedures (e.g. trimming of beak, toes, or comb) and

administration of vaccines through injections may provide additional means of entry for staphylococci.

2.  Another type of damage to bird's defence occurs following Gumboro disease, chicken infectious anaemia, or possibly Marek's disease virus infection. In these diseases, the bursa of Fabricius or thymus is injured and the immune system is functionally handicapped. Under these circumstances, septicaemic staphylococcal infection (i.e. blood infection) can occur and cause sudden death. Gangrenous dermatitis caused by *S. aureus*, along with *Clostridium septicum*, can be seen following early Gumboro disease virus infection (see **'gangrenous dermatitis'**).

3.  Environmental stress, and accompanying or earlier infections with other disease-producing organisms, may result in lowered resistance to this organism. For example, infection with reovirus may predispose to tenosynovitis in which staphylococci are involved.

## Disease

### Arthritis and Tenosynovitis

**'Arthritis'** is inflammation of a joint, and **'tenosynovitis'** inflammation of a tendon and its sheath (covering). A tendon is that portion by which a muscle attaches itself to a bone. **In broiler breeders** stress caused by an uneven feed distribution or coccidiosis, may predispose to an increase in cases of staphylococcal infections.

The affected joints, usually the hocks, are hot, swollen and painful and affected birds are usually depressed, lame, and unwilling to walk. When the phalangeal joints (joints of fingers or toes in feet) are affected, staphylococcal abscesses may occur under the skin in the sole of the feet. The condition is called **'bumble foot'**. There is some necrosis (death of tissue) and the exudate (inflammatory material) may later become caseous (i.e. like cheese). If the bird survives, the condition becomes chronic with the formation of fibrous tissue.

### Gangrenous Dermatitis

This occurs in birds of all ages, but is most common in broiler chickens. The wing tips and the dorsal pelvic region are the sites most frequently affected. The affected sites are dark, moist and gangrenous (decaying) in appearance with crepitation (a crackling sound). Staphylococci are usually associated with *C. perfringens* **type A** which may be the main disease-producing organism. Immunosuppression (suppression of the natural immune responses) from damage to the bursa of Fabricius may predispose to gangrenous dermatitis in young growing chickens (see **'gangrenous dermatitis'** given at some other place).

## Yolk Sac Infection

See 'yolk sac infection' under 'colibacillosis'.

## Subdermal Abscesses

'Subdermal abscesses' are the abscesses which occur under the skin. They usually affect the feet (bumble foot) and sternal bursa (a small pouch or sac on sternum) and usually occur in mature birds, particularly those of the heavy breeds. There is abscess formation with swelling, heat and usually some pain. This leads to lameness. In bumble foot, the under-surface of the foot is first affected, and the lesion (change) may then spread to involve the whole foot. There is caseous (cheesy) and necrotic (dead) tissue and some haemorrhage (bleeding). The sternal bursa may be similarly affected, but less commonly and less severely.

## Spondylitis and Osteomyelitis

'Spondylitis' is inflammation of one or more vertebrae, and 'osteomyelitis' infection of the bone and bone marrow. *S. aureus* can cause abscesses in the bodies of the fifth to seventh thoracic vertebrae with inflammation of the fibrous membrane covering the vertebrae (periostitis) and of the bone marrow (osteomyelitis). The resulting pressure on the spinal cord may cause paresis (slight paralysis) or paralysis. The head of the femur and sometimes other bones may also be affected with inflammation of the bone marrow (osteomyelitis). The femur head usually separates from the shaft by a fracture through the neck when hip joint is disarticulated ('femoral head necrosis'). Affected joints are swollen and filled with inflammatory exudate (material).

## Staphylococcal Septicaemia, Endocarditis and Granuloma

'Staphylococcal septicaemia' is invasion of the blood by staphylococci. It usually occurs from a primary local staphylococcal focus. That is, from a local seat of infection. It is relatively rare and may result in sudden death with marked congestion of the carcass. Or, first there may be depression and appearance of haemorrhages and necrotic foci (areas of dead tissue) in the liver (Fig. 14), lungs, kidneys, spleen, and heart. **Staphylococcal septicaemia causing sudden deaths in laying birds is prevalent in hot weather and resembles fowl cholera.** In chronic cases, these foci may develop into granulomas (small nodules) with loss of weight. Endocarditis (inflammation of the internal lining of heart) may also be a sequel and vegetations (abnormal growths), particularly affecting the valve between left atrium and left ventricle of the heart (see 'avian heart'), are seen at postmortem.

## Symptoms

Early symptoms include ruffled feathers, limping on one leg, drooping (hanging downwards) of one or both wings, and fever. This may be followed by severe depression

159

and death. Birds surviving the acute disease have swollen joints, sit on their hocks and keel bones, and are unwilling or unable to stand. Signs of septicaemic staphylococcal infection and gangrenous dermatitis occur in birds in good condition, and may become noticeable only because of increased mortality in the flock.

Following mild injury, gangrenous dermatitis lesions develop on the wing tips of birds infected with chicken infectious anaemia virus. This condition has been called **'blue-wing disease'** (see **'chicken infectious anaemia'** and **'blue-wing disease'**).

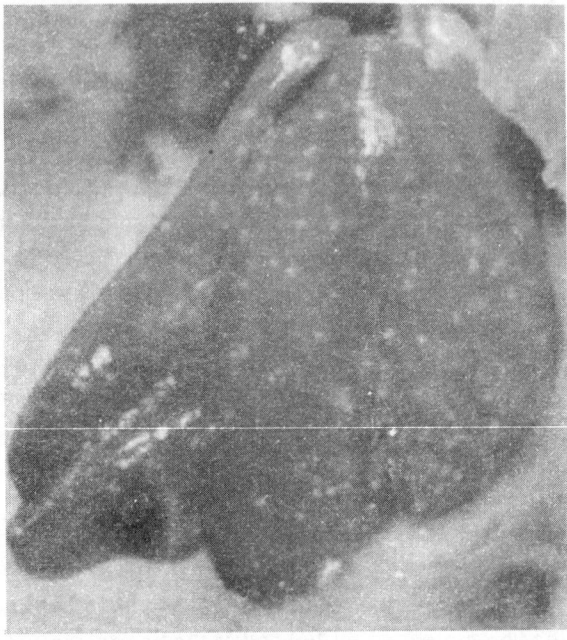

**Fig. 14.** Multiple areas of dead tissue (white foci) in the liver of a layer chicken following blood infection with staphylococci.

## Diagnosis

The history, symptoms, if any, and postmortem findings may be helpful, but as other organisms, such as *E. coli, Salmonella gallinarum, Pasteurella multocida, Mycoplasma synoviae* and reoviruses may cause some of these disease conditions, it is necessary to isolate and identify *S. aureus* to confirm diagnosis.

## Treatment

*S. aureus* infection can be successfully treated, but sensitivity tests should always be performed, **because antibiotic resistance is common.** Drugs used successfully for treatment include penicillin, tetracyclines, streptomycin, erythromycin, suphonamides, lincomycin, and spectinomycin. However, advanced and chronic cases do not respond well to therapy.

## Control

1.  Because wounds are a route of entry for *S. aureus* into the body, anything reducing the chance of injury will help prevent infection. Sharp objects, such as splinters, stones with pointed and sharp edges, or metal edges that cut or puncture feet, should be eliminated from areas where poultry are reared. **Maintenance of good litter quality will reduce foot pad ulceration.** Particular attention should be

given to **hatchery management and sanitation.** *S. aureus* is found everywhere, and conditions in incubators and hatchers are ideal for bacterial growth.

2. Prevention of early infection with Gumboro disease virus and chicken infectious anaemia virus will also help prevent staphylococcosis.

# STREPTOCOCCOSIS

Streptococcosis in poultry is worldwide in distribution. It occurs both as an acute septicaemic infection (i.e. blood infection), and also as a chronic infection, with mortality ranging from 0.5% to 50%. Infection is considered secondary since **streptococci form part of the normal intestinal flora of poultry,** including wild birds. Among the streptococci, *Streptococcus zooepidemicus* is the species most commonly associated with disease. *S. zooepidemicus* occurs usually in mature chickens. Streptococci are Gram-positive bacteria. They are present everywhere in nature and are often found in various poultry environments.

## Spread

**Spread of streptococci occurs usually through oral (by mouth) and respiratory routes.** Spread can also occur through skin injuries, especially in caged layers. Respiratory infection of *S. zooepidemicus* results in acute septicaemia (blood infection) in chickens.

## Symptoms

The disease may occur in **two distinct forms: acute or chronic. In acute form** of the disease, in birds of any age, death may occur without any preceding symptoms. Symptoms are related to septicaemia and include marked depression, ruffled feather, pale comb and wattles, fine head tremors, and a decrease in egg production. Droppings are fluid (diarrhoea), and there is rapid loss of weight. Mortality can vary, but may be as high as 50% of the flock. In hatching eggs, there is late embryo mortality with resulting reduced hatchability.

In the **chronic form,** the symptoms include loss of body weight, lameness, diarrhoea, fever with temperature up to $110^0$ F, occasional head tremors and torticollis (twisting of the head to one side).

## Postmortem Findings

Postmortem findings in the **acute form** include presence of fluid mixed with blood under the skin and in the pericardial sac (below covering of the heart), peritonitis (inflammation of peritoneum) and enlargement of the liver, spleen and kidneys. Small necrotic foci (areas of dead tissue), from pinpoint to 1cm in diameter, may be seen in liver and they may vary in colour from white to dark brown.

Postmortem findings in the **chronic form** include dehydration, emaciation, arthritis (inflammation of a joint), deformed ova, peritonitis (inflammation of peritoneum, a membrane in the body cavity), endocarditis with vegetations on the heart valves (i.e. inflammation of the internal lining of the heart with growths on the valves), pericarditis (inflammation of the covering of heart), and pneumonia (inflammation of the lungs). The heart may be dilated and there may be mild ascites (accumulation of fluid in the abdominal cavity).

## Diagnosis

Clinical symptoms and postmortem findings indicate streptococcal infection, but other disease-producing organisms, such as staphylococci, **Erysipelothrix**, **Pasteurella**, and some strains of *E. coli* may produce similar conditions.

Diagnosis depends on demonstration of the causal organism. A tentative diagnosis may be obtained by the demonstration of Gram-positive cocci in smears from the blood, liver, or spleen. Culture and identification of the organism by biochemical and serological means is necessary to confirm diagnosis. Because the organisms are present everywhere and are found in the faeces of normal poultry, it is essential that material for examination is not contaminated.

## Treatment

Treatment includes use of antibiotics, such as penicillin, erythromycin, oxytetracycline, chlortetracycline, tetracycline, or nitrofurans in acute and subacute infections. Affected birds respond well in the course of the disease. As the disease progresses within a flock, treatment efficacy decreases. Dietary bacitracin decreases the incidence of streptococci in young chickens. Certain streptococcal strains develop resistance after exposure to antibiotics, such as tylosin. Isolates should be subjected to sensitivity tests in support of treatment.

## Control

1.  Proper cleaning and disinfection can reduce environmental streptococcal load and reduce exposure.

2.  Use of **formaldehyde** reduces the total count of streptococci in the hatchery by as much as 85.7%.

3.  Control requires reducing stress and preventing immunosuppressive diseases and conditions (i.e. diseases and conditions which suppress development of immunity).

## CAMPYLOBACTERIOSIS

Campylobacteriosis is a chronic (i.e. of long duration and less severe), contagious bacterial disease of chickens. Also known as **'avian vibrionic hepatitis'**, campylobacteriosis causes liver disease, unevenness in young growing flocks, and reduced egg production in older birds. Special attention should be given to this disease because of its **association with intestinal disease in humans and consumption of poultry products.**

## Cause

Campylobacters are Gram-negative bacteria. There are many species of **Campylobacter.** The three main species of poultry are *C. jejuni, C. coli* and *C. lari*, the main species being *C. jejuni.* Campylobacters are found in the intestinal tracts of a wide variety of animals and birds often without causing disease. **It is believed that all the three species exist in the intestinal tract of poultry as harmless commensals.** That is, existing in a relationship in which they obtain food or other benefits from the chickens, without damaging or benefiting them.

## Prevalence

**Broiler flocks** usually become infected without showing symptoms, when the chicks are 3-5 weeks old. Within 3-7 days of initial infection, 80-100% of the flock becomes infected and remains carrier until slaughtered at 6-7 weeks of age. Poultry serve as primary reservoir hosts of campylobacters. Up to 90% of broilers may be infected. **Prevalence of infection in broiler breeder flocks has been found to be as high as 80%,** but campylobacters are rarely isolated from hatcheries or newly hatched chicks.

## Spread

1.  *C. jejuni* is shed in the faeces. **Spread is by ingestion of the organism, directly, or through contaminated feed or water.** Affected birds shed the organisms for weeks to months.

2.  Contaminated feed can introduce infection to young chicks. **Drinking water may also act as a means of infection for growing broiler chickens.** Campylobacters survive well in cold water. Chlorination of the water supply has been shown to reduce the prevalence of *C. jejuni* in flocks supplied with water from a borehole. Whenever the drinking water is chlorinated, it should be ensured that header tanks and drinkers are kept clean because chlorine is rapidly inactivated by organic matter.

3.  **Insects (cockroaches)** have been shown to be carriers of *C. jejuni.* It has been shown that houseflies can transmit *C. jejuni* to chicks in the laboratory, but it is not known how important this transmission is in the field.

4.  *C. jejuni* is also commonly carried by domestic and other animals found on farms, including cattle, pigs, dogs, rodents (rats, mice), domestic sparrows and wild birds. Unless strict control measures are adopted, most poultry sites harbour a large rodent population. **Rodent droppings** can be a particularly important source of campylobacter infection for flocks, especially if rodents enter into poultry houses or feed stores.

5. Infection may be spread by movement of people between broiler houses or farms. Campylobacters have been recovered from the **shoes of poultry farm workers** and surface water near poultry houses. Thorough cleaning and disinfection of broiler sheds after disposal is very important to prevent this source of infection and subsequent flocks becoming infected.

6. Transmission of infection through eggs from breeder flocks seems unlikely since eggs and newly hatched chicks from infected breeder flocks have been found to be free of campylobacter. As campylobacters are extremely sensitive to drying, drying will destroy organisms on the surface of clean eggs within a short period following laying. Moreover, *C. jejuni* does not penetrate the eggshell.

## Symptoms

Symptoms are usually limited to depression and diarrhoea. In growing broilers, reduced weight gain and poor feed efficiency are observed. Layers show decreased egg production. There is no specific clinical disease in poultry that can be said to be caused by these bacteria. **Large numbers of campylobacters can be present in the intestinal tract of poultry without producing any gross changes.**

## Postmortem Findings

In chicks postmortem findings include distension of the intestinal tract extending from the duodenal loop to the bifurcation of the caecum. Accumulation of mucus and watery fluid occurs, and haemorrhages may be present. The newly hatched chicks may show red or yellow mottling of the liver. These discoloured patches reflect areas of dead tissue (necrotic lesions).

## Diagnosis

Clinical disease can be diagnosed from symptoms, postmortem findings, and identification of the organism by culture of bile in the laboratory.

## Treatment

Erythromycin, doxycycline, chloramphenicol, furazolidone, and gentamicin have been found to be effective.

## Control

1. Sanitization of drinking water (preferably chlorination) and improved hygiene on farms are recommended.

2. Unrestricted movement of people, recycling of litter, and the entry of flies, vermin, and possibly wild birds all contribute to infection, and must therefore be prevented.

3. Thorough decontamination, including removal of litter and disinfection of equipment and buildings, followed by a rest period of at least 7 days, will effectively eliminate

residual campylobacters in poultry houses.

4. High-quality sanitation programme and biosecurity should be practised to prevent introduction of the organism.

# TUBERCULOSIS

Tuberculosis of chickens is a contagious disease caused by the bacterium *Mycobacterium avium.* The disease is characterized by its **long course**, persistence in a flock when once established, and tending to produce emaciation, decreased egg production, and finally death. Mortality over a short period may not be important, but loss of adult birds from time to time (particularly if valuable breeding stock is involved), culling (removal) of poor quality birds, and drop in production can cause serious economic loss.

Tuberculosis in chickens occurs throughout the world. Its persistence within the flocks is mainly due to keeping stocks older than the first laying period, and under conditions where cleanliness and hygiene in management are not properly followed. At one time the disease was widely prevalent in India, but is now rare because of improved rearing and management practices.

Avian tuberculosis is less prevalent in young chickens, not because the younger birds are more resistant to infection, but because in older birds the disease has a greater chance to become established through a longer period of exposure.

## Cause

The cause of avian tuberculosis is *Mycobacterium avium,* an acid-fast organism. It usually appears beaded under the microscope. *M. avium* is relatively resistant to a number of disinfectants. However, the unprotected organism is killed by direct sunlight. **Outside the body it can survive for many years (up to 4 years).**

## Spread

1. The most important source of the organism is the **infected chicken.** A large number of organisms are discharged from the ulcerated lesions in the intestine. **These are passed in the faeces,** creating a constant source of infection. Although other sources of infection exist, none equals **infective faecal material** in the spread of avian tuberculosis. Faecal discharges may contain organisms from lesions of the liver and lining of the gallbladder. The respiratory tract can also be a source of infection, especially if lining of the trachea is involved.

2. Then, because of the long survival of *M. avium* outside the body of the host, items contaminated with the droppings and faeces of the infected birds, are the second most important source of the organism. These items include litter, contaminated pens and pasture, equipment and implements that come into contact with infected

birds, and the hands, feet and clothing of attendants. Organisms may be carried by persons whose shoes have been soiled with faecal matter.

3. The contaminated environment containing soil and litter loaded with bacteria is a very important factor in the spread of disease to uninfected birds. The longer the premises have been occupied by infected birds and the more concentrated the population, the more prevalent the infection is likely to be.

4. Other sources of the spread of organism are carcasses of birds that die of the disease, and offal (internal organs) from chickens dressed for food. Even cannibalism may play a role in spread.

5. Wild birds and pigeons may be infected with *M. avium* and are therefore capable of spreading the organism to poultry flocks.

6. Egg is only of minor importance in the spread of avian tuberculosis.

## Symptoms

The disease is usually **chronic**. That is, it has a long course and symptoms may spread over a period of weeks or months before death. There is usually progressive but slow loss of condition, accompanied by lack of energy. Although the appetite remains good, there is loss of weight with marked wasting of the breast muscles. As a result, the keel bone (breast bone) becomes very prominent, deformed, or even **'knife edged'**. The face and comb become pale and sometimes jaundiced, and the comb is shrunken. In extreme cases, in the end, most of the fat disappears and the face of the affected bird appears swollen than normal. If the affected bird is greatly emaciated, one may detect nodular masses along the intestine by palpation of the abdomen. Persistent diarrhoea with soiling of the tail feathers is usually seen.

An occasional bird may show hopping, jerky type of movement caused by tubercular changes in the bone marrow of the leg bones or joint changes. Some birds may adopt a sitting position.

Affected birds may die within a few months or live for many months, depending on severity or extent of disease. A bird may die suddenly as a result of haemorrhage from rupture of the affected liver or spleen.

## Postmortem Findings

Gross changes are usually seen in the **liver, spleen, intestine** and **bone marrow**. These are **irregular, greyish-yellow or greyish-white nodules (tubercles),** varying in size from pinpoint to large masses of fusing tubercular material. When cut through, the nodules are firm and caseous (cheese-like) and centres may have a pale yellow colour, particularly those from the bone marrow. The **spleen** and **liver** are often markedly enlarged and sometimes rupture with resulting blood in the body cavity. The smaller nodules in these organs may be easily removed from the surrounding tissue, particularly when they project from the surface. (This is in contrast to lymphoid leukosis, in which somewhat similar lesions cannot be removed from the surrounding tissue.) The projection of nodules from the surface of the spleen gives it an irregular **'knobbly'** (i.e. lumpy) appearance.

**The wall of the intestine also always contains similar lesions,** varying in size from a millimetre to several centimetres in diameter. They usually involve entire thickness of the intestinal wall and finally ulcerate into the lumen of the intestine. This results in the discharge of bacilli (bacteria) into the lumen, constituting the major source of infection in the droppings. The bone marrow of the long bones of the legs usually contains tubercular nodules. These can be seen if the bones are split longitudinally. They are pale yellow in colour and vary in size and number. This is one of the characteristic features of tuberculosis in the chicken. The lungs are less commonly affected. Tubercle bacilli have been isolated from some cases of arthritis affecting the phalangeal joints (**'bumble foot'**).

## Diagnosis

1. The symptoms and postmortem findings strongly indicate avian tuberculosis. Demonstration of acid-fast tubercle organisms in smears of infected liver, spleen or other organs, or in crushed lesions, supports the diagnosis. There is rarely any difficulty in demonstrating the organisms, which are usually present in very large numbers, particularly in young nodules and those from the bone marrow.

2. Cultural examination is also necessary for isolation and identification of the causal agent.

3. Immunological tests are also of value in the diagnosis of infected birds during life. They include the tuberculin test, an agglutination test, and ELISA.

## Treatment

Antibiotics are not used to treat tuberculosis in chickens. Also, *M. avium* is more resistant to antibiotics compared to the tubercle bacteria of humans and animals.

## Control

In the control of tuberculosis in poultry there are certain basic facts that must be considered.

1. The main sources of infection are infected chickens, live or dead. Anything might be contaminated by their excretions and faeces. Therefore, the resistance of the organism outside the body of the chicken must be kept in mind. Other poultry, wild birds, pigs and other mammals may also be important as reservoir of infection.

2. Infection can be detected from symptoms, postmortem findings, or serological means.

3.   Neither drug treatment nor vaccination is economically possible.

4.   Greatest losses occur in flocks older than 18 months of age.

5.   On some premises it may not be possible to eliminate the infection.

   **Control may be achieved by:**

(i)   Removal of infection, or

(ii)  Living with reduced infection

   **For removal of infection, and later freedom from infection, the requirements include:**

(a)   Premises that are free of infection with *M. avium.*

(b)   A source of tuberculosis-free birds, such as day-old chicks or older stock, considered to be free because of absence of symptoms and any postmortem findings and negative serological tests.

(c)   The prevention of entry of the infection to the flock, and

(d)   Monitoring the flock to confirm, when considered appropriate, that it is free from infection. Such monitoring is valuable for flocks on premises which have been cleaned and disinfected following previous infection with this agent.

## Living with Reduced Infection

   Under circumstances in which it is not possible to remove the infection, the harmful effects of the disease can be reduced by:

1.   Not keeping the flocks longer than the first laying season.

2.   Monitoring the infection.

3.   Removal of the positive reactors, and practising all possible hygienic precautions to prevent entry of the infection.

## AVIAN CELLULITIS

   Avian cellulitis is a bacterial infection which occurs under the skin and affects the **broiler chickens**. Also known as **'coliform cellulitis'**, **'inflammatory process'** and **'infectious process'** avian cellulitis is characterized by the accumulation of sheets of fluid containing fibrin, blood, and cheesy material (exudate) under the skin. These lesions (changes) are called **'plaques'**.

   Cellulitis is usually associated with a skin injury or a traumatic wound, which enables a variety of bacteria to enter the wound and grow under the skin. *Escherichia coli* is the most commonly involved organism, but a variety of other bacteria may also be associated. Overcrowding and poor quality litter are factors which contribute to avian cellulitis. It occurs more commonly in males than females. Older birds are more likely to develop the disease.

Avian cellulitis affects the akin over the abdomen, or between the thigh and midline. The lesions are usually discovered at processing and have been an important cause of carcass condemnation. Cellulitis lesions are mainly unilateral and located on the abdomen or thigh. Skin colour changes from normal to red-brown and the skin is swollen at the site of inflammation. Below the skin, there is accumulation of fluid (oedema) and muscle haemorrhage. **A fibrinous (containing fibrin) to caseous (cheese-like) plaque between the muscle and the tissues below the skin is the characteristic lesion.**

**A positive association between cellulitis and ascites has been shown.** Ascites is a common condition in broilers characterized by an abnormally large abdomen. Because most cellulitis lesions are located in the abdominal area, it may be that **ascites becomes a predisposing factor for cellulitis.** Also, it is possible that both conditions may show common risk factors, such as rapid growth.

**There is no treatment for avian cellulitis, and control of the disease is difficult because of the widespread presence of** *E. coli.*

Chapter **5**

# Mycoplasmal Diseases

ycoplasmas are the smallest organisms. In contrast to bacteria, they have no cell wall but are bounded by a plasma membrane. Of the 22 species of mycoplasma recovered from birds, only two produce disease in chickens. These are *Mycoplasma gallisepticum* and *M. synoviae*.

## MYCOPLASMOSIS

### *MYCOPLASMA GALLISEPTICUM* INFECTION

Commonly known as **'chronic respiratory disease, or CRD'**, *M. gallisepticum* (MG) infection is found everywhere and is extremely **important both in broilers and layers.** While not a great killer, the disease is of great economic importance. Laying flocks positive for *M. gallisepticum* have been shown to produce as many as 20 less eggs per year than MG-negative flocks. **Also, it is an important egg-transmitted disease.** *M. gallisepticum* infection is a serious problem in India.

The disease is characterized by abnormal respiratory sounds, coughing, and nasal discharge. Symptoms are usually slow to develop and the disease has a long course. The disease is of particular importance in the respiratory group of diseases along with other disease-producing micro-organisms, since it affects the growth in broilers and egg production in layers. **'Complicated CRD (CCRD)'**, also known as **'airsac disease'**, is a severe airsacculitis (inflammation of airsac) which occurs when *M. gallisepticum* infection gets complicated by *Escherichia coli* and some respiratory virus infections. In addition, the disease causes reduced hatchability in chickens, and rarely, may be associated with arthritis (inflammation of a joint) and salpingitis (inflammation of oviduct). Most of the commonly used chemical disinfectants are effective against *M. gallisepticum.*

### Spread

1. **Infection is usually transmitted through the hatching egg (vertical transmission). This is the major means of spread.**

2. **Carrier birds** (i.e. birds which carry the infection without showing symptoms) are responsible for transmitting the disease. *M. gallisepticum* rarely survives for more than a few days outside the bird; therefore carrier birds are essential in the spread of disease. Direct contact of susceptible birds with infected carrier chickens causes

170

outbreaks of the disease. In some flocks it may be quite rapid, but in others it may take weeks. Walls between the houses may form partial barriers and may slow the spread of the organism. All the same, on continuous production sites spread of infection is difficult to control.

3. **Through the air:** Spread may also occur by **contaminated dust, droplets, or feathers carried through the air.** The organisms may travel short distances through the air. This is enough to cause infection of birds within a pen, but is not of much importance in their transfer from house to house. **Infection occurs through the respiratory tract and conjunctiva.**

4. **People are important carriers.** It is believed that 60% of cross-contamination between houses is the result of organisms being transported by people on clothing and the equipment they use.

5. An increase in the bird density increases the rate at which lateral spread occurs.

# Disease

Disease caused by *M. gallisepticum* is influenced by the disease-producing power (virulence) of the organism, the number of organisms, the age of the bird, simultaneous infection with other disease-producing micro-organisms (pathogens), and stress factors.

The infection usually affects almost all birds in a flock, but it varies in severity and duration. It is more severe and of long duration in the cold months, and **affects younger birds more severely than mature birds.** However, **in mature birds, there is considerable loss from reduced egg production.**

Infection may last from a few weeks to 18 months, or longer. **The organism is fragile (easily destroyed) outside the body of the bird and survives only for a few days,** or even less when present under usual poultry house conditions. **However, if protected** by exudates (inflammatory material) and/or a cold environment, **the organism may survive longer.** The commonly used chemical disinfectants are effective against *M. gallisepticum.*

While *M. gallisepticum* is the main cause of **'chronic respiratory disease'**, usually other organisms cause complications. Severe airsac infection, commonly called **'complicated CRD (CCRD)'** or **'airsac disease'** is the condition mostly seen in the field. Ranikhet disease or infectious bronchitis may precipitate outbreaks of *M. gallisepticum* infection. *Escherichia coli* has been found to be the most common complicating organism. **However,** *E. coli* **cannot readily infect the airsacs unless they are previously invaded by** *M. gallisepticum* **alone, or in combination with infectious bronchitis or Ranikhet disease virus.**

Mortality is negligible in adult flocks, but there may be a reduction in the number of birds in production. In broilers mortality may range from low in uncomplicated disease to as much as 30% in complicated outbreaks, and especially during the colder months.

Infection results in an immune response, which may provide some degree of protection.

## Symptoms

The most characteristic symptoms in adult flocks are abnormal respiratory sounds, nasal discharge, sneezing, coughing, and breathing through the open beak. Feed consumption is reduced and birds lose weight. In laying flocks, **egg production decreases,** and the disease is usually more severe during winter. In broilers most outbreaks occur between 4 and 8 weeks of age.

However, the appearance of disease depends, as already mentioned, on the presence at the same time of other disease-producing organisms, or stress factors. **Uncomplicated infections usually cause no symptoms, or cause mortality only in the very young.** The other pathogens include the viruses of Ranikhet disease and infectious bronchitis (including the live vaccine strains), Gumboro disease, disease-producing strains of *E. coli*, and *Haemophilus paragallinarum* (cause of infectious coryza). Stress factors include excessive ammonia, dust, nutritional deficiency and the stress associated with intensive management (overcrowding, etc.).

## Postmortem Findings

The postmortem findings include inflammatory material (exudate) in nasal passage, trachea, bronchi, and airsacs. **Airsacs usually contain cheese-like inflammatory material**. Some degree of pneumonia (inflammation of the lungs) may be seen. In severe cases of airsac disease, there is pericarditis (inflammation of pericardium, covering of the heart) and perihepatitis (inflammation of liver surface) along with massive airsacculitis (inflammation of airsac).

In disease which is made worse by other disease-producing organisms, the changes are more severe and prolonged, giving rise to **chronic condition**. With *E. coli* infection in young chickens of 4-10 weeks of age, colisepticaemia may result in pericarditis, perihepatitis, and disease of the respiratory tract, including airsacculitis (see **colisepticaemia**). The rare cases of tenosynovitis (inflammation of a tendon and its sheath) and arthritis (inflammation of a joint) resemble the condition caused by *M. synoviae* (see '*M. synoviae* infection', described next). (A tendon is that tissue by which a muscle is attached to the bone.) In salpingitis, cheesy material (caseous exudate) occurs in the oviduct.

## Diagnosis

1.   There are no symptoms or postmortem findings which are characteristic of *M. gallisepticum* infection in chickens.

2. Demonstration of the organism is the most certain method of confirming the infection. For isolation, samples can be taken from live birds, fresh carcasses, or dead-in-shell embryos, or chicks which have broken the shell but failed to hatch. From freshly killed and dead birds swabs may be taken from the nasal cavity, trachea, airsacs, and lungs.

3. If mycoplasmas are isolated, identification can be made by using specific sera for immunofluorescence.

4. There are a number of serological tests which are used for the demonstration of specific antibody. Enzyme-linked immunosorbent assay (ELISA) has emerged as a sensitive and more specific test for *M. gallisepticum* antibodies. Commercial ELISA test kits are now being used increasingly as a screening test for flock monitoring and serological diagnosis.

## Treatment

1. *M. gallisepticum* is susceptible to several antibiotics. These include streptomycin, oxytetracycline, chlortetracycline, tiamulin, kanamycin, neomycin, gentamicin, tylosin, erythromycin, spiramycin, lincomycin, and spectinomycin, and more recently, the fluoroquinolones (enrofloxacin, danofloxacin). Some isolates, however, are somewhat resistant to streptomycin, erythromycin, spiramycin, and tylosin.

2. Use of oxytetracycline or chlortetracycline at 200 g/tonne of feed for at least 8-10 days has given good results.

3. **Tylosin is an antibiotic specific for the treatment of *M. gallisepticum*.** It has been injected subcutaneously (below the skin) at 3-5 mg/lb body weight, or given at 2-3 g/gallon of drinking water for 3-5 days. Inclusion of very low levels of tylosin in feed reduces egg production losses.

4. Tiamulin, and tiamulin plus salinomycin, are also effective treatments.

5. Administration of streptomycin, oxytetracycline, chlortetracycline, erythromycin or tylosin to breeder flocks reduces the rate of transmission of *M. gallisepticum* through eggs. However, it is not adequate to obtain completely infection-free flocks.

6. **Egg-dipping** with a temperature or pressure differential has been used as a means of getting antibiotics into hatching eggs to remove egg-transmitted *M. gallisepticum*. Tylosin or gentamicin solution is used for treating hatching eggs. In general, these methods are effective, but sometimes do not eliminate completely the possibility of egg transmission. However, egg-dipping in antibiotic solution has made it possible to obtain sufficient *M. gallisepticum*-free flocks to provide the poultry industry with means for producing clean progeny on a large scale. This has resulted in *M. gallisepticum*-free breeder flocks.

## Control

1.  Treatment is only a temporary solution and is usually quite expensive. Removal of infection is the most satisfactory means of control, and where spread of infection can be limited, this must be done.

2.  Since *M. gallisepticum* can be transmitted through eggs, maintaining chicken flocks free of *M. gallisepticum* infection is only possible by obtaining replacement flocks that are known to be free of the infection, and rearing them in strict isolation to avoid introduction of the disease.

3.  Control measures are to be started from the breeding stock, and include the following:

    (a)  Treatment of hatching eggs to reduce spread of mycoplasma through the embryo and progeny.

    (b)  Maintenance of the progeny flocks during the eradication period in groups of 200-300 birds. Each group must be kept separate because the whole flock has to be rejected if mycoplasma infection is found on monitoring.

    (c)  Monitoring the progeny periodically for infection with mycoplasma.

4.  **Infected female parents must be removed as a source of infection. Unlike pullorum disease, control of *M. gallisepticum* is difficult for three reasons:** (1) It is so contagious that only one or two infected birds in the pen can infect almost all others in a very short time. (2) An infected bird continues to be a carrier, and passes the organism through the eggs. Thus, if any infected birds are found in the breeding pen, all the birds in the pen must be removed as a source of hatching eggs. **There is no such thing as testing and retesting, as with pullorum disease.** (3) Breeder flocks may remain clean (no infected birds) for long periods, but suddenly break with infection. **Removal at the breeder level is the best method of handling the disease.**

## Treatment of Hatching Eggs

1.  Infection of hatching eggs with mycoplasma can be reduced by treating them with drugs, or by heating, or both, before incubation. Antimicrobials (drugs which destroy or prevent the growth of micro-organisms) can be introduced into hatching eggs by two ways:

    (i)  Injection into the albumen at the pointed end of the egg, and

    (ii)  Dipping of the egg in a solution of antimicrobial (tylosin or gentamicin), and creating a pressure differential so that the solution passes through the shell into the egg. This is refereed to as **'egg-dipping'**.

2.  Heat treatment of eggs for reducing infection involves gradually heating them to

$46^0$ to $47^0$ C over a period of 11-14 hours and then allowing them to cool to room temperature. Although this is an effective method of reducing infection, some strains of mycoplasma may show resistance. Moreover, it might cause embryo mortality of about 5-10%.

## Monitoring of Progeny Flocks

This includes cultural and/or serological examination. For cultural examination swabs may be taken from dead embryos at candling, or from dead-in-shell at hatch, and from chicks that die over the first few weeks of life. Older birds may also be swabbed during life at any age, but particularly at the time of laying. Serological examination is made at several intervals in the life of the bird, including the time of laying. All the birds in a flock should be subjected to at least one serological test.

Flocks may be considered uninfected with mycoplasma only when serologically negative progeny have been obtained from negative parent birds and hatching eggs. Also, neither generation should have been subjected to anti-mycoplasma treatment. By these methods mycoplasma-free breeder flocks have been produced, and their progeny are hatched free of mycoplasma infection.

Antibiotic treatment is also of value in the face of disease, and for egg treatment to reduce infection in the hatching egg.

## Vaccination

It is virtually impossible to control mycoplasma infection on continuous production (multi-age) sites. Also, antimicrobial treatment is very costly. As such vaccination can be very useful in the control of mycoplasma infection. A number of vaccines have been produced, both live and killed.

**Live vaccines** are of relatively low virulence (i.e. have very low disease-producing power) for chickens. The F-strain gives protection to broilers when vaccinated by eye drop or aerosol at 10 days of age. **Killed vaccines** have been used particularly for reducing drop of eggs in layers, but vaccinated birds do not produce as many eggs as similar hens uninfected with mycoplasma. Live vaccine is also used in breeders. The vaccine, both in layers and breeders, is administered to healthy birds at least 3-4 weeks before production starts.

**Note:** For a list of commercially available vaccines against *M. gallisepticum*, refer to Chapter 19 under **"Mycoplasma vaccines"**.

## *MYCOPLASMA SYNOVIAE* INFECTION

Also known as **'infectious synovitis'**, this infection was originally associated with joint changes and lameness. As a result it caused **reduced growth in broilers and growers. The disease is most common in broilers.** Although this condition is still seen, the infection usually results in either no symptoms, or in only a mild upper respiratory disease, or in a more severe respiratory condition when combined with Ranikhet disease, infectious bronchitis, or both. It may be associated with a **reduction in egg production.** *M. synoviae* **is an important egg-transmitted disease.** The organism has only a **single serotype.**

The ability of *Mycoplasma synoviae* (MS) to survive outside the body of the bird is similar to that of *M. gallisepticum,* **and within the bird infection may last for several years.** Although not studied in as much detail as for *M. gallisepticum,* similar predisposing factors play an important part in aggravating disease, particularly of the respiratory system.

## Spread

Spread of infection is also similar to *M. gallisepticum,* except that it is **more rapid**. Transmission through eggs (**vertical transmission**) occurs, and plays a major role in the spread of *M. synoviae.* After infection, breeders shed the organisms between 14 to 40 days. **Lateral spread** occurs readily by direct contact. Spread between cages in the same room occurs through air. Infection occurs via the respiratory tract. **Birds are infected for life and remain carriers.** Transmission also occurs on clothing, trucks and equipment over long distances. *M. synoviae* spreads through blood and produces infection mainly of **joints** and **respiratory tract.**

## Symptoms

Natural infection may occur as early as within one week, but acute infection is usually seen when chickens are 4-16 weeks old. Infection may occur without any symptoms. When symptoms occur they may take a **respiratory or joint form. Chronic infection follows the acute phase and may persist for the life of the flock.** The chronic stage may be seen at any age.

In the **joint form**, there is marked depression, paleness of the face and comb, rapid loss of condition and swelling of the joints. The feet and hock joints are particularly affected, with accompanying lameness. In the **chronic form** swelling of the joints occurs with lameness, but without severe systemic disturbance.

In the **respiratory form**, which can occur independently of the joint form, there may be mild respiratory sounds and coryza (nasal discharge). Morbidity (number of birds affected) varies but averages about 10%. More severe respiratory conditions are seen when *M. synoviae* infection is associated with viruses, bacteria, and other predisposing factors as described for *M. gallisepticum.*

## Postmortem Findings

Postmortem findings in the **respiratory form** are similar to those of *M. gallisepticum* infection. Changes involving the **joints** include accumulation of fluid (oedema) and thickening of the tissues surrounding the joints. The feet and hock joints are usually affected, but others may also be involved. This change also occurs in bursa. For example, the sternal bursa (a pouch or sac on the keel bone) gets enlarged and thickened. The inflammatory material (exudate) becomes cheesy and is usually orange to brown in colour. In some chickens the spleen is enlarged, the liver swollen and green or dark red in colour, the kidneys are swollen and pale, and the bursa of Fabricius and thymus are greatly reduced in size (atrophied).

## Diagnosis

1. Neither the respiratory symptoms nor the postmortem findings are characteristic. However, a tentative (presumptive) diagnosis may be made on the basis of pale combs, leg weakness, enlarged hock joints, and enlarged spleen, liver, or kidneys.

2. Confirmation of diagnosis depends on the isolation and identification of the organism or demonstration of the antibody by serology. The trachea, lungs, airsacs and joints are the best sites for isolation of *M. synoviae.*

3. For serological diagnosis, enzyme-linked immunosorbent assay (ELISA) is now commonly used as a diagnostic test. ELISA kits are available commercially.

4. Recently, direct detection of *M. synoviae* in tissues using DNA probes has been described, but its sensitivity is not adequate. On the other hand, polymerase chain reaction (PCR) is a simple, rapid and highly sensitive method of detecting *M. synoviae* DNA in tissues, and PCR kits are commercially available.

## Treatment

1. *M. synoviae* is sensitive to several antibiotics, including chlortetracycline, danofloxacin, enrofloxacin, lincomycin, oxytetracycline, spectinomycin, spiromycin, tetracycline, tiamulin, and tylosin. In contrast to *M. gallisepticum, M. synoviae* isolates appear resistant to erythromycin. Antibiotic medication does not eliminate *M. synoviae* infection from the flock.

2. Chlortetracycline (50-100 g/tonne of feed) given continuously provides satisfactory control of infectious synovitis in chickens. Higher concentrations (about 200 g / tonne) are required to control synovitis after infection has occurred.

3. Soluble lincomycin-spectinomycin (2 g/gallon of drinking water) is useful in preventing respiratory tract infection (airsacculitis) in broilers.

4. Tiamulin in the drinking water (0.006-0.025%) has been shown to be effective in preventing airsacculitis and synovitis in chickens.

## Control

1. The methods of control are similar to those for *M. gallisepticum. M. synoviae,*

however, is more resistant to antimicrobials. Vaccines are not available for the control of *M. synoviae*.

2.   **Effective biosecurity measures** should be used to prevent introduction of the infection (see **'biosecurity'**).

3.   **Control of disease at the farm is rather difficult.** This is because some birds do not produce antibodies against the organisms quickly and therefore the presence of *S. synoviae* cannot always be detected by the blood test.

4.   **Antibiotic treatment of breeders is not effective in eliminating *M. synoviae*,** although the level of egg transmission may be reduced.

# Chapter 6

# Fungal Diseases

**F**ungi (plural of 'fungus') are larger than bacteria with thick cell walls. These thick walls make fungi detectable under the microscope in tissues, even in the presence of dead tissue. Moreover, their shape can be characteristic enough for tentative identification of the species of fungus under the microscope. However, usually cultural isolation is required for identification. Immunosuppressive drugs (i.e. drugs that suppress the immune responses) favour fungal infections of all varieties.

## ASPERGILLOSIS

Also known as **'brooder pneumonia'** and **'mycotic pneumonia'**, aspergillosis involving respiratory system is common in poultry. Whenever aspergillosis is mentioned in poultry, it is usually in the context of lungs. Although the primary target of the agent is the respiratory system, other manifestations of the disease also occur in poultry. **Newly hatched chicks are highly susceptible to infection.** Stress of cold, high ammonia and dusty environments increase the incidence and severity of infection, as also conjunctivitis produced by Ranikhet disease vaccination. Older birds are constantly exposed from the environment, but due to their increased resistance, rarely develop new infections. In adults infection occurs only when the organism is present in sufficient quantities to establish disease, or when the bird's resistance is damaged by factors such as environmental stress, immunosuppressive compounds (i.e. drugs that suppress the immune responses); or infectious, nutritional, or toxic disease.

### Cause

Aspergillosis is caused by various species of the fungus **Aspergillus**. The two most common species in chickens are *A. fumigatus* and *A. flavus*. These organisms are distributed worldwide. Although *A. fumigatus* is found commonly, it does not always produce disease in young broiler chicks. Both the species of **Aspergillus** usually occur in decaying vegetative matter, soil and feed grains. Their reproductive structures (conidia) occur in the air of most environments. **Contaminated poultry litter is usually the source of infection.** Both fungi are quite resistant to chemical agents, and produce toxins that are involved in the development of the disease.

### Spread

1.  **Infection occurs by inhalation of spores.** A spore is that form of fungus which

is very tough and resistant, and is therefore difficult to destroy. Spores usually originate from infected eggs that are opened during incubation or hatching, releasing large numbers of spores and contaminating other chicks of the same hatch (hatch mates).

It has been suggested that **fungus may penetrate through the eggshell during incubation and thus newly hatched chicks get infected.** Egg embryos are quite susceptible to infection by *A. fumigatus* during incubation.

2.  Infection within the hatchery may also occur from contaminated air ducts or other equipment. After infection in the hatchery, lateral spread after placement is not usually an important source of new infections.

3.  Aspergillosis can also be produced by **inhalation of spores from contaminated feed or poultry house litter.** Fungal growth in wet litter produces large numbers of spores. These spores disperse as suspended particles in air as wet litter dries. In such instances, new cases continue to appear some time after placement.

## Development of the Disease

Fungi carried through the air get deposited on conjunctival (in eye), nasal (in nose), tracheal (in trachea, windpipe) and airsac lining, and start producing **nodules (granuloma)** at these places. These nodules gradually expand and fungi tend to grow within them. They rarely invade neighbouring tissues in birds whose immune responses are normal. Sometimes aspergillosis-induced inflammatory material gets lodged in the trachea or syrinx and produces severe respiratory distress in chronically infected birds. (Syrinx is vocal organ of birds. It is a special modification of the lower part of trachea.)

**After inhalation, spores are rapidly spread through blood circulation to other tissues.** This is the route through which lesions (changes) are produced in the brain, pericardium (covering of the heart), bone marrow, kidney, and other soft tissues.

## Symptoms

Within the first 3-5 days **newly hatched chicks** infected in the hatchery show very rapid and difficult breathing, and **start breathing with an open mouth ('gaspers')** due to the gradually developing obstruction of the airway. When the symptoms are associated with other respiratory diseases, such as infectious bronchitis and infectious laryngotracheitis, they are usually accompanied by gurgling and rattling noises, whereas in aspergillosis there is usually no sound.

**Survivors may become dull and stunted,** show sleepiness, lack of appetite, emaciation, increased thirst, develop eye swelling or blindness, and show torticollis (twisting of the neck to one side) and other central nervous system abnormalities. Other birds may remain subclinically affected (i.e. affected without showing symptoms) for some time, but they later slowly develop breathing problems. This is because their increasing body weight puts demands on the reduced functional capacity of the lungs. They may also suffer from a lack of oxygen due to blockage of the syrinx or the trachea.

**Infected poultry flocks usually show mortality in two phases in aspergillosis.** **Acute** (sudden and severe) **respiratory disease** may cause 5-50% mortality in the first 1-3 weeks of age. Those which survive usually develop **chronic disease** (i.e. less severe and prolonged) with up to 5% mortality due to gradual loss of lung function, ascites, blindness, or spread of fungus to nervous system.

## Postmortem Findings

**Nodules** (granulomas) may be present in the lining of eye, nasal passages, trachea, lungs, and airsacs. They appear as distinct (separate) 1-5 mm diameter **white plaques or nodules**. They are composed of dead (necrotic) centres containing fungi. Older nodules in air-filled cavities may appear green to black due to development of pigmented fungal conidiophores (i.e. stalks supporting conidia. Conidia are spores of fungi.) Sometimes **lungs** are just diffusely greyish yellow, and **caseous exudate** (cheese-like inflammatory material) may be present in the syrinx in infected birds.

## Diagnosis

1.  Aspergillosis is usually diagnosed at postmortem examination. This is based on finding **white caseous nodules in the lungs or airsacs.**

2.  Although symptoms of respiratory disease in the first 2 weeks of life and postmortem findings of nodules in the lungs or airsacs are highly suggestive, they are not specific for aspergillosis. This is because difficult breathing and plugs of inflammatory material (exudate) in the trachea can be produced by severe respiratory virus vaccination reactions, or even by poor air quality in the hatchery or brooder house. Moreover, nodules in the lungs or eyes cannot be grossly differentiated from those produced by some other fungi, *E. coli*, staphylococci, or salmonella infections.

3.  Diagnosis depends on the demonstration in the nodules of fungus **Aspergillus**, and also by its cultural isolation and identification. Fungus can be seen microscopically in smears of lesions after the addition of one or two drops of 10% potassium hydroxide (KOH) and then heating it to clear. Fungus is routinely seen in H & E stained tissue sections, but special stains may be required in some cases.

4.  Serological tests are of limited value due to non-specific nature of the antigens

## Treatment

**There is no treatment for aspergillosis.** While certain drugs have been used for treatment of aspergillosis in mammals, they are not cost-effective (economical) in poultry. Therefore, prevention is at present the best means of control.

## Control

1.  As there is no treatment for aspergillosis, control depends on reducing exposure to the fungus and risk factors.

2.  *A. fumigatus* in young chicks has been somewhat controlled by **hatchery sanitation.** Media are available to monitor air in hatcheries. Mouldy litter or feed should be avoided to prevent outbreaks of aspergillosis. Examination of premises, or materials used for feed or litter, usually reveals the source of infection. It is advisable to treat the poultry house and litter with antifungal compounds.

3.  Any mouldy feed should be removed, bulk feed containers cleaned, old litter removed from the house and replaced with new, and drinkers and feeders cleaned and disinfected.

4.  Eggs for hatching should be collected and stored so as to reduce sweating and exposure to spore-loaded dust. Hatching equipment and air ducts should be cleaned, disinfected and monitored by periodic cultures.

5.  Areas around feeders and drinkers are fertile areas for growth of fungi. Therefore, frequent moving of feed troughs and watering places is advisable.

6.  In the brooding house, wet or previously wet litter or soil and mouldy or dusty feeds, should be avoided.

7.  A thorough cleaning of the brooding premises will eliminate the source of infection for future flocks.

8.  Daily cleaning and disinfection of feed and water utensils help in eliminating infection. **In outbreaks, a 1:2000 aqueous solution of copper sulphate for all drinking water may be used to prevent spread of aspergillosis.** Also, feed and water lines should be disinfected, and when possible the surrounding soil should be decontaminated.

9.  Increased ventilation within poultry houses reduces the fungi carried through the air. Therefore, this could be used as a preventive measure in controlling aspergillosis. Natural ventilation appears better than forced-air ventilation.

## CANDIDIASIS (THRUSH)

**Candidiasis or thrush is a fungal infection of the digestive tract.** The fungus involved is *Candida albicans*. Infection caused by *Candida albicans* is also called **'moniliasis'.** This fungus may cause infection of the mouth, oesophagus (food pipe), or crop. Of these, the more common is infection of the crop and is called **'crop mycosis'.** (**'Mycosis'** means a **'fungal infection'**).

Candidiasis of mouth, oesophagus, or crop is quite common, but only rarely causes symptoms. It is usually associated with other diseases existing at the same time, or immunosuppression, or altered bacterial population of the digestive tract. Candidial infections are usually opportunistic rather than primary infections.

## Cause

*C. albicans* is widespread in the environment and **is usually present in the upper digestive tract of normal birds.** The most common factor associated with the excessive growth of this fungus is **administration of antibiotics over a long period.** This suppresses normal bacterial flora and competition for nutrients, and thus allows candida to grow. Other risk factors include highly contaminated drinkers or feeders, eating litter, concurrent immunosuppression, environmental stress, or nutritional disease.

## Disease

Infections are more common in birds under 3 weeks of age. This suggests acquired or age resistance. Mortality directly due to candidiasis is low to nil, and most of the symptoms are due to other concurrent diseases or reduced feed intake.

**Candida is acquired by ingestion** and becomes part of the normal bacterial population of the mouth, oesophagus, and crop. With inhibition of competing bacteria or immunosuppression, **Candida** grows on the surface and invades superficial layers. This invasion stimulates growth (proliferation) of lining epithelial cells and a false membrane (a pseudo-membrane) or a true membrane (diphtheritic membrane) is formed. It appears grossly as a thick covering or a pad of white cheesy (cheese-like) material in the crop, and less commonly in the oesophagus and pharynx. Candidial coverings and membranes are usually adherent and cannot be washed away like normal accumulations of mucus (a digestive tract secretion). Inflammatory response to candidial infection of mucosa (i.e. digestive tract lining) is mild unless formation of ulcers occurs.

## Symptoms

Infections are common, but symptoms are present in only severely affected birds. Symptoms are not particularly characteristic. Birds with superficial infections of the mouth, oesophagus or crop may fail to gain weight, remain stunted, show roughness of feather, and become dehydrated. In rare cases there is systemic invasion, and symptoms of disease of nervous system, kidney, or intestine may be present.

## Postmortem Findings

Changes (lesions) are most common in the **crop** and consist of thickening of the lining (mucosa) with formation of whitish circular, raised ulcers. **Crop is greatly thickened by a soft, yellow-white to grey irregular false membrane. It has a curd-like appearance, and its surface tends to fall off in thin layers**. The mouth and oesophagus show ulcer-like patches. When the proventriculus is involved, it is swollen. Its inner lining (mucosa) is haemorrhagic and may be covered with inflammatory material

183

and dead tissue. The oesophagus, crop and proventriculus show an ulcerated and scaly condition.

## Diagnosis

1. **False or true membranes in the crop, oesophagus and mouth are highly suggestive of candidiasis.** However, such membranes can be produced after ingestion of caustic substances and mycotoxin trichothecene.

2. Demonstration of fungus under the microscope in either scrapings or tissue sections will confirm candidiasis. Identification of the species requires culture on Sabouraud dextrose agar or other fungal culture media, but many normal birds may be positive.

## Control

1. Since fungal infections of the digestive tract are related to unhygienic, unsanitary and overcrowded conditions, these should not be allowed to exist, or should be corrected.

2. Crop mycosis is best prevented by controlling the use of antibiotics, and also by controlling immunosuppressive diseases like Gumboro and chicken infectious anaemia. Strict observation of cleanliness and sanitation is most helpful in controlling crop mycosis.

3. Candidiasis can be controlled temporarily by adding gentian violet (8 mg per kg of feed), or nystatin (142 mg per kg of feed).

## MYCOTOXICOSIS

Growing fungi (moulds) produce a large number of chemicals as by-products and secrete them into surrounding substances. Some are toxic to birds. These toxic by-products are called **'mycotoxins',** or **'fungal toxins'.** ('**Myco**' is a Greek word meaning **'fungus'** and **'toxin'** means **'poison'**). Thus, mycotoxins are toxins secreted by fungus, and **'mycotoxicosis' is poisoning which results from consumption of mycotoxins. Mycotoxicosis is a major problem in poultry industry.**

Growth of fungus is necessary for mycotoxin production in grain. However, this growth may or may not produce visible damage. Fungi can infect and grow in grains before harvest, during storage, or after getting into finished feeds. Many mycotoxins are stable during grinding and crushing in a mill and also during feed storage. Therefore, toxins can be present in grains **after the fungi that produced them are dead.** Even with the best system, contamination of grain and feedstuffs is thus unavoidable; and despite all efforts in controlling mycotoxicoses, **mycotoxins always creep into the feed.**

Hundreds of mycotoxins are now recognized. The type of fungus, temperature, moisture and grain determine whether the toxin will be produced and in what amounts.

## How do moulds contaminate the feedstuffs?

Moulds reproduce by forming spores. These spores are carried by air and insects, and are routinely found in the soil. They thus contaminate the grain and other feedstuffs. Spores may enter the crop at any stage, such as during processing, storage, feed manufacturing, delivery to the farm and while feeding the poultry. It is estimated that 25% of the world grain is contaminated with mycotoxins (fungal toxins).

## It is said that mycotoxins act in synergism? What does this mean?

Individual fungus usually produces more than one toxin. **It is uncommon to find a single mycotoxin occurring under field conditions. Usually they occur in combination of two or more.** These toxins therefore often act in synergism. This means that **their combined effect is much more damaging than that of the individual mycotoxin.** For example, in feed, even if aflatoxin content is very low, its harmful effect is greatly increased by the presence of ochratoxin, even though present in low level. Therefore, naturally occurring mycotoxicoses can occur with only one-tenth the levels required to reproduce poisonings in the laboratory with individual purified mycotoxin. This should be kept in mind when deciding acceptable toxin levels in grains used in poultry feeds. **Fast-growing broilers are more susceptible than commercial layers. The degree of damage does not only depend on the level of mycotoxin, but also on the duration of exposure.**

## What are the harmful effects of mycotoxins?

1. Poor growth and weight gain

2. Decreased egg production and shell quality

3. Immunosuppression

4. Feed refusal

5. Leg weakness

6. Damage to organs

7. Infertility

8. Mortality

9. Toxin residues in meat and eggs

**Net result: Great economic loss.**

**Aflatoxicosis, ochratoxicosis and trichothecene mycotoxicosis are the most commonly seen mycotoxicoses in poultry.** Other mycotoxicoses are less common. **Under hot and humid Indian conditions, with poor storage facilities, mycotoxicoses are widespread.** Various mycotoxicoses will now be discussed, briefly.

## 1. AFLATOXICOSIS

**Aflatoxin** is the most common and also the most important mycotoxin likely to be consumed by poultry. **Aflatoxins are highly toxic mycotoxins** produced by various species of fungi **Aspergillus**. The fungus *Aspergillus flavus* produces most of the aflatoxin and also gives this toxin its name. ('A' from Aspergillus and **'fla'** from **'flavus'** = **afla-toxin** = **aflatoxin**). However, aflatoxin is also produced by *A. parasiticus* and *Penicillium puberulum*. Both fungi are widespread in the environment and produce aflatoxin in warm (30⁰ - 35⁰C), high humidity conditions. Mould growth occurs more rapidly when moisture content is more than 10% and at 28⁰ - 30⁰C. **Aflatoxins can withstand extreme environmental conditions and are highly heat stable.** Aflatoxin contamination is therefore more common in grains grown or handled in a tropical country like India. Handling or storage of grains in these conditions anywhere will also stimulate production of aflatoxin. Poultry feed and ingredients are easily prone to fungal growth and aflatoxin formation. Pelleting feed may eliminate fungi, but does not reduce or eliminate aflatoxin. Aflatoxin is found in **maize**, groundnuts, rice, cottonseed, millet, sorghum and other feed grains. Field levels are 20-100 ppb and may even be up to 500 ppb. **High moisture content in fresh maize and grain damage favour mould growth.** For example, compared to whole grain, mycotoxin may get 30-50 times more concentrated in the broken grain.

Naturally occurring aflatoxins contain aflatoxin **B1, B2, G1** and **G2**. Designations **B** and **G** are given after their **blue (B)** or **green (G)** colour reaction to fluorescent light. **Of all, alfatoxin B1 is usually found in the highest concentration, and is also the most toxic. It damages mainly liver.** Aflatoxin is stable once formed in grain, and is not destroyed during normal grinding and crushing in the mill and storage.

Aflatoxin-producing fungi and aflatoxin-contaminated poultry feedstuffs occur worldwide and cause harmful effects on poultry production. **Young birds are more sensitive to aflatoxin than are adults.** There are also large species differences, ducks being 10 times more sensitive than chickens.

## Development of the Disease (and Postmortem Findings)

After ingestion, aflatoxin B1 undergoes a biological change into a number of metabolites (products of metabolism). Metabolites bind to DNA and RNA, reduce protein synthesis, **and decrease both antibody-mediated and cell-mediated immunity (i.e. immunosuppression).** (To understand these two types of immunity, refer to chapter 32: **The avian immune system**). The metabolic changes lead to liver, kidney and spleen enlargement, and a decrease in the size of bursa of Fabricius, thymus, and testes. With high-dose exposure, fat accumulates inside the cells of liver as clear vacuoles. As a result, **liver is greatly enlarged, yellow, and friable (easily broken).** Small haemorrhages may occur following injury due to decreased clotting factor synthesis and increased fragility (easy breakage) of minute blood vessels. This leads to a condition known as **'bloody thigh syndrome'**. Aflatoxin is rapidly excreted in the bile and urine and does not accumulate or persist in the body tissues. This explains the rapid recovery of egg production and hatchability after ingestion of toxin has stopped.

## Harmful Effects of Aflatoxin

Aflatoxicosis causes **loss of egg production** (layers); anaemia (deficiency in blood of red cells, haemoglobin, or total volume), haemorrhages, liver damage, paralysis and lameness, and poor performance and feed efficiency (in broilers); increased mortality from heat stress (in broiler breeders); and increased susceptibility to infectious disease both in broilers and layers. Aflatoxin affects egg production by reducing synthesis and transport of yolk precursors in the liver. Egg size, yolk weight, and yolk as percent of total egg size, are decreased. Cases of aspergillosis and aflatoxicosis occurring together confirm that **Aspergillus** species in the feed, litter, and environment are a threat to poultry production.

**Aflatoxicosis affects weight gain, feed intake, feed conversion efficiency, pigmentation, egg production, and male and female reproductive performance.** Even **less than 100 ppb** (parts per billion), **in broilers**, can result in poor feed conversion and reduced weight gain, which may be due to liver damage and reduced nutrient absorption. Once the damage has been done, birds may not fully recover even if they return to toxin free ration. Some effects of aflatoxin are direct, while others are indirect, such as from reduced feed intake.

## Immunosuppression

**Aflatoxicosis suppresses the immune response. As a result, aflatoxicosis is associated with increased susceptibility to infectious disease.** In chickens, aflatoxicosis increases susceptibility to, or severity of caecal coccidiosis, Marek's disease, **E. coli** infection, salmonellosis, inclusion body hepatitis, and Gumboro disease. Vaccination failures are emerging as a result of aflatoxicosis in chickens (see **'vaccination failures'** under chapter 34).

Aflatoxicosis induced immunosuppression is due to **reduction in the size of bursa of Fabricius, thymus and spleen.** Aflatoxin is toxic for B-lymphocytes in the late stage of embryo (i.e. developing chick). The clearance functions of blood phagocytes (a type of protective blood cell known as 'monocyte'), and also those in the tissues (known as 'macrophages'), are damaged. Aflatoxin affects both number and activity of phagocytic cells (macrophages). That is, they are lower in number than normal, and also their movements are reduced. The condition is called **'lazy leukocyte syndrome'**. Such phagocytic cells will produce very poor immune response. Serum complement activity is reduced in broilers. Cell-mediated immune responses are decreased. (To understand the role of bursa, B-lymphocyte, cell-mediated immune responses and phagocytes (like macrophages) in the production of immunity in the chicken, refer to **Chapter 32: 'The avian immune system').**

**Immunosuppression in breeders can be serious as it reduces the passive maternal immunity** (see Chapter 32, for **'maternal immunity').** Decreased level of maternal immunity, combined with stress and highly infectious environment, have devastating effects on chicks in the early part of their life.

## Other Effects

Aflatoxin causes anaemia, young birds being more susceptible. Aflatoxicosis also affects blood clotting, more than either ochratoxicosis A or T-2 toxin, but the effects of ochratoxin A last longer.

## Symptoms

Aflatoxin usually does not cause mortality directly, although high levels (more than 10.0 ppm) may cause death. Economically the most important effects of aflatoxicosis in growing birds are **decreased growth and poor feed conversion** (more than 1.0 ppm). There is also a **marked decrease in the resistance of birds to infections,** such as salmonellosis, coccidiosis, Gumboro disease and candidiasis due to **immunosuppression** (more than 0.5 ppm). **Affected hens have decreased egg production** and the hatchability of those eggs that are produced is reduced (more than 2.0 ppm). In adult breeder males weights of testes and sperm counts are reduced. Insemination of hens with semen from affected males has shown decreased fertility in some studies.

Level of aflatoxin B1up to 0.38 ppm may be considered as relatively safe. Field levels of aflatoxins are between 20-100 ppb and may be even up to 500 ppb.

## 2. OCHRATOXICOSIS

Ochratoxicosis is caused by the mycotoxin **'ochratoxin'.** Its name is derived from the fungus *Aspergillus ochraceus,* the first fungus shown to produce it. Ochratoxicosis is less common in poultry than aflatoxicosis, **but is much more harmful.** Although aflatoxin B1 is the most potent of all aflatoxins, **ochratoxin is three times more harmful.** Thus, ochratoxins are among the most toxic mycotoxins for poultry. **They damage mainly kidney.** Apart from *A. ochraceus*, five other species of **Aspergillus** also produce it. However, most naturally occurring cases have been associated with ochratoxin produced by *Penicillium viridicatum*, but six other species of **Penicillium** produce it as well. **Ochratoxins** are formed on numerous grains and feedstuffs, and are of four types **A, B, C** and **D. Of these, ochratoxin A is the most toxic, most common,** also produced in greater quantities, and is relatively stable. Ochratoxin occurs in **maize,** rice, most small grains and in animal feeds. It readily forms in poultry feeds under conditions of high temperature and high moisture. Field levels are between 20-200 ppb, but may be even up to 2.0 ppm. **In the naturally occurring disease, ochratoxin A is the main toxin**

**involved.** Ochratoxin B and C occur only with high concentration of ochratoxin A. **Contamination, at the same time, of feed with both ochratoxin and aflatoxin is common.**

**Young birds are most sensitive to ochratoxin ingestion.** Severe (acute) ochratoxicosis causes **deaths due to kidney failure.** In those that survive there is immunosuppression and slow growth.

## Development of the Disease

Ochratoxin A prevents protein synthesis, **produces degenerative changes in the kidneys,** and prevents normal secretion of uric acid from the kidneys. Affected kidneys are white to yellowish-brown, swollen, hard and may have white pinpoint urate crystals. If damage is extensive enough to cause **kidney failure,** there is dehydration, increased amount of uric acid in the blood and deposition of urate in organs. **Pasty white urates are deposited on heart, liver (visceral gout) and in joints (articular gout)** (see 'gout').

In addition to changes in the kidney, there is mild to moderate fatty change and glycogen deposition in liver cells. This results in the **livers being yellow and enlarged.**

## Harmful Effects of Ochratoxin

Ochratoxicosis **in broilers** causes mortality and failure to gain weight. Growth rate, feed conversion and pigmentation are affected. Ochratoxicosis **in growers** delays sexual maturity. The unwillingness of hens to eat feed contaminated with ochratoxin leads to reduction in body weight, egg production and egg weight. Ochratoxin can reduce egg size and interior quality. **Immunosuppression** by ochratoxin A is mainly due to reduced size of thymus, although all lymphoid organs are affected. Cell-mediated immunity is significantly damaged in broilers. Antibody-mediated immunity is affected after depletion of antibody-containing cells in lymphoid tissues. **As a result, vaccination responses are severely damaged,** and the severity of concurrent coccidiosis and salmonellosis is increased. (For information on 'cell-mediated and antibody-mediated immunity', refer to Chapter 32).

## Symptoms

**Affected birds** are depressed, dehydrated, usually pass more urine, and **die from kidney failure.** Those that survive are stunted, poorly feathered and have anaemia and immunosuppression (ochratoxin level more than 0.6 ppm). There may be reduced weight gain (ochratoxin level more than 2.0 ppm). Laying hens may have delayed sexual maturity, or develop wet droppings causing increased numbers of stained eggs. There is also a decrease in egg production and hatchability (ochratoxin level more than 2.0 ppm), and poor performance in progeny derived from affected hens.

## 3. TRICHOTHECENE MYCOTOXICOSIS

Trichothecene mycotoxins are produced mainly by the fungus **Fusarium** and other related fungi. These common soil and plant fungi are found worldwide. Of the 100 trichothecene mycotoxins, more than one-half are produced by **Fusarium. Trichothecene toxins include T-2 toxin, diacetoxyscirpenol (DAS), nivalenol, and deoxynivalenol (DON, vomitoxin).**

Trichothecene mycotoxins occur usually in **maize**, rice, wheat, barley, oats, rye, and sorghum and safflower seed worldwide. DON is the most prevalent and is usually associated with aflatoxin, zearalenone, and other mycotoxins.

Trichothecene mycotoxicosis at naturally occurring levels usually does not cause mortality. Losses instead are due to reduced feed intake, decreased growth, and **immunossuppression**. Trichothecene-producing fungi grow at many temperatures. The greatest toxin production occurs with high humidity and temperatures of 6-24°C. Trichothecene mycotoxins are therefore associated with winter season, or when infected grain has been stored in cold conditions.

### Harmful Effects

**In broilers** T-2 toxin reduces growth, produces vesicles on the feet and legs, and ulcers in the mouth. There may also be digestive disturbances, rickets, nervous disorders, abnormal feathering, pigmentation defects and haemorrhages.

**In hens,** T-2 toxin decreases egg production, causes depression, feed refusal, and bluish discoloration of the comb and wattles. There may also be ulcers in the mouth making closure of the mouth difficult. Feathers are uneven and poorly formed. Experimental trichothecene mycotoxicosis in broiler chickens causes haemorrhages and yellow discoloration of the liver. Field level of T2 toxin is up to 1.0 ppm.

### Symptoms

Chickens develop ulcers at the commissures (angles) of the mouth, on the hard palate near the beak and on the upper surface of the tongue. Ulcerative stomatitis (i.e. inflammation of the mouth associated with ulcer formation) leads to decreased feed intake, reduced weight gain, and decreased feed efficiency.

Affected birds have poor feathering. Birds become anaemic, immunosuppressed, and have reduced growth rates. Adult birds are more resistant, but develop oral ulcers and decreased egg production, shell quality, and hatchability.

### Other Mycotoxicoses

**Several other mycotoxicoses have been described in poultry, but are rare, and their economic importance is also not much.** These include:

## 1.   Citrinin Toxicosis

This mycotoxin is produced by many species of fungi **Penicillium** and is natural contaminant of **maize**, rice, and other cereal grains. **In broilers**, citrinin causes wet droppings and reduced weight gain. **This toxin damages kidneys.** At postmortem, kidneys are swollen and the gizzard lining is discoloured and fissured.

## 2.   Oosporein

**This mycotoxin also acts on kidneys. It is capable of causing gout and high mortality in poultry** (see **'gout'**). Oosporein has been isolated from **maize**, groundnuts, rice, and a number of other feeds and grains.

Oosporein mycotoxin in very young chickens causes **gout** in abdominal organs and joints. Effects are particularly **severe in chicks less than one week old** and lead to **deposition of urates on abdominal organs and joints and mortality up to 20%.** This is due to the damage caused to the kidneys, which results in increased concentration of uric acid in blood. Water consumption increases and faecal droppings become fluid (**wet droppings**). At postmortem, kidneys are swollen, carcass is dehydrated, and there are **white uric acid deposits on liver, heart, and kidneys.** In less severe cases, gout in organs is not prominent, or may even be absent, but joint gout, characterized by white uric acid deposits, is common.

Oosporein reduces both feed consumption and egg production at doses capable of causing kidney damage and gout.

## 3.   Moniliformin

Moniliformin is produced by the fungus *Fusarium moniliforme* and other **Fusarium** species. **This fungus occurs in unharvested maize, and may be involved in advanced decay of stored high-moisture maize.** The fungus also occurs in soyabeans, wheat, sorghum, and barley.

This mycotoxin has an effect on the heart and kidney, and can cause death in chickens. Decreased feed intake and reduced body weights are seen in **broiler chicks** fed 100 ppm. In layers, the mycotoxin causes reduced rate of laying and delays peak production.

## 4.   Fumonisins

*Fusarium moniliforme* also produces mycotoxins **'fumonisins'**. They are more harmful to horses and pigs. **Poultry are more resistant.**

## 5.   Fusarochromanone

This toxin is also produced by **Fusarium** species, but is rarely found. It causes leg deformities in chicks.

## 6. Zearalenone

Also known as **F-2**, zearalenone occurs in **maize**, wheat, barley, oats and other grains. Chickens are more resistant than turkeys. In fact, zearalenone is **relatively non-toxic to chickens** but is capable of causing harm. Its presence indicates that other toxins are also present.

## 7. Ergotism

The fungus (**Claviceps** species) which forms this mycotoxin occurs in cereal grains, such as wheat, rice, barley, and oats. Ergotism reduces feed intake and growth, causes death of tissues of the beak, comb and toes, and diarrhoea. There may be vesicles and crusts on the comb and wattles, face and eyelids. Combs and wattles are permanently reduced in size. Laying hens show reduced feed consumption and egg production.

## Diagnosis

1.  Clinical history, symptoms and postmortem findings would point to mycotoxicoses affecting poultry. Confirmation requires identification of the level of toxin capable of producing the observed effects.

    However, testing the feed for some particular toxin may not give a clear picture, as there could be a number of other toxins. **Under field conditions, it is rare to find a single mycotoxin.** As a result, **the damage caused by the combination is more severe.**

    Therefore, the analytical capability of the diagnostic laboratory is also a factor. Analysis for aflatoxin may be available, **but analysis for other mycotoxins is usually not available.** This is possible in only a few laboratories.

2.  **If a mycotoxin is suspected, a complete diagnostic investigation is necessary in addition to feed analysis.** Other diseases may be occurring along with mycotoxicosis and may affect the production. A flock rarely experiences a single disease stress. A mycotoxicosis may be suspected, but not confirmed by feed analysis. However, a complete laboratory examination can exclude other diseases. Birds that have died recently and those sick should be selected for submission.

## Sampling

Proper sampling of feed for mycotoxin testing is most important to get reliable results. It is believed that 90% of the error in mycotoxin assay (testing) is associated with errors in sampling. Therefore, while taking samples, remember that:

(i)   Mycotoxins are present in very small quantity (ppb, i.e. parts per billion).

(ii)  Mycotoxins need to be evenly distributed in the feed.

(iii) Mycotoxin content is not related to the amount of mould present.

(iv) **Absence of one mycotoxin does not mean absence of others. Usually laboratories test aflatoxin first, and if it is positive, they stop analyzing further. However, aflatoxin is usually associated with other toxin(s) and the combined effect is more severe.**

1. Therefore, samples from suspected feed should be properly collected and sent to a diagnostic laboratory for chemical analysis without delay. Mycotoxin formation may not be uniform in a batch of feed, and multiple samples from different places increase the chances of confirming mycotoxins. Samples should be collected from all possible places in the chain of feed storage, feed manufacture and transport, feed containers, and feeders within the poultry houses. Samples of 500 g (1 lb) should be collected and submitted in separate containers. Clean paper bags, properly labelled, are adequate. Sealed plastic or glass containers are suitable only for a short storage and transport because grain rapidly gets spoiled in airtight containers.

2. Collect the samples of the following feedstuffs/whole lot of feed in the amounts indicated for a meaningful representation, and to get reliable results.

    (i)   Intermediate particle type          3 kg
          (Ground meals, flours,
          compounded feed)

    (ii)  Small grains                        5 kg
          (Wheat, rice, sorghum, barley)

    (iii) Intermediate grains                 10 kg
          (Maize, cottonseeds/cake)

    (iv)  Large grains                        20 kg
          (Groundnuts/cake)

3. Collect at least 100 small samples from the whole lot. For example, from a truck of 100 bags of maize, collect 100 g maize from each bag to obtain a total sample size of 10 kg. Then, get about 50-100 g of sub-sample from the total sample. **The sub-sample thus collected can be subjected to analysis.**

## Testing

1. Analytical techniques for testing mycotoxins include chromatography (thin-layer, gas, liquid), mass spectrometry, and monoclonal antibody-based technology.

2. Rapid on-site screening tests for several mycotoxins (aflatoxin, T-2 toxin, deoxynivalenol, fumonisin, ochratoxin, and zearalenone) are now available in **monoclonal antibody-based detection kits.**

3. Confirmation of mycotoxicoses can also be achieved by feeding trials with the suspect feed to reproduce the field toxicosis.

## Treatment

1. Toxic feed should be removed and replaced with uncontaminated feed. **Poultry usually recover from most mycotoxicoses soon after an uncontaminated feed is available.**

2. Increase the dietary levels of protein. As the mycotoxins affect protein and amino acid metabolism, increasing the dietary level of proteins can minimize the ill effects especially when contaminated with **aflatoxin. Increase also the vitamin supplementation.**

3. Supply of **methionine** and other sulphur-containing amino acids, over and above the requirement, can protect the chicks from growth depressing effects of aflatoxin.

4. Treatment of bacterial or parasitic diseases, occurring at the same time, will reduce additional interactions.

5. **Poor management** is particularly harmful to poultry stressed by mycotoxins and **should be improved.**

6. **Liver tonics** may be given (see Chapter 19 for a list of commercially available 'liver tonics'). Additional amount of lipotropic agent like **choline** helps in minimizing liver damage.

7. **Mycotoxins are free radical generators and therefore challenge the antioxidant responses within the poultry.** Therefore, increase the supplementation of **vitamin E, vitamin C and selenium.** Vitamin E and C are natural antioxidants, and selenium is involved in the formation of enzyme glutathione peroxidase which is vital for cellular detoxification. Such antioxidant mechanisms of vitamin E and selenium partially neutralize the effects of aflatoxin, ochratoxin, and T-2.

8. **Vitamin D3** supplementation can minimize the adverse effect of aflatoxins, such as leg weakness, and poor eggshell quality.

## Control

Occurrence of mycotoxins in grains is extremely common, and therefore requires a programme for controlling their ill effects in poultry. As with most poultry diseases, **prevention is more economical than treatment.**

1. **Purchase a clean feedstuff.** Check the ingredients before purchase. Prevention of mycotoxicoses largely depends on getting mycotoxin-free feedstuffs, and application of feed manufacturing and management practices which prevent fungal growth and mycotoxin formation. A proper sample drawn from a lot should be analyzed for the presence of mycotoxins. But this is not always possible in practical feeding situation. It requires availability of a good laboratory with capability to confirm

the purchase of ingredients free of mycotoxins, proper storage of ingredients, and feed processing and handling procedures to minimize mycotoxin formation.

2. Discard the grains suspected of contamination, that is, mouldy and caked feed.

3. Keep the moisture of grains less than 12%.

4. **Sun drying is the best method to prevent mould growth. However, it does not destroy the toxin.**

5. Store the feed and ingredients in well ventilated dry place, which is water, insect, and rodent proof. Adequate ventilation of poultry houses to reduce humidity removes moisture available for fungal growth and mycotoxin formation in feeders.

6. Avoid storage of feed for more than a week.

7. Mycotoxins form in decayed, crusted feed in feeders, feed mills, and storage containers. **Therefore, regular inspection of feed containers is essential.** Inspection of containers and their cleaning between flocks to ensure absence of feed residue is important. **Minimum feed residence time is important, even under cool, dry conditions.**

8. **Withdraw toxin contaminated feed immediately.**

9. Pelleting feed destroys fungal spores and decreases fungal burden. The combination of pelleting and an antifungal agent has additional effectiveness.

10. **However, despite all the precautions, mycotoxins do get into the feed. Therefore, to deal with this difficult problem, the most practical way is to use effective mould inhibitors and scientifically tested broad-spectrum toxin binders** (see Chapter 22: "Mould Inhibitors and Toxin Binders").

**The most common approach has been chemical inactivation of mycotoxins. This is because the mould inhibitors added to feeds to prevent fungal growth have no effect on toxin already formed.** Therefore, destruction of toxin (detoxification) is another approach in utilizing mycotoxin-contaminated feeds and also preventing mycotoxicosis. For this purpose various compounds that inactivate the toxins by binding **(toxin-binders)** are used (see Chapter 22). Zeolytes, silica-containing compounds, are practical and economical feed additives that can reduce the effects of certain mycotoxins, especially aflatoxin. Hydrated sodium calcium aluminosilicate (HSCAS) binds aflatoxin B1 in the digestive tract, and reduces toxicity. **This applies mainly to aflatoxin, because zeolytes are ineffective against ochratoxin A and diacetoxyscirpenol (DAS).** Sodium aluminosilicate added to poultry ration at 0.5%, binds aflatoxin and prevents its absorption. Ammoniation is particularly effective in decontaminating feeds and grains for aflatoxin. Copper sulphate is a poor mould inhibitor for poultry feeds. Certain cultures of **Lactobacillus** prevent aflatoxin absorption from the small intestine.

Feed preservatives and antifungal agents may be added to prevent fungal growth in storage containers or finished feeds.

**Note:** For more information on 'mould inhibitors and toxin-binders', refer to Chapter 22; and for a list of commercially available **'mould inhibitors and toxin binders'**, see Chapter 19.

# Chapter 7

# Chlamydial Disease

Chlamydiae (plural of 'chlamydia') are minute bacteria. However, in contrast to other bacteria, they multiply only within the cells. Chlamydiae are large enough and can be seen with a light microscope using selective stains. All chlamydiae are Gram-negative, but the Gram stain is of no practical value in identifying organisms within the cells.

## AVIAN CHLAMYDIOSIS

Also known as **'psittacosis'** and **'ornithosis'**, chlamydiosis in poultry is caused by *Chlamydophila psittaci. C. psittaci* causes disease both in birds and humans. **In humans,** since the disease was first contracted from parrots, it was called **'parrot fever'.** Chlamydiosis is referred to as **'psittacosis'** when it affects humans, mammals, and psittacine birds (e.g. parrots, parakeets, etc.). The disease is called **'ornithosis'** when it affects birds other than psittacines. However, the two diseases are currently considered to be the same. Chlamydiosis in poultry is worldwide in distribution. In birds, it usually involves various body systems and is sometimes fatal. **Chickens, although susceptible, are rarely affected.**

Factors that contribute to the development of the disease, or increase its severity, include **stress** due to movement of birds, crowding, change of diet or environment, and concurrent infections with other organisms, such as salmonella or *Pasteurella multocida* (cause of fowl cholera).

## Spread

1. Spread of infection occurs directly when birds are in close contact, and indirectly through chlamydia-contaminated substances (fomites). **Infection occurs by inhalation or ingestion of contaminated material.**

2. The sources of infection are birds in incubation, sick birds and carriers (birds carrying infection without showing symptoms), and infected inanimate (not living) material.

3. **Elementary bodies** (i.e. infective form of chlamydia) are found in faeces and also in respiratory excretions of sick birds. Spread occurs mainly through the inhalation of infected, contaminated dust.

4. **Egg transmission is not known to occur.**

5.    The role of insects in the spread of chlamydiae is uncertain.

## Development of the Disease

After entry into the body, **mainly by inhalation**, the organisms multiply in the lungs, airsacs and pericardium (covering of the heart). They later spread through blood circulation to liver, spleen, and kidneys where further multiplication and production of elementary bodies occur.

## Symptoms

**Chickens are rarely affected.** Chickens appear to be relatively resistant to disease caused by *C. psittaci*. Acute infection progresses to disease and mortality occurs only in young birds. The incidence of actual outbreaks is low. **Most infections in chickens are not noticeable and short-lived.** However, clinical cases with conjunctivitis (inflammation of the conjunctiva of eye), pericarditis (inflammation of pericardium), perihepatitis (inflammation of the liver surface) and airsacculitis (inflammation of the airsac) have been reported.

**Symptoms** include dullness, fever, abnormal excretions, nasal (from nose) and eye discharges, and reduced egg production. Mortality varies from 0% to 30% of affected birds.

## Postmortem Findings

Postmortem findings vary and depend on the severity of the disease. There may be pericarditis, peritonitis (inflammation of the peritoneum, a membrane in the body cavity), congestion of the lungs, cloudiness of airsac walls and enlargement of the liver and spleen. Both liver and spleen may show small foci of dead (necrotic) tissue and haemorrhages.

## Immunity

**Immunity to chlamydia is generally poor and short-lived.** As birds become older, however, they become more resistant to clinical disease, even though infection may occur.

## Diagnosis

1.    Symptoms and postmortem findings are helpful, but confirmation depends on demonstration of chlamydia, or on its isolation and identification, or on serological examination of blood (serum).

2.    Demonstration of chlamydia is done by several ways. One easy method is by direct smear examination. Impression smears are made from exudate (inflammatory material), lesions, or surface of the liver or spleen, or cloacal, tracheal or conjunctival swabs. They are stained by modified Ziehl-Neelsen method. **Elementary bodies**

stain red while the background is blue-green. Other staining methods include Giemsa, Machiavello, Castanada and an iodine technique.

3.  Isolation and identification of chlamydia is one of the reliable methods of diagnosis, and involves isolation of organism in cell culture or embryonated eggs.

## Treatment

Treatment of infected birds with broad-spectrum antibiotics (tetracyclines, chloramphenicol, and erythromycin) for several weeks is effective in reducing infection and may eliminate it in some cases. Chlortetracycline has been most commonly used in the drinking water. The treatment has to be continued for up to 45 days.

Doxycycline, a semi-synthetic tetracycline derivative, is also useful. It is rapidly and almost completely absorbed from the digestive tract, and its absorption is less interfered with by calcium than chlortetracycline. It has a longer serum half-life and provides greater tissue concentration. Quinolones (enrofloxacin, etc.) are also effective against chlamydial infections in birds.

## Control

1.  **Hygienic precautions** are important to minimize spread of infection to other birds and human attendants. These include restriction on movement of flock and people, cleaning and the use of appropriate disinfectants, such as iodophores or formaldehyde. In particular, attention should be given to minimize the spread of infected dust. Movement of people should be restricted so that visitors do not have a free entry to premises having birds.

2.  There are no commercial chlamydial vaccines that produce long-lasting protective immunity against chlamydia. Live and killed vaccines (bacterin) have been found to be protective. But live vaccines may result in carriers (birds carrying infection without showing symptoms), whereas several injections of the killed vaccines are necessary to induce protection. There are no commercially available vaccines for the protection of poultry against chlamydiosis in India.

Chapter **8**

# Parasitic Diseases

## A. HELMINTHIC DISEASES

**Helminths** are commonly known as **'worms'**. A great variety of worms infect birds. However, in poultry, worms are usually not a major cause of disease or economic loss because rearing inside a building prevents their contact with intermediate hosts and also because of the relatively short life-span of broilers.

Helminthic diseases are caused by three different types of worms. These are: (1) Flukes (Trematodes), (2) Tapeworms (Cestodes), and (3) Roundworms (Nematodes). **Of the three, roundworms constitute the most important group of worms of poultry.** The amount of damage done by them is far more than that of flukes and tapeworms.

### 1. FLUKES (Trematodes)

A number of flukes have been described in birds. They are flat leaf-like organisms. **Most have low disease-producing ability.** All require intermediate hosts. **Oviduct fluke** has caused economic losses to poultry farmers by reducing egg production. Sometimes they are enclosed within a hen's egg and later discovered by a complaining customer. However, flukes are virtually of no importance in modern poultry operations.

### 2. TAPEWORMS (Cestodes)

A large number of tapeworms have been described in birds. Different species differ in their disease-producing power. **Most have low disease-producing ability.** All species require intermediate hosts, and are of not much importance in modern poultry operations. However, the common tapeworm to occur is **Raillietina.**

Tapeworms are flattened, ribbon shaped, usually segmented worms. Most are quite large, up to 4 inches in length and several millimetres in width. They are easily seen with the naked eye. They are found more frequently in warmer seasons, when intermediate hosts are abundant. Many species of tapeworms are now rare in intensive poultry-rearing systems because the birds do not come in contact with intermediate hosts. The intermediate host may be an insect (beetle, housefly), earthworm, snail, or leech depending upon the species of the tapeworm. Birds become infected by eating an intermediate host that had fed on the faeces of infected chickens. **Small intestine is the usual site of tapeworm's attachment.**

200

## Harmful Effects

Some of the larger tapeworms may completely **block intestine** of the infected bird. One species produces **nodules** in the small intestine (nodular disease of chickens). **Symptoms** of tapeworm infestation include emaciation, weight loss, ruffled feathers and slow movements, breathing difficulties, decrease in egg production, paralysis and death.

## Diagnosis

Detection of tapeworms in the faeces, or at postmortem examination, establishes diagnosis. Eggs or individual segments (proglottids) recently shed in faeces, or collected from the intestine during postmortem, may be examined under a microscope. Wet-mount preparations of the eggs or segments may be examined under a coverslip with x100 or higher magnification. Microscopic examination does not only help in establishing the diagnosis, but it also identifies the different species of chicken tapeworms.

## Treatment

1. If a tapeworm infection appears during a postmortem examination, a farmer usually asks for a drug for removal of the worms. However, expulsion of the parasite is a very short-term means of solving the problem, **if the intermediate host as a source of infection is still present.**

2. Mebendazole and butynorate (dibutyltin dilaurate) are effective drugs for treating tapeworms in poultry.

## Control

Prevention of contact with the intermediate host is the most important step that should be taken in the control of tapeworm infection.

## ROUNDWORMS (Nematodes)

**Roundworms are the most important worms of poultry.** Regarding the extent of damage done, it is far greater than that of flukes and tapeworms.

Roundworms of poultry have either a direct or an indirect type of development. In roundworms with direct life cycles, the chicken becomes infected by eating eggs containing larvae, or free larvae. For those with indirect life cycles, the intermediate host ingests the eggs containing larvae or free larvae, and retains the larvae within the body tissues. The chicken becomes infected by eating the infected intermediate host. In poultry, roundworms infect the intestinal and respiratory tracts, **intestinal worms being more important.**

## INTESTINAL ROUNDWORMS

Only three types of intestinal roundworms are important: (1) **Ascaridia,** (2) **Capillaria** species, and (3) **Heterakis.**

## 1. ASCARIDIA

**Ascaridia are the largest roundworms of birds.** They are also the **most common of all roundworms in poultry.** The adults live in the lumen of the small intestine, but the larval stages invade the intestine.

*A. galli* is the species found in chickens. Its life cycle is direct. Therefore serious infestations can sometimes occur in birds on litter, **especially if the litter is reused in the case of broilers. *A. galli* are found in the small intestine.** The male is 50-76 mm and female 60-116 mm in length.

### Harmful Effects

*A. galli* infection causes **poor bodily condition and weight loss.** The extent of damage is related to the number of worms present. It has been observed that weight loss is greater with high dietary levels of protein (15%) than with low levels (12.5%). **In severe infections intestinal blockage can occur.** Chickens infected with a large number of worms suffer from loss of blood, reduced blood sugar content, retarded growth, enteritis (inflammation of the intestine), and greatly increased mortality. *A. galli* can also have harmful effects through interactions (combined effect) with other diseases, such as coccidiosis and infectious bronchitis. *A. galli* has also been shown to contain and transmit ovarian reoviruses. Sometimes, *A. galli* is found in the hen's egg. It is believed that worms migrate up the oviduct through the cloaca, and later get included in the egg. Infected eggs can be detected by candling.

### Immunity

Chickens 3 months or older show a lot of resistance to infection with *A. galli*. In older birds, larvae are recovered that have undergone little or no development since coming out of the egg. The nutritional state of the bird also affects the development of immunity. Diets consisting mainly of animal proteins, with no plant protein, help the chicken in building resistance to infection. Birds getting a diet consisting mainly of animal protein develop fewer worms than those getting a diet low in animal protein. Diets high in vitamin A and B complex increase the fowl's resistance to *A. galli*, and diets low in these vitamins favour infection. Increased levels of dietary calcium and lysine decrease the length and number of worms recovered.

### Diagnosis

At postmortem examination, worms are found in the small intestine.

## 2. CAPILLARIA

**Capillaria are the smallest of the roundworms.** A number of species infect different chickens. Different species affect different parts of the intestinal tract. They can be very harmful when present in large numbers. The most common and harmful in modern units is *Capillaria obsignata*. It has a direct life cycle and can be a problem in birds on litter. **It is found in the small intestine and caecum.**

Chickens heavily infected with *C. obsignata* show emaciation, reduced weight gain, diarrhoea, haemorrhagic enteritis, and death. However, the most important effect of infection from a practical point of view is the **less efficient utilization of feed and poor weight gains.**

*C. contorta* is another disease-producing species in chickens. It occurs in the oesophagus and crop. The roundworms can be extremely harmful. In light infections, the wall of the crop and oesophagus becomes slightly thickened and inflamed. In heavy infections, there is a marked thickening and inflammation. The crop may become non-functional. Infected birds become dull, depressed, weak, and emaciated.

## Diagnosis

At postmortem, worms are found by careful examination of mucosal washings under dissecting microscope.

## 3. HETERAKIS

**This roundworm is found in the caeca of chickens.** It is not much harmful. In heavy infections, **nodules** form in the caeca.

## Treatment

## 1. Ascaridia

**Piperazine compounds** have been widely used for treatment against **Ascaridia** infection, since they are non-toxic. Piperazine may be given to chickens in the feed (0.2-0.4%), water (0.1- 0.2%), or as a single treatment (50-100 mg/bird.) A high concentration of piperazine in contact with the worms at a given time is very important for maximum removal. Therefore, to be more effective, piperazine should be consumed by birds in a period of few hours. Piperazine in drinking water is the best method of administration. Since piperazine is available as a wide variety of salts, the level should be calculated on the basis of milligrams of active piperazine. Piperazine compounds have a sleeping effect on the worms. This enables worms to be expelled by means of the naturally occurring successive waves of contractions in the intestine (peristalsis). The worms are expelled alive.

**Fenbendazole** at 8-10 mg/kg for 3 or 4 days is also effective. Fenbendazole given **in the feed** at the level of 30 ppm for 4 days, or 60 ppm for 3 days, is reported to be 100% effective against *A. galli* in chickens.

## 2. Capillaria

**Fenbendazole** is more than 97% effective in removing **Capillaria** infection.

## 3. Heterakis

**Fenbendazole** has 100% efficacy in treating **Heterakis** infection.

## Control

1. Modern poultry practices, especially confinement rearing of broilers and growers and caging of laying hens, have greatly reduced roundworm infections in poultry. **Roundworms, in large part, can be prevented by raising birds in cages.**

2. Worms usually cannot build up in broiler chickens with a short life-span. However, for species which produce highly resistant eggs, e.g. **Ascaridia**, the reuse of litter may allow a gradual build-up of potentially harmful numbers.

3. **For most roundworms, control measures consist of sanitation and breaking the life cycle, rather than treatment with drugs.** Confinement rearing on litter prevents infections with roundworms that use outdoor intermediate hosts, such as earthworms or grasshopper. On the other hand, roundworms with direct life cycles or those that use indoor intermediate hosts, such as beetles may prosper. Treatment of the soil or litter to kill intermediate hosts is useful.

4. Litter may be treated with suitable insecticides. Changing of litter can reduce infections.

5. Extreme care should be taken to ensure that feed and water are not contaminated.

**Note:** For a list of commercial preparations available in the market against worms, refer to Chapter 19 under **"Anthelmintics"**.

# B. PROTOZOAL DISEASES

Protozoa are single-celled organisms like bacteria. However, they are animals, and are similar to higher forms of life, except that all the functions are carried out within a single cell. In the host, they live within the cell and eventually destroy it. Of the various diseases caused by protozoa in poultry, the most important is **coccidiosis.**

## COCCIDIOSIS

### Introduction

**Coccidiosis is one of the most important diseases of poultry worldwide,** and is characterized by bloody diarrhoea and high mortality. It is one of the most devastating of poultry diseases. Coccidia grow in the intestinal tract and cause damage, resulting in defective digestion and absorption, dehydration, blood loss, and increased susceptibility to other infectious agents.

**In India, coccidiosis is a serious problem and is one of the biggest causes of economic losses to poultry. It inflicts heavy mortality each year mainly in**

**broilers and also in growers raised on deep litter.** Most coccidia in poultry belong to the genus **Eimeria.**

Coccidiosis mainly occurs under conditions of overcrowding, which favour build-up of the parasite in disease-producing numbers. Thus, coccidiosis is especially important under intensive poultry operations. Apart from causing disease and losses, **sub-clinical infections** (i.e. mild infections without showing symptoms) cause **defective feed conversion.** Since feed expenses form some 70% of the cost of producing broiler chickens, **the economic impact of coccidiosis can be immense.**

**Coccidiosis is largely a disease of young birds** because immunity quickly develops after exposure and gives protection against later outbreaks. However, chickens of all ages and breeds are susceptible to coccidiosis. Outbreaks are common between 3-6 weeks of age and are rarely seen in flocks of less than 3 weeks. **There is no cross-immunity (cross-protection) among the seven species of Eimeria and later outbreaks may be the result of different species.** Growers are at the greatest risk if they are kept on litter. **Coccidiosis rarely occurs in layers and breeders because of prior exposure to coccidia resulting in immunity.** The short direct life cycle and high reproductive ability of coccidia increases the chances for severe outbreaks of disease in the modern poultry house where as many as between 15-30,000 chicks may be reared together.

Coccidiosis may be mild, resulting from ingestion of a few oocysts and thus may go unnoticed, or it may be severe as a result of ingestion of millions of oocysts. Most infections are mild, but can turn into serious outbreaks, **causing great financial loss.** Therefore, all young chickens are given continuously anticoccidial drugs at low levels to prevent infection. Immunity is not important in broiler chickens, which are kept only for 6-8 weeks before marketing, as in layers, which are kept much longer. Vaccines against coccidiosis have met with limited success and have been used mostly in breeder pullets.

**Coccidiosis still continues to be one of the most expensive and common diseases of poultry in spite of the advances in treatment, management, nutrition, and genetics.** Therefore, to understand this disease better and to appreciate its full impact on poultry industry, let us begin with a consideration of coccidia's life cycle.

## Life Cycle

First, the infectious form of coccidia (sporulated oocysts, explained later) is ingested by the bird. **(Fig. 15** shows the life cycle of *Eimeria tenella*, which is typical of all coccidia.) After ingestion, mechanical and chemical factors in the intestine release sporocysts and sporozoites from the sporulated oocysts. The released sporozoites enter into the cells lining the intestine. They grow within the cells. First, they grow by an asexual multiplication called **'schizogony'.** This results in the formation of schizonts and merozoites. After at least two generations of this type of asexual growth, sexual multiplication called 'gametogony' occurs. **With some species (*E. tenella, E. necatrix*), the maximum tissue damage occurs when second generation schizonts rupture to release merozoites. Other species have small schizonts which cause little damage.** Sexual multiplication leads to the development of sexual form of the parasite known as 'gametocytes'. These differentiate into **macrogametocytes** and **microgametocytes**. The macrogametocyte develops into a single macrogamete, whereas microgametocyte releases many **microgametes**. The motile microgamete finds out a macrogamete and unites with it (**fertilization**). The union between the two results in the formation of a **zygote** which develops into an **oocyst**. Oocysts are then released from inside the cells into the intestinal lumen **and passed out in the faeces.** The entire process takes 4-7 days, depending on the species.

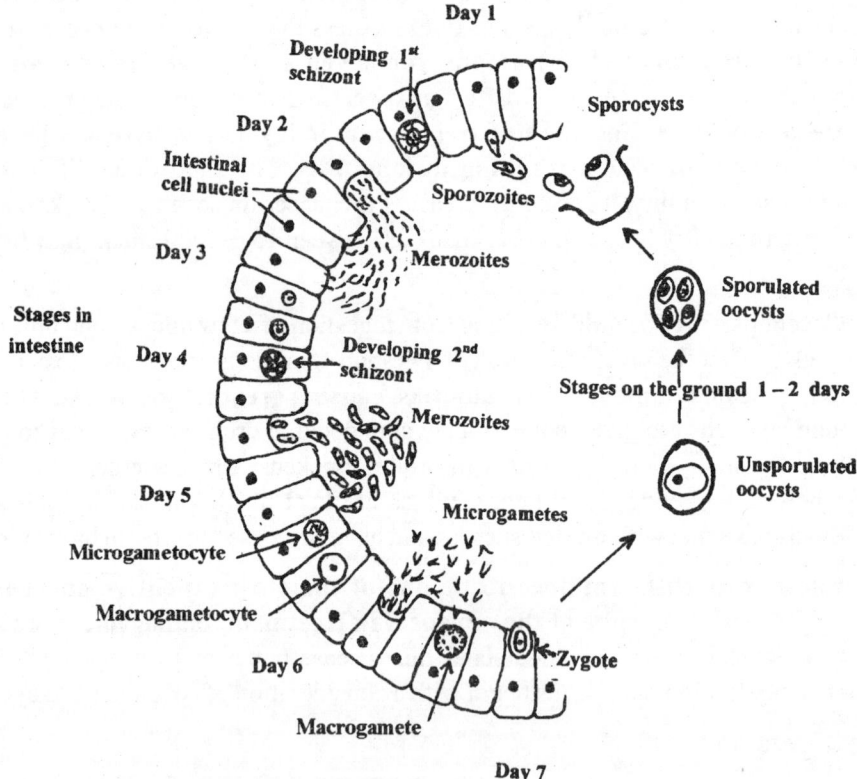

**Fig. 15.** The 7-day life cycle of *Eimeria tenella*, typical of the genus **Eimeria**.

In the case of *E. tenella*, the life cycle is **of seven days**, with a prepatent period of only 4-5 days. Prepatent period is the interval between ingestion of the infective form (sporulated oocysts) and the appearance of oocysts in the faeces. This period varies slightly with different species of coccidia. During this period there is tremendous multiplication of coccidia within the intestinal cells. This also varies with the species, but usually results in the production of not thousands but millions of oocysts from just one ingested oocyst.

A teaspoonful of faeces from a bird with severe coccidiosis contains several million oocysts. These are easily transferred to a new location by shoes, feed trucks, crates, pets, rodents (rats, mice), and moving equipment. Once sporulated (discussed next), the oocysts soon cause an outbreak of coccidiosis in the new premises. Consumption of as few as 10,000 sporulated oocysts (i.e. infective form) will produce coccidiosis.

## Sporulation

When oocysts are passed in the faeces, they are not capable of producing the disease. They become infective only after undergoing the process of 'sporulation'. Explained simply, sporulation is conversion of a non-infective form of oocyst into an infective form, and requires three conditions: warmth, moisture (20-30%), and oxygen. Between temperatures of $25^0$ - $30^0$ C, it takes 1-2 days. Sporulated oocysts, that is, the infective form of oocyst, are protected by the thick oocyst wall. They are therefore resistant to many environmental conditions, and are able to survive for months or even years. This is an extremely important factor in the occurrence of coccidiosis. Only temperatures above $56^0$C can kill them as well as desiccation (drying), but oocysts are able to tolerate most disinfectants. Only compounds like ammonia and methyl bromide kill them, but as these are very harmful gases, they are of no practical use.

## Immunity

Day-old chicks usually do not get maternal antibodies from the hen as protective immunity. Therefore, birds of any age are susceptible to coccidiosis. In fact, most chicks get infected in the first few weeks of life and this infection produces a good immunity. In most cases this immunity persists for life due to frequent low-grade re-exposure to infection. But in the absence of infection, immunity may decrease gradually. An important feature of the immunity is that it is species specific. Thus, for example, immunity against *E. maxima* does not give complete protection against *E. tenella* and so on.

Immunity is best produced by repeated exposure to low numbers of oocysts. This is known as 'trickle infection'. This is the usual situation in the field. Immunity leads to a reduction in tissue damage and a marked decrease in oocyst output. The mechanisms of immunity are not fully understood, but cell-mediated immune responses appear to be extremely important. Secretory IgA may also contribute to protective immunity, but circulating antibodies (IgM, IgG), although produced in response to infection, play only minor roles. (To understand cell-mediated immune responses and the role of different antibodies, refer to Chapter 32.)

## Occurrence

The severity of disease depends on the species of coccidia and the number of infective oocysts ingested as well as on the immune status of the bird. **It is impossible under farm conditions to produce a coccidia-free environment.** Occysts remain in the building from previous crops of birds and are also carried on feet of people, or possibly by other agencies (animals, birds, and insects). From whatever source, **chicks brought into the building quickly become infected.** Due to the short prepatent period (explained under life cycle) of the parasite and its high biotic potential (i.e. coccidia's inherent capacity to reproduce and survive), the number of oocysts in the litter rises rapidly. A dynamic interaction occurs between development of flock immunity by repeated exposure to low numbers of oocysts (i.e. '**trickle infection**', see under '**immunity**') and an increase in the parasite population.

Usually immunity develops without clinical disease occurring, oocyst output is reduced and numbers of oocysts in the litter fall rapidly. However, if this balance is disturbed by factors which favour the parasite, such as an initial high degree of contamination by oocysts or conditions that favour sporulation, such as wet litter, then a large number of infective oocysts, that can cause disease, are ingested by non-immune birds **and disease occurs**. In chickens on litter, this usually occurs between 3-6 weeks of age. However, it can also occur in older birds, especially with certain species, e.g. *E. necatrix*, or under conditions in which immunity has decreased, or has never been fully acquired. This can happen, for example, when floor-reared birds are caged for laying. This prevents re-infection and birds are later re-exposed to infection.

Certain anticoccidials are so effective in preventing infection that they do not allow the development of immunity. Thus, after drug withdrawal, birds may remain fully susceptible at an age when they are expected to be immune. **For this reason, many outbreaks of coccidiosis occur after mistakes in the inclusion of preventive doses of anticoccidial drugs in the feed.**

**To conclude, the most important factors in the occurrence of coccidiosis are:**

1. Oocysts continue to exist in the environment.

2. There is no maternally-derived protective immunity in chicks.

3. The parasite has a short prepatent period and a high biotic potential (discussed under 'life cycle' and 'occurrence').

4. Disease depends on the dose of oocysts and species.

5. Immunity is acquired by infection and maintained by periodic re-infection.

## Spread

1.  **Ingestion of the infective form of oocysts (sporulated oocysts) is the only natural method of spread.** Infected chickens may shed oocysts in the faeces for several days or weeks. As discussed, the oocysts become infective through the process of sporulation within two days. Susceptible birds in the same flock may ingest the oocysts through the litter-pecking activities common in chicks, or through ingestion of contaminated feed or water.

2.  **Oocysts can be spread mechanically** by animals, insects, contaminated equipment, wild birds, and dust. They are resistant to environmental extremes and to disinfection. Oocysts may survive for many weeks in soil, but their survival in poultry litter is limited to a few days because of the ammonia and the action of moulds and bacteria.

3.  Spread from one farm to another is facilitated **by movement of people and equipment between farms** and by the migration of wild birds, which may spread the oocysts mechanically. New farms may remain free of coccidia for most of the first batches of chickens until the introduction of coccidia to a completely susceptible flock. Such outbreaks, which are more severe than those experienced on older farms, are called **'the new-house coccidiosis syndrome'.**

4.  Threat of coccidiosis is less during hot dry weather (summer) and greater in cooler wetter weather (rainy and winter seasons).

## Harmful Effects of Coccidia

**Of the seven disease-producing species, *E. tenella, E. necatrix* and *E. brunetti* are the most harmful and cause high morbidity** (number of birds affected) **and high mortality** (number of deaths caused). *E. tenella* affects caeca and *E. necatrix* middle portion and *E. brunetti* lower portion of the small intestine.

*E. maxima* and *E. acervulina* are moderately harmful. *E. maxima* affects middle portion of the small intestine, and *E. acervulina* mainly upper portion, that is, duodenum.

*E. mitis* and *E. praecox* are least harmful and both affect duodenum.

Usually infections with *E. tenella, E. maxima* and *E. acervulina* are seen between 3-6 weeks of age and *E. necatrix* between 8-18 weeks of age. **Concurrent infection with two or more species of coccidia is common.** The tissue damage and changes in the intestinal tract function may allow growth of various harmful bacteria, such as *Clostridium perfringens*, **leading to necrotic enteritis.**

## Symptoms

**Symptoms vary with the species of coccidia.** *E. tenella* causes **'caecal coccidiosis'. It is a severe** disease associated with blood droppings, high mortality, reduced weight gain, and emaciation. **The losses caused make this species one of**

**the most harmful in chickens.** Most of the mortality occurs between 5 and 6 days following infection.

*E. necatrix* is associated with severe weight loss, morbidity and mortality. It causes **'intestinal coccidiosis' in relatively older birds.** Droppings of affected birds usually contain blood, fluid, and mucus. **Like *E. tenella*, this species is also most harmful.** Naturally occurring infections have caused more than 25% mortality in commercial flocks.

*E. brunetti* is less serious than *E. tenella* and *E. necatrix*, but is still capable of producing moderate mortality, loss of weight gain, poor feed conversion and other complications.

*E. maxima* is moderately harmful and causes poor weight gain, diarrhoea, and sometimes mortality. There is usually extreme emaciation, roughening of the feathers, and loss of appetite.

*E. acervulina* is also moderately harmful. There is reduction in the rate of weight gain. Heavy infections sometimes cause mortality. Egg production may be reduced in laying birds.

*E. mitis* and *E. praecox* are least harmful and may cause reduced weight gain and poor feed conversion.

## Postmortem Findings

**Again, these vary with the species of coccidia involved.**

*E. tenella*: **The caeca may be greatly enlarged and distended with clotted blood.**

*E. necatrix*: **The middle portion of the small intestine is usually distended to twice its normal size (ballooning) and the lumen may be filled with blood (Fig. 16).** Changes may extend throughout the small intestine in severe infections. From the surface, foci of infection appear as small white plaques and tiny red haemorrhages. That is, the infection is seen as white or red foci.

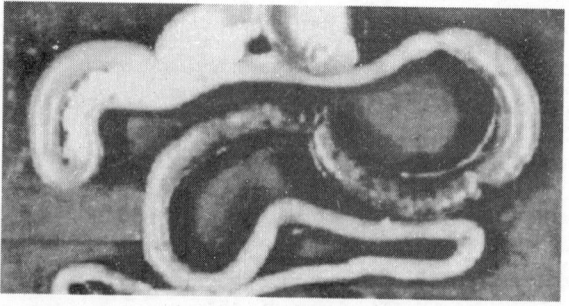

Fig. 16. Intestinal coccidiosis caused by *Eimeria necatrix*. Note ballooning in the middle portion of the small intestine.

*E. brunetti*: The lining of the small intestine is covered with tiny haemorrhages. The clotted blood and mucosa are seen in droppings. The mucosa may be swollen and thickened.

*E. maxima*: The middle portion of the small intestine may be loose and filled with fluid, containing mucus and blood (**ballooning**).

*E. acervulina*: Changes can usually be seen from the surface of the duodenum and small intestine. The mucosa may be covered with white plaques, which tend to arrange in transverse fashion and cause a ladder-like appearance because of the striations.

*E. mitis* and *E. praecox*: The changes are very slight and can be easily missed.

## Diagnosis

1.  **The presence of faeces with blood, dysentery and diarrhoea suggests coccidiosis.** However, with less harmful coccidia, the only symptoms are reduced growth and poor feed conversion. On the other hand, the earliest symptoms with the most harmful species may be a sudden increase in daily mortality.

2.  **Postmortem examination is necessary to confirm diagnosis.** A few sick birds should be sacrificed for this purpose so that fresh material is available. Lesions (tissue changes) can be seen from the external surface, but the internal (mucosal) surface should be examined carefully. In fact, the entire intestinal tract should be examined properly.

3.  **Microscopic examination:** It is important to demonstrate the parasite along with lesions by microscopic examination of the mucosal scrapings. A small amount of mucosal scraping should be diluted with saline on a slide, then covered with a coverslip and examined under a microscope with appropriate light.

    Many stages of coccidia can be seen in smears taken from suspected lesion. **Oocysts** are very easily seen (**Fig. 17**), but in many cases the lesion is caused by **schizonts** (**Fig. 18**). Presence of groups of large schizonts, **without oocysts**, in the middle portion

    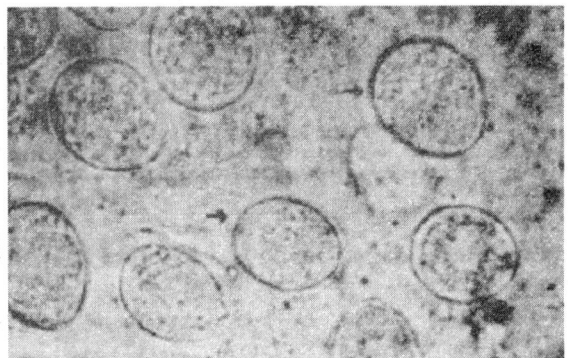

    Fig. 17. Wet smear of caecal scrapings showing oocysts (arrows) of *Eimeria tenella*.

    of the small intestine is typical of *E. necatrix* infection, while the presence of both schizonts and oocysts in the caeca indicates *E. tenella* infection.

4.  The findings of a few oocysts by microscopic examination indicate presence of infection, but not diagnosis of the disease. This is because coccidia are usually

present in the intestine of 3-6 weeks old birds in most flocks. **The infection should be diagnosed as coccidiosis only when gross lesions are serious and associated with mortality.**

**Note:** In birds receiving preventive anticoccidial medication, investigation of an outbreak of disease should also include the submission of feed samples for drug assay. Samples should be representative of the feed used 5-10 days before the outbreak. This analysis will show whether, or not, the outbreak was because the drug was by mistake not included, or that it was included at a low dose, or whether drug resistance is taking place.

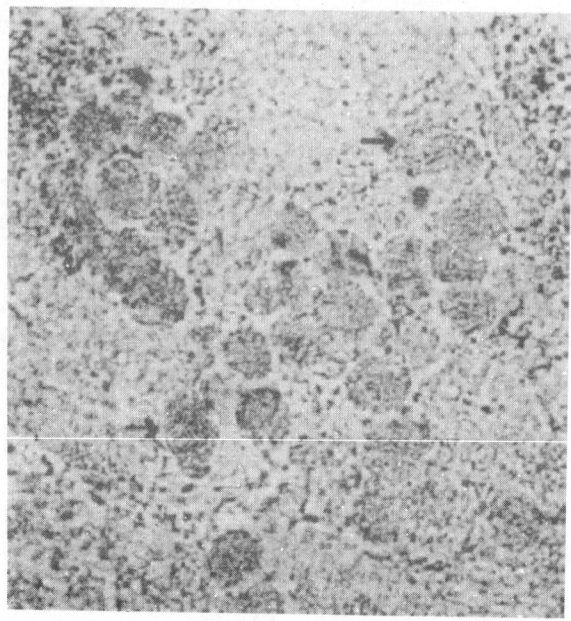

**Fig. 18.** Wet smear of caecal scrapings showing schizonts of ***Eimeria tenella*** (arrows).

## Treatment

Outbreaks of coccidiosis are usually treated with water-soluble drugs, such as sulphonamides, amprolium, and the more recently introduced diclazuril and toltrazuril. Water medication is convenient and can be rapidly given. **In broiler operations, the cost of an outbreak of disease is considerable, even if treatment is effective. Therefore, control measures should be strongly followed.**

**Note:** For a list of commercial drugs available at the market for treating coccidiosis, see Chapter 19 under **"Anticoccidials"**.

## Control

**Coccidiosis is far more easily prevented than treated.** Control depends mainly on drugs, although an effective vaccine is now available for breeder or layer replacements. Drugs have been very important in controlling coccidiosis but the emergence of **coccidial drug resistance** has affected the usefulness of the drugs. The possibility that drugs may not always be relied upon to control coccidiosis has led to an interest in **other means of control.** Thus, control is discussed under four headings: (1) **Drugs**, (2) **Hygiene**, (3) **Vaccine**, and (4) **Genetics**.

## 1. Drugs

The earlier approach was to treat outbreaks of coccidiosis with sulphonamides or other compounds. Soon, the concept of preventive medications came with the realization that most of the damage is done once coccidiosis occurs in a flock. **Today almost all the broiler flocks throughout the world receive preventive medication, and treatment is used as a last resort.**

**Drugs are used mainly for prevention.** The term **'coccidiostat'** means a compound that inhibits its life cycle but does not kill the parasite, whereas a **'coccidiocide'** is a compound that kills the parasite. The term **'anticoccidial'** is preferred to describe all drugs that act against coccidia. Most anticoccidials are formulated as feed additives, and broiler feed almost always contains an anticoccidial agent. Apart from preventing the disease, inclusion of these drugs usually works out economically beneficial due to the **control of subclinical coccidiosis.** The inclusion rates of anticoccidials in feed are very important to ensure their effectiveness and also to prevent any toxicity. It is important that the instructions printed on the anticoccidial premix bags are strictly followed.

The main drugs currently used are:

| | |
|---|---|
| **Ionophores** | Maduramicin, salinomycin, monensin, lasalocid, narasin |
| **Thiamine analogues** (i.e. compounds similar to thiamine) | Amprolium |
| **Sulphonamides** | Diclazuril, toltrazuril |
| **Carbanilide** | Nicarbazin |
| **Pyridones** | Clopidol |
| **Quinolones** | Decoquinate |

**The most widely used drugs are the ionophores.**

## Features of Anticoccidial Drugs

1. A drug may be effective against one or several of the species of coccidia, **but very few drugs are equally effective against all.**

2. Each class of anticoccidial is unique in the type of action exerted on the parasite, and even on the developmental stage of the parasite. The coccidia are prone to attack by drugs at various stages of development in the host.

3. Some drugs kill the parasite (**coccidiocidal**), but others only arrest development (**coccidiostatic**). When coccidiostatic treatment is stopped, arrested parasites continue to develop and contaminate the environment with oocysts. In such cases,

coccidiosis can come up again. In general, the coccidiocidal drugs have been more successful than those that are coccidiostatic.

4. An anticoccidial should prevent infection from as many species of **Eimeria** as possible. It should not interfere with egg production, be non-toxic, stable, and economically affordable.

## Effects of Anticoccidials on the Chicken

Most compounds used in poultry feeds are toxic to coccidia, but are non-toxic to birds. However, drugs can be toxic and have side effects on the birds in case mistakes in formulation lead to **overdose**. For example, the **ionophores** (maduramicin, salinomycin, monensin, lasalocid, narasin) **are very toxic at higher doses**. They cause a temporary paralysis in mild overdoses, but a permanent paralysis and deaths in more severe cases. With slight overdoses, **most of the ionophores decrease weight gain.** Symptoms of toxicity include loss of appetite, depression, weakness, and from unwillingness to move to complete paralysis. Some birds may lie down with neck and legs extended. **Death may be due to respiratory failure or from dehydration**. Mortality varies but may be greater than 70%.

## Anticoccidial Drugs in Broilers

**In broilers,** the purpose is usually to produce the maximum growth and efficiency with minimum of disease, while **in layers** or **breeders** the purpose may be immunization. Often a single drug is used in broilers from day one to slaughter. But, **with time, coccidia become tolerant to that particular drug** and birds are not protected against coccidiosis. This is the most serious problem about the effectiveness of anticoccidials. Surveys show that this **drug resistance** is widespread. Although coccidia develop less resistance to some drugs than others, long-term exposure to any drug will produce a loss in sensitivity, and eventually, resistance. Drug resistance is a genetic phenomenon, and once established in a line of coccidia, remains for many years. To overcome this problem, **shuttle programmes** and frequent rotation of drugs may be practised. These are discussed next.

## Shuttle Programme

The use of one anticoccidial in the starter and another in the grower feed is called a **'shuttle programme'.** The shuttle programme is meant to improve coccidiosis control. For example, intensive use of the ionophore drugs for many years has produced strains of coccidia that have 'reduced sensitivity' for the ionophores. It is a common practice to use another drug in either the starter or grower feed to strengthen the programme of control against coccidiosis, and to take some pressure away from the ionophore. **The use of shuttle programme has been found to reduce drug resistance.**

## Rotation of Drugs

It is very useful to make changes in the use of anticoccidial drugs. Rotation of drugs may improve productivity. This is because the new drug will be effective against the build-up of coccidia that had reduced sensitivity against the previous product that had been used for a long time. Farmers usually find an increase in productivity for a few months after a change of anticoccidial drugs.

## 2. Hygiene

**It is impossible under commercial farming conditions to prevent infection.** The major source of infection is the residual environmental contamination from previous lots, and it is impossible to eliminate oocysts from a farm environment by drugs. **Good hygiene, however, can greatly reduce the numbers of oocysts contaminating the environment.** Moreover, good hygiene ensures that litter is kept dry so that it does not provide good sporulation conditions. Attention should be given to prevent overflow in drinkers and leaking water pipes. By maintaining birds on perforated floors, coccidial infection is greatly reduced. This may not be possible for broilers, but layers are usually kept on wire floors without access to litter. Sometimes this can be disadvantageous in that any immunity acquired while on litter may decrease.

## Disinfection and Sanitation

The older recommendations of preventing outbreaks of coccidiosis through sanitation and disinfection may not be of much help for the following reasons:

1. There have been too many failures in such programmes.

2. Oocysts are extremely resistant to common disinfectants.

3. Complete house disinfection is never complete, and

4. An oocyst-free environment for birds maintained on floors can prevent development of early immunity and allow late outbreaks.

## 3. Vaccines

Two types of vaccines have been used to obtain immunity (protection) against coccidiosis.

## Live Vaccines

All seven species of coccidia are included in these vaccines after destroying their disease-producing power. Although their disease-producing power has been destroyed, they retain their immunity-producing capacity. Birds are vaccinated through drinking water between the age of 5 and 9 days. The vaccines have been found effective. (For a list, see Chapter 19 under **'Coccidiosis vaccines'**).

215

## Killed Vaccines

A killed vaccine is also commercially available.

## 4. Genetics

This is a theoretical plan, and is not of practical use. It has not been possible to develop strains of chickens that are less susceptible to coccidiosis.

# C. ARTHROPOD DISEASES
# (ECTOPARASITES, INSECTS)

Arthropod diseases are those diseases which are caused by **insects** (lice, fleas, mites, ticks, etc.). **Insects are common external parasites of birds.** Since insects live on the outer surface of the body, they are also known as **'ectoparasites'. Of the various diseases caused by insects in poultry, infestation by lice is the most common.**

## Lice

Lice are common external parasites of birds. Several species of biting (chewing) lice may infect poultry. More than 40 species have been reported from the chicken. Fortunately for the poultry farmer, all the species are controlled by the same methods. Although there are many species of bird lice, only a few are commonly seen. **Lice infestations tend to increase in winter.**

## Symptoms

Infestation with lice in poultry may lead to **weight loss and low production**. Lice may irritate nerve endings. Thus, they interfere with the rest and sleep so necessary for young birds. Lice infestation is usually associated with of poor health.

## Diagnosis

Lousiness is diagnosed by finding the straw-coloured lice on skin or feathers of birds.

## Control

1.  **Good hygiene** and the **use of chemicals** form the basis of control.

2.  **Lice tend to increase during winter**. Therefore, flocks should be examined for lice on a regular basis, at least two times per month, and treated, if required.

3.  If treatment (spraying) is required, the birds should be treated two times on a 10 day interval. Only the mature and immature forms will be controlled. This is because **none of the available chemicals kill eggs.**

4.  A second treatment (spraying) is necessary to control the lice that will hatch after

initial treatment.

5. Spraying of birds is the best method of control.

6. A variety of chemicals are available, including organophosphorus compounds (malathion, coumaphos). Malathion is very safe in poultry and may be applied to houses in the presence of birds (1% - 3% solution).

**Note**: For a list of commercial disinfectants that can be used to kill the lice, see Chapter 19 under **"Disinfectants"**.

# Fleas

Several species of fleas have been reported to infest poultry. Fleas are parasites in the adult stage, but are free-living as larvae. Fleas breed away from the bird and keep infesting the environment for many months. Adults possess piercing-sucking mouth parts and long legs suitable for jumping. **Fleas** are brown to black and **suck blood from birds.** They are worldwide in distribution.

## Harmful Effects

Irritation and blood loss caused by fleas may damage poultry seriously, especially young birds in which death may occur. Production is lowered in older birds.

## Control

1. The most important control measures are removal of infected litter and thorough house spraying to kill immature fleas.

2. Fresh litter should be put in the house. House should be treated to kill adult fleas on birds and also those that drop into litter.

3. Sunlight, hot dry weather and excessive moisture prevent development of fleas.

# Mites

**Mites can be a serious problem in poultry due to their blood-sucking habits.** Heavy infestations can cause reduced egg production and anaemia (deficiency in blood of red cells, haemoglobin, or total volume).

Mites are widely distributed throughout the world. The three common mites of poultry are: (1) **chicken mite (red mite)**, (2) **northern fowl mite**, and (3) **tropical fowl mite.** They are **blood suckers** and can run rapidly on skin and feathers. Of lesser importance are members of many other mite families that burrow into the skin, or infect various internal passages and organs.

## 1. Chicken Mite

The chicken mite, also called **'red mite'**, or **'poultry mite'** is found worldwide and is particularly important in tropical countries, like India. It is a **non-burrowing mite.**

**This mite can transmit fowl cholera.**

These mites may not only produce anaemia, and thus seriously lower production and increase feed consumption, but actually kill birds, particularly chicks and laying hens.

## 2. Northern Fowl Mite

Northern fowl mite is also **a non-burrowing mite**. It sucks blood. Of greater importance is the economic impact of this mite on **egg production** from infested caged layers. Northern fowl mite is also harmful to male birds. Extremely dense infestations cause reduced semen production, anaemia and even death. **Northern fowl mite may harbour the viruses of fowl pox and Ranikhet disease after feeding on infected chickens.** However, the proof of spread is lacking.

## 3. Feather Mites

These mites live on the feathers of birds, or in the quills. They cause reduced egg production and feather loss in mite-infested body regions. Feather mites in India have been reported to cause weakness, and poor laying performance.

## 4. Quill Mite

The quill mite occurs inside quills of poultry. These mites cause partial or complete loss of feathers.

## 5. Scaly-Leg Mites

These are usually found on older birds that should ordinarily be removed from flocks. Infected birds spread the infection to non-infested birds by contact. Lesions (changes) are produced on non-feathered portions of the bird's legs and sometimes on skin of the comb and wattles. These are **burrowing mites** and bore tunnels in the skin, causing formation of scales and crusts. Affected birds are unable to walk if the infestation is severe.

## 6. Depluming Mite

These mites are more prevalent in summer, at which time infestation spreads rapidly by contact. Mites burrow into shafts of feathers. Intense irritation forces the bird to pull out body feathers. Some affected birds lose weight and show reduced production.

## 7. Cyst Mite

The cyst mite infests the skin and is usually found in the underlying loose subcutaneous (under the skin) tissue, muscles, and the abdominal organs. These mites do not appear to affect the health of the infested birds.

## 8. Airsac Mite

Airsac mite is found in bronchi, lungs, airsacs, and bone cavities of chickens. Heavy infestations have been associated with weakness and serious loss in weight.

## Diagnosis

Diagnosis is confirmed by examination of skin scrapings, cleared in 10% potassium or sodium hydroxide, under the microscope.

## Control

1. Monitor all birds and houses. Proper monitoring will reduce the spread of mites from farm to farm on service personnel (people), repair personnel, egg trays, replacement birds, and equipment that carry live birds.

2. All egg trays and cases should be checked if they are coming from an infected farm. Farms that use plastic trays should ensure that they are washed with hot water and detergent before being re-delivered to another farm. Farms that use fibre trays and cardboard cases should ensure their inspection before sending them back to the farm.

3. Birds can be treated with any of the standard insecticides. **Pyrethroid permethrin spraying** has been found to be most effective, its effect lasting up to nine weeks after treatment when applied at 0.05%. Red mites can be controlled by treating both the birds and the house.

**Note:** For a list of commercial insecticides effective against lice and mites, refer to Chapter 19 under **"disinfectants"**.

## Ticks

Ticks are large mites. They are widely distributed in tropical areas. **Soft ticks are the most important ticks of poultry,** and of these the most important is *Argas persicus*. However, fowl ticks are rarely found in modern, large commercial cage-layer operations.

## Harmful Effects

Birds suffer from attack of these ticks mainly during the warm dry season. Loss of blood may be so great that the anaemia caused can lead to death of the bird. If death does not occur, the anaemia leads to emaciation, weakness, weight loss, slow growth, and decreased egg production. Ruffled feathers, poor appetite, and diarrhoea are the symptoms that suggest tick infestation. Fowl ticks have been reported to transmit *Pasteurella multocida* (cause of fowl cholera) in some regions of the world.

## Control

Control requires treatment of premises, because adult and nymphal ticks are on birds only for a short time, and then hide in the surroundings. Their litter, walls, floors, and ceiling must be sprayed thoroughly, forcing spray into cracks and behind nest boxes.

**Note:** For a list of commercial disinfectants that can be used against ticks, see Chapter 19 under **"Disinfectants"**.

## Houseflies

**Flies produced on farms are a health and sanitation problem**. Intensive modern poultry farms produce a tremendous amount of manure. It must be properly managed to ensure that it does not attract flies for breeding, and that it does not cause an unpleasant smell problem.

## Control

1.  Fly control on poultry farms should be based on manure management, and through insecticides.

2.  Manure should be maintained in a moisture range of less than 60%. Manure moisture of 60 to 90% is ideal for fly development. Sufficient airflow should be provided over the manure to help in its drying. Airflow over manure is very important. It keeps manure dry and will not support fly breeding.

3.  **High salt levels** in water and feed increase water consumption and, in turn, increase the amount of water in manure. **Wetness makes the manure more suitable for fly breeding.** The water supply should be tested and the salt levels determined so that diets can be adjusted to maintain proper salt content.

4.  **The use of insecticides for fly control is very important.** Insecticides that are meant for use in poultry buildings for fly control are the only insecticides that should be used to avoid residues in eggs or meat.

5.  Insecticides can be applied as sprays. Sprays should be applied early in the morning or late in the evening when most of the flies will be resting within the building.

6.  Control of fly larvae in the manure is done with a larvicide. **Larvicide is an agent that kills a larva.** Larvicides can be applied as a liquid, dry, or in the feed of the birds. Use of a larvicide should only be done on a spot-treatment basis where large numbers of larvae are seen.

**Note:** For a list of commercial preparations used for the control of houseflies, refer to Chapter 19 under **"Miscellaneous drugs"**.

## Mosquitoes

Many species of mosquitoes feed on poultry and transmit disease. Some 140 species have been described. **A number of these are known to suck chicken blood.** The female possesses long mouth parts for piercing the skin. The male does not suck the blood, but feeds on plant juices.

Mosquitoes may attack poultry in large numbers. **Several species of mosquitoes transmit fowl pox virus.** One species can infect birds up to 39 days after contacting the virus of fowl pox.

## Control

1.  **The best approach is to prevent mosquito development.** The farm should be surveyed for all water areas that may produce mosquitoes, including ponds, stagnant pools, and water-filled containers of all types. Mosquito production can be stopped by removal of such containers.

2.  If needed, breeding areas can be treated with larvicides using effective chemicals.

# Chapter 9

# Nutritional Diseases

M ore than 36 nutrients are absolutely essential and must be included in the diet to enable poultry to make the best expression of their genetic potential. That is, **to grow and reproduce.**

**Food substances important in poultry nutrition are:**

1.  Proteins and amino acids

2.  Carbohydrates

3.  Fats

4.  Vitamins

5.  Essential mineral elements, and

6.  Water

**Nutritional diseases, or deficiencies, can occur in several ways, such as:**

1.  Dietary insufficiency. **Errors in the formulation or feed mixing may sometimes result in deficient or toxic levels of one or more nutrients.**

2.  Inhibition of absorption or utilization, or

3.  Metabolic abnormality

A specific mineral or trace element deficiency usually produces characteristic symptoms, pointing to a specific metabolic function. Serious effects may be caused by the unavailability of minute amounts of these nutrients.

In making a diagnosis of nutritional deficiency, care must be taken to rule out other possibilities. It is very common to jump to a conclusion that a clinical condition, which does not fit the pattern of some known disease, must be caused by the feed. Similarly, because a problem disappears when a different feed is tried, does not necessarily mean that the disorder was nutritional.

It must be remembered that nutritional deficiencies seen in the first week or so after hatching, **usually point to the food reserves in the yolk,** derived from the hen's diet, **rather than the nature of the starter feed.**

Liberal supplements of vitamins and trace elements are usually included in the feed to meet essential requirements with a suitable margin of safety. This also takes care of the poor bioavailability of some trace elements, and for the losses that can occur in feed processing and storage.

## NUTRIENT DEFICIENCIES

Today, simple uncomplicated nutrient deficiencies are rarely seen in practice. Experience, however, teaches us not to remain too confident, for example in the light of fatty liver and kidney syndrome in fast-growing broilers.

Sustained genetic advancement in poultry breeding continues year after year, as measured by various performance criteria. **However, metabolic limits are being reached in maintaining this performance;** for example, the ascites/circulatory problems in meat chickens (see 'ascites') and various leg and skeletal problems in broilers as well as in layers at the end of laying.

## PROTEINS AND AMINO ACIDS

Protein requirement means a collective **need for 10 absolutely essential amino acids,** namely, arginine, histidine, isoleucine, leucine, lysine, methionine, phenylalanine, threonine, tryptophan, and valine; two amino acids cysteine and tyrosine that can be synthesized from essential amino acids; two amino acids that are essential for young chicks (glycine or serine, proline); plus amino acids to satisfy the nitrogen requirement for synthesis of non-essential amino acids.

Certain ingredients are poor in one or more amino acids. For example, maize and wheat are deficient in **lysine.** In rations composed of soyabean meals as the source of protein, **methionine** supplementation is usually necessary.

In contrast to the specific symptoms that may occur as a result of vitamin or mineral deficiencies, the effects of essential amino acid deficiencies are non-specific and include **reduced growth, reduced feed consumption, decreased egg production and egg size, and loss of body weight in adults.**

When birds are given dietary protein in excess of their requirements, the surplus protein is catabolized (broken down), and the nitrogen released is converted to uric acid. **A large excess of protein may cause hyperuricaemia** (increased level of uric acid in blood) **and gout** (see 'gout'), **particularly in birds that are genetically susceptible.**

Excess of individual amino acid due to **feed mixing errors** is especially toxic. **Methionine is the most toxic of the amino acids** and also the amino acid likely to be supplemented in the poultry feed. Oxidation of excess methionine results in the release of sulphate, which generates two moles of acid. Oxidation of phosphorylated and dibasic amino acids also contributes to metabolic acidosis. Thus, **high levels of dietary proteins**

**or of methionine** cause **metabolic acidosis** and this may lead to a variety of problems in poultry, such as **poor bone mineralization, thinning of eggshells, and poor growth.**

## CARBOHYDRATES

This food component is the main source of metabolizable energy in poultry diets.

## FATS

Fats are included in the diets of poultry as concentrated sources of energy and to supply the **essential fatty acids, linoleic acid and arachidonic acid. Linoleic acid cannot be synthesized but can be converted to arachidonic acid by poultry.** Both fatty acids are important constituents of cell membranes, cell organelles and adipose (fat) tissue. Lack of these fatty acids in the diet of young chicks results in **poor growth and enlarged fatty livers.** Essential fatty acid deficiency **in laying hens results in reduced egg production, egg size, and hatchability.**

**Unsaturated fatty acids may undergo oxidative rancidity with several effects:**

1. Essential fatty acids are destroyed.

2. Aldehydes that are formed react with free amino groups (NH2) in proteins reducing amino acid availability, and

3. The active peroxides generated during rancidification may destroy activities of vitamin A, D, and E, and water-soluble vitamins, such as biotin.

**Addition of synthetic antioxidants to poultry feeds protects vitamin A and other essential nutrients.**

## VITAMINS

The term **'vitamins'** refers to a group of **fat-soluble (A, D, E, K)** and **water-soluble (B group and C)** chemical compounds essential in nutrition that have no structural or functional relationship to each other. **All vitamins, except vitamin C, are dietary essentials for poultry.** Although amounts of various vitamins needed in poultry diets vary from parts per million (ppm) to parts per billion (ppb), each is required for normal metabolism and health.

**Deficiency of a single vitamin in the diet of a chick results in breakdown of the metabolic process in which that particular vitamin is involved.** This causes a vitamin-deficiency disease, which in some cases shows characteristic symptoms and postmortem findings. Sometimes, a particular disease may result from a deficiency of any one of several nutrients. For example, **chondrodystrophy** (earlier known as **'perosis'**), occurs in young chicks when the diet is deficient in manganese, but it can also occur from the deficiency of any one of these vitamins, namely, choline, nicotinic acid, pyridoxine, biotin, or folic acid. **Chondrodystrophy** is a structural deformity of long bones in young chickens, which is characterized by enlargement of the hock joints and short, thick, and usually deformed long bones. **If both legs are affected, death usually. results since the chick cannot get food and water.** Analysis of the feed is the only way to find out which specific nutritional deficiency is responsible for the condition.

Vitamin A, D and riboflavin (vitamin B2) are most likely to be deficient if special attention is not given to provide them when feed is formulated. Poultry rations are usually formulated to contain more than adequate amounts of all vitamins, providing margins of safety to compensate for possible losses during feed processing, transportation, and storage, and environmental conditions.

## Fat-Soluble Vitamins

**Fat-soluble vitamins (A, D, E, and K)** are absorbed with the fat of the diet. This is helped by bile salts. Any factor which interferes with normal fat absorption may induce a fat-soluble vitamin deficiency.

Antagonisms (opposite actions) can occur between different fat-soluble vitamins due to competition at the site of absorption. Therefore, excessive levels of any particular vitamin should be avoided.

If the dietary fat contains a high proportion of polyunsaturated fatty acids, more vitamin E will be required.

## Water-Soluble Vitamins

**Water-soluble vitamins (B group and C)** are primarily needed for the transfer of body energy. Chickens require all the known water-soluble vitamins in their diet, **except vitamin C.** Although vitamin C is produced by chickens, there are situations such as **heat stress** that may create an increased requirement. When feed contains more water-soluble vitamins than the bird needs, excesses of all except one are excreted in the urine. **Vitamin B12 has the capacity of being stored.** Those not stored must be included in the daily diet. The bird has no reservoir on which to draw.

B vitamins act in the regulation of metabolism, and overlapping of some of the metabolic pathways occurs. For example, choline, cobalamin (vitamin B12) and folic acid interact directly in the metabolism of methyl groups, and a deficiency in one of these vitamins can lead to an increased requirement for the others. In other cases, an excess of some vitamins can cause a deficiency of others. For example, the biotin level of the chick is decreased by over-supplementation with a wide range of other B vitamins. Excessive choline supplementation has a similar effect on biotin requirements. Moreover, high levels of choline chloride in feed supplement products can increase the rate of loss of other constituent vitamins during product storage.

## VITAMIN A

Vitamin A is essential in poultry diets for growth, good vision, and integrity of mucous membranes. Since epithelial linings of the digestive, respiratory, urinary, and genital systems are composed of mucous membranes, these are the tissues in which alterations of vitamin A deficiency are mostly observed. **From a nutritional point of view, vitamin A is the most challenging of all the vitamins, because it is most likely to be deficient in poultry.**

Vitamin A is a group of related natural and synthetic chemicals that exert a hormone-like activity or function, the most important and active being **retinol**, an alcohol. Oxidation of retinol in the body yields the aldehyde, **retinal**, and the acid **retinoic acid**, also having a vitamin A activity. Vitamin A is transported in the body in the form of retinol and stored mainly in the liver as **retinyl ester. More than 90% of the body's vitamin A reserves are stored in the liver.** The term **retinoids** refers to both naturally occurring and synthetic form of vitamin A. Plants do not contain vitamin A as such, but have a variety of **carotenoids**, which can be converted to active vitamin A in the body. The most important of these is **beta-carotene**, which consists of two linked molecules of retinol. In animal tissues, vitamin A exists mainly as retinol, retinal, retinoic acid and retinyl esters.

Retinol, retinyl esters and retinal can be inter-converted, and can be used to synthesize retinoic acid. Thus, the vitamin A requirement can be met with by retinol or retinal.

## Functions

Vitamin A has two very different metabolic functions in cells: (1) the hormone-like regulatory action of retinol and retinoic acid, and (2) the photoreception action of retinal. In addition, **vitamin A increases immunity against infections.**

## 1. Regulatory action of retinoic acid

This is due to the interactions of retinol and retinoic acid with cytoplasmic and nuclear-binding proteins. In particular, retinoic acid binds to specific nuclear receptors and induces expression of the genes that regulate cell proliferation, differentiation and pre-programmed cell death.

**Explained simply**, vitamin A is concerned with the maintenance of epithelial structures (mucous membranes) and their function. For example, retinoic acid brings about the differentiation of epithelial basal cells into the cuboidal, columnar, and goblet cells characteristic of the lining epithelial cells in the mucous membrane of respiratory and gastro-intestinal tracts. In the absence of vitamin A, the basal cells of the respiratory tract, mouth, oesophagus, cloaca, ureters, bursa of Fabricius, oviduct, and the conjunctiva of the eye differentiate into keratinizing cells (these are dead cells), which form a hard, dry squamous epithelium characteristic of the skin. This change is known as **'squamous**

**metaplasia'** and leads to secondary infection, particularly of the respiratory and intestinal tracts.

## 2. Photoreception Function

This function of vitamin A is involved in maintaining normal vision in reduced light. Vitamin A-dependent photoreception is only useful to the bird when light is dim and the rods of the eye are utilized. Vitamin A deficiency damages the function of the rods in the eyes, causing **night blindness.** In conditions of bright light, this system is inactivated and cones, which do not utilize vitamin A, are active.

## 3. Increasing Immunity against Infection

**Vitamin A plays an important role in bird's resistance to infections.** This is due to its ability to stimulate immune system, possibly through the formation of a recently discovered metabolite (i.e. a product of metabolism) called **14-hydroxyretinol.** In addition, during infections the bioavailability of vitamin A is reduced. The acute phase response (see Chapter 33 for more information) that accompanies many infections reduces the formation of retinol-binding protein in the liver. This results in the reduction of circulating retinol levels, which in turn leads to reduced tissue availability of vitamin A. **Therefore, supplementation of vitamin A during the course of disease improves bird's resistance to infections.**

For more information on the role of vitamin A in immunity, refer to Chapter 33: **"Impact of nutrients on avian immunity".**

## Causes of Deficiency:

1.  Low levels of vitamin A in the feed

2.  Oxidation of vitamin A in the feed

3.  Errors in mixing

4.  Intercurrent disease, for example, coccidiosis, worm infestation

## Deficiency Symptoms

**Chicks from hens getting the diets high in vitamin A have sufficient amount in the yolk to meet the requirements for 2-3 months,** if diet is lacking in vitamin A. Chicks from hens getting diet slightly adequate in vitamin A have low stores, and may begin to express deficiency symptoms soon after hatching.

**Deficiency symptoms include** loss of appetite, poor growth, ruffled feathers, drowsiness (sleepiness), and weakness. **Deficient chicks are very susceptible to infections,** due to inadequate antibody production because of keratinization of the bursa **(squamous metaplasia)** and poor differentiation of B-lymphocytes. T-lymphocytes are also affected. (For information on B- and T-lymphocytes, see Chapter 32). Aggravating the situation, infections are more common due to loss of integrity of the mucous membrane lining respiratory and gastro-intestinal tracts. Also, **secondary infections are more likely. Death from infections may occur** before gross symptoms that are diagnostic of vitamin A are seen.

**In adult chickens,** the first alteration of vitamin A deficiency appears **in the pharynx and oesophagus,** where the normal mucous epithelium is replaced with stratified squamous (keratinizing) epithelium. This condition (**squamous metaplasia**) blocks the ducts of mucous glands and necrosis (death) of their contents causes the development of **small white pustules (raised spots).** That is, the blocked ducts of the mucous glands cause them to become distended with secretions and necrotic (dead) materials. The **pustules** are easily visible to the naked eye and are a **characteristic lesion of vitamin A deficiency. Egg production decreases sharply** and hatchability is also reduced. The incidence and severity of **blood spots in eggs** is increased in vitamin A deficiency. The mucous epithelium of the intestine does not become keratinized but the number of goblet cells in the intestine decreases, reducing mucus secretion. This causes enteritis and increased infection.

Inappropriate differentiation of the kidney tubules causes diminished uric acid excretion, crystallization of urates in soft tissues, and **gout** (see 'gout').

Vitamin A deficiency damages the function of the rods in the eyes, causing **night blindness.** More severe deficiencies result in keratinization of the conjunctiva and inadequate lubrication of the cornea. Subsequent infections cause irreversible loss of sight. This condition is known as **xerophthalmia** (dryness of eye) and is characterized by the accumulation of white inflammatory material in the eye and discharge of thick fluid (exudate), which often causes the eyelids to stick together. At this stage of the disease, eyes fill with white exudate to such an extent that it is impossible for the chicken to see unless the mass is removed. In many cases, the eye is destroyed. A sticky exudate is also discharged from the nostrils if they become infected.

Vitamin A deficient cocks have decreased sperm counts, reduced sperm motility, and a high incidence of abnormal sperms.

**Grossly excessive levels of vitamin A are toxic,** affecting body structure and performance.

## Treatment of Deficiency

Poultry found to be severely deficient in vitamin A should be given a stabilized **vitamin A preparation at a level of about 10,000 IU** (International Units) **vitamin A per kg of feed.** Absorption of vitamin A is rapid. Therefore, chickens not in advanced stages of deficiency should respond promptly, except for blindness which may be permanent.

## To prevent deficiency:

1.  Use stabilized vitamin A in poultry feed.

2.  Add adequate levels of antioxidants in feed.

3.  Provide adequate storage for feed and feed ingredients.

## VITAMIN D

This vitamin has several forms, but **D2** and **D3** are the most important. Vitamin **D3** (cholecalciferol) is utilized by birds, humans and animals, while **D2** is of value to humans and animals. **Thus, D3 is essential for poultry. Vitamin D3 helps in the absorption of calcium and phosphorus from the intestinal tract.**

**Vitamin D is required by poultry for proper metabolism of calcium and phosphorus** in the formation of normal bones, hard beaks and claws, and **strong eggshells.**

Birds can synthesize vitamin D3 from 7-dehydrocholesterol in the skin under the influence of ultraviolet rays of sunlight. **However, it is not sufficient to satisfy the requirements of chicken under the conditions of modern poultry farming.** The chickens are closely confined to houses with no irradiation from the sun. Even glass does not allow the ultraviolet rays to pass. **Therefore, vitamin D3 supplements must be added to the feed.**

## Metabolism

Metabolism of vitamin D can be outlined as follows:

1.  First, there is absorption of vitamin D from the intestine, or synthesis in the skin.

2.  Vitamin D is then bound to D-binding protein in the blood and transported to liver.

3.  In the liver, vitamin D (D3, cholecalciferol) is enzymatically converted to 25-hydroxycholecalciferol.

4.  25-hydroxycholecalciferol in the kidney is then enzymatically converted to **1, 25-dihydroxycholecalciferol. Biologically this is the most active form of vitamin D** than the other two forms, namely, vitamin D3 and 25-hydroxycholecalciferol.

## Functions

1.  The most important function of vitamin D is the **maintenance of normal levels of calcium and phosphorus in the blood.** It does this by its action on intestines, bones and kidneys. Vitamin D regulates calcium metabolism by stimulating the intestinal absorption of calcium and phosphorus. That is, **it controls absorption of calcium and phosphorus from the intestine** and then its transfer through blood. Vitamin D helps to form a protein in the intestinal tract to keep the calcium in

solution so that it can pass the intestinal wall and reach the cells.

Vitamin D thus regulates calcium and phosphorus balance in the body, **mineralization in the bone**, and **eggshell formation**. As such, vitamin D is considered to be a hormone as well as a vitamin. (A hormone is a product (a protein) of cells that circulates in blood and produces a specific effect on the activity of cell, away from its site of origin).

2.  Vitamin D works jointly with parathyroid hormone (i.e. hormone of parathyroid gland) in the removal of calcium from the bone.

3.  Vitamin D stimulates parathyroid hormone dependent re-absorption of calcium in the kidneys.

## Causes of Deficiency

1.  Lack of adequate amounts of vitamin D (vitamin D3) in poultry feed, especially in confinement rearing.

2.  Sulpha drugs in the feed may interfere with vitamin D3 absorption.

## Deficiency Symptoms

1.  When dietary intake is insufficient, **deposition of minerals (calcium and phosphorus) in the bones is defective.** This gives rise to a disease called **'rickets'** in the young chickens, and **'osteomalacia'** in adult birds. Rickets is due to reduced deposition of minerals in the bones, whereas osteomalacia due to loss of minerals from the bones.

2.  The **deformities in rickets** (caused by inadequate dietary calcium, phosphorus or vitamin D3, or calcium:phosphorus imbalance) **develop** especially **in the legs, producing painful, hard joint swelling and lameness. The hock joints are enlarged.** This deformity is very clearly seen in the structure of the proximal tibio-tarsus. The **head of the ribs may be enlarged** (see **Fig. 24**) and sometimes also the costo-chondral junctions. This **'beading'** of the ribs at their junction with the spinal column, and formation of well-defined knobs on the ribs at the costo-chondral junction (**rachitic rosary**), are the most characteristic internal changes of vitamin D deficiency in chicks. **The bones, beaks, shanks, and claws become soft and rubbery.** That is, they are pliable and **can be bent or twisted easily without breaking. Growth is retarded.** Feather development is poor, and there is general unthriftiness.

3.  **In the laying birds, egg production decreases** with **thin and soft-shelled eggs** and reduced hatchability. Osteomalacia gives rise to brittle (easily broken) bones of reduced density and strength (**osteoporosis**). Such bones are light, porous, and fragile (breaking easily). Individual hens show **extreme leg weakness.**

Very high levels of vitamin D3 (4 million IU or more per kg of feed) cause kidney damage from calcification. A moderate excess of vitamin D increases eggshell pimpling, which is characterized by excessive localized calcareous deposits (i.e. containing calcium carbonate) on and within the eggshell.

## Treatment of Deficiency

**Feeding a single very large dose of 15,000 IU of vitamin D3 by mouth cures rickets more quickly compared to when significant levels of the vitamin are added to the feed.** This single dose by mouth protects cockerels against rickets for 8 weeks and layer chicks for 5 weeks. In giving a very large dose to chicks suffering from rickets, it should be remembered that **excess vitamin D can be harmful.** The dose should be adjusted according to the degree of deficiency, and excessive amounts of vitamin D should not be added to the feed.

**In advanced cases, injection of a single dose of vitamin D3** may produce a better response than generous levels in the feed. Suggested dose for young chickens is 50 IU per kg body weight and double this level for hens. Following injection, adequate levels of vitamin D3 should be maintained in the feed. Injections may be given either by intramuscular or subcutaneous route.

**To prevent deficiency,** add adequate levels of vitamin D3 in the feed. Excessive levels of vitamin D3 given for long period will cause kidney damage, due to deposition of calcium.

## VITAMIN E

Vitamin E consists chemically of a group of closely related alcohols, called **tocopherols.** There are at least 8 different tocopherols having vitamin E activity. Of these **alpha-tocopherol** is the most active and most widely available and therefore the most important. As acetate, it is used as a dietary supplement, which is converted to tocopherol during digestion and absorption. Vitamin E is necessary for maintaining the integrity of cellular membranes.

## Functions

1. **The most important function of vitamin E is that it acts as an antioxidant,** preventing oxidation of unsaturated lipids within cells. Its deficiency leads to abnormal formation or accumulation of lipid hydroperoxides, with resulting cell damage. The more active the cell, the more lipids are required for activity and the more risk of damage. The protective action of vitamin E ensures the stability of red blood cells and integrity of minute blood vessels.

   For more information on the role of vitamin E as an antioxidant and the mechanism of its action, refer to **'Vitamin E'**, under Chapter 33.

2.    **Vitamin E prevents degenerative changes in muscles and liver.**

## Requirements and Related Aspects

1.    Most oilseeds, green plant material and cereal germs are rich in tocopherols, which are easily oxidized in air. Or, they may be oxidized by peroxides of polyunsaturated fatty acids, formed when fat (for example, in feed) becomes rancid. Therefore, the amount of fat or oil (particularly polyunsaturated fatty acids) present in feed plays a part in deciding the amount of vitamin E that should be included. **Vitamin E can be called a naturally occurring antioxidant.**

2.    An important factor that has a bearing on the inclusion of vitamin E in feed is the amount of selenium (see **'selenium'**). **There is a close working relationship between vitamin E and selenium in their functions within tissues.** It is said that selenium spares vitamin E.

      **Selenium is a constituent of glutathione peroxidase,** the enzyme that removes active peroxides from cells, before they oxidize unsaturated fatty lipids, which are protected by tocopherols (see **'selenium'**). To a small extent, vitamin E and selenium are mutually replaceable.

3.    **Most grain storage leads to loss of natural vitamin E, and therefore increases the supplementation requirement.** Also stressful conditions, such as overcrowding, transportation, poor ventilation and disease, increase the requirements of vitamin E.

4.    Inadequate vitamin E levels give rise to several conditions in poultry. These may occur separately or together, depending on age, degree of deficiency, and other factors.

## Deficiency Symptoms

1.    Vitamin E deficiency may give rise to several disease conditions. As a fat-soluble antioxidant inside the cells, the main function of vitamin E is a protective effect on cell membranes. Therefore, its deficiency results in damage to blood vessels and changes in capillary (minute vessels) permeability. Deficiency in breeders may give rise to early embryonic mortality associated with changes in blood vessels (usually around 4th day of incubation).

2.    **In young growing birds,** deficiency conditions include: (1) **encephalomalacia,** (2) **exudative diathesis,** and (3) **nutritional muscular dystrophy** (or **myopathy**).

## 1. Encephalomalacia (Crazy Chick Disease)

      **Encephalomalacia is a nervous disorder**. It is seen in birds, usually in good condition, up to the age of 5 weeks (often between 2 and 3 weeks). Symptoms include muscular weakness, progressive muscular incoordination with frequent falling, backward or downward retraction of the head, and/or rapid contraction and relaxation of the legs, torticollis (twisting of the neck) and finally paralysis and death.

## Postmortem Findings

Changes in the blood vessels give rise to oedema (accumulation of fluid characterized by **swelling**), and **minute** (petechial) **and larger haemorrhages on the surface of the cerebellum (one part of the brain).** Such gross changes seen in cerebellum in association with appropriate clinical symptoms **are almost diagnostic.** The reason why cerebellum is affected and not cerebrum (a different part of the brain) is that increased polyunsaturated fatty acid levels occur in the second and third weeks in the cerebellum, **but not in the cerebrum.**

## Treatment

The usual treatment is **vitamin E given through drinking water.** The condition is prevented by ensuring the availability of adequate vitamin E. Selenium is said to have some preventive effect.

## 2. Exudative Diathesis

**Exudative diathesis is an oedema of the subcutaneous tissue (i.e. accumulation of fluid under the skin).** Changes in the walls of the minute blood vessels cause leakage of fluid (plasma). This fluid accumulates under the skin, particularly **over the breast and under the wings.** It also accumulates in the pericardial sac (i.e. under the covering of the heart) and between the muscles.

**In severe cases,** chicks stand with their legs far apart as a result of accumulation of fluid under the ventral skin. This green-blue viscous (thick and sticky) fluid is easily seen through the skin, because it usually contains some blood from slight haemorrhages that appear throughout the breast and leg muscles, and in the intestinal walls. Distension of the pericardium (covering of the heart) and sudden deaths have been observed.

The condition is prevented by, and also responds to, vitamin E and selenium. **The usual treatment is vitamin E through drinking water.**

## 3. Nutritional Muscular Dystrophy (or Myopathy)

This condition occurs with exudative diathesis. It occurs when vitamin E deficiency is accompanied by a deficiency of sulphur-containing amino acids (methionine and cysteine) in chicks.

Thrombosis (kind of blood clotting) of smaller blood vessels causes blockage, which gives rise to degeneration and necrosis (death) of muscle fibres. This is seen as pale (white) streaks (long thin lines) mainly in breast and thigh muscles.

**Prevention and treatment are by vitamin E supply.**

## 4. Sterility in Males

Vitamin E deficiency may cause sterility in males and non-production in the females. **Hens stop laying on diets low in vitamin E,** but cessation is not permanent. Addition of vitamin E to the diet restores the bird to normal egg production.

### Excess Vitamin E

Vitamin E has a low level of toxicity for poultry, and levels greater than 100 times the requirement, are well tolerated. High levels of dietary vitamin E may cause a deficiency of other fat-soluble vitamins.

## VITAMIN K

It is interesting to know that **vitamin K was discovered in chickens** by Henrik Dam in 1943, who was awarded the Nobel Prize.

Vitamin K consists of a group of compounds that exhibit anti-haemorrhagic activity. Vitamin K is indispensable for blood coagulation (clotting). It is synthesized by bacteria. Microbial synthesis in the chicken occurs in the caeca and rectum. **Among fat-soluble vitamins, only vitamin K is synthesized in the intestinal tract.** This may not take place if there is oral (by mouth) administration of antibacterial drugs **(antibiotics). Sulpha drugs also act against vitamin K activity.**

### Functions

1.  Vitamin K is required for blood coagulation. **In its absence blood cannot clot.** This is because vitamin K is required for synthesis of prothrombin. In the absence of vitamin K, an abnormal type of prothrombin is released into the blood by the liver. Since prothrombin plays an important role in blood-clotting mechanism, deficiency of vitamin K results in markedly prolonged blood-clotting time. **An affected chick may bleed to death from a slight bruise or other injury.**

2.  Among the fat-soluble vitamins, vitamin K is unique in that it functions solely as a cofactor for an enzyme involved in the formation of certain factors required for blood clotting.

### Requirement

The storage of vitamin K in the body is small and its tissue turnover is relatively rapid compared to the other fat-soluble vitamins. Despite this, however, the dietary requirements for vitamin K are relatively low. This is because the enzyme for which vitamin K acts as a cofactor, is in low concentration in the body of chicken. Moreover, its formation in the intestine by bacteria and availability from **coprophagy** (i.e. through eating of faeces) further decrease the need for dietary vitamin K in many species. **The faeces of chickens contain levels of vitamin K that are more than ten times the amount in the diet. Therefore, coprophagy is a quantitatively important dietary**

**source in this species.**

## Causes of Deficiency

1. Factors which increase the requirement for vitamin K include infectious diseases, specific vitamin K antagonists (i.e. substances which act against the activity of vitamin K, such as sulpha drugs), antibiotics, and conditions that prevent its absorption (e.g. high dietary levels of vitamin E and A). **Presence of sulpha drugs in the feed or water interferes with vitamin K activity.**

2. The therapeutic (curative) use of **antibiotics** depletes intestinal microflora and increases the need for a dietary source of vitamin K.

3. In the absence of above complicating factors, vitamin K deficiencies are rarely observed in the chicken.

4. Inadequate levels of vitamin K in feed, or loss of vitamin K potency in feed during storage.

5. Poor absorption from the intestine due to diseases, or dietary factors.

## Deficiency Symptoms

1. When vitamin K is low or lacking, the blood vessels rupture, causing excessive bleeding. **Large haemorrhages** appear on areas that are prone to be damaged from rubbing or scraping, such as breast, legs and wings, and in the abdominal cavity.

2. Internally, petechial (pinpoint or minute) haemorrhages in the liver, and erosion of the lining of the gizzard may occur.

3. With a severe deficiency, even minor trauma may lead to internal bleeding and death.

4. The amount of vitamin K transferred to the egg is related to the dietary supply, although yolk stores do not reach very high levels. Embryos from vitamin K deficient chickens have high mortality, due to bleeding late in incubation.

## Treatment of Deficiency

Within 4-6 hours after vitamin K is administered to deficient chicks, blood clots normally. However, recovery from anaemia or disappearance of haemorrhage, takes some time.

**For prevention,** supply adequate levels of vitamin K in the feed, and administer antibiotics and sulpha drugs with great care.

## VITAMIN B1 (Thiamine)

It is interesting that **vitamin B1 (thiamine) was also discovered in chickens,** in 1929, by Christian Eijkman who received the Nobel Prize.

## Functions

Vitamin B1 **plays an important role in carbohydrate metabolism,** through several enzyme systems.

## Causes of Deficiency

1.  Inadequate levels of vitamin B1 in the feed.

2.  High carbohydrate-based feed, low in vitamin B1.

## Deficiency Symptoms

**Loss of appetite** is usually the first symptom of deficiency and can become very severe, causing **loss of weight, emaciation and weakness.** Other signs that follow include a group of symptoms known as **'polyneuritis'** (inflammation of many nerves), **leg weakness, unsteady gait,** tremors, paralysis, and convulsions. The chicken characteristically sits on its flexed legs and draws back (retracts) its head, called **'stargazing or opisthotonus'** (Fig. 19). Retraction of the head is due to paralysis of the anterior muscles of

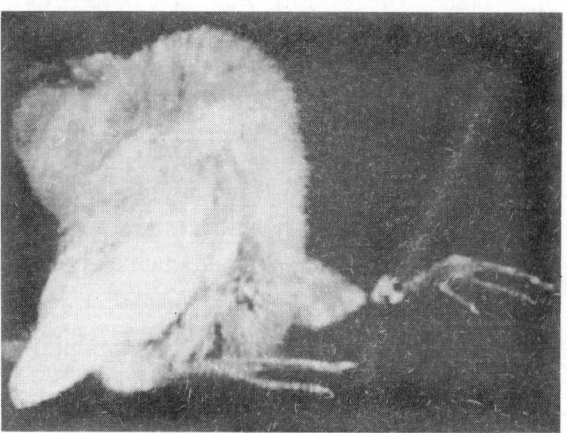

**Fig. 19.** Typical stargazing pose shown by a chick suffering from vitamin B1 deficiency.

the neck. Stargazing was the symptom that led to the discovery of vitamin B1. **The chicken soon loses the ability to stand or sit upright, and it falls on the floor,** where it may lie with the head still drawn back.

## Treatment of Deficiency

Chickens suffering from thiamine deficiency respond within a few hours to oral administration of vitamin B1. Since thiamine deficiency causes severe loss of appetite, supplementation of the feed with vitamin is not a reliable treatment. Feed supplementation should be given only after chickens have recovered from acute deficiency. Recommended dose rate for young chickens is 5-10 mg per day, and for older birds 10-50 mg per day.

# VITAMIN B2 (Riboflavin)

**Vitamin B2 is essential for growth and health.** It is synthesized in the adult bird (not in the young chick) by bacteria in the caeca and large intestine. However, as the absorption of vitamin B2 occurs from the small intestine, this is of no use to the bird. Therefore, **coprophagy** (eating of faeces) appears to be the useful source. The bacterial content and vitamins are especially high in **caecotrope** (caecal faeces). Preferential eating of caecal faeces over rectal faeces, that is, **'caecotrophy'**, is common in chickens.

The vitamin is not stored in the body but it is stored in the eggs, particularly the yolk. Absence of body storage means that daily supply is required in the feed.

## Functions

**Vitamin B2 is a cofactor (coenzyme) in many enzyme systems in the body.** A very large number of enzymes (more than 50) involved in oxidation and reduction reactions require riboflavin as a cofactor. These enzymes participate in the metabolism of carbohydrate, amino acid and fat, and the regular cellular metabolism. **Therefore, vitamin B2 is essential for growth and health.**

## Causes of Deficiency

1.  In chickens, high levels of dietary fat or protein increase the riboflavin requirement, since many of the enzymes responsible for the oxidation of these nutrients require riboflavin cofactors.

2.  The use of high-energy poultry diets, with ingredients low in B2, requires additional feed supplementation.

3.  Inadequate levels of vitamin B2 in the feed.

4.  Presence of antagonists of vitamin B2 in the feed, such as **mycotoxins**, mainly **aflatoxin**. These interfere with absorption or body transport.

5.  Riboflavin is sensitive to light and pH.

High levels of dietary riboflavin do not increase tissue levels, or provide significant protection against a future dietary deficiency.

## Deficiency Symptoms

Riboflavin deficiency affects all tissues of the body, and **symptoms are first seen in young birds** as **reduced growth rate** and **poor efficiency of food utilization.** A severe deficiency causes degeneration of the peripheral nerves, particularly affecting the sciatic nerve. The sciatic (and brachial) nerves are swollen four times their normal size. The resulting continuous stimulation causes muscle contractions, sometimes leading to leg paralysis and inability to extend the digits, producing the condition called **'curled-toe paralysis'.** Toes are curled inward while both walking and resting **(Fig. 20).**

**Breeders are particularly susceptible to marginally low levels of riboflavin, which is required for good hatchability.** There is a greater requirement of vitamin B2 for hatchability than for egg production. Reduced egg production occurs in severe deficiency, but with slightly low deficiency there is greatly reduced hatchability, with peak embryonic deaths around mid-incubation (dead-in-shell). **Hatched chicks may be dwarfed with shortened limbs, poor feathering, and leg**

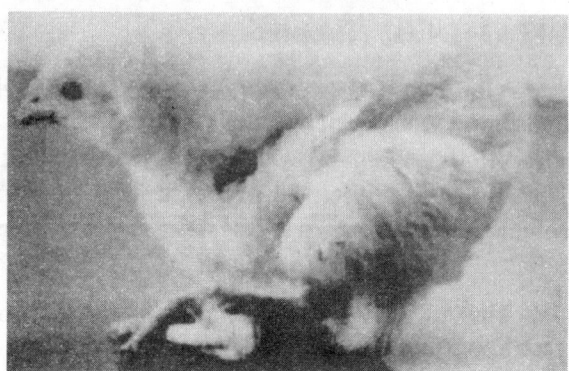

**Fig. 20.** Curled-toe paralysis in a chick, typical of vitamin B2 deficiency. The chick is unable to stand or walk, sits on hocks and toes are curled inward.

**paralysis (curled-toe paralysis).** The chick is unable to stand or walk, sits on hocks and toes are curled inward **(Fig. 20).** There is improper growth of the down (very fine soft feathers), giving it a blunted appearance (club-shaped appearance), known as **'clubbed down'.**

## Treatment of Deficiency

In adults, deficiency symptoms can be reversed with supplemental riboflavin, but with growing birds this becomes less likely. To prevent deficiency, incorporate an adequate level in the ration. Suggested oral dose of vitamin B2 is 5 mg per chicken and 15 mg per hen per day.

## VITAMIN B6 (Pyridoxine)

Vitamin B6 is the general term and includes three naturally occurring substances: **pyridoxine, pyridoxal,** and **pyridoxamine.** All have similar vitamin activity, and are collectively referred to as **pyridoxine.** The main forms vary among foods of plant and animal origin. Plant tissues contain mostly pyridoxamine, whereas animal tissues contain a mixture of pyridoxal and pyridoxamine.

## Functions

**This vitamin plays a part in protein, carbohydrate, and fat metabolism.** It forms a part of several enzymes. B6 is particularly involved in amino acid metabolism through numerous enzymes.

## Causes of Deficiency

1. Diets high in total protein, or containing unbalanced protein, markedly increase the requirement for vitamin B6. This is because more number of vitamin B6-dependent

238

enzymes is required to metabolize the excess of amino acids. Fortunately, most foods that have high levels of proteins also contain high levels of vitamin B6, and **therefore deficiencies of this vitamin are rare.**

2.    Inadequate levels of vitamin B6 in the feed.

## Deficiency Symptoms

Due to a large number of metabolic functions performed by vitamin B6, wide-ranging effects may be produced in deficiency. **Chicks show reduced appetite, slow growth, weakness, poor feather growth, anaemia, inability to coordinate muscle movements (ataxia), chondrodystrophy** (see **'chondrodystrophy'**), and characteristic **nervous symptoms.** They show jerky, nervous movements of the legs when walking and usually undergo convulsions (i.e. abnormal violent and involuntary contractions of the muscles) that usually end in death. During these convulsions, chicks may run aimlessly, flap their wings and fall to their sides, or roll completely over on their backs, where they perform rapid jerking motions with their feet and heads.

**In adult birds**, pyridoxine deficiency causes marked reduction of egg production and hatchability, as well as decreased feed consumption, loss of weight, and death.

Vitamin B6 is not particularly toxic when fed at high levels.

## NICOTINIC ACID (NIACIN)

Nicotinic acid in food occurs mainly in bound forms. In many foods of plant origin, these complexes are not digested and are unavailable to birds.

Niacin is synthesized by bacterial action in the caecum and rectum, but because there is no absorption beyond this level, this is not of much use. In chicken, a certain amount is synthesized from the amino acid **tryptophan**. Chickens are able to synthesize about 1 mg of nicotinic acid from 45 mg of dietary tryptophan.

## Functions

Nicotinic acid is the vitamin component of two important enzymes, nicotinamide adenine dinucleotide (NAD) and nicotinamide adenine dinucleotide phophate (NADP). These enzymes are extensively involved in carbohydrate, fat, and protein metabolism. They are especially important in metabolic reactions that supply energy.

## Causes of Deficiency

1.    Inadequate levels of nicotinic acid in the feed.

2.    Insufficient absorption.

3.    Stress conditions requiring high levels.

4.    Errors in mixing.

## Deficiency Symptoms

Symptoms usually develop **in** severely deficient **chicks** and include **loss of appetite, poor growth,** skin and feather disorders, inflammation of the mouth (oral cavity), dermatitis (inflammation of the skin), poor feathering, and enlargement of the hock joints of the legs. **In young growing birds**, nicotinic acid is one of the primary nutritional deficiencies, along with that caused by manganese, zinc, choline, biotin, folic acid, and pyridoxine. All these deficiencies cause **chondrodystrophy** - a generalized disorder of the bone resulting in short, thick and usually deformed long bones, along with enlargement of the hock joints.

## Treatment of Deficiency

1.  Supplement the deficient feed with required amounts of nicotinic acid. Pure nicotinic acid can be used at the dose rate of 40-50 mg per chicken.

2.  To control deficiency in young chickens, supply well balanced feed with adequate levels of nicotinic acid.

## PANTOTHENIC ACID

Pantothenic acid has been referred to as **'chick anti-dermatitis factor'.** (Dermatitis is inflammation of the skin). Pantothenic acid is an unstable hygroscopic (readily taking up and retaining moisture) oil, and is widely distributed in plant and animal tissues. In combination with coenzyme A, pantothenic acid is important for metabolism of protein, carbohydrates and fats required by all cells. **The requirements of young and growing chicks for pantothenic acid are high.**

## Functions

Pantothenic acid is an essential part of coenzyme A. Coenzyme A is a vital element of energy and **participates in the metabolism of carbohydrate, fatty acids and amino acids;** in antibody formation; and in the function of nerves. It is also precursor of cholesterol and thus of steroid hormones.

## Causes of Deficiency

1.  Low pantothenic acid in breeder feed.
2.  Inadequate levels in chick starter feed.

## Deficiency Symptoms

**Severe deficiencies are rare,** due to the wide distribution of pantothenic acid. Mild deficiencies may occur in birds consuming diets based on cereal grains. Mild deficiencies cause **slow growth, poor feathering, and weakness.** More severe deficiencies include incoordination of muscular movements (ataxia), skin lesions at the corners of the mouth, swollen and encrusted eyelids; and cracks and later haemorrhages in the skin of the feet and toes. Internal changes include fatty liver, and atrophy (reduction in size) of thymus and bursa.

Pantothenic acid-deficient hens do not show any significant decrease in egg production, but embryos from their eggs have high mortality, characterized by oedema, haemorrhages, and poor feathering. Excess pantothenic acid is rapidly excreted in the urine, and high dietary levels are not known to be toxic.

## Treatment of Deficiency

Pantothenic acid deficiency can be completely cured, if not very advanced, by oral treatment or injection with the vitamin. This should be followed by restoration of an adequate level in the diet. Suggested dose rate is 10-20 mg per chick per day.

## BIOTIN

Biotin is believed to be a member of vitamin B group. Biotin is synthesized by bacteria in the caeca and large intestine, but this supply is inadequate. It supplies only up to about 10% of growing bird requirement. Biotin from the food, and also that obtained by coprophagy (from eating of faeces), is absorbed through the small intestine. Coprophagy seeds the digestive tract with beneficial bacteria. The bacterial content and vitamins are especially high in caecotrope (caecal faeces). Preferential eating of caecal faeces over rectal faeces, that is 'caecotrophy', is common in chickens. **However, in the chicken, only one or two caecal faeces are evacuated per day, compared with 15 or more rectal droppings per day.** In the chicken, the entire process of defaecation takes less than four seconds.

Most feed components contain biotin, but again, **most of it is organically bound and biologically unavailable to the bird.** It is bound to proteins and many sources of protein-bound biotin are resistant to digestion. **Therefore, biotin is one of the least available of the vitamins.** Thus, in many foods of either plant or animal origin, less than half of the biotin is available. Moreover, such availability of biotin to poultry differs greatly between feed ingredients. For example, from maize it is 100%, from wheat only 5%.

## Functions

In general, **biotin is essential for growth, food utilization, bone development, reproduction, and maintenance of skin.**

Biotin is a cofactor (coenzyme) for several carboxylase enzymes. A carboxylase enzyme is one that either removes the carboxyl group (COOH) (de-carboxylation), or adds the carboxyl group (carboxylation). Two of the most important carboxylase enzymes are: (1) **pyruvate carboxylase,** and (2) **acetyl coenzyme A carboxylase.**

**Pyruvate carboxylase** is involved in **gluconeogenesis**, that is, formation of glucose from non-carbohydrate sources, such as proteins and fats. It occurs in the liver under conditions of low carbohydrate intake, or starvation. The enzyme **acetyl coenzyme A carboxylase** is involved in **lipogenesis**, that is, in the formation of fat. **Biotin is therefore essential in carbohydrate and fat metabolism, as well as in protein synthesis.**

## Causes of Deficiency

1.  Conditions which decrease intestinal synthesis, such as **antibiotics** and **diarrhoea. Antibiotics in chickens may kill those bacteria which synthesize biotin in the intestine.**

2.  Presence of **biotin binders** and antagonists in feed, such as **mycotoxins**, mainly **aflatoxin.**

3.  Inadequate levels of biotin in the feed.

## Deficiency Symptoms

**Biotin deficiencies are relatively rare**, except when diets are based on grains with very low biotin bioavailability, or when biotin binder/antagonists, **such as aflatoxin,** are present in the feed.

**In growing chickens,** the first symptoms of biotin deficiency occur in skin. There is **defective feathering**, periocular dermatitis (inflammation of skin around the eyes), encrustations (formation of crusts or hard coatings), and fissures in the angles of the beak and eyelids and on the foot pads and toes. Severe deficiency leads to **reduced growth**; dry, encrusted, fissured, haemorrhagic skin on the feet, poor feathering, deformed 'parrot' beak, and sometimes, bone abnormality (**chondrodystrophy**), resulting in shortened, bowed legs with enlarged hocks. The occurrence of chondrodystrophy in the young bird is influenced by the biotin level in the egg, which in turn is influenced by the dietary status of the hen. High levels have a good or delaying effect.

Dietary biotin content is not considered to be important in egg laying flocks, but **in breeders** very severe deficiency leads to **reduced egg production. Even slight deficiency will affect hatchability,** deform the chick embryo and result in parrot beak. Biotin present in the egg (mainly yolk) is most important for hatchability and chick viability. These conditions improve with higher levels of biotin in the egg.

Diets slightly deficient in biotin cause a metabolic disorder known as '**fatty liver and kidney syndrome' (FLKS)**. It can cause death in young broilers and sometimes growers, usually between 10-30 days of age. FLKS responds to biotin treatment (see **'fatty liver and kidney syndrome'**).

**To conclude,** inadequate biotin can have two very different manifestations **in young chickens**: (1) clinical **skin and bone changes**, or (2) the **fatty liver and kidney**

**syndrome.** The balance between these two forms is determined by the balance between the metabolic requirements for different biotin-dependent enzymes. This balance in turn depends on the dietary content of other nutrients, mainly protein and fat.

## Treatment of Deficiency

Injection or oral administration of a few micrograms of biotin is sufficient to prevent biotin deficiency symptoms in chicks. Administration of biotin through drinking water, followed by adequate levels in the feed, provides complete recovery.

## Control

To prevent biotin deficiency:

1. Supply adequate levels of biotin in the feed.

2. Avoid excessive use of antibiotics.

3. Eliminate biotin antagonists where possible.

4. Assay feed samples to determine the levels of biotin at frequent intervals.

## FOLIC ACID (Folacin)

**Folic acid is a complicated chemical compound.** Several related compounds with similar activity in amino acid metabolism are grouped under this heading. Folic acid is necessary for growth, muscle formation, blood formation, and feather growth. Diets are rarely low in this vitamin.

## Functions

1. Folic acid is a part of the enzyme system involved in single-carbon metabolism. **It is involved in the synthesis of methyl groups ($CH_3$) of such important metabolites as choline, methionine, and thymine.**

2. Folic acid is therefore required for normal nucleic acid metabolism and formation of the nucleoproteins **required for cell multiplication.**

3. **The nutritional importance of various interactions of folic acid involved in single-carbon metabolism is greater in birds than mammals,** because of the bird's high rate of uric acid synthesis for nitrogen excretion, combined with a very high methionine and cysteine requirement. **Uric acid synthesis requires single-carbon units from several sources.**

## Causes of Deficiency

1. Inadequate levels of folic acid in the feed.

2. Solvent extracted soyabean meal is low in folic acid content.

3. Stability of folic acid is poor particularly through the pelleting process.

## Requirement

1. High dietary levels of protein increase the folic acid requirement. This is because of a greater need for uric acid synthesis for nitrogen excretion.

2. Inadequate levels of other methyl donors (methionine, vitamin B12, choline, betaine, and amino acid serine) also increase the requirement.

3. Antibiotics and other mediators that act against intestinal synthesis, increase the dietary requirements.

## Deficiency Symptoms

Deficiency of folic acid results in defective synthesis of DNA and RNA, **resulting in reduced cell division.** Tissues that depend on high rates of cell division are the first to be affected and therefore the symptoms in the beginning include **anaemia** (decrease of red blood cells, haemoglobin, or total blood volume) and leukopaenia (decrease of white blood cells). This is followed by **poor appetite and growth**, and very poor feathering. With greater deficiency, a severe anaemia develops caused by reduced red blood cell formation. Growth stops and defective feather development and pigmentation occur. **Leg deformities** appear due to **chondrodystrophy**, a generalized disorder of bones, resulting in short, thick and usually deformed long bones, along with enlargement of the hock joints. Folic acid is one of the many nutrients (other being manganese, zinc, choline, biotin, folic acid and pyridoxine) whose deficiency may lead to this condition.

**In hen**, folic acid deficiency damages the oviduct's response to oestrogen (female sex hormone) and ability to form albumen.

## Treatment of Deficiency

Addition of folic acid in the diet results in complete recovery of the affected chickens. A single intramuscular injection of 50-100 µg of pure folic acid provides good recovery from anaemia. Addition of 500 µg folic acid per 100 g feed causes recovery similar to that obtained with injection of the vitamin.

**To control the deficiency**, provide adequate levels of folic acid in the feed.

## VITAMIN B12 (Cobalamin)

**Of all the vitamins, vitamin B12 has the most complex structure.** Vitamin B12 deficiency is rare in chickens raised on the litter. This is because vitamin B12 is synthesized by the bacteria in the intestine, and also in the litter.

This vitamin is associated almost entirely with ingredients of animal and fish origin. Plant products contain little or no vitamin B12. Bird's own droppings are a source of vitamin B12. **Therefore, birds raised on wire are more likely to show a deficiency than those kept on a litter floor.**

## Functions

1.  Vitamin B12 is involved in the metabolism of protein, carbohydrate, and fat. In this action it is closely associated with folic acid.

2.  Vitamin B12 is also involved in nucleic acid and methyl group synthesis, along with folic acid.

## Causes of Deficiency

1.  High-protein diets increase the demand for vitamin B12 for use in amino acid-metabolizing enzymes, thus increasing the requirements.

2.  Inadequate levels of vitamin B12 in the feed.

## Deficiency Symptoms

Symptoms of vitamin B12 deficiency include **slow growth, decreased efficiency of feed utilization, mortality, and reduced egg size and hatchability.** **Chondrodystrophy** (a bone disorder, earlier known as 'perosis') may occur in vitamin B12-deficient chicks when their diets lack choline, methionine, or betaine as sources of methyl groups (see **'chondrodystrophy'**). Addition of vitamin B12 may prevent chondrodystrophy under these conditions because of its effect on the synthesis of methyl groups.

Vitamin B12-deficient embryos (developing chicks) have maximum mortality on the 7th day of incubation, reduced size of muscles in the legs, diffuse haemorrhages, chondrodystrophy, and fatty liver. **If laying birds are deficient, hatchability may drop to zero in about 6 weeks.**

## Treatment of Deficiency

1.  Intramuscular injection of 2 µg vitamin B12 per hen increases hatchability of eggs within one week.

2.  Addition of 4 mg vitamin B12 per tonne breeding ration is sufficient to maintain maximum hatchability. It also produces chicks which have enough stores of this vitamin to prevent any deficiency during the first few weeks of life.

3.  Similar injections in young chicks followed by supplementation of the chick ration will also correct the deficiency.

## CHOLINE

Choline is at times classed as an accessory substance, rather than a vitamin. This is because vitamins are needed in traces, **whereas choline is required in large amount in the diet** (greater than 1% of the dry matter). This high level is similar to the amounts of essential amino acids and fatty acids required by birds. Choline forms a part of the actual cell structure (in lecithin), and is therefore required in considerably greater quantities than vitamins. Choline can be synthesized to a minimal extent by chickens. It is synthesized in the liver from the amino acid serine.

**The chick's requirement for choline is high.** Choline may be synthesized by the chick, but the amounts are small and usually inadequate. Lesser amounts of dietary choline are required as the chick ages.

## Functions

Choline has **four main functions** in birds.

1. **Structural:** The primary role of choline is as a component of lecithin and other lipids. Lecithin is a main component of cell structure. As such **choline is needed for the structure of cell membranes.**

2. **Neurotransmitter:** In tissues, choline forms the important neurotransmitter acetylcholine. Acetylcholine plays an important role in the transmission of nerve impulses in the body.

3. **Methyl donor:** Choline is also oxidized to betaine. **Betaine is an important donor of methyl groups (CH3)** for conversion of homocysteine to methionine **(Fig. 21).** This pathway is particularly important for saving methionine, when methionine is deficient in diet.

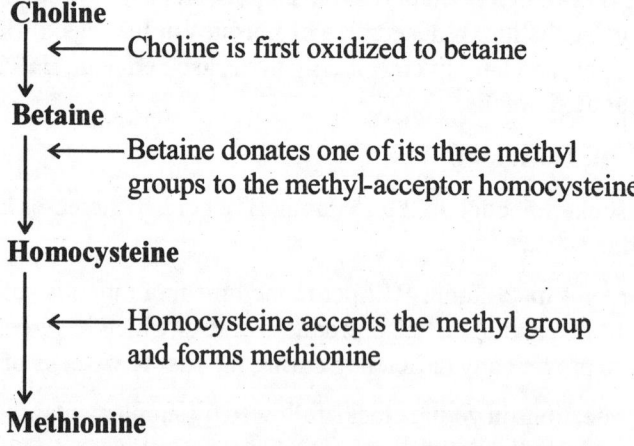

**Choline**
↤ Choline is first oxidized to betaine

**Betaine**
↤ Betaine donates one of its three methyl groups to the methyl-acceptor homocysteine

**Homocysteine**
↤ Homocysteine accepts the methyl group and forms methionine

**Methionine**

**Fig. 21.** Formation of methionine in the chicken.

4. **Choline has essential roles in fat metabolism.** In liver, for transformation of neutral fat (triglycerides) to phospholipids, choline is needed. In egg-laying hens, during choline deficiency triglycerides in liver are not converted into very low density lipoproteins. These triglycerides then accumulate in the liver causing a condition called **'fatty liver'** (hepatic steatosis). Choline is therefore called a **'lipotropic**

**factor'** or **'lipotrope'**, because it promotes the mobilization of lipids out of the liver. **Methionine, vitamin B12 and folic acid have lipotropic activity by participating in the synthesis of choline in the body.**

## Causes of Deficiency

1.    Inadequate choline levels in the diet.

2.    **Requirement for choline is increased when the dietary level of protein is high.** This is probably due to the additional need for methyl groups (CH3) to synthesize and excrete **uric acid.** The requirement of choline can be reduced by giving excess of either of the methyl donors - **methionine or betaine.** Dietary methionine in excess of that required for protein synthesis can spare the choline requirement effectively in adult chickens, **but its conversion to choline is limited in young chicks.** Betaine effectively spares choline in both young chicks and older birds. However, betaine can only replace the methyl donor functions of choline, and it cannot be used to synthesize choline to perform choline's structural and neurotransmitter functions. Thus, **dietary betaine can only substitute for about one-third of the choline requirement.** This point is discussed here because commercial betaine preparations are making their entry in poultry industry. Excess of choline in the diet than its requirement can improve marginal deficiencies of methionine, folic acid, and vitamin B12.

3.    Lack of choline synthesis by the chicken.

## Deficiency Symptoms

**In chicks,** apart from **poor growth**, the most important symptom of choline deficiency is **chondrodystrophy** (a bone disorder, earlier known as 'perosis'). Chondrodystrophy is first characterized by pinpoint haemorrhages and a slight swelling around the hock joint, followed by short, thick, and bowed legs typical of the disease.

**In egg-laying hens,** choline deficiency causes fatty liver, that is, the percentage of fat in the liver increases. In livers of choline-deficient chickens, **fat content is higher in females than males. Choline deficiency, however, is rare in adult chickens.** Eggs from hens fed low-choline diets may be smaller, but do not contain low levels of choline. High levels of additional choline, as choline chloride, depress growth.

## Treatment of Deficiency

If choline deficiency is noticed in chicks before severe symptoms of chondrodystrophy have developed, the deficiency can be cured by supplementing the ration with sufficient choline to meet the requirements. Once severe chondrodystrophy has developed, the damage is irreparable.

**Choline chloride** is the usual feed supplement. It contains 25 to 50% choline.

## VITAMIN C (Ascorbic Acid)

Most animals and **birds can synthesize sufficient amounts of vitamin C from glucose,** because they possess the required enzymes. Therefore, animals and birds do not normally need a dietary source of vitamin C. Humans, monkeys, and guinea-pigs lack this enzyme, and so cannot synthesize vitamin C. These species therefore require a dietary source; otherwise they quickly develop deficiency symptoms.

**Chickens do not normally require vitamin C, as they can synthesize it from glucose. Chickens synthesize vitamin C only in the kidneys, and not in the liver.** The site of synthesis varies with the species. Most birds synthesize vitamin C in the liver. It is interesting that **whereas chickens synthesize ascorbic acid only in the kidneys, sparrows synthesize it only in the liver, and crows both in the liver and kidneys.**

## Functions

1. **As an antioxidant,** ascorbic acid prevents damage to proteins from the free radical hydrogen peroxide ($H_2O_2$). Moreover, being a water-soluble antioxidant, it can inactivate (destroy) free radicals directly in the fluid portion of the cell - cytosol (see Chapter 33).

2. Vitamin C is also involved in protecting cellular membranes indirectly by regenerating the antioxidant form of vitamin E.

3. Vitamin C is a cofactor in the hydroxylation of amino acids lysine and proline of collagen fibres. This is necessary for the proper folding, structural stability and strength of mature collagen. **In chickens, vitamin C is especially important in the formation of collagen during wound repair.**

4. Dietary ascorbic acid promotes the bioavailability of dietary iron. It therefore decreases the iron requirement.

## Causes of Deficiency

1. Severe stress, such as **heat** and physical trauma.

2. Infections.

3. Consumption of some types of purified diets.

**Even the high rate of synthesis of vitamin C in the chickens may be inadequate during periods of severe stress of heat and physical trauma, and infections.** Also, there are no stores of vitamin C that are able to protect against prolonged dietary deficiency. Moreover, in the chicken, vitamin C is not transported to the egg, **but it is synthesized by the young embryo** (developing chick). Blood levels of ascorbic acid increase with increasing dietary ascorbic acid.

## Requirement

Vitamin C is useful to the young growing chickens during the **periods of stress from environment or infections.** Dietary levels of between 50 and 150 mg / kg dry matter are most effective. Higher levels sometimes cause reduction in growth rates, or efficiency of feed conversion in non-stressed poultry. Ascorbic acid supplementation of grain-based diets has been reported to **improve resistance** to a variety of infectious diseases and to improve wound healing.

**Vitamin C is relatively non-toxic.** High dietary levels of vitamin C are absorbed by the intestine and then excreted by the kidneys. Very high levels of vitamin C (more than 1%) cause slight diarrhoea and gastroenteritis (inflammation of the stomach and intestine).

**Note:** For a list of commercial preparations of all vitamins available at the market, see Chapter 19 under **"Vitamins".**

## ESSENTIAL MINERALS

**Essential minerals are as important as amino acids and vitamins in the maintenance of life, well-being, and production in poultry.** They enter into composition of bones and give the skeleton the rigidity and strength required to support the soft tissues. Minerals combine with protein, lipids, and other substances that make up the soft tissues. They take part in the maintenance of osmotic pressure and acid-base balance (i.e. pH). Minerals are also necessary for activation of many enzymes of the body.

The minerals essential for chickens are the **macro-minerals** calcium, phosphorus, magnesium, potassium, sodium, chlorine, and the **trace elements (micro-minerals)** manganese, iron, copper, zinc, iodine, molybdenum, and selenium. Fluorine in small amounts is a constant constituent of several tissues, particularly bones. However, there is no direct evidence of its beneficial effect in poultry. Analyses of individual mineral constituents in the body of chickens show that major portions of calcium, phosphorus, magnesium and zinc are present in bones. Other minerals are distributed mainly in muscles, other soft tissues, and body fluids.

## CALCIUM AND PHOSPHORUS

**Calcium is the most common mineral in the body,** and is required in the diet in a greater amount than any other mineral. Calcium is also one of the most metabolically active minerals. It constitutes more than a third of the total mineral content of an adult bird. **About 98% of body calcium and 85% of the phosphorus are present in the bones** (skeleton), which not only give bones their strength, but also act as a mineral reserve. Calcium and phosphorus are closely associated in metabolism, particularly in bone formation. **Calcium is primarily required for bone and eggshell formation.** It is deposited in bone mainly as calcium phosphate, but there is also some calcium carbonate. **Eggshells are almost entirely calcium carbonate.**

## Functions

1. The major portion of dietary calcium is used for **bone formation in growing chicks** and for **eggshell formation in laying hens.**

2. Calcium and phosphate perform important functions as electrolytes in body fluids.

3. Calcium ions activate several enzymes and act in nerve cell stimulation, neuromuscular transmission, muscular contraction, and blood clotting.

4. Phosphate is a component of nucleic acids, phospholipids, certain proteins and enzymes. It is also a part of acid-base balance (pH) and other biochemical processes, such as metabolic energy transfer, protein synthesis, and carbohydrate metabolism.

## Requirement and Related Aspects

1. **Laying hens** require at least 50% of their calcium as a less soluble large particle (limestone or oyster shells) to provide calcium during the dark hours when layers are forming eggshells. The larger particles of calcium stay in the gizzard until the acid from the proventriculus dissolves the calcium particles.

2. Except for animal products, such as meat meal, bone meal, the ingredients of poultry feed are low in calcium. Therefore, supplementation, for example with limestone, is included.

3. Phosphate is present mainly in cereals and other plant products, largely as phytate, that is, bound by phytic acid. It is therefore poorly utilized, especially by young birds. (For more information on this, refer to **'phytic acid'** in Chapter 23 on **"Enzymes"**).

4. **Phytate or phytic acid also binds calcium strongly and inhibits its utilization** (see **Fig. 28**). Calcium in plants usually exists in complexes with phytic acid or oxalate which reduce its digestibility. One mole of phytic acid can bind up to 6 moles of calcium to form insoluble phytates at the pH of the intestine. **Phytic acid forms complexes with cations** (i.e. positively charged ions), **such as calcium ($Ca^{++}$), magnesium ($Mg^{++}$), manganese ($Mn^{++}$), iron ($Fe^{++}$), zinc ($Zn^{++}$), and potassium ($K^+$), and reduces their availability.**

5. Phosphorus found in animal by-products is completely available, but plant phosphorus has a low biological availability for poultry. This is because only a small part of the total phosphorus is present in the inorganic form, which is fully available to birds; **but the majority, some 60-70%, is in the phytic form, which is unavailable to birds.** For more information on this, refer to Chapter 23 on **"Enzymes"** under **'Phytase'**.

6.  The availability of phytic phosphorus decreases with increasing calcium content. For example, at high levels in layer feeds (4% calcium) and feeds for very young chicks (about 1% calcium), phytic phosphorus is virtually unavailable to these birds. **There is a lack of enzyme phytase in bird's intestine, especially in young chicks,** but phytase is present in some grains. For these reasons, poultry feeds require supplementation with phosphate.

7.  High levels of dietary calcium decrease the absorption of phosphorus by forming precipitates in the intestines. Not only is phosphorus availability affected by calcium present, but calcium also affects other dietary nutrients, mainly **vitamin D**, which **largely controls absorption of calcium in the intestine** through formation of calcium-binding protein. This protein keeps the calcium in solution so that it can pass the intestinal wall and reach the cells.

8.  The total calcium and available phosphorus ratio present in feed for growing birds is formulated as 1.5 - 2:1. This is similar to the ratio of calcium and phosphorus present in bone as calcium hydroxyphosphate.

9.  **Calcium requirement in the layer depends on production.** Therefore, calcium is increased in the formulated feed as production increases. In layer feeds (with a calcium content of more than 4%), care must be taken to ensure that separation (sedimentation) of heavier mineral ingredients, particularly calcium, does not occur during and after transportation. This separation can occur quickly in mash feed, particularly if the calcium particle size is large. **This leads to reduced calcium intake by birds, resulting in poor or soft-shelled eggs.**

10. **The absorption of calcium and phosphorus depends on the presence of an adequate amount of vitamin D in the diet.** In vitamin D deficiency, the deposition of these minerals in bones of growing chickens is reduced, bones become depleted of minerals, and the quantity of calcium in eggshells is decreased.

11. The requirement of phosphorus is highest in the growing chicks and gradually decreases as skeletal growth subsides.

12. **The phosphorus requirement increases during egg laying.** It is much greater than the amount of phosphorus present in the egg. This is because the higher demand for calcium to synthesize eggshells causes bone to be mobilized. **The ratio of calcium to phosphate in bone (2.5:1) is much lower than that in eggshell (20:1),** and much of the excess phosphate that is liberated is excreted by the kidneys. This internal loss results in an increase in the phosphorus requirement. The phosphorus requirement of birds of any age is increased by high dietary calcium levels, or a vitamin D deficiency.

13. There are a large number of interactions or inter-relationships between major mineral

elements, namely, calcium, phosphorus, magnesium, sodium, and potassium. **Certain bone abnormalities may be partly due to these relationships.**

## Deficiency Symptoms

1.  When dietary supplies of calcium and/or phosphorus are inadequate, the bones are depleted. As a result, the most common signs of deficiency of either nutrient are seen in the **bones**, in the form of **'rickets'** in the young growing bird (see **'rickets'**), or as **'osteoporosis'** in the grown or layer bird (see **'osteoporosis'**).

    A calcium deficiency may occur due to a low dietary level of calcium, or to excess dietary phosphorus. Insufficient vitamin D may cause a secondary calcium deficiency by interfering with calcium absorption and bone formation.

2.  Growers, deprived of calcium, show increased general activity and pecking. An early sign of calcium deficiency **in the laying hen is reduced egg production and production of thin or soft-shelled eggs.** The average shell thickness of normal eggs is 330 μm in chickens. In the chicken the shell contains 2.0 - 2.2 g calcium. This amount remains the same throughout laying. Therefore, as eggs become larger as laying progresses, calcium becomes more thinly spread, and there are increasing shell quality defects.

3.  **'Cage layer fatigue'** is seen in caged hens in good bodily condition. They suddenly lie down, sometimes paralyzed, with legs extended. The bones are brittle (easily broken), ribs and sternum are usually deformed, and bone fractures are common. These problems are due to osteoporosis (reduction in the quality of fully formed structural bone), which arises from a generalized loss of cancellous bone throughout the skeleton.

    **There are two types of bone in laying hens: (1) Structural, cancellous, compact or cortical bone,** which is responsible for the strength of bones, and (2) **Medullary bone,** which acts as a reserve of calcium for shell formation. **It does not contribute to strength.** At the onset of sexual maturity, hens deposit medullary bone in the cavity of their long bones, under the influence of sex hormones oestrogens and androgens, released by maturing ovarian follicles. **Medullary bone supplies calcium for eggshell formation during periods when dietary supply is insufficient.** In hens, calcium in the medullary bone is accumulated in the morning and used in the night. When egg production stops, medullary bone disappears in the next week.

    **During egg laying, there is a continuous turnover of medullary bone with removal of existing bone and formation of new bone.** However, structural bone cannot be formed when hens are in laying, but the continuing process of bone removal means that the amount of structural bone decreases during the laying period. This leads to older hens becoming severely depleted in the amount of structural bone, **which then develop osteoporosis.** In other words this means that in calcium deficiency, first there is complete removal of calcium from the medullary bones, followed by a gradual removal from the structural bone. Ultimately, bones become so thin that spontaneous fractures may occur, especially in vertebrae, tibia and femur. This condition may be associated with **'cage layer fatigue'.**

## Control

The relative inactivity of caged birds accelerates these processes. If birds are given more exercise, this greatly improves bone quality. Nutrition, on the other hand, is not very effective in preventing osteoporosis. However, poor nutrition, such as deficiencies of calcium, phosphorus, or vitamin D can quicken the onset of osteoporosis.

## Excess Calcium

Excess calcium in the feed of young broilers or growers, (especially between 6-12 weeks of age) will give rise to disease of kidneys. Feeding of growers on layer rations (i.e. about 4% calcium instead of about 0.8%), or a mixing error, will lead to **visceral gout.** Low levels of dietary phosphorus during the rearing period aggravate the effect of excess calcium.

## SODIUM CHLORIDE

Among minerals in the diet, sodium ($Na^+$) and potassium ($K^+$) are the main cationic (positively charged) electrolytes and chloride ($Cl^-$) is the main anionic (negatively charged) electrolyte. All three are important in maintaining ionic balance in body fluids.

**Sodium ($Na^+$) and chloride ($Cl^-$) ions in the body play a vital role in the maintenance of osmotic pressure, and water and acid-base (pH) balance.** The **sodium ion** is the main cation of the fluid present outside the cells (in extra-cellular fluid), and is involved in metabolite transfer across membranes. The **potassium ion** is the main cation of the fluid present inside the cells (in intra-cellular fluid), and is involved in maintaining intra-cellular fluid volume and osmotic pressure. **Chloride ($Cl^-$)** is the main anion present mainly outside the cells and also plays a role in maintaining fluid volume and ionic balance. It also occurs as hydrochloric acid (HCl) in the secretions of proventriculus. Deficiencies of these ions therefore produce widespread disturbances in function of the cells and water distribution. Depending on the degree of deficiency, symptoms will include retarded growth, reduced egg production, dehydration, neuromuscular dysfunction, and death.

## Requirement

Poultry feeds must be supplemented to meet sodium requirements. This is usually done by adding common salt (sodium chloride) and/or sodium bicarbonate. In feed formulation for poultry, minimum sodium level is around 0.15%, the minimum requirement being about 0.12%. Below this level, for example at 0.10%, broiler chicks fail to grow to their best. **However, it is undesirable to add too much salt,** that is, more than 0.12%. This will cause increased water consumption, and therefore wet droppings. This is not only undesirable in caged layers, but even more so in broilers. In broilers, wet litter gives rise to carcass downgrading (reduction in quality/volume) due to breast blisters and hock lesions. **Additions over 8% cause deaths.**

In commercial layer feeds the balance between potassium, sodium and chloride ions is very important in working out the best egg laying performance, and also shell formation and quality. **The bicarbonate ion is most important in shell formation and quality.** Therefore, today some amount of sodium in layer feed may come from sodium bicarbonate, and also in the broiler feed to limit chloride intake, again to reduce water consumption (see above). In such cases, the salt addition is limited to a maximum of 0.37%. That is, 3.7 kg per tonne of feed.

## Deficiency Symptoms

1. Birds receiving diets deficient in sodium fail to grow, develop softening of bones, show poor food utilization, and decreased fluid volumes. Cardiac (heart) output drops, and a state of shock occurs that may terminate in death.

2. **Chicks show retarded growth with decreased efficiency of feed utilization.** When frightened, they fall forward with their legs outstretched behind them and lie paralyzed for several minutes. Then appear quite normal until frightened again.

3. **Sodium deficiency in laying hens causes a sudden drop in egg production with reduced egg size.** Actually, a low-sodium diet has been suggested as a means of inducing a pause in egg production.

4. However, if the deficiency is only marginal (slight) and some laying continues, the drop in production is accompanied by increased bird activity, **with greatly increased pecking behaviour and intense cannibalism** (see 'cannibalism'), especially at the everted cloaca (cloaca turned inside out) of other birds while laying eggs.

5. Diarrhoea, and other gastro-intestinal disturbances, increase the excretion and decrease the absorption of electrolytes. This greatly increases the requirement of electrolytes. **Electrolyte replacement treatment is a common component of the care given to birds suffering from intestinal infections.**

6. **Both deficiencies and excesses of salt are very harmful to poultry, and problems of this nature are quite common.**

## Signs of Toxicity

**Large amounts of salt in the ration are toxic to chickens.** The lethal dose, that causes death, is about 4 g / kg body weight. Young chicks appear to be more susceptible to toxic effects of salt than older birds, and also if drinking water is restricted.

**Signs of toxicity include** diarrhoea, intense thirst, loss of appetite, pronounced muscular weakness, inability to stand, convulsions and death. **Excess sodium results in ascites** (accumulation of fluid in the body cavity) **in broiler chickens** (see **'ascites'**). High level of salt also causes the excretion of dilute urine and wet litter.

Severe kidney damage occurs in young birds, with renal failure (i.e. kidney failure) and death. **Postmortem findings** include **visceral gout** (see **'gout'**) and impaction of ureters with urates. Older birds are more tolerant of increased salt levels, provided adequate water is available. However, the feed intake and egg production are depressed by 5% sodium chloride in laying hen diets.

Electrolytes in the water are much more toxic than similar levels in the feed.

# POTASSIUM

**Potassium is found mainly inside the cells of the body.** Soft tissues of the chicken contain three times more potassium than sodium. As a major cation (positively charged ion) within the cells, potassium plays an essential role in the maintenance of cellular fluid balance.

Potassium participates in a large number of biochemical reactions. It is necessary for normal heart activity, reducing contractility (power of contraction) of the heart muscle and favouring relaxation.

## Deficiency Symptoms

The main effect of potassium deficiency is overall muscle weakness, characterized by weak extremities, poor intestinal tone with distensions, cardiac (heart) weakness, and weakness of the respiratory muscles and their ultimate failure. Severely affected birds may show convulsions (constant muscular contractions) followed by death.

Low levels of potassium in layer's diet cause decreased egg production and eggshell thinning. High temperature results in increased loss of potassium in the urine.

# MAGNESIUM

Magnesium is essential for carbohydrate metabolism and for activation of a large number of enzymes. Magnesium ions in the blood are taken up by all cells of the body, and like potassium, have a high concentration inside the cells. **Magnesium is essential for bone formation, about two-third being present in bone. Eggshells contain about 0.4% magnesium.** Calcium is poorly utilized in the absence of magnesium.

## Causes of Deficiency

**Magnesium deficiencies are rare,** because most foods have concentrations which are well above the requirement. The most common cause of deficiency is high dietary calcium or phosphorus levels. However, most calcium and phosphorus supplements are

255

high in magnesium. Therefore, such a possibility is unlikely.

## Deficiency Symptoms

**In chicks**, signs of magnesium deficiency include slow growth, dullness, brief convulsions, accompanied by gasping, and finally periods of coma, sometimes ending in death.

## Excess Magnesium

Excess of magnesium than the body's requirement is stored in the bone. Further excesses of magnesium are excreted through the kidney. Most of the magnesium in eggs is found in the shell and becomes available to the developing embryo (chick) as it withdraws calcium.

An excess of magnesium in the feed is as harmful as too little. Excess magnesium interferes with calcium absorption and metabolism and symptoms are similar to a calcium deficiency, that is, poor bone mineralization and thin eggshells. Excess magnesium also acts as a laxative and causes wet droppings. High dietary calcium and phosphorus levels reduce magnesium toxicity.

## MANGANESE

Manganese is required for normal growth and reproduction, and prevention of chondrodystrophy, a bone disorder resulting in shortening of the long bones.

**The greatest concentration of manganese is in the bones (skeleton).** Birds are much more susceptible to deficiency than mammals because their requirement is much higher (up to 100 times in some cases). This is due to relatively poor duodenal absorption. Absorption is prevented by excessive dietary calcium and phosphorus, phytic acid, and fibre.

## Functions

1.  Manganese is an activator of several enzymes. It is necessary for formation of normal bones. Manganese deficiency interferes with the growth of bones.

2.  Manganese is also necessary for maximum eggshell quality, egg production, and hatchability.

## Deficiency Symptoms

1.  **Skeletal deformities occur and eggshells become thin, porous and soft,** when manganese intake is inadequate.

2.  **In young growing birds,** growth is retarded and there is deformity of bone growth called **'chondrodystrophy',** earlier known as **'perosis'.** This condition results in short, thick, and usually deformed long bones, and is often associated with an

enlargement of the hock joints. **The affected birds show lameness.** Apart from manganese, a number of nutritional deficiencies can cause chondrodystrophy, which include choline, biotin, nicotinic acid, folic acid, zinc, and pyridoxine.

3. **In the laying or breeder bird,** manganese deficiency causes **a marked drop in egg production, eggshell thinning,** and greatly **reduced hatchability** (even up to 50%) in incubated eggs. Embryos (developing chicks) usually die in the last third of incubation, showing gross skeletal and other defects. In newly hatched chicks, muscular incoordination and head retraction (drawing back) may be seen.

Manganese is considered to be one of the least toxic trace minerals, and dietary levels of 1000 mg per kg are tolerated.

Since all diets composed of normal feedstuffs are deficient, manganese is added to the feed as manganese sulphate, or manganous oxide. A 70% feeding grade is commonly used. From 30 to 50 g of manganese are added to a tonne of feed to prevent chondrodystrophy (perosis) and 50 to 75 g to increase eggshell strength.

# IODINE

Traces of iodine are required for normal functioning of the thyroid in poultry. Iodine is an essential part of the thyroid hormones. No other metabolic functions have been described in birds. **Thyroxine,** an iron-containing hormone of the thyroid gland, contains about 65% iodine, and acts as an important regulating agent in body metabolism. Besides being a part of many metabolic functions in growing and adult birds, iodine is needed by the developing embryo (i.e. chick).

## Deficiency Symptoms

Iodine deficiency results in an enlargement of thyroid gland (goitre) and, in some cases, lower body weight in growing chicks. Other symptoms include mortality late in incubation. Hatching time is delayed. Embryo size is reduced and yolk sac resorption is retarded.

## Treatment

Use of 0.25% iodized salt (iodine added as potassium iodide) in chicken should prevent development of iodine deficiency. This would supply 0.175 ppm in addition to that contained in the diet.

Iodine deficiency in poultry has been largely prevented by widespread use of iodine either in iodized salt, or as part of the trace mineral premix.

# COPPER

Copper deficiency in chickens results in anaemia. (Anaemia is a condition in which blood is deficient in red blood cells, in haemoglobin, or in total volume). Most of the absorption of dietary copper occurs in the proventriculus and duodenum. High levels of dietary calcium, phosphorus, phytic acid, and oxalate decrease copper absorption by forming insoluble complexes in the intestine.

Copper in excess of immediate requirement is stored in the liver and other tissues. Further excesses of copper are excreted through the bile.

**Young growing birds have a higher copper requirement than adults, and are more likely to show a deficiency.**

## Functions

1. Copper is a component of a variety of enzymes that participate in redox (oxidation-reduction) reactions in the body.

2. **Copper is essential for formation of haemoglobin.** Haemoglobin is an iron-containing pigment of red blood cells that functions in oxygen transport to the tissues, and transports back carbon dioxide to the lungs, after giving away its oxygen. Its deficiency results in **anaemia.**

3. In the absence of copper, although dietary iron is absorbed and deposited in the liver and elsewhere, but haemoglobin synthesis does not occur. Copper is necessary for iron utilization when haemoglobin is formed. **Therefore, if copper is absent from the diet, anaemia results.** The amount of copper and iron needed in the diet is quite specific. Excesses may be toxic. **About 5 to 10 times as much iron as copper is required.** Usually, only small amounts, if any, are added to commercial feeds.

4. Most of the blood copper is found as a component of **ceruloplasmin**, a copper-binding protein with enzymatic activity. Ceruloplasmin is necessary for iron transport and also plays a role in the acute phase of the immune response. **It protects the bird by reducing the formation of free radicals.** The need to synthesize ceruloplasmin during an infection increases copper requirement of the bird. (For more information on ceruloplasmin, see Chapter 33 under 'acute phase proteins'.)

## Deficiency Symptoms

1. Copper deficiency symptoms include anaemia, haemorrhages, lameness, and poor feather pigmentation. Anaemia is due to low levels of ceruloplasmin, which causes poor iron utilization.

2. **In laying hens**, deficiency of copper causes reduced egg production, infertile eggs, increased egg size, and abnormal eggshell calcification. Eggshell abnormalities include shell-less eggs, misshapen (deformed) eggs, wrinkled eggshells, and reduced eggshell thickness.

Excess dietary levels of copper have been reported to cause abnormalities of the gizzard.

# IRON

Iron is an essential component of **haemoglobin**, and is also an essential component of several enzymes.

## Deficiency Symptoms

Iron deficiency results in **anaemia**. A deficiency in laying hens also causes anaemia in the developing chick embryo and reduced hatchability. Chicks that survive incubation are weak and without energy or vitality. However, they recover when given supplemental iron.

# ZINC

**Zinc is an essential trace element for poultry.** In birds, zinc affects growth, development, reproduction, and because of its involvement in many enzymes, it plays a role in almost every metabolic function.

**Zinc has a very large number of functions and is an activator, or a cofactor, of more than 200 enzymes. It is among the most metabolically active of the trace minerals.** Its deficiency affects all metabolic pathways, regulation of gene expression, and cell division.

## Requirement

A daily supply is required due to its utilization and excretion. Zinc absorption is decreased by high dietary levels of **phytic acid** due to formation of an insoluble zinc complex. (For more information on this refer to Chapter 23 under 'phytase' and 'phytic acid'.) Also, high calcium, phosphorus, and copper levels reduce the availability of **phytate-bound zinc.** Calcium and phosphate form insoluble precipitates with zinc in the intestinal lumen. In addition, high calcium levels in feed intensify the effects of zinc deficiency. The main reserves in bone can be mobilized for metabolic use even when calcium intake is high. In chickens, stores last for only about 4 days. Bone stores last a few days longer, but a zinc deficiency soon develops.

Of the raw materials commonly used in poultry feeds, the richest sources of zinc are animal protein ingredients, such as meat and fish meals. To ensure adequate intake, supplementation with a zinc compound has long been a standard practice in feed manufacturing.

As feedstuffs are generally low in zinc, this mineral is usually added to the ration as zinc carbonate (about 57% zinc), or zinc oxide (about 80.5% zinc). Normally, from 15 to 30 g of zinc are added to 1 tonne of feed.

## Deficiency Symptoms

1. Zinc is required mainly for **skeletal growth and development**, for epithelial tissue

formation and maintenance, and for egg production.

2. Deficiency gives rise to **poor growth and appetite**, poor feathering, infertility, scaly skin especially on the legs and feet, and in young growing birds, to the generalized bone disorder called **'chondrodystrophy'**. Chondrodystrophy results in short, thick, and usually deformed long bones, often accompanied by an enlargement of the hock joints.

3. There is also **reduced egg production and hatchability** is affected. Embryonic mortality is highest around mid-incubation.

4. **Zinc deficiency affects immunocompetence of the birds.** That is, their ability to produce immunity. For example, chickens maintained on a zinc-deficient diet are unable to produce antibodies against T-cell-dependent antigens, even though lymphocytes are capable of antibody production. To understand this, and for more information on the role of zinc in the production of immunity in chickens, refer to Chapter 33: **"Impact of nutrients on avian immunity"**.

## Excess of Zinc

1. In chickens, toxicities have not been reported at the level of 1 g per kg of feed, and levels above 2 g per kg of feed are usually tolerated by adults. Birds can tolerate relatively high levels of dietary zinc. Excess zinc is excreted through pancreatic secretions and bile.

2. Excessive dietary levels of zinc, such as 20, 000 ppm as zinc oxide, induce moulting in laying hens and stop egg laying. High dietary zinc increases the requirement of selenium, iron, and copper.

**Note:** 1. For advantages of organic zinc over inorganic, refer to Chapter 33.

2. For a list of commercial preparations available at the market containing zinc, refer to Chapter 19 under **"Minerals"**.

## SELENIUM

Selenium was shown to be an essential mineral element in 1957. About this time, it was also shown that certain diseases of livestock caused by deficiencies of vitamin E responded to dietary supplies of selenium. Among these conditions was **'exudative diathesis'** of poultry, which is caused by vitamin E deficiency.

## Functions

Metabolic role of selenium was found in 1973, when it was shown to be a constituent of the cell enzyme **glutathione peroxidase** (GSH-Px). This enzyme destroys peroxides (free radicals) as they are formed in the cells, and is important in protecting tissues against oxidative damage caused by peroxides. (For more information on the protective role of selenium against free radicals, refer to Chapter 33 under **'selenium'**). Thus, there is a close relationship between selenium and enzyme glutathione peroxidase. **Vitamin E is also an important antioxidant and both vitamin E and glutathione peroxidase work together to reduce the oxidative damage.** This **complementary nature of selenium and vitamin E** is the basis for their mutual sparing effect on requirements. High levels of vitamin E partially reduce the need for glutathione peroxidase and decrease the selenium requirement. Chickens fed diets high in vitamin E have a selenium requirement that is at least five times less than those fed low vitamin E. Large amounts of selenium are stored in the body tissues when intake is high, and these stores take care of mild dietary deficiencies.

The connection between the biochemical roles of selenium and vitamin E was found to be that cell damage by lipid hydroperoxides could be prevented either from removal of the already formed peroxide by glutathione peroxide, or from the antioxidant activity of vitamin E preventing hydroperoxide formation. **Both the functions are required when cells have heavy loads of oxygen-derived free radicals, or unsaturated fatty acids. (Lipid hydroperoxides** are formed by the action of active peroxides on unsaturated fatty acids present in the phospholipids of the cell membrane. Vitamin E binds with the unsaturated fatty acids and prevents hydroperoxide formation). For more information on this, refer to Chapter 33 under **'selenium'.**

The adequate dietary level of selenium is 0.1 ppm for chickens up to 16 weeks of age. Sodium selenite is a compound that can supply selenium; 464 g to 1,023 kg of ration will supply 0.1 ppm.

## Deficiency Symptoms

1.  Deficiency of selenium reduces production and function of glutathione peroxidase. This leads to lipid hydroperoxide production in oxygen-loaded cells which then causes cell wall damage.

2.  **In poultry**, selenium deficiency leads to **nutritional muscular dystrophy, exudative diathesis**, and **encephalomalacia** (for information on these conditions, refer to **'Vitamin E'**).

    **Exudative diathesis** is caused by oxidative damage to the capillaries (minute blood vessels) and by the leakage of fluids. This results in gelatinous oedema (swelling) which is usually seen under the skin of the breast and abdomen. Small haemorrhages cause the accumulation of blood in the fluid, giving it the characteristic green-blue colour. **Exudative diathesis responds to selenium supplementation in the presence of adequate vitamin E.** In fact, selenium prevents development of exudative diathesis in young chickens.

3.  Chicks severely deficient in selenium show poor growth and feathering, and also poor fat digestion.

4.  **Deficiency of selenium affects the immune status of the bird.** For its role in the production of immunity, refer to Chapter 33).

## Toxicity of Selenium

Selenium becomes toxic to birds at levels 5-20 mg per kg dry matter. That is, about 50 times higher than the requirement. **Thus, selenium is the most toxic of the trace minerals,** and has the lowest margin between deficient and excess dietary levels. The exact dietary level that is toxic depends on the chemical form. Organic selenides are the most toxic.

Excess selenium interferes with sulphur metabolism, due to the formation of sulphur-selenium complexes. This reduces protein synthesis. The developing embryo (chick) is particularly affected by high selenium. **The toxicity of selenium is reduced by high levels of dietary methionine.**

The amount of selenium added to diets is very small and the margin between the bird's requirement and the toxic level is narrow, **so selenium supplementation must be done carefully.**

**Note:** 1. For advantages of organic selenium over inorganic, refer to Chapter 33.

2. For a list of commercial preparations available in the market containing various minerals, including selenium, refer to Chapter 19 under **"Minerals".**

## Nutrition in Relation to Immunity and Disease

The functioning of the **immune system** is damaged by a variety of nutritional deficiencies. On the other hand, supplementation with higher than normal levels of certain vitamins, for example of vitamin A and D, increases the ability of poultry to mount an effective immune response. **Stress increases the need for a number of vitamins. For example, vitamin C which is not normally a dietary requirement, improves the effect of heat stress in broilers and layers.** A large number of nutrients have a marked influence on the immune system of poultry, and therefore on the production of effective immunity. For more information on this vital aspect of poultry farming, refer to Chapter 33: **"Impact of nutrients on avian immunity".**

## WATER

Water holds a unique position in nutrition, mainly due to its physiological properties.

1.  Because of its solvent (dissolving) properties, it acts as a transport medium for other nutrients and products of metabolism, and increases cell reactions.

2.  Because of its high specific heat, it can absorb the heat of reactions produced in the oxidation of carbohydrates and fats with little rise in temperature. Water evaporates readily, removing any calories from the body as latent heat of vaporization. These

and many other functions explain why the bird is able to exist much longer without food than without water.

**Unlike larger farm animals, chickens must have a continuous water supply, because they drink only small amounts of water at a time. An insufficient amount results in decreased growth and egg production.**

# Chapter 10

# Metabolic Diseases

**M**etabolic diseases result from a disturbance of the normal metabolic processes.** They have their own economic importance in the modern poultry industry. Their importance is on two accounts.

**Firstly,** having largely controlled most of the infectious diseases with the help of very effective vaccines, antibacterial agents and anticoccidials, our most serious problems now relate to metabolic diseases. Metabolic diseases are responsible for a great deal of morbidity (sickness) and mortality (deaths) in both broilers and layers. **They affect birds with the greatest growth rate, or the highest egg production.** Conditions, such as ascites and sudden death syndrome in broilers, now probably account for 30% of the total mortality.

**Secondly,** they are **extremely common,** the reason being that **their origin usually lies in the mistakes of management.** For example, simple dehydration due to lack of water, or inadequate number of drinkers, can lead to an outbreak of gout in chicks. Likewise, poor ventilation, faulty brooding, or ammonia formation may later result in ascites. Rickets may occur from calcium, phosphorus, and/or vitamin D3 deficiency, or their imbalance.

This chapter deals with metabolic diseases of poultry, **highlighting causes associated with the lapses of management,** and gives special emphasis on their effective control.

## GOUT

Gout is a condition in which high levels of uric acid in the blood (hyperuricaemia) lead to deposition of urates on the surfaces of various internal organs, or various joints, especially the hock joint. **Gout is not a disease condition, but a clinical sign of severe kidney dysfunction.** The dysfunction occurs from kidney damage, and results in hyperuricaemia. Gout is a common finding during postmortem examination of poultry, and can be **a source of great economic loss to farmers. Birds usually die from kidney failure.**

**Gout occurs in two distinct forms: (1) Visceral gout, and (2) Articular gout. The current concept is that visceral and articular gout are two separate diseases, as shown below:**

| Visceral gout | Articular gout |
|---|---|
| 1. It is usually an acute condition | 1. It is usually a chronic disease |
| 2. It is very common | 2. It is rare |
| 3. Occurs at one day and above | 3. Occurs at 4-5 months and above |
| 4. Occurs in both males and females | 4. Occurs mostly in males |
| 5. Kidneys are always involved and look abnormal due to deposition of white, chalky, precipitates | 5. Kidneys are usually normal |
| 6. Liver, heart, spleen and peritoneum are usually involved | 6. These organs are rarely involved. At times, urate precipitates can also be seen in the comb, wattles, and trachea |
| 7. Soft tissues around the joints are mostly not involved | 7. Soft tissues around the joints are always involved. They are white due to urate deposition |
| 8. Occurs due to failure of urate excretion (kidney failure) | 8. Occurs due to a metabolic defect in the secretion of urates by the kidney probably due to high protein in the diet |

## Visceral Gout

Visceral gout is characterized by **deposition of monosodium urates in the kidneys,** mesentery, and peritoneum (a membrane in the abdominal cavity). In some cases, surfaces of muscles and synovial sheaths (coverings) of tendons (a tendon is a tough tissue that attaches muscles to bones) and joints may be involved, and deposition may also occur within the liver and spleen. **The deposits on the surfaces of heart, liver, airsacs, and peritoneum appear as white chalky coating.**

## Articular Gout

Articular gout is characterized by **tophi. Tophi** (singular is 'tophus') **are deposits of urates around joints, particularly those of the feet.** The joints are enlarged, and feet appear deformed. When these joints are opened, the periarticular tissue (i.e. tissue surrounding a joint) is **white due to urate deposition**. White semifluid deposits of urates may be found within the joints.

Articular gout is an occasional individual bird problem, and is not of much economic importance.

## Causes

A number of factors may be involved in the production of gout in poultry. These include:

1.  **The basis of gout is kidney dysfunction (abnormal function).** Deposition of urates in organ is usually due to a failure of urinary excretion. This may be due to kidney damage, dehydration (lack of water), or obstruction of ureters. The abnormal function of kidney results in inadequate excretion of uric acid and therefore leads to **hyperuricaemia** (excess uric acid in the blood). The level of uric acid in the blood is increased in both visceral and articular gout.

2.  **Dehydration**, due to lack of water, or inadequate number of drinkers, is a common cause of visceral gout in poultry.

3.  **Excess of dietary calcium, or calcium: phosphorus imbalance** (see 'calcium'). That is, excess of calcium in relation to phosphorus, or low intake of phosphorus in relation to calcium.

4.  **Vitamin A deficiency** can also cause outbreaks of visceral gout in poultry.

5.  **Increased intake of protein** may result in increased uric acid production, especially in older birds. As articular gout can be produced by feeding high-protein diets, it has been suggested that it results from excessive production of uric acid, particularly in birds that are genetically susceptible. Thus, **a large excess of protein may cause hyperuricaemia and articular gout.**

6.  Generally **excessive amount of salt (sodium chloride)** causes severe kidney damage in young birds, with visceral gout, urate impacted ureters, kidney failure, and death.

7.  **Infection with nephrotropic/nephropathogenic** (i.e. affecting kidneys) **strains of infectious bronchitis virus in young chickens.** Infection with such strains causes outbreaks of renal (kidney) gout, in which kidneys are enlarged and usually distended with urates.

8.  **Mycotoxins** (fungal toxins) may be involved. Many of the mycotoxins (ochratoxins, aflatoxins, oosporein, etc) found in poultry feed can directly or indirectly influence kidney function. Of these, **oosporein is the most damaging to kidneys,** and is capable of causing extensive visceral gout.

9.  **An electrolyte excess or deficiency.** This is because diet electrolytes can influence water balance and kidney function. **Since salts of uric acid are very insoluble, they are precipitated when water is in short supply.** In most cases, when the birds become dehydrated the ureters are distended with urates.

10.  Treatment with sodium bicarbonate.

11.  Certain antibiotics.

12.  Urolithiasis.

13.  Obstruction of ureters.

## Development of the Disease

**Birds** are prone to gout because they are **uricotelic**. That is, in them, the waste product of protein metabolism (i.e. excretion of nitrogen) is mainly in the form of **uric acid**. This is because they lack the enzyme uricase, which converts uric acid into allantoin. Moreover, **uric acid is water insoluble.** Therefore, any injury or damage to bird's kidney, from whatever cause, interferes with the elimination of uric acid, which then accumulates in the blood (**hyperuricaemia**) and leads to **visceral gout**, that is, deposition of urate crystals on the surfaces of the internal organs. **Uric acid is produced in the liver.**

**Mammals**, on the other hand, are **ureotelic.** That is, in them the waste product of protein metabolism is mainly in the form of **urea**, and mammals are therefore not prone to gout like birds. Also, **urea is water soluble.**

Excess dietary calcium, particularly if associated with low available dietary phosphorus, results in the deposition of fine **crystals of calcium sodium urate** in the kidneys. It is believed that deposition of calcium sodium urates is due to high levels of urinary calcium and **more alkaline urine**. Dietary acidification with ammonium chloride, ammonium sulphate, or methionine has been shown to decrease deposition of calcium sodium urates in urolithiasis (i.e. stone formation in kidneys) induced experimentally with high-calcium diets. Ammonium chloride, however, is not recommended for use in the field, because it causes increased water consumption, urine flow, and wet litter. Ammonium sulphate is more effective than the two forms of methionine.

## Postmortem Findings

In the **visceral gout**, kidneys are swollen and congested and greyish white in colour with a soft consistency. Apart from the kidney, heart, proventriculus, and lungs are the main sites of urate deposition. The deposits on the surfaces of these organs appear as **white chalky coating**. One or both of the ureters may be distended with white material.

In the **articular gout,** when joints are opened, the **tissue surrounding the joints is white due to urate deposition.** White semifluid deposits of urates may be found within the joints.

## Diagnosis

Diagnosis is based on typical postmortem findings.

## Treatment and Prevention

1.  Gout poses a real problem in laying hens fed high levels of calcium in advance of sexual maturity. Therefore, **avoid feeding high levels of calcium.** No more than 1% calcium should be fed to Leghorn birds before maturity.

2.  High level of crude protein increases blood uric acid levels which can lead to gout. Therefore, **reduce the high level of protein, increase maize, and formulate the feed accordingly for a few days to get over the problem.**

3.  Kidney dysfunction is associated with an increased loss of water and electrolytes. Therefore, **give plenty of water containing electrolytes.**

4.  **Use urine acidifiers,** such as methionine hydroxy analogue (MHA), or even supplemental DL-methionine. Acidified urine results in increased calcium solubilization (dissolving) in the urine. It can even dissolve urate deposits already formed in mature birds.

## UROLITHIASIS

Urolithiasis is the formation of calculi (abnormal concretions, stony or hard masses) in the urinary tract. **It is mainly seen in layers, and causes increased mortality and decreased egg production.** Urolithiasis is characterized by severe reduction in the size (atrophy) of one or more kidneys, distended ureters often containing uroliths (hard masses), and varying degrees of gout in kidneys and abdominal organs.

### Causes

1.  **Excess dietary calcium**, if combined with low dietary phosphorus, can cause urolithiasis.

2.  **Nephropathogenic strains of infectious bronchitis virus** (i.e. affecting kidneys), after a high-calcium laying ration, increases the incidence of urolithiasis.

3.  **Water deprivation.**

4.  **Mycotoxins** which are nephrotoxic, that is, damaging to the kidneys such as oosporein, ochratoxin, etc.

### Symptoms

Mortality in affected flocks may be above 2% for several months and, at times, may be very high. Urolithiasis is mainly a disease of laying birds. **Layers die suddenly and may be in good condition and in full lay.** The uroliths may cause sudden death by plugging ureters, but this is probably secondary to kidney damage.

### Postmortem Findings

**Kidneys are markedly reduced in size (atrophied) and ureters are dilated.** There may also be diffuse urate deposits on the abdominal organs. Reduction in the size of kidney is usually more severe in anterior lobes and is unilateral, but it may be bilateral. The surviving lobes on the same side, or on the opposite side, may be enlarged. The **ureters** coming from the reduced lobes are **dilated** and **full of white irregular**

**concretions** (masses) or **uroliths**. These uroliths are composed of crystals of **calcium sodium urate.**

## Control

Dietary acidification with ammonium chloride, ammonium sulphate, or methionine decreases the incidence of urolithiasis caused by high-calcium diets. However, ammonium chloride is not used because it causes increased water consumption, urine flow, and manure moisture. The other compounds do not have this disadvantage. Ammonium sulphate is more effective than the two forms of methionine.

## ASCITES

**Ascites is accumulation of fluid in the abdominal cavity of chickens. It is not an infection,** but is caused by a series of complex events that affect the supply of oxygen to the tissues. Also called **'pulmonary hypertension syndrome'** and **'water belly'**, ascites has emerged as **a major source of economic loss in the broiler industry.** In extreme situations, up to 25% mortality is seen. However, 5-12% is the most common.

## Past Background and Present Status

Ascites for many years has resulted in **significant mortality in broilers raised at high altitudes**. In fact, the disease was first reported from high altitudes in 1968 in the growing broiler chickens from the South American country of Bolivia, followed by its reporting in flocks at high altitudes in Peru, Mexico and South Africa. The high incidence of ascites at high altitudes was due to **hypoxia**, that is, from a lack of an adequate amount of oxygen in the inhaled air.

However, in the past 15 years ascites has also been reported in flocks reared at low altitudes from a number of countries, including India. **Moreover, its incidence has increased over the years.** This is on account of the continuing genetic and nutritional improvement in the rate of growth and feeding efficiency.

But before we go any further into the discussion of ascites, as to how it develops, it would be helpful if first we acquaint ourselves with the avian heart.

## The Avian Heart

The bird's heart is cone-shaped (see **Fig. 24A, left heart**) and is proportionately larger, longer, and narrower than that of the mammals. It is a hollow muscular organ with chambers and valves. It works as a pump, and is enclosed in a membranous sac (a covering), the pericardium.

**Avian heart has four chambers:** two upper chambers are called right and left atrium; and the two lower chambers right and left ventricle. The right side has no communication with the left. The right atrium receives impure blood from the tissues, and on contraction, passes the blood into the right ventricle. On contraction of the right ventricle, blood flows through the pulmonary artery into the lungs. It is oxygenated in the lungs, and through the pulmonary vein it goes into the left atrium. On contraction of the left atrium, blood flows into the left ventricle, and on contraction of the left ventricle, oxygenated blood is pumped into the systemic circulation to meet oxygen requirements of the tissues. Thus, the **atria** (plural of 'atrium') **are the receiving chambers, and ventricles, the pumping chambers.**

**The left ventricle in the bird is very thick-walled compared to that in mammals.** The chamber is small. The right ventricle is thin-walled and is not as long as the left ventricle. The atria are large and thin-walled. The right atrio-ventricular (AV) valve is a muscle flap between right atrium and left ventricle. The thin-walled right ventricle is meant to work as a volume pump, and not as a pressure pump. This means that it responds very rapidly to an increased workload or pressure by dilatation, thickening, and enlargement (hypertrophy). For example, in the case of raised blood pressure within the pulmonary artery (pulmonary hypertension), as occurs in ascites, right ventricle gets dilated, thickened, and enlarged. The right AV valve also thickens. This leads to failure of the valve to close properly (valvular insufficiency) and makes the avian heart very much prone to right ventricular failure (i.e. failure of the right ventricle to perform its normal function). **This change is fundamental and forms the very basis of ascites,** as would be discussed later.

## How do heart muscles respond to increased workload?

Like other muscles, the heart muscles respond to increased workload **by undergoing enlargement (hypertrophy).** The enlarged heart has increased muscle mass. These changes occur in two forms:

1. If the enlargement is caused by an increased volume of blood, as in the case of increased oxygen requirements (e.g. in ascites), the chambers enlarge causing the whole heart to enlarge. The mass of the heart increases, **but the muscle wall does not become thicker.**

2. If the enlargement is caused by pressure overload, as in the case of systemic or pulmonary hypertension (discussed later), **the ventricles react individually. The ventricular wall becomes thicker.** Heart enlargement is minimal but the chamber becomes smaller. Increased volume and pressure may occur together, as for example, if the volume of blood requires more pressure to force it through the vessels, or if the pressure overload results in valvular insufficiency as occurs in ascites **(pulmonary hypertension syndrome)** in broilers. This is discussed later.

## What then are the factors responsible for ascites in poultry?

There are **certain basic important differences in the respiratory system of birds and mammals.**

1. **Lungs of birds cannot expand like mammalian lungs.** This is because they are rigid and cannot enlarge, and also because they are fitted tightly into the thoracic cavity.

2. **The minute blood vessels of bird's lungs** (capillaries) can enlarge (dilate) very little. Therefore, they cannot accommodate increased blood flow like the mammalian lungs. In other words, they **have restricted space for blood flow.**

3. **The lungs of chickens grow slowly compared to the rest of the body.** The slower growth of lungs, compared to whole body growth, makes chicken prone to ascites.

## Why is ascites confined to broilers?

**The modern broiler chicken is susceptible to ascites because of its rapid growth rate, high feed efficiency, and a large breast muscle mass, which require a high demand for oxygen.** The metabolic rate of fast-growing broiler chicken is very high. Thus, an imbalance between oxygen supply and the oxygen required to sustain rapid growth rates and high food efficiencies, causes ascites in broiler chickens.

Moreover, the modern broiler has a small lung volume: body growth ratio. In other words, **the modern broiler has small lungs compared to body size,** which make its respiratory system unable to meet the broiler's increased oxygen requirements. Together, these factors create a deficiency of oxygen in the blood (**hypoxaemia**), and make the modern broiler victim of developing hypoxaemia. Thus, **hypoxaemia (insufficient oxygen in blood) is the major factor in the development of ascites.** This is further discussed under development of the disease.

**In addition**, the following factors also contribute to the development of ascites in broilers.

1. **The red blood cells of broilers are more rigid than those of layers.** That is, they are less flexible and cannot change shape.

2. **Broiler has a thicker blood-gas barrier than that of layers.** That is, the partition in the exchange of oxygen between the air capillaries of the lung and the blood capillaries (minute vessels) is thicker. This makes oxygenation of lungs less efficient in broilers. (Note that in birds, the air which is inhaled, flows within minute channels inside the lungs called **'air capillaries'**, and not in the air cavities (airsacs, alveoli), as is in mammals.)

3. Saturation of haemoglobin with oxygen in broilers is less efficient than in layers.

4. **More recently,** it has been reported that in the lungs and liver of **broiler chickens affected with ascites, there are lower levels of antioxidants.** This means that broilers are more prone to the harmful effects of **'free radicals'** produced in the

body. In other words, they are more prone to **'oxidative stress'**. Recent work has also shown that **increased levels of antioxidants, such as vitamin E and selenium in the diet reduce mortality in ascites** (see vitamin E, selenium, and chapter 33).

## Causes

Several factors, alone or in combination, may cause ascites. These include:

1. Rapid growth rate and a smaller lung capacity.

2. **Cold**. Cold is an important factor. **It increases metabolic rate, and therefore causes an increased demand for oxygen.** This, in turn, increases the incidence of ascites.

3. Pelleted feed. The incidence of ascites is lower in broiler chicken fed mash diets than those given pelleted feed.

4. High energy diets.

5. More feed. Feed restriction at an early age decreases ascites, but also reduces breast muscle growth.

6. Certain feedstuffs may increase the demand for oxygen and the incidence of ascites. Also anything that increases the metabolic rate of the bird.

7. Overcrowding.

8. **Poor ventilation**. That is, **insufficient ventilation in the poultry houses.**

9. Faulty brooding.

10. **Ammonia formation and dust.**

11. **Sodium toxicity causes ascites.** This is because it is the most important cause of hypervolaemia in commercial chickens. **Hypervolaemia** is a great increase in the blood volume, which contributes to pulmonary hypertension and thus results in ascites. Apart from increasing blood volume, excess sodium decreases flexibility of red blood cells. They tend to become rigid.

12. Continuous versus intermittent lighting. Continuous lighting increases cases of ascites.

13. Heat. Heat also causes an increased demand for oxygen, and thereby increases the incidence of ascites.

14. Aspergillosis (a fungal infection). Also, infectious respiratory diseases.

15. Strain differences.

16. High altitude.

17. High sodium and low phosphorus.

18. Vitamin E/selenium deficiency.

19. Furazolidone.

20. Mycotoxin, hepatotoxin (liver toxin).

21. Stress

## Development of the Disease

Since several different mechanisms are involved in the development of ascites, for a better understanding, it would be helpful if we first discuss ascites as it occurs at high altitude.

## HIGH-ALTITUDE ASCITES

**At high altitudes, there is reduced amount of oxygen in the air.** Therefore, the bird does not get enough oxygen due to low oxygen tension in the inhaled air **(hypoxia) (Fig 22 A).** As a result, haemoglobin of red blood cells is not fully saturated with oxygen during breathing. This leads to deficiency of oxygen in the blood **(hypoxaemia)**, and body tissues do not get enough oxygen.

**Hypoxaemia** (insufficient oxygen in the blood) stimulates production of more red blood cells, so that blood can carry more oxygen for tissues in the haemoglobin of red cells. Hypoxaemia in birds stimulates kidneys to produce the hormone **erythropoietin** which, in turn, stimulates the production of red blood cells in the bone marrow. Even a moderate altitude (1000 metre) stimulates production of more red cells in fast-growing broiler chickens. The excess of red blood cells **(polycythaemia) (Fig. 22A)** makes the blood more viscous (thick and sticky), and then it does not flow that easily. Moreover, the newly produced red cells are larger and more rigid. These cells have difficulty in passing through minute vessels (capillaries) of the lungs. **All these lead to an increased resistance to blood flow (Fig. 22A).** As a result, heart finds it difficult to pump viscous blood through the lung. Moreover, capillaries of the bird's lungs are rigid and cannot enlarge much. As a result, resistance to the flow of blood develops quickly. Viscosity of the blood has its maximum effect on the capillaries. It all leads to a very peculiar situation. For example, on the one hand, the high oxygen demand by tissues makes heart pump more blood to the lungs, but on the other, restricted space in the lungs, viscosity of blood and rigid capillaries provide **resistance to the flow of blood**. This resistance to the flow is most important in the development of **pulmonary hypertension** in broiler chickens, as is explained next.

### A. High-Altitude Ascites

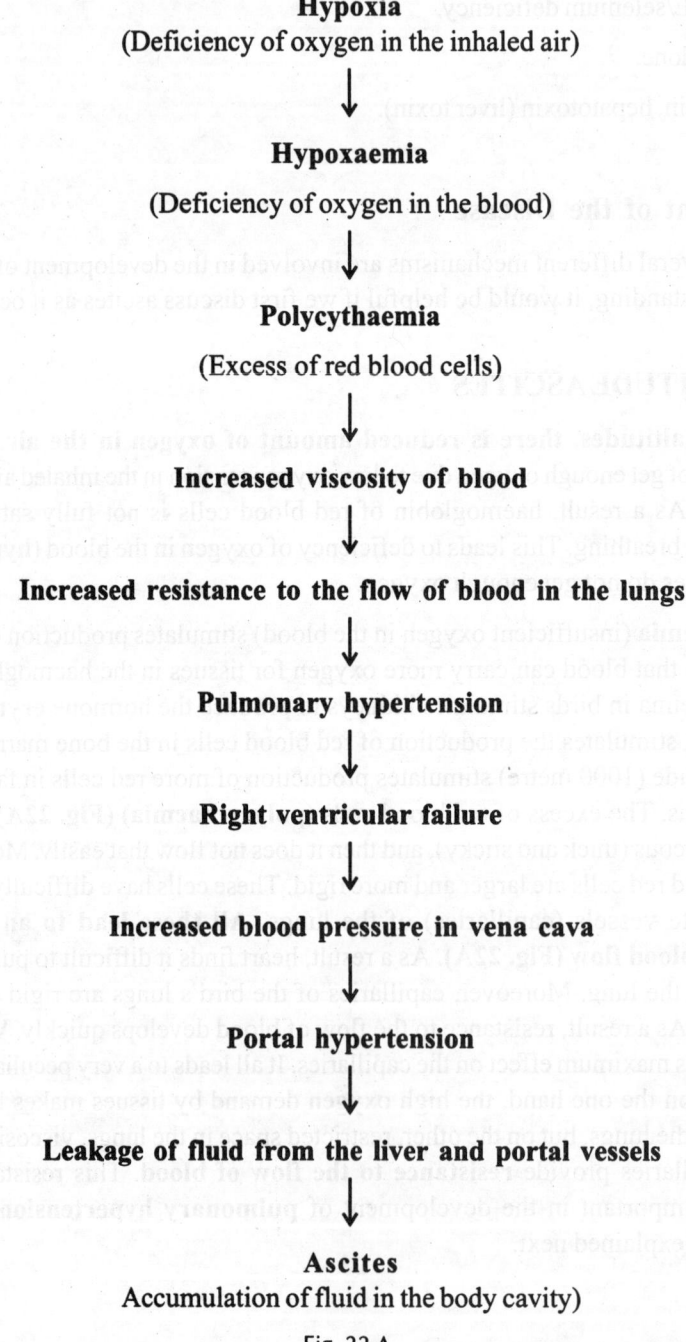

**Hypoxia**
(Deficiency of oxygen in the inhaled air)

↓

**Hypoxaemia**
(Deficiency of oxygen in the blood)

↓

**Polycythaemia**
(Excess of red blood cells)

↓

**Increased viscosity of blood**

↓

**Increased resistance to the flow of blood in the lungs**

↓

**Pulmonary hypertension**

↓

**Right ventricular failure**

↓

**Increased blood pressure in vena cava**

↓

**Portal hypertension**

↓

**Leakage of fluid from the liver and portal vessels**

↓

**Ascites**
Accumulation of fluid in the body cavity)

Fig. 22 A.

## B. Low-Altitude Ascites

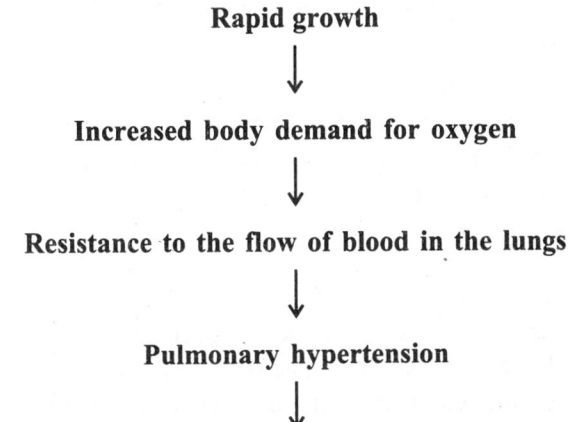

**Rapid growth**

↓

**Increased body demand for oxygen**

↓

**Resistance to the flow of blood in the lungs**

↓

**Pulmonary hypertension**

↓

**Remaining events are the same as shown for the high-altitude ascites**

**Fig. 22 B.** Summary of events involved in the development of ascites.

As stated earlier, on contraction of the heart, blood from the right ventricle flows through the pulmonary artery to lungs. When heart tries to pump more blood into the lungs, in an attempt to meet high oxygen requirements, it puts an extra stress on the right ventricle. Moreover, on account of the resistance in the lungs to blood flow, back-pressure is built up, and the blood pressure within the pulmonary artery rises. This is known as **'pulmonary hypertension' (Fig. 22A). Pressure within the pulmonary artery may even be doubled.** To overcome this abnormally high pressure, the right ventricle begins to pump more forcefully. However, soon it tires itself out and undergoes dilatation, thickening and enlargement (hypertrophy), and fails in its attempts to pump blood adequately. This is the stage of **'right ventricular failure' (Fig. 22A).** Under normal conditions, the right ventricle is relatively small, **but in right ventricular failure its size is doubled.**

When right ventricle gets dilated, thickened and enlarged, soon its atrio-ventricular (AV) valve (valve between the right atrium and right ventricle) also thickens, and is then unable to close the valvular opening effectively. This is called **'valvular insufficiency'.** As a result, when right ventricle contracts, some blood passes in the reverse direction into the right atrium. That is, a volume of blood re-enters the atrium with each heart beat. In the normal course, all the blood goes into the lungs through the pulmonary artery. Thus, due to the back flow of blood, pressure rises in the vena cava **(Fig. 22A).** Vena cava is the main blood vessel that brings impure blood of the body to the heart and opens into the right atrium. This increased blood pressure in the vena cava, in turn, leads to **'portal hypertension' (Fig. 22A).** Portal hypertension is an increase in the blood pressure within **hepatic vein**, a vessel that carries impure blood from the liver into the vena cava, and also within that vessel which brings blood to liver from the abdominal organs known as **portal vein.** In other words, there is a gradual increase in the blood pressure within both portal and hepatic veins, and as a result within the blood spaces of the liver, the sinusoids.

**The net result of all these complex events is that,** because of the increased pressure within sinusoids, **there is leakage of fluid (plasma) through the surface of the liver and also from the portal vessels, which then accumulates in the abdominal cavity (ascites). This is the way ascites develops in broilers.**

## LOW-ALTITUDE ASCITES

**At the low altitude,** it is not lack of oxygen in the air that causes the increased pulmonary arterial pressure (pulmonary hypertension). **In fact, oxygen is rarely low even in poorly ventilated houses.** Also, dust or harmful fumes in the houses are not important because they reduce growth rate, and reduced growth rate does not cause ascites.

The **most important factor** in the development of ascites at low altitude is **an extremely high metabolic demand of oxygen by the tissues due to the rapid growth in the modern broiler (Fig. 22B),** combined with restricted space for the blood flow through the blood vessels of the lungs. The high oxygen demand causes increased blood flow, whereas the restricted space causes resistance to flow within the lungs. This results in **pulmonary hypertension (Fig. 22B).** Rest of the mechanisms involved in the accumulation of fluid in the abdominal cavity and development of ascites are the same as discussed for high-altitude ascites.

## Symptoms

**Ascites may show itself as sudden death.** The peak incidence of ascites occurs in the 5th or 6th week of the growing period. **Mortality is greatest after four weeks.** Symptoms do not develop until right ventricular failure occurs. Affected birds are smaller than normal and depressed with ruffled feathers. This is because the growth stops once right ventricular failure occurs. They have a pale head and a shrunken comb, and in white chickens the feathers lose their bright white sheen (shining condition). **Severely affected birds show abdominal distension.** The abdominal skin may be red and the vessels congested. Birds may be reluctant to move, show difficult breathing, even panting, and are cyanotic (i.e., slightly bluish).

## Postmortem Findings

Postmortem examination shows the presence of **a large amount of clear yellow fluid in the body cavity.** More than 300 ml of fluid, with or without fibrin clots, may be present. **This explains the abdominal distension (Fig. 23).** Some birds may die before ascites develops. **The heart is markedly enlarged (Fig. 24).** The enlargement is due to dilatation of both right atrium and right ventricle **(Fig. 24)** and also from enlargement of the right ventricular wall. **Hydropericardium** (accumulation of fluid under the covering of the heart) may be present. The **liver** may be **swollen and congested, or firm and shrunken** with an irregular surface. The **lungs** are extremely congested and oedematous (i.e. contain fluid). The intestines are severely congested.

**Not all birds that die from ascites show accumulation of fluid in the abdominal cavity.** Death may occur before symptoms are observed, and affected broilers usually die on their back. On postmortem there may be a swollen liver, enlargement of the heart as well as marked lung congestion and oedema. Death in such cases is from respiratory failure. Heart changes differentiate such deaths from sudden death syndrome (see **'sudden death syndrome'**).

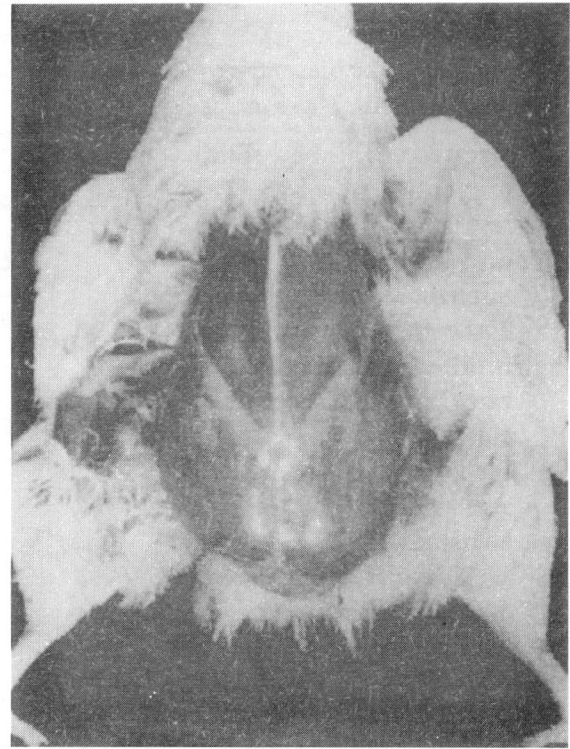

**Fig. 23.** Ascites in a broiler chicken. Note abdomen is distended with fluid.

## Diagnosis

Diagnosis is based on typical postmortem findings.

## Treatment

**There is no effective treatment for ascites,** and once birds show symptoms, death occurs fairly quickly. Frusemide, a diuretic (an agent that increases the flow of urine) reduces mortality in ascites. This is because it causes reduced fluid and electrolyte retention, and also because it reduces pulmonary vascular resistance, **as frusemide acts as a vasodilator** (i.e. causes dilatation of blood vessels).

**Vitamin C, vitamin E and organic selenium** are effective in reducing mortality from ascites. This is because oxidative stress and formation of free radicals are involved in the development of ascites. Reduced mortality may be due to their antioxidant effect (see vitamin C, vitamin E, and selenium).

## Control

Ascites can be prevented by a number of methods. These include:

1. Ascites can be totally prevented through feed restriction, or through the use of very low energy feed throughout the entire cycle. **Therefore, reduce feed intake to slow metabolic rate.** This can be done by skip-a-day feeding, or by restricting feed, or the time feed is available each day (i.e. 8-10 hours each day from 7-21 day age). Restrict the daily amount of feed by 20-40% during the early growing period. **But this may affect growth rate of the entire flock.**

2. Use mash rather than pelleted feeds.

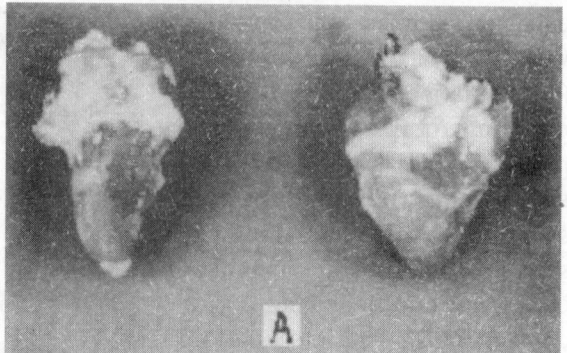
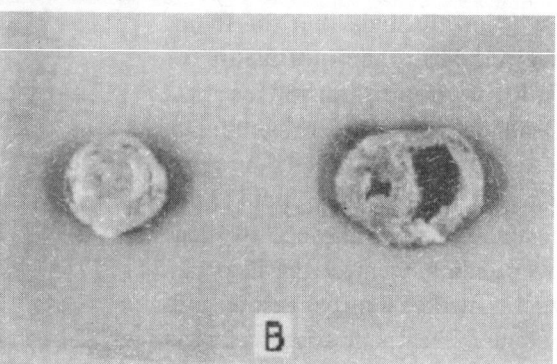

**Fig. 24.** Ascites in a broiler chicken. **A.** Enlarged heart (right) along with a normal heart (left). **B.** Cut section of the enlarged heart (right) showing dilation and enlargement of the right ventricle compared with a cut section through the normal heart (left).

3. **Prevent chilling, that is, exposure to cold.** Avoid night-time cold stress. This is particularly **important in the first two weeks of life, when chicks are especially susceptible to cold stress.**

4. Ensure **adequate ventilation.**

5. **Avoid dust and ammonia.** They are major lung irritants and damage the lungs, and thus contribute to ascites. Litter management and water management are the major factors that affect ammonia levels (see **'litter'** and **'water management'**).

6. **Sodium in feed should not exceed 2000 ppm.** Excess of sodium increases blood volume, which leads to pulmonary hypertension and thus contributes to the development of ascites.

7. Intermittent lighting, or lighting programmes with increasing photoperiods, have proved successful in reducing the incidence of ascites without affecting broiler performance. The benefits of reducing day length are due to slower early growth rates.

8. Environmental temperature, humidity and air movement should be controlled to prevent excessive body heat loss.

9. **Minimize toxin contamination of feed**. Feed free of mycotoxins and other toxins will prevent ascites, as they are toxic to liver.

10. Addition of 1% sodium bicarbonate to a broiler feed causes alkalosis (increased alkalinity of blood and tissues) and reduces ascites in experimental birds. This is based on the concept that the pulmonary constriction is mediated by hydrogen ion concentration (pH).

11. Also, **supplemental L-arginine** (an essential amino acid) reduces mortality from ascites in experimental broilers. This is because L-arginine is required as a substrate for the production of **nitric oxide (NO),** a powerful vasodilator. **Nitric oxide relaxes the tone of the main resistance vessels, thereby permitting increased blood flow.**

12. **Increased vitamin E in the diet and organic selenium** reduce mortality in ascites. Recently, it has been shown that in order to prevent mortality caused by ascites, high levels of vitamin E and selenium are required. **Organic selenium is more effective than the inorganic.** Selenium forms a part of the enzyme glutathione peroxidase. **Both vitamin E and glutathione peroxidase are excellent antioxidants, destroy toxic free radicals, and thus reduce oxidative stress** (see vitamin E and selenium, and also chapter 33 for more information on vitamin E and selenium on their role as antioxidants). Earlier it was mentioned that in the lungs and liver of broiler chickens, affected with ascites, there are lower levels of antioxidants. This suggests a deficiency in the control of oxidative stress.

## RICKETS

**Rickets is a condition in which there is a failure or inadequate deposition of minerals in the bones.** This results in the abnormalities of shape and structure of bones. Rickets causes increased bone flexibility and deformity resulting in **lameness.** It is usually seen in rapidly growing young chicks. **Birds under four weeks of age are most susceptible, but the condition may occur at any age.**

## Causes

1. Calcium, phosphorus and/or vitamin D3 deficiency, or imbalance (see 'calcium and 'phosphorus' and 'vitamin D').

2. Faulty mixing of feed ingredients.

3. Intercurrent diseases influencing vitamin D3 and mineral absorption.

## Development of the Disease

Rickets is characterized by a thickened and poorly mineralized growth plate and poorly mineralized bone. Growth plate is that site of long bones where cartilage is produced to be replaced by bone. Poor mineralization of bone is caused by calcium, phosphorus and/or vitamin D3 deficiency, or imbalance.

## Symptoms

Affected chickens show poor growth, symptoms of muscular incoordination, stiff-legged gait (walking), and progressive lameness. They have a tendency to remain squatted (sitting). Severely affected birds when forced to move appear to be walking in pain. The hock joints are enlarged. **The beak and shanks in young chicks are soft and flexible.** As the condition progresses, feathers become ruffled, there is loss of condition, and dehydration becomes noticeable. Morbidity (number of birds affected) in an untreated flock may reach 100%, **and mortality (deaths) up to 50% has been observed.**

## Postmortem Findings

Apart from varying degrees of emaciation, the beak and bones are soft. **Characteristically, bones do not break with a snap (a sudden sharp sound) because they become soft and rubbery from poor mineralization.** In birds with severe rickets, the keel bones

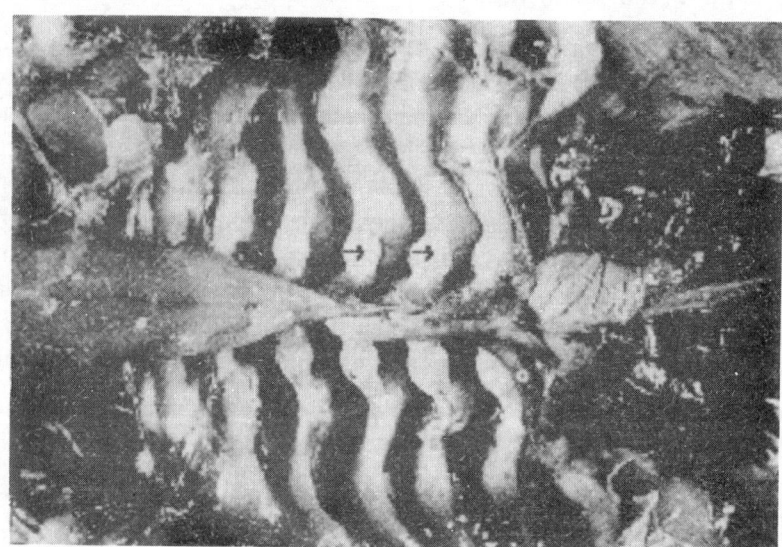

Fig. 25. Rickets. Note heads of the ribs (arrows) are enlarged.

are crooked (not straight, but twisted, bent, or curved), ribs are **'beaded'** (i.e. heads of the ribs are enlarged as nodules) **(Fig. 25)**, the legs are bowed (bent), and the ends of the long bones enlarged. When rickets is due to calcium or vitamin D3 deficiency, the parathyroids are likely to be enlarged.

## Diagnosis

Flock history, symptoms and typical postmortem findings are usually enough for field diagnosis.

## Treatment

1.  Administer vitamin D3 2-3 times the recommended level through drinking water.

2.  Additional calcium and phosphorus should be supplied *ad libitum* (i.e. without restriction) for 5-7 days.

3.  Replace the suspected feed with the known well balanced and properly mixed feed.

## Control

1.  Ensure adequate supply of vitamin D3 and calcium and phosphorus in 2:1 ratio in the feed.

2.  Mineral premixes should be properly mixed in the feed for even distribution.

## FATTY LIVER AND KIDNEY SYNDROME

Fatty liver and kidney syndrome (FLKS) is a metabolic disorder **causing death of young broilers,** and sometimes growers. It usually occurs between 10-30 days of age. Although FLKS responds to biotin, it is not just simple biotin deficiency. Of course, it is **often associated with diets that have low levels of biotin,** but there are no signs of true biotin deficiency (see 'biotin').

Since **FLKS is a complicated metabolic disorder,** and its development involves interactions of a number of factors, it would be helpful if first we understand the mechanisms involved in its development. This would be followed by a discussion of its causes. Although the mechanisms involved are not entirely clear, the current concepts are as follows.

## Development of the Disease

There are two enzymes closely associated with carbohydrate and fat metabolism. First is **pyruvate (pyruvic) carboxylase. It is a biotin-containing enzyme,** and its role is to form glucose in the liver from non-carbohydrate sources, such as protein and fat. The process is known as **"gluconeogenesis",** and occurs under conditions of low carbohydrate intake, or starvation. The second enzyme is **acetyl coenzyme A (CoA) carboxylase.** This enzyme is involved in the formation of fat. The process is known as **"lipogenesis"** (fat formation). **Biotin is a cofactor for both these enzymes.** Here, it is important to mention that acetyl CoA carboxylase has a greater access to biotin than pyruvate carboxylase. This means that in case of competition between the two for biotin, when biotin is deficient, acetyl CoA carboxylase will succeed in getting biotin, whereas pyruvate carboxylase will suffer. In other words, fat formation (lipogenesis) will continue as usual, but glucose formation (gluconeogenesis) will suffer. This will lead to **hypoglycaemia** (decrease of glucose in the blood).

**When feed is high in fat content,** fat formation in the body is not required. Therefore, requirement of acetyl CoA carboxylase for biotin is decreased. As a result, biotin is available for pyruvate carboxylase to form glucose, and **there is no hypoglycaemia.** However, **when feed is low in fat,** formation of fat is required. Therefore, acetyl CoA carboxylase comes into operation, and, as already mentioned, it has a greater approach. to biotin than pyruvate carboxylase. As a result, formation of glucose from non-carbohydrate sources (gluconeogenesis) suffers. Therefore, if normal fat intake is interrupted for even a short period of time, **hypoglycaemia develops.** The condition is worsened by the very low glycogen reserves of the young chick.

**In response to the low blood glucose level,** there is mobilization of free fatty acids into the liver, from body tissues, for fat formation. The purpose being that fat so formed can be utilized to produce glucose to correct the low blood level. However, as pyruvate carboxylase is a biotin-containing enzyme, its activity is decreased in biotin deficiency. **Biotin deficiency therefore prevents conversion of fat into glucose.** This leads to increased conversion of pyruvate to fatty acids. **The net result is marked accumulation of fat in the liver.**

## Causes

Thus, whereas birds suffer from fatty liver and kidney syndrome due to nutritional factors, the sudden onset of the disease is believed to be brought about by the environmental factors. **The syndrome involves an interaction of nutritional, environmental, stress, and maternal factors.** These may act as follows:

1. **Biotin** is the single, most important nutritional factor.

2. **High levels of fat in the feed offer protection,** because then there is not much need for fat formation. Decreased fat formation means that more biotin is available for the action of pyruvate carboxylase to form glucose from non-carbohydrate sources.

3. Other vitamins, at higher levels, increase the incidence of fatty liver and kidney syndrome.

4. Pelleted feed. More rapid growth occurs with pelleted feed than with mash feed.

5. Floor rearing. Faecal biotin is available on floor rearing, but not so on wire floors, such as, in cages.

6. High house temperature, light failure, excessive noise and transport all increase stress.

7. Starvation and stress deplete glycogen (glucose) reserve.

8. Age and biotin status of parent. Eggs from older hens have more biotin.

9.  Other diseases cause stress and reduce intestinal absorption of biotin.

10. Biotin is rapidly destroyed by oxidizing agents, for example, rancid fat.

11. **Aflatoxin (a fungal toxin) is a biotin binder and causes biotin deficiency.**

## Importance of Biotin

**Inadequate biotin can have two very different manifestations in young birds.** (1) Clinical skin and bone lesions (changes), or (2) fatty liver and kidney syndrome (see 'biotin').The balance between the two forms is determined by the balance between metabolic needs for different biotin-dependent enzymes. This balance, in turn, depends on the dietary contents of other nutrients, namely, fat.

## Symptoms

Symptoms are sudden in onset. Well-grown birds become dull and depressed, lose appetite, and lie down. Mortality may range between 5-30%.

## Postmortem Findings

**Liver and kidneys are enlarged, pale, and fatty.** Adipose tissue is pink due to congestion of blood vessels. Crop and intestines usually contain blackish fluid due to blood content. The paleness of the liver and kidneys is due to the presence of excessive amounts of fat (**two to five times the normal**). This is mostly neutral fat (triglycerides).

## Treatment

1.  **Addition of biotin and choline in drinking water for one day may prevent new cases.** Biotin should be dissolved in ethyl alcohol, before adding water. The mixture should be added to choline. The following mixture has been used with success.

    | | |
    |---|---|
    | Biotin | 100mg/1000 birds |
    | Choline 70% | 19 g/1000 birds |

2.  Elimination of stress factors is important for effective treatment.

## Control

1.  Eliminate stress factors, such as starvation, cold, etc.

2.  **Maintain adequate biotin levels in the diets of all chicken and breeder flocks.**

## FATTY LIVER - HAEMORRHAGIC SYNDROME

Fatty liver-haemorrhagic syndrome (FLHS) is a metabolic disorder **characterized by a very fatty liver, accompanied by haemorrhages.** The condition is **seen** sometimes in **older laying hens kept in cages, particularly in hot weather.** There is usually a fall in egg production in the affected flock. Death occurs occasionally and is due to massive liver haemorrhage.

## Causes

1.  Feed, especially high carbohydrate, low-fat feed given *ad lib* (i.e. without restriction). That is, **high energy diets for increased egg production.** These lead to fattiness. Linoleic acid and selenium deficiencies aggravate occurrence.

    **Explained simply,** excessive consumption of high-energy diets in birds, whose exercise is restricted in cages, results in excessive fat deposition. This is aggravated by hot weather.

2.  Nutritional imbalances.

3.  High temperature. This discourages movement that would reduce heat loss.

4.  Lack of exercise. For example, in caged birds.

5.  Deficiency of nutrients that mobilize fat from the liver (lipotropic agents), such as choline.

6.  Stress; toxins; high egg production.

7.  Hormonal (endocrine) imbalances, such as high oestrogen (female sex hormone), low thyroid blood hormone levels.

8.  Strain of bird. **The average liver fat in differen' strains of layer may vary from about 25% to about 50%.** (Note that high fat level has no link with increased egg production.).

9.  Low levels of dietary calcium may result in increased feed consumption, liver fat, and haemorrhage. Laying hens, however, can have high levels of fat in their livers without haemorrhage.

    **The higher percentage of liver fat** (i.e. fatty liver) **is not in itself sufficient to cause fatty liver-haemorrhagic syndrome, but it does predispose liver to haemorrhage.** The haemorrhage usually occurs in heavier birds in the latter half of the laying period.

10. Recent studies have revealed greatly **increased blood oestrogen, calcium,** and **cholesterol** in chickens having fatty liver-haemorrhagic syndrome. This suggests that **the syndrome may be due to a hormonal imbalance.**

## Development of the Disease

Although the exact cause of excessive fat deposition in the liver is not known, **it is now well established that the disease is of nutritional origin.**

There are very important basic differences in carbohydrate and fat metabolism between birds and mammals. In birds, glucose levels are several times (3-4 times) higher than mammals. Mammalian embryos obtain glucose through the placental circulation, whereas the chicken embryo develops on yolk nutrients, **the energy source being almost all fat, not carbohydrate.** The chicken embryo must therefore contain high levels of gluconeogenic enzymes. These enzymes form glucose from substances other than carbohydrates, such as proteins and fats. The enzymes decrease after hatching as carbohydrate intake becomes available. Moreover, in contrast to mammals where fat formation (lipogenesis) is mostly in adipose tissue (i.e. fat tissue), in birds, it nearly all occurs in the liver. Fat formation increases in the first week or two after hatching from almost zero in the embryo (due to high fat yolk content) to much higher levels.

As hens approach sexual maturity and start laying, there is a further and much more striking increase in liver lipogenesis (fat formation). There are very high blood fat levels available to supply the developing ova in the ovaries; and liver **fat storage enormously increases at this time.**

It is this fat-forming (lipogenesis) function of the liver in the birds that forms the basis for the occurrence of conditions which involve excessive accumulation of fat in the liver. These conditions are fatty liver and kidney syndrome in young broiler birds (already discussed earlier in this chapter), and the present fatty liver-haemorrhagic syndrome in older laying hens.

**Fatty-liver haemorrhagic syndrome is characterized by very fatty liver accompanied by haemorrhages.** The fat content of liver is usually greater than 40% dry weight and may reach 70%. The proportion of oleic acid in the fat is increased. The cause of haemorrhage is not known. Excessive fat may damage structure of the liver and this results in weakening of the blood vessels in the liver.

## Symptoms

The syndrome appears only in good-laying flocks. **Most birds appear in good physical condition.** For this reason, there is no indication of the disease until egg production drops between 10% and 40%, that is, a sudden drop; or the flock fails to have a high peak of egg production. Hens may be overweight, with large pale combs and wattles. Body weight increases from 20% to 25% are observed. The problem is more serious with birds housed in cages than with those housed on the floor.

There is usually **an increase in mortality,** and birds in full production are found dead with pale heads. Birds die, especially following stress, such as hot weather, handling, transportation, or fright. Mortality varies from 2% to 10%.

## Postmortem Findings

Dead birds have pools of blood, or large blood clots, in the abdomen. Usually the clots partly cover the liver, and also originate from it. **The liver is enlarged, fatty, is of light greyish brown to yellow colour, very friable** (easily broken), and **may show** subcapsular (i.e. under the surface) **haemorrhages**. There is an increased fat content. The fat content is sometimes more than 70%. **Death** only occasionally occurs and **is due to massive liver haemorrhage.** Liver may have smaller haematomas (collection of clotted blood) inside. When cut with a knife, these haematomas may be recent and dark red, or older and green to brown. Large amounts of fat are present in the body cavity and around the organs. The kidneys are pale and swollen. **Dead birds are in full production** and usually have a developing egg in the oviduct.

## Diagnosis

Flock history and postmortem findings are usually adequate for field diagnosis.

## Treatment

1. Various nutritional supplements have been tried with mixed results.

2. Addition of the following supplement to the feed has been shown to significantly improve the condition in some laying flocks, but not all. This is because the syndrome is not a single-source problem. It involves complex nutritional and possibly environmental interactions that are still unknown.

   Add to a tonne of regular feed:

   | | |
   |---|---|
   | 10,000 IU | Vitamin E |
   | 1,000 g | Choline chloride |
   | 12 mg | Vitamin B12 |
   | 900 g | Inositol |

## Control

1. **Reducing energy intake**, either by feed restriction, or by lowering the metabolizable energy, is helpful.

2. Therefore, controlled feeding programme during rearing, and well balanced diet during production to prevent fattiness, are recommended.

3. Addition of choline and inositol to the feed has given variable results.

4. Avoid use of mouldy feed or feed ingredients in the poultry diets.

5. **High levels of selenium, vitamin E and other antioxidants reduce the peroxidation of lipids in the liver and may reduce the incidence of fatty liver- haemorrhagic syndrome.**

# CAGE LAYER FATIGUE

Cage layer fatigue is the most important disease of bones in modern chickens used for egg production. As the name suggests, **it is due to the poor bone structure in laying hens kept in cages.** It is well known that the breaking strength of bones of layers kept in cages is less than that of the birds reared on a litter floor. **Poor bone strength, due to the lack of exercise in cages,** is considered to be the single greatest factor responsible for cage layer fatigue. The major economic loss is due to the bone breakage when birds are processed. The market value of the spent hens is seriously reduced, often to the point that the birds cannot be sold.

The bones in laying hens are prone to fractures because the bones are osteopenic. That is, they have a reduced quantity of normal bone tissue. **Osteopenia**, a reduction in the quantity of normal bone tissue, usually occurs from **osteoporosis**. Osteoporosis is reduced quantity of fully mineralized (fully formed) structural bone. Osteoporosis, which is the basic factor responsible for cage layer fatigue, may be caused by:

1. Loss of bone due to **oestrogen** (female sex hormone) **activity** coinciding with the onset of laying. Oestrogen activity is greatly increased at this time.

2. Osteoporosis/cage layer fatigue may be precipitated during egg laying due to **inadequate amounts of calcium in the feed** (see 'calcium and phosphorus').

## Causes

1. Confinement of laying hens in cages. This reduces their bone strength significantly.

2. Low-phosphorus, low-calcium and vitamin D-deficient diets.

3. The modern laying hen has a very active calcium metabolism, and high egg production may result in cage layer osteoporosis (fatigue). Marginal nutritional deficiencies may result in severe osteoporosis and clinical signs.

4. Feed low in calcium and very high in phosphorus.

5. High environmental temperature, limiting the food intake.

## Development of the Disease

**The laying hen possesses two types of bone: (1) Structural (compact, cancellous, cortical) bone, which is responsible for the strength of bones, and (2) Medullary bone, which acts as a reserve of calcium for eggshell formation.** It does not contribute to strength. **At the onset of sexual maturity**, hens deposit **medullary bone** in the cavity of their long bones, under the influence of sex hormone oestrogen, released by maturing ovarian follicles. Medullary bone supplies calcium for eggshell formation during period when dietary supply is insufficient. **In hen,** calcium in the medullary bone is accumulated in the morning and used in the night-time. When egg production stops, medullary bone disappears in the next week.

**During egg laying, there is a continuous turnover of medullary bone with removal of existing bone and formation of new bone.** However, structural bone cannot be formed when hens are in laying, but the continuing process of bone removal means that the amount of structural bone decreases during the laying period. This leads to older hens becoming severely depleted in the amount of structural bone, which then develops **osteoporosis**. This means that in calcium deficiency, first there is complete removal of calcium from the medullary bones, followed by its gradual removal from the structural bones. Ultimately, bones become so thin that spontaneous fractures may occur, especially in the vertebrae, tibia and femur. This condition is the **"cage layer fatigue"**.

## Symptoms

**Cage layer fatigue is seen in caged hens in good bodily condition.** Hens may suddenly lose control of their legs and lie on their sides, sometimes paralyzed, with legs extended, and die from dehydration. However, the egg production does not seem to be greatly affected. Some birds die suddenly. **The paralysis gave rise to the term fatigue.** The bones are brittle (easily broken), ribs and sternum are usually deformed, and bone fractures are common.

## Postmortem Findings

Paralyzed or dead birds have **bones that are easily broken. Fractures** may be found in leg and wing bones, and in the thoracic spine. Sternum is often deformed, and there is characteristic infolding (folding inside) deformation of the ribs at the junction of the sternum and vertebrae. Parathyroid glands are enlarged. Many birds have small ovaries and are dehydrated, while some others have an egg in the oviduct. These may have died suddenly.

## Diagnosis

Flock history, characteristic symptoms and postmortem findings are usually sufficient to recommend corrective measures.

## Treatment

1. There is no recognized treatment.

2. If paralyzed birds are removed from their cages and given adequate balanced feed and water, they usually recover.

3. Supply additional calcium with the feed, for example, oyster shell. Also add extra vitamin D.

## Control

1. Formation of strong structural bone and adequate medullary bone before egg

production is helpful in reducing cage layer fatigue.

2.  Increased calcium in the ration before egg production may be necessary.

3.  The relative inactivity of caged birds quickens the process of cage layer fatigue. **It occurs only in birds kept in cages.** Confinement of laying hens in cages reduces bone strength significantly. If birds are given more exercise, this improves bone quality.

4.  Nutrition is not very effective in preventing cage layer osteoporosis (fatigue). However, poor nutrition such as deficiencies of calcium, phosphorus, or vitamin D can quicken the onset of osteoporosis.

# SUDDEN DEATH SYNDROME

Also known by several other names, such as **'acute death syndrome', 'heart attack', 'died in good condition', 'flip-over disease'** and **'lung oedema'**, sudden death syndrome **is a condition in which healthy broiler chickens die suddenly** for no visible or understandable cause. Mortality occurs in apparently healthy, fast-growing broilers, which die suddenly with a short, wing-beating, convulsive attack. Most affected broilers die on their back, hence the name **'flip-over disease'**. (To **'flip over'** means to turn over on one's back with a sudden sharp movement). **More than 70% of the losses due to sudden death syndrome are in males.**

## Incidence and Distribution

**Sudden death syndrome is seen in broilers due to increased feed intake and more rapid growth.** Mortality may start within 72 hours of hatching and may continue up to 12 weeks of age, with **peak mortality from 2 to 3 weeks.** This coincides with the age at which feed conversion is maximum. However, flocks in which there is restricted growth during the first three weeks may experience higher than normal losses after 3-4 weeks. Mortality may be from 0.5% in a low-prevalence flock to 2% in a high-prevalence flock. Since **about 75% of the affected birds are males,** mortality as high as 4% can occur in all male flocks. In a well managed flock, sudden death syndrome is the major cause of death.

## Development of the Disease

Since there are no specific gross or microscopic changes, sudden death syndrome is considered to be **a metabolic disease**, in which an imbalance of metabolites (i.e. products of metabolism), or electrolytes, results in an irregularity of the heart. It is not known whether all broilers are susceptible to sudden death syndrome, or the low incidence indicates a genetic predisposition to the condition. It has been observed that genetic, nutritional and environmental factors may affect the incidence. **Overcrowding** can increase the occurrence of sudden death syndrome.

## Symptoms

Affected chickens show **no clinical signs** or unusual behaviour until less than a minute before death. **Death occurs within 1-2 minutes.** Majority of the birds keep eating and drinking till two hours before the attack. **Birds dying from sudden death syndrome are healthy,** fast-growing broilers moving about normally before the convulsive attack. Birds may give a loud high-pitched cry during the attack, characterized by the loss of balance, convulsions, and violent flapping (wing-beating). (A convulsion is a sudden violent body movement that cannot be controlled. It is caused by contraction of muscles.) **Most birds die on their backs** with one or both legs extended or raised, but some may die on their keel bones, or sides. Birds may show signs of respiratory distress or they convulse and die.

## Postmortem Findings

**There are no specific gross changes.** Affected birds appear healthy, are well fleshed, and usually have feed in their digestive tract. Livers are enlarged, pale, and friable (easily broken). Usually the gallbladder is empty. Kidneys may be pale. Lungs are often congested and oedematous.

## Diagnosis

Diagnosis of sudden death syndrome is difficult since there are **no specific postmortem findings.** The supine position (i.e. lying on back) is important when present, and broilers that die are always well fleshed, and usually have ingesta (eaten material) in the crop and gizzard. In young broilers, the liver is large and usually pale and fatty, and the gallbladder is small or empty (less common after 5 weeks). The lungs are congested and usually oedematous (i.e. contain fluid). Small haemorrhages may be present on the liver and kidney. The bursa is large and normal, which again indicates that the bird was healthy immediately before death.

## Control

1.  Lower carbohydrate energy intake by changing feed texture (mash), or density.

2.  Apply management methods, such as feed restriction.

3.  Long dark periods may be effective in reducing the number of deaths in broilers from sudden death syndrome. Increased mortality is usually associated with unusual activity or bright light, particularly sunlight. Therefore, low-intensity light is recommended, and the flock should be disturbed as little as possible. It has been suggested that **intermittent light may decrease the incidence of sudden death syndrome.**

4.  **Addition of biotin** to broiler rations may reduce the incidence of sudden death syndrome, but this has not been confirmed. Biotin will prevent fatty liver and kidney

syndrome (see 'biotin'). It has been suggested that an abnormality occurring as a result of fatty liver and kidney syndrome may contribute to the initiation of sudden death syndrome (see **'fatty liver and kidney syndrome'**).

5.  There is circumstantial evidence that **ionophore anticoccidials** are in some way involved with sudden death syndrome. The condition seems to be more prevalent when ionophore anticoccidials are used.

6.  Recently it has been suggested that thiamine (vitamin B1) may influence the incidence of sudden death syndrome.

# CHONDRODYSTROPHY

Earlier known as **'perosis'**, chondrodystrophy is a failure of growth plate cartilage proliferation, **resulting in the shortening of the long bones.** Explained simply, it is a generalized disorder of the growth plate of bones **characterized by shortening of the leg bones.** (A growth plate is the site from where a long bone grows. Here, first a cartilage is produced which is later replaced by bone.) **Chondrodystrophy is different from rickets** in that mineralization (deposition of minerals) is not interfered with.

The term **'perosis'**, once used for this and other conditions, is confusing and not clearly defined, and therefore should not be used.

## Causes

1.  **Manganese deficiency** results in chondrodystrophy. In addition, **deficiencies of choline, nicotinic acid, biotin, folic acid and pyridoxine,** contribute to the development of chondrodystrophy.

2.  **Mycoplasma infection.** Mycoplasma interferes with the supply of nutrients to the growth plate cartilage. However, mycoplasmas as a cause of chondrodystrophy are more important in the turkey than in chickens.

## Symptoms

**The long bones are short, thick, and usually deformed.** There is often **enlargement of the hock joints.** If both legs are affected, death usually occurs since the chick cannot obtain food and water.

## Control

1.  Ensure adequate amounts of the concerned, as well as all other minerals, in the feed.

2.  Add anti-mycoplasmal drugs in the feed to check **Mycoplasma** infection.

**Note:** For a list of anti-mycoplasmal drugs, refer to Chapter 19 under **"Anti-mycoplasmal drugs".**

# Chapter 11

# Miscellaneous Diseases / Conditions

This chapter describes those diseases and conditions of poultry that could not be placed elsewhere.

## HEAT STRESS

Also known as **'heat stroke'**, or **'heat prostration'**, heat stress is that condition in which the body temperature is so high that it interferes with normal body functions, and if continued, leads to exhaustion and death. **Heat stress is an important cause of mortality in our country.**

Summer is associated with high environmental temperatures. This leads to heat stress. All classes of poultry experience heat distress when **high temperatures,** accompanied by **high humidity,** rise above their comfort zones. **Birds, unlike mammals, do not have sweat glands.** When the environmental temperatures are between 28° C and 35° C (82° F and 95° F), birds use **non-evaporative cooling** as the major means of heat loss. They achieve non-evaporative cooling in two ways: (1) by increasing the surface area by relaxing the wings and hanging them loosely at their sides, and (2) by increasing the peripheral blood flow. But when the environmental temperature reaches the body temperature of the bird (41° C or 106° F), the rate of respiration increases and the bird breathes through open mouth to increase **evaporative cooling** or water evaporation. If this **open-mouth breathing (panting)** fails to prevent their body temperatures from rising, birds become listless, go into a state of deep unconsciousness, and soon die from respiratory, circulatory, or electrolyte imbalances.

## Causes

1.  In a tropical country like ours, heat stress is due to **high environmental temperature,** which in some areas is caused by hot dry winds.
2.  Inadequate water supply.
3.  Inadequate ventilation.
4.  Overcrowding.
5.  Very low ceiling of the poultry house.
6.  Absence of vegetation or trees or creepers to cool the air in and around the poultry house.

7.   In temperate (cold) climates, heat stress may be caused by ventilation failure in houses containing large numbers of birds.

A number of factors can influence the effect of high environmental temperatures on poultry. **These include:**

1.   Genetic constitution of the bird. In general, **broiler breeds are more susceptible than layers.**

2.   Influence of the rate of metabolism. **Laying hens and rapidly growing male broilers are more prone to heat stress.**

3.   High stocking density. That is, **overcrowding.**

4.   High-energy, high-protein rations make birds more susceptible to heat stress.

5.   **An inadequate supply of drinking water** may further intensify the reaction of birds to high temperatures.

6.   Age is important. **Chicks up to about 3 weeks of age are more tolerant than older birds.**

7.   **High humidity** has a highly adverse effect on cooling.

## Symptoms

Symptoms include **panting** (i.e. an increase in respiration rate characterized by short, quick breaths in a laboured manner), increased thirst, reduced appetite, **fall in egg production** and size of eggs, thinning of shells, **reduced growth in broilers**, birds standing with wings outstretched, and eventually, prostration (lying down in exhaustion) and death. The temperature of affected birds may be as high as $42^0$ C ($107.6^0$ F), or more. Mortality may vary from 5% to 50%, and sometimes may go even up to 100%.

## Harmful Effects of Heat Stress

1.   Increased respiration rate alters the acid-base balance because the carbon dioxide ($CO_2$) concentration in the blood decreases. The higher blood pH reduces the amount of calcium in the blood, which is needed for eggshell formation. As a result, in laying flocks, there is **an increase in the number of thin-shell eggs.**

2.   Panting or open-mouth breathing in heat-stressed birds may lead to an **increased incidence of respiratory infection.** This is because the natural filters of the nasal passages are by-passed.

3.   Another symptom of heat stress in a flock is **reduced feed intake.** In growing birds, **fasting will decrease growth rate.**

4.   **In laying flocks,** the reduction of feed intake will result in the **reduction of egg size, egg production, and egg quality.**

## Postmortem Findings

The carcasses of birds that have died of heat stress are markedly dehydrated and congested. The breast muscles are particularly affected. They lose their normal red colour and become pale to white and present a **'cooked meat appearance'. This is characteristic of heat stress.** There is often mucoid (mucus-like) exudate in the nostrils and the mouth.

## Treatment

1.  Immediately make available **adequate cool drinking water.**

2.  Air movements, in the form of ventilation and fans, or sprinklers and foggers, facilitate heat loss. **Increase air circulation** in the house by running ventilation equipment at full capacity.

3.  **Give vitamins** in increased amounts, particularly vitamin C (see **'Vitamin C'**). Heat stress decreases food intake and may increase losses of body's vitamins. This, in turn, increases the vitamin requirement. Addition of vitamin and electrolyte supplements in the drinking water helps to restore the minerals and correct the acid/base balance.

4.  **Give electrolytes,** as heat stress creates electrolyte imbalances. For a list of commercial electrolyte preparations, see Chapter 19 under **'Electrolytes'.**

5.  Some drugs, such as virginiamycin, may reduce heat distress.

6.  Recently, several diet manipulations have been tested in heat-stressed birds. The addition of **vitamin E** in the diet has shown a beneficial effect in layers. However, responses to the addition of **vitamin C** in the diet have varied from no effect to substantial reductions in the harmful effects of heat stress.

7.  Cooling the air inside the house can be achieved by using sprinklers, or spraying on the floor, walls, ceilings, and outside roof with cool water during times of extremely high temperatures.

8.  An attempt to cool the bird can be made by dipping them in water, or by spraying.

9.  Cooling of the air can also be achieved by using a hose to wet the floor, walls, ceiling, and outside roof.

## Control

1.  Control should be aimed at providing the best environment for survival and production, and reducing the rate of metabolism.

2.  To ensure the best environment, houses should be of proper height and width to provide adequate ventilation.

3.   The roof should be insulated and the outside painted white, by using white or aluminium paint, to minimize the effect of radiation. Planting of creepers to cover the roof of the poultry houses may be helpful.

4.   **Water sprinklers** may be provided for the roof, and perhaps, the ground around the house.

5.   **Foggers** may be provided for inside cooling, preferably without the birds themselves becoming wet.

6.   Evaporation coolers, through which the air is drawn into the building, have also been shown to be very effective in cooling. **The air movement is very important.**

7.   **The birds should be provided with adequate cool water in the summer and a ration with a reduced protein: energy ratio. Water increases bird's resistance to heat stress.**

8.   The stocking density should be reduced both on floors and cages to about 80% of that tolerated in cooler conditions. In other words, **avoid overcrowding.**

## Remarks

**It is very important to control heat stress.** Otherwise, apart from the direct losses, on account of the lowered resistance from heat, such a flock may also suffer from infectious diseases like colisepticaemia (*E. coli* infection), infectious coryza, mycoplasmosis (chronic respiratory disease, CRD), and even coccidiosis. **This, in turn, will increase damage and ruin the economy.**

## VICES

**'Vice' means a bad, or an evil habit. In poultry,** it is an abnormal and undesirable behaviour that is harmful to its health, or usefulness. Vices are usually brought about by some aspect of management, or environment. Once started by individual birds, a vice is copied by others, and may become quite widespread. Its control then poses a great problem. The resulting injuries may often lead to death, or to devaluation of carcasses in the case of meat birds, and loss of eggs in layers. **Thus, vices can cause a huge loss to the poultry farmer.** The vices include:

## I. CANNIBALISM

**'Cannibalism' is the abnormal habit of feeding on the flesh of its own species.** In poultry, it is a condition in which birds in a flock attack their pen mates and eat their flesh. The resulting injuries can cause death and may result in heavy mortality. The condition is always recognized by blood around the vent (cloacal opening), through which much of the intestine has been removed by the cannibal birds. **Poultry farmers must remain vigilant to prevent cannibalism as there is no treatment.**

## Causes

1. **Overcrowding.** This gives less opportunity for exercise and the less active birds pick up vices.

2. Cannibalism starts particularly when non-debeaked chickens are placed together in high density. Feather follicles and feet of young birds usually shine under bright, especially red light, which attracts the attention of other birds. Being very curious, birds pick on feet or feather follicles, resulting in drawing of blood. **Once blood is drawn, this will attract more and more chickens, till the victim is dead.**

3. Insufficient feeders and drinkers. Also, insufficient feeding or drinking space.

4. Too much heat during brooding. That is, high brooding temperature.

5. Excessive light in pens and cages.

6. Haemorrhages in the cloacal region, due to the laying of large eggs by new hens, attract other birds. **Once the birds develop a taste for blood and meat, they pick up the habit of cannibalism.**

7. Lack of ventilation.

8. Feeding only pellets, or compressed feed, will usually cause an outbreak, particularly in birds in cage-rearing systems and in laying cages.

9. **Unbalanced feed.** For example, less protein in the feed, or excess of maize in the ration can be important factors. **Deficiency of amino acids, such as arginine and methionine, may be responsible for development of cannibalistic activity. Deficiency of salt (sodium chloride) and minerals** as well as **low protein** may also lead to this condition.

10. Being without feed and water too long.

11. Irritation from external parasites. Loss of feathers from the body, or haemorrhages from the skin due to parasitic infection (lice, mites) may predispose to cannibalism.

12. Wounds caused by fighting between the birds may also serve as a stimulus for cannibalistic activity.

13. Fearfulness.

14. Accelerated sexual maturity.

15. Increased egg production.

16. Low humidity.

17. Idleness, boredom and vent pecking.

**Cannibalism in chickens occurs in many forms. These include:**

## 1. Vent Pecking

Pecking of the vent (cloaca), or region of the abdomen several inches below the vent, **is the commonest and also the most severe form of cannibalism.** It is usually **seen in layer flocks in high production.** The problem usually starts in growers as they come into lay, and is sometimes caused by the straining associated with the passage of unusually large eggs. The resulting damage to the skin of the vent and the lining of the cloaca encourages attack by another bird, and usually leads to complete removal of the intestines and death of the victim. The presence of blood, and the taste of it, leads to rapid spread of the vice.

## 2. Feather Pecking or Fea '.er Pulling

This is a **milder form of cannibalism.** It is usually seen in flocks kept in close confinement resulting in lack of sufficient exercise. **Overcrowding**, as broiler reach slaughter age, is usually followed by an outbreak of feather and tail pecking, often leading to serious downgrading of the carcasses of the affected birds. **Nutritional and mineral deficiencies** may be the contributing factors. Also, it may be provoked by the bullying of a weak or sick bird.

## 3. Toe Picking

Toe picking is usually **seen only in young birds** during rearing and is often **initiated by hunger**. It is usually the result of feeding errors, or failure by the birds to find the feed in the litter. Chicks may not find feed because feeders are too high, or too far from the heat source. Feeder space may be inadequate, and the smaller or more timid chicks may be prevented from eating by aggressive birds. **If the chick cannot find feed, it may pick at its own, or a neighbour's toe.** In serious outbreaks the pecking continues until most of the affected toe has been removed. It is good practice to put feed on chick box covers, or trays, and place them under the hover the first few days of brooding.

## 4. Head Picking

Head picking usually **follows injuries to the comb or wattles caused by fighting among males.** A different form of cannibalism is now being seen in beak-trimmed (debeaked) birds kept in cages. The area around the eyes is black and blue due to subcutaneous (under the skin) haemorrhage, wattles are dark and swollen with oozed blood, and ear lobes are black and necrotic (dead). Even though birds have trimmed (cut) beak and are kept in separate cages, they will reach through the wire and peck at a neighbour. Or, they may grasp its ear lobes, or wattles, and shake their heads in much the same way as a cat shaking a rat.

## Prevention

Cannibalism can best be prevented by paying attention to the predisposing and contributing factors. These include:

1. Prevention through **proper management and good nutrition** is the best control of cannibalism.

2. **Avoid overcrowding.**

3. **Debeaking is necessary to prevent cannibalism.** In cages, where high-density rearing is practised, it is necessary to trim the beaks before housing. Debeaking involves removal of one-third of the beak, by cautery, usually when the chicks are about a day old (see **'debeaking'** under Chapter 42).

4. Reduce light intensity.

5. **Provide adequate feed and water space,** and do not allow birds to go without feed for long periods. **Feed must be available in sufficient quantity at all times.**

6. Careful attention to ventilation and light intensity may prevent an outbreak of cannibalism.

7. **The quantity of salt, minerals and vitamins may be slightly increased in poultry ration.** Likewise, **increasing** the amount of **methionine** may be helpful to prevent this habit **in layers.**

8. Laying nests must be built. This is because, following laying, the congested external genitalia (genital organs) of layers attract other birds for cannibalism. Provision of red bulbs near laying nests may help during the period of the problem.

9. Birds involved in cannibalism must be isolated. **Wounded birds should also be segregated and given proper treatment.**

## II. Egg Eating

Sometimes birds develop a tendency to **eat their own eggs.** It may start due to the presence of cracked eggs or accidental breaking of eggs; and **once the birds develop taste for them, they start breaking their own eggs.** It then becomes quite difficult to prevent this vice. Factors responsible for breaking of eggs, or cracking of eggs, are thin or soft eggshells or lack of sufficient bedding material in the laying area. Presence of eggs for long period in the pens may also encourage the birds to start egg eating.

## Prevention

1. Isolate the birds which have developed this habit.

2. Egg eaters may then be kept in cages in which eggs roll away. Thus, the egg will be beyond the reach of the bird after laying.

3.  The quality of limestone and protein may be increased in the diet, after proper consultation.

4.  Debeaking is also helpful in reducing this tendency (see **'debeaking'**).

5.  Darkness in the laying area may prevent this habit.

6.  Egg collection interval should be reduced.

## III. Pica

Birds may start eating materials which are not fit for consumption, such as feathers, litter material, threads, etc. It is less commonly found in modern poultry farm. Phosphorus deficiency, parasitic infestations, new litter material, etc., may predispose the birds to pica. **Good managemental care and balanced diet** are recommended for the prevention of pica.

## EFFECTS OF AMMONIA

Most commercial poultry today are kept in total confinement. Therefore, the health and well-being of these birds are greatly influence by the **air quality.** Air pollutants such as **ammonia** and **dust** have been associated with an **increased incidence of respiratory diseases**. The incidence of respiratory diseases is higher in **winter**, when less ventilation results in more air pollution.

**Ammonia production in a poultry house depends on:**

## 1. Inadequate Ventilation

Improper ventilation can lead to **wet litter**. Ammonia fumes develop in wet litter and droppings. If ventilation is poor and fumes accumulate, they may reach to a high concentration which may prevent growth and performance, cause eye changes, and **aggravate respiratory infections.**

## 2. Wet Litter (Increased Moisture)

When litter moisture is maintained between 20-25%, ammonia is usually not produced. Ammonia production starts when moisture exceeds 30% and increases further as the temperature rises. **Wet litter exposes to more coccidiosis.** This is because wet litter favours the survival and development of coccidial oocysts. Wet litter also results in soiling of birds and eggs, and in poor performance.

## How is ammonia produced?

When litter is wet (high moisture content), **urate-splitting bacteria present in the litter,** produce fermentation of the urates in faeces under warm, moist conditions. This leads to the production of ammonia in the house. Ammonia concentrations are increased by moisture, high temperatures, overcrowding, and poor ventilation. In most cases, **excess ammonia in a broiler house is due to wet litter and insufficient ventilation.**

## How does ammonia produce the harmful effects?

Ammonia ($NH_3$) is a gas. **It is highly soluble in water.** When it comes in contact with the lining (mucous membrane) of the respiratory tract following inhalation, or in contact with the eyes, it dissolves in the liquid (i.e. mucus of the respiratory tract) to produce **ammonium hydroxide** ($NH_3 + H_2O = NH_4OH$) [ammonium hydroxide], that is, solution of ammonia gas in water. **Ammonium hydroxide ($NH_4OH$) is an irritating alkali and is responsible for the damage caused.** It destroys cilia (minute hair-like processes) of the respiratory tract.

## What are the harmful effects of ammonia?

**Ammonia levels should be less than 25 ppm** (parts per million), but in poorly ventilated litter-type houses, ammonia may exceed 100 ppm.

1. **When concentration of ammonia is greater than 25 ppm** it may have the following effects:

    (i) **Ammonia damages the respiratory system and predisposes to infections,** such as colibacillosis (i.e. *E. coli* infection), infectious coryza, and Ranikhet disease.

    (ii) **Depresses growth rate by 4 to 8%.** This increases feed conversion ratio by 3 to 6% in broilers.

    (iii) **Reduces appetite.**

2. **When concentration is greater than 50 ppm.**

    (i) Ammonia, actually the **ammonium hydroxide** that is formed, destroys cilia of the upper respiratory tract of birds. Each lining cell of the respiratory tract possesses around 250 of these cilia on its surface. The cilia are minute short hair-like processes. They beat continuously at approximately 1000 strokes per minute and push forward mucus (a liquid secretion) in the nasal passages and trachea at the speed of about 20 mm per minute. Rapid and powerful movement of the cilia creates a series of waves. **The purpose is to push forward any trapped disease-producing micro-organisms in the mucus and throw them out.** This is the most important protective mechanism of the respiratory system against infectious agents. By destroying cilia ammonia also destroys this natural mechanism of bird of physically removing the deposited particles, or dissolved toxic gases, from the respiratory tract. **Once this defence mechanism is destroyed, the birds become most susceptible to respiratory infections.** For example, the inhaled *Escherichia coli* are then able to establish themselves, grow, and produce disease. Or, it predisposes to more severe respiratory diseases associated with a variety of respiratory pathogens (i.e. disease-producing organisms).

(ii)  Ammonia also reduces body weight and feed efficiency.

3.  **When concentration of ammonia is greater than 75 ppm:**

Ammonia reduces food consumption and growth rate. Egg production could also be affected. At levels of 75-100 ppm, there may be **haemorrhages in trachea and bronchi.**

4.  **When concentration of ammonia is greater than 100 ppm:**

Ammonia, in concentration of 150 ppm and above, sometimes causes **'ammonia blindness'**, also known as **'ammonia burn'** (kerato-conjunctivitis) **in broilers.** It is caused by ammonia fumes coming out from poorly managed litter in an ill-ventilated house.

**Affected birds keep their eyes closed, stand dejectedly** with ruffled feathers, and are reluctant to move. They may rub their head and eyelids against their wings. The eyelids are swollen and cornea may be ulcerated. The condition usually affects both eyes. Affected birds do not eat and become weak. Recovery is often rapid, once the excess ammonia is removed. However, in extreme cases corneal ulceration (i.e. ulceration of the cornea of eye) may cause permanent damage and impaired vision. Prevention is based on proper ventilation and litter management (see **'litter management'**). **The ammonia fumes are formed in wet litter.**

**The human nose is able to detect ammonia levels at around 20 ppm.** Ammonia **concentrations of just 5 ppm** (undetectable by the human nose) have been shown to **irritate and injure the protective lining of the chick's respiratory tract, causing increased susceptibility to respiratory disease.** If one waits until levels are high enough to detect by sense of smell before taking steps to control ammonia, some damage has already occurred.

As a general principle, the concentration of ammonia in a poultry house sufficient to cause irritation of the human eye may cause lesions in chickens, if the exposure is prolonged **(Table 2).**

## Prevention

1.  **Keep the ammonia level of the poultry house less than 25 ppm.** When litter moisture is maintained between 20-25%, ammonia is usually not produced.

2.  **Ensure proper ventilation.** Perhaps the most difficult aspect of broiler management to understand is ventilation. This is because it is not possible to 'see' good ventilation. It is difficult, by seeing, to determine the volume and direction of fresh air being brought into the broiler house. During cold weather and during the

**Table 2.  Effects of Ammonia on People and Chickens**

| Ammonia (ppm) | Chickens | | | | |
|---|---|---|---|---|---|
| | People | Drop in egg production | Weight loss lesions | Respiratory lesions | Eye |
| 20 | Very slight smell | No drop | No loss | Slight | No changes |
| 25-30 | Very slight smell | No drop | No loss | Slight | No changes |
| 50-60 | Increasing smell | No drop | + | + | + |
| 100 | Eye and nose irritation | + | ++ | + | + |
| 200 | Eye and nose irritation | ++ | +++ | ++ | ++ |

brooding period the main function of ventilation system is to remove ammonia and moisture from the broiler house. **Many farmers underestimate the harmful effects of ammonia.**

3.  **Ensure proper litter management** (see **'litter management'**). Litter dries better, if it is stirred frequently. But in spite of all efforts, it may remain wet in rainy season and, to some extent, also in winter. If wetness and excess ammonia concentration persist, litter should be changed and ventilation improved.

   **The key to reduce ammonia problem and ensure good air quality is to control moisture in the poultry house. Adequate ventilation** to remove moisture and reduce humidity levels in the poultry house is the most effective method of ensuring good air quality.

## DEHYDRATION

   **'To dehydrate'** means to deprive the body or tissues of water. Chicks can survive several days without water, but will die from the 4th or 5th day. Mortality reaches its peak during the 5th or 6th day and stops suddenly if the water is provided. Chicks which are not drinking would have died by this period, and survivors are those that have found the water and are drinking. **Laying birds need a constant water supply otherwise production will drop and even stop if the water restriction is severe.**

## Causes

1.   Complete lack of water, or failure to provide adequate amount of water.

2.   Drinkers in cool zones.

3.   Failure of birds to find water.

4.   Inability of birds to reach the water.

5.   In some cases due to a deterring factor in the water. That is, something present in the water discourages the bird from drinking the water. In other words, **unpalatable water**.

6.   Intercurrent disease.

7.   Inaccessible drinkers.

## Symptoms

Symptoms include insufficient weight of chicks for size and age, and dehydrated and wrinkled skin on the shanks. They appear weak with sunken eyes.

## Postmortem Findings

The chickens are emaciated and dehydrated. Skin is tough and dry and the beak shows blue discoloration. The breast muscles are dry and dark and there is no food in the crop, or the food in the crop is dry. Kidneys are dark, ureters show accumulation of urates, and there is visceral gout and darkening of the blood.

## Dehydration in Older Birds

Symptoms and postmortem findings in older birds are similar to those in chicks, and weight loss is much more noticeable.

## Control

Ensure adequate supply and distribution of fresh clean water.

## SMOTHERING

'**To smother**' means to kill through lack of air. That is, to kill birds by making them unable to breathe. In other words, **to suffocate them**.

Smothering is usually caused by **crowding** or **piling** (getting one on top of the other) of birds in a corner. **The history of the case usually indicates that mortality occurs only at night, and the flock in general looks healthy.**

## Causes

1.   Inadequate heat supply.

2. Insufficient space under the brooder.

3. Presence of draughts (i.e. flow of cold air) in the brooding area. That is, when young birds get chilled.

4. Poor lights inhibiting bird movement.

5. Overheating below the brooder.

6. Mechanical and electrical failures.

7. Piling may occur when birds are frightened.

8. Piling may also occur when birds are moved to new sheds/houses/quarters.

9. Smothering of baby chicks can occur in chick boxes that are piled too high without an air space between each box. Smothering can also occur if boxes do not have sufficient ventilation holes, or in boxes placed in a closed compartment, such as the boot (luggage compartment, trunk) of a car.

## Symptoms

Chicks appear to be huddling and chirping (i.e. making a sharp sound) in corners. Early symptoms are dehydration, off feed and laboured breathing and, at later stages, drooped (fallen) wings, prostration (lying stretched out on the ground), and death. Temperature exposure below $15^0$C is usually regarded as lethal (i.e. able to cause death).

## Postmortem Findings

Postmortem examinations of chicks which have died from smothering usually do not show much gross changes to make a positive diagnosis. However, a thorough examination will rule out other possible causes of death. In broilers and older birds that have smothered, there is **congestion of trachea and lungs.** The crop is without feed, yolk sac is unabsorbed and kidneys are pale with some urates in the tubules. Feathers are removed where birds have been trampled (i.e. crushed and injured).

## Diagnosis

Adequate flock history, symptoms, postmortem findings, and negative bacteriology confirm the diagnosis.

## Prevention

1. Adequate supply of heat and proper management of chicks during the brooding period.

2. Smothering of chicks in the brooder house can be prevented by putting a circle of cardboard (chick guards) around the hover during the first week, and gradually widening the diameter as chicks get older. This will prevent piling in a corner during

night (see **'brooding management'**).

3.  When birds are moved to new quarters, the use of a dim light or lantern for the first few nights will decrease the possibility of smothering.

4.  Birds transferred to new quarters should be checked late in the evening for signs of piling.

5.  Frequent observation of the flock is very important during the first few days after getting a batch of new chicks.

# SWOLLEN HEAD SYNDROME

Swollen head syndrome is a condition that affects chickens of all types, **but mainly broilers and broiler parents.** It is caused by an **avian pneumovirus**, but bacteria may be involved as secondary invaders.

## Symptoms

**In broilers,** the main symptom is **swelling of the head** which is more severe than in breeders. It gives the face a puffy (swollen) appearance caused by subcutaneous oedema (i.e. accumulation of fluid under the skin) around the eyes which extends over the head, and down into the intermandibular tissue (i.e. between the jaw) and wattles. Respiratory symptoms include coughing and sneezing. Many affected birds have a severe tracheitis (inflammation of the trachea) and usually die from secondary septicaemia (blood infection) caused by *Escherichia coli.* Although morbidity (i.e. number of sick birds in a flock) is usually low, the **condition is aggravated by poor ventilation and high levels of ammonia and dust.** If affected birds are removed from the poultry house in the early stages of the disease, they usually recover within 24 hours.

**Affected broiler breeders** sit with neck arched so that the head rests on the back **(opisthotonus).** There is usually swelling around the eyes and over the top of the head. Affected birds usually have green, foul-smelling diarrhoea which causes soiling around the vent. Birds showing clinical symptoms usually die. In general only females are affected, but sometimes a small number of males show similar symptoms. The disease usually occurs at, or around peak laying (between 26 to 30 weeks), but can be as late as 52 weeks of age. There is usually a drop in egg production.

## Postmortem Findings

Puffiness of the skin is seen over the head. Gelatinous fluid and inspissated (thickened) pus are observed subcutaneously. Removal of the skin over the head shows yellow, oedematous subcutaneous tissue.

## Treatment and Control

1.  It is often beneficial to administer broad-spectrum antibiotics through water, followed

by medication in the feed to control secondary bacterial infections (see chapter 19 for a list of commercial antibiotic preparations).

2. Vaccination with TRT (turkey rhinotracheitis) vaccines has been successful.

3. Control of other disease-producing organisms, particularly respiratory viruses such as infectious bronchitis virus and Ranikhet disease virus, which predispose to swollen head syndrome, is essential.

4. **Good ventilation is essential to minimize the amount of ammonia and dust in the air,** which predispose to secondary *Escherichia coli* infection.

## EGG-BOUND CONDITION

It is a condition in which an egg is lodged in the cloaca, but cannot be laid.

## Causes

1. Inflammation of the oviduct.

2. Partial paralysis of the muscles of the oviduct, or

3. Production of an egg so large that it is physically impossible for it to be laid.

However, the exact cause of the condition is not known.

Young hens laying an unusually large egg are more prone to the problem.

## Postmortem Findings

At postmortem, an egg is found lodged in the cloaca and fails to be laid. The egg is unusually large.

## BIG LIVER AND SPLEEN DISEASE

It is an infectious, transmissible disease caused by a **virus**. The virus so far has not been identified. The disease is characterized by decreased egg production, a slight increase in mortality, and enlargement of the liver and spleen of mature chickens. It is especially seen in **broiler breeders** and, less commonly, egg layers. The disease was first recognized in Australia in 1980.

Sick birds show paleness of combs and wattles, depression, loss of appetite and soiled vent feathers or pasty droppings. There may be a drop in egg production that could reach 20%. This is accompanied by increased mortality up to 1% per week for 3-4 weeks. During the period flock is affected, eggs produced are thin-shelled.

**Postmortem findings include an enlarged spleen (2-3 times normal size) and liver.** Typical clinical signs with enlarged liver and spleen are sufficient for a presumptive diagnosis.

# FEMORAL HEAD NECROSIS

Disintegration (decomposition) of the proximal femur (head of the femur) **in broilers** is a common postmortem finding, and an important cause of **lameness**. The condition is known as **'femoral head necrosis'** or **'proximal femoral degeneration'**.

## Causes

Proximal femoral degeneration is usually the result of a bacterial chondritis and osteomyelitis. That is, inflammation of the cartilage (chondritis) and bone marrow (soft tissues in the cavity of long bones) or of the bone and marrow (osteomyelitis) caused by a focal bacterial infection. Extensive changes are often caused by a small bacterial focus. **Mostly the following bacteria are involved.**

1. **Staphylococci** are the most commonly involved bacteria, the species being *Staphylococcus aureus*. **Staphylococci**, mainly *Staphylococcus aureus*, are ubiquitous organisms (i.e. commonly present) in broiler and broiler breeder environment. Staphylococci may be found in litter, on feather and fluff (soft feathers on birds) samples, and on particles in the air in broiler houses.

2. *Escherichia coli* **is** also involved. Like *S. aureus, E. coli* is also present everywhere. The strains commonly found in poultry in the 'normal' intestinal flora are usually harmless, but they can become pathogenic (disease-producing) in the intestine, or in other sites. This may occur if there is concurrent (simultaneous) viral infection, or immunosuppression (suppression of immunity). Under these conditions, *E. coli* colonizes (i.e. grows in) unusual sites, and specific strains with increased disease-producing power, or liking for a particular tissue, come to dominate.

3. **Salmonella** bacteria may also be involved, though their involvement is rare.

4. Besides the above three types of bacteria, viruses known as **'reoviruses'** may also sometimes be involved mainly in broilers between 4 and 8 weeks of age (see **'avian reoviruses'**). However, they have been also recorded in younger birds.

5. Bacterial osteomyelitis and chondritis, which lead to femoral head necrosis, are also seen in some isolated birds with a generalized septicaemia (i.e. blood infection caused by bacteria).

6. **Non-infectious lesions** (changes) **in the proximal femur** (e.g. from trauma/ injury) **may provide focus for bacterial infections.** Also, non-bacterial lesions may cause lameness in some birds.

## Symptoms

Femoral head necrosis occurs **in broilers** usually **between 25 and 50 days of age.** The affected birds can be identified by a characteristic trembling gait (way of walking). They often use a wing for support while moving and also while sitting down.

Some affected birds give a loud harsh cry when middle portion of the proximal femur is palpated.

## Postmortem Findings

The femoral head usually separates from the shaft by a fracture through the neck when hip joints are separated. **Both head and proximal portion of the femur show marked degeneration.**

## Treatment/Control

It is advisable to mix an effective broad spectrum antibiotic in the feed. Refer to chapter 19 for a list of commercially available antibiotics under **'Antibiotic growth promoters'.**

## BUMBLE FOOT (ENLARGED FOOT PADS)

Bumble foot is an abscess in the foot pad. It is a common infection in mature chickens. Bumble foot leads to massive swelling of the foot and lameness. It is caused by **staphylococci bacteria.**

Some males develop **enlarged foot pads (bumble foot).** These usually become inflamed, and as a result the male does not mate. Wire and slat floors, and wet litter, are instrumental in causing an increase in this condition. If a male is seriously affected, it should be removed from the pen, because such a bird seldom recovers.

## INTUSSUSCEPTION

Intussusception is the invagination (insertion) of one segment of intestine into another. It is a relatively rare condition in poultry. Intussusception is seen in young chickens usually involving lower part of the small intestine. The affected portion soon becomes necrotic (dead), with adhesions to neighbouring tissues. Death of the bird occurs from peritonitis (inflammation of the peritoneum, a membrane present in the body cavity) and toxaemia (presence of toxic substances in the blood).

Sometimes minor outbreaks occur with a few birds being found dead daily. In such cases there is usually an enteritis (inflammation of intestine), or parasitic infestation, such as worms or coccidiosis, which may have caused spasmodic anti-peristaltic movement in the intestine. That is, sudden involuntary muscular contraction of the intestine against its normal, advancing, wavelike movement (i.e. peristalsis). Sudden movement in the **opposite direction** leads to intussusception.

## VOLVULUS

Volvulus occurs when there is **torsion (twisting) of the intestine around itself,** or the root of the mesentery. It is a relatively rare condition in poultry. In young birds, volvulus of the small intestine may be caused by twisting around the yolk sac. Volvulus may be secondary to enteritis (inflammation of the intestine), or abnormal peristalsis caused by worms or coccidial infection. **Symptoms** include loss of appetite and progressive weight loss. Death occurs in a few days. **At postmortem**, the affected and distal portion of the intestine are severely congested due to compression of circulation.

# IMPACTION OF THE CROP, GIZZARD AND SMALL INTESTINE

Impaction means firm packing. Impaction of the crop or gizzard is sometimes seen in poultry. It occurs mainly in young birds which eat indigestible fibrous tissue, such as tough grass, straw, or string. It is more common in birds on free range, or may even be seen while on deep litter. Such impaction may continue into the upper small intestine. Impaction of the small intestine may also sometimes occur with very large numbers of ascarid worms (see *'Ascaridia galli'*).

# GIZZARD EROSION

Gizzard erosion is a condition in which lining of the gizzard is eroded (gradually destroyed) and darkened. It is a condition seen usually in **broiler chickens**. The cause is uncertain, but it is associated with dietary factors, and especially with certain types of fish meal. Economically the condition is important because there is some reduction in weight gain.

# PROLAPSE OF THE OVIDUCT

The failure of the hen to pull back the outer end of the oviduct after laying an egg is known as **prolapse**. It can be put back, but tends to recur. It is seen in layers, and first occurs due to the effect of oviposition (egg laying). The appearance of the oviduct leads to cannibalism, and the problem is difficult to solve (see **'vices'**). **In many cases, the prolapse becomes so serious that such birds are pecked to death by their cage mates.**

The tendency for flocks to have prolapse is inherited, but its expression is more common in cages than with regular nests, where the birds are not exposed during the time the oviduct is being pulled back. Growers that are overweight, or carry too much fat at the onset of egg production, can also experience increased prolapse. Feeding a high fibre diet, or starting management practices to reduce egg production, will help the flock to return back to normal.

# VENT GLEET

'Vent' is another name for **cloaca**, the external opening of the rectum (large intestine). **Vent gleet is an inflammatory condition of the cloaca,** and is also therefore known as **'cloacitis'** (inflammation of the cloaca).

Vent gleet generally affects **laying hens**, and sometimes, males. Usually a very few birds in a flock are affected. It begins as a red area around the cloaca which becomes swollen and covered with a yellow, moist, necrotic (i.e. composed of dead tissue) membrane. **Vent gleet is associated with a sharp, characteristic, unpleasant smell.** Treatment is usually not necessary, but the application of antiseptic or antibiotic ointments may be helpful.

## FOREIGN BODY IN PROVENTRICULUS

Sometimes chickens may accidentally ingest nails, pieces of wire, stumps of feathers, or pieces of sticks. They cause obstruction or proventriculitis (inflammation of the proventriculus). Rupture of the proventriculus may result in peritonitis (inflammation of the peritoneum, a membrane in the body cavity) and death of the bird.

## BLUE-WING DISEASE

Blue wing disease is a condition that affects **broilers. It is caused by a synergistic effect between chicken anaemia virus and a reovirus.** Birds infected with both viruses have significantly lower weight gain and more severe damage in several tissues. The disease may inflict up to 10% mortality.

In chickens infected with chicken infectious anaemia virus, if there is mild trauma then gangrenous dermatitis lesions begin to develop on the wing tips of affected birds (see **'gangrenous dermatitis'**). This condition has been referred to as **'blue-wing disease'.**

Characteristic lesions of blue wing disease are haemorrhages and oedema (accumulation of fluid in the skin's underlying tissue and muscles), accompanied by atrophy (reduction in size) of thymus, spleen, and bursa of Fabricius. A large number of **reoviruses** and **chicken infectious anaemia virus** have been isolated from chickens affected with blue wing disease (see **'chicken infectious anaemia'**).

## RODENTS

Rodents (**rats** and **mice**) are very common pests in and around poultry houses. They cause a tremendous amount of damage if an effective control programme is not carried out. Rodents eat or contaminate feed, which increases feed costs and affects feed conversions. They may also carry a variety of diseases and ectoparasites (i.e. insects). Rats are usually seen in layer and breeder houses, while mice are problems in all types of houses. If present in large numbers, they may attack birds.

## RATS

Rats eat almost any type of food, including eggs and poultry feed. However, they prefer fresh food. A population of 200 adult rats may consume 25 pounds (11.35 kg) of feed daily. **A single rat can eat 25 pounds (11.35 kg) of grain in a year,** and in the process contaminate 10 times that amount of poultry feed by defaecating and urinating.

**Most rat activity, including feeding, occurs at night.** Rats seen outside their shelters during the day indicate a large population. **Rats have a high rate of reproduction.** This can lead to large numbers of rats in a fairly short period of time. A single pair of rats and their offspring could produce as many as 1500 rats in one year, if all the offspring survived. Rats will breed at an age of 3-5 months, and give birth approximately 3 weeks after mating. Four to seven litters, with each litter having 6-12 young, are produced in one year. A litter is a group of young rats produced at one time. The female rat breeds again 1-2 day after giving birth. **Breeding occurs all year.**

## MICE

Mice eat almost any kind of food. Mice require much less water than rats and are capable of extracting water from the food they eat. Mice are able to reproduce at an age of 6-8 weeks. They give birth to 5 or 6 young about 3 weeks after mating. Two to four days after giving birth, the female mouse can breed again. Usually, 5 to 8 litters are produced in a year. **Mice breed regularly throughout the year.**

## Control

There are **three aspects to rodent control.** They are **rodent-proofing, sanitation,** and **rodent killing.**

1. **Rodent-proofing** can be an effective long-term measure. It is, however, impractical, if not impossible, to rodent-proof a poultry house.

2. **Sanitation** involves cleaning up around the poultry building. Rodents are secretive creatures. They do not like to move about in open areas. Therefore, mowing (cutting) the grass and weeds on a regular basis creates a less favourable place for living. Removing heaps of old wood, nests, or any rubbish helps to make the area less attractive to rodents, and makes early detection possible.

3. After sanitation, **a rodent-killing programme** should be implemented. Rodent killing includes baiting (baiting means putting a poisonous material at a place where it will be eaten by the rat with a purpose to kill it), fumigating, trapping, or even shooting. **Usually, a properly conducted baiting programme is the easiest and most effective means for killing rodents.**

**There are many products on the market that will kill rodents.** The **first group** of safe and commonly used baits (poisonous materials) are the multiple-dose anticoagulants, such as warfarin. Multiple-dose anticoagulants must be consumed for several days to be lethal (i.e. able to cause death). The **second type** of rodenticide (an agent that kills rodents) includes the single-dose anticoagulants, such as bromadialone. A single feeding is sufficient to kill a rodent. The **last category** includes acute single-dose rodenticide, such as zinc phosphide. These chemicals are very effective and useful for a quick destruction of a large rodent population. These chemicals are highly toxic.

**Precautions** for carrying out rodent-killing programme include:

1.  For any killing programme to be effective, **rodents must consume the poisonous material (bait), and they need to consume a lethal amount.** To achieve this, care must be taken in placing the bait. Random placing of bait around a poultry house, does not work. Always remember that rodents will not go out of their way to eat poisonous bait, if they have food readily available. Therefore, placing the bait in or closer to their shelters (places of living), than their regular food source, is important. One of the best and safest places to put the bait is down in the active rodent burrow. It will save bait, time and money if we first find out which burrows are active before starting baiting. This can be done by filling in all the burrows around the poultry house with soil or newspaper. These burrows should be re-checked next day and all burrows that have been re-opened should be baited.

2.  When using a multi-dose rodenticide, **be sure to put bait in all active burrows daily until the bait is no longer consumed.** When bait is no longer taken, remove the uneaten bait and fill in the burrow.

3.  When a single-dose anticoagulant is used, **the active burrows should be baited** for two successive days, and 4 or 5 days later, all of the burrows should be filled, and any that are active baited for 2 more days.

4.  **When baiting for mice, always remember that mice live in the upper areas of a poultry house.** When this occurs, baiting at ground level will be ineffective. Therefore, put out a small amount of bait in many places rather than putting out a large quantity of bait in a few places. The bait can be placed on the sill (ledge at the bottom of a window or door), in the feed rooms, or spread in the attic area if the house has a drop ceiling.

     **To conclude, a rodent control programme must be a continuing effort, if it is to be effective.** Usually control programmes are implemented only when there is a severe problem. At that time, control requires a great deal of effort and money; and when most of the rodents are killed, the control effort stops until the rodents become a serious problem again. **This type of control programme is a waste of time and money.** It is much easier and less expensive to control, or totally eliminate, a small rodent population. This can be achieved by **checking the poultry houses for rodent activity on a regular basis,** even after the control programme has killed most of the rodents. Look for rodent signs both inside and outside the poultry houses at least every two weeks, and start baiting as soon as any activity is observed.

# Section II

# DISEASE DIAGNOSIS

# Chapter 12

# Introduction

After becoming familiar with various diseases and ailments of poultry, the next step is to get their diagnosis as soon as possible. This is because the course of action will depend on the nature of the disease. One should not delay the diagnosis for any reason when a disease threatens, otherwise it may get out of hand before diagnosis is made. Therefore, **getting a diagnosis as quickly as possible is of the greatest importance.** It is not always possible to treat a disease or check its harmful effects, but to plan effectively for the future, it is important to identify all diseases that occur.

A multi-pronged approach is made in this section to arrive at a diagnosis. A key to good disease diagnosis is **'to see the forest as well as the trees'**. That is, to diagnose the most important flock problems(s), rather than getting too much occupied with individual bird disorders. **The best approach is to begin with history.** Get a complete history of the disease and all the related events leading to the outbreak. The more information is collected, the more easily one can proceed at solving the problem. The next chapter therefore begins with the topic **'How to carry out a field investigation'**.

# Chapter 13

# How To Carry Out a Field Investigation

**W**hile carrying out a field investigation, one must always remember that **common things occur commonly.** Therefore, one should concentrate on probabilities (i.e. what is more likely) rather than possibilities. The following basic points must be borne in mind.

1.  The problem lies at the farm rather than in the laboratory.

2.  The diagnosis should indicate the major production problem, rather than just an obvious cause of mortality.

3.  The preliminary diagnosis may require only good observation and scissors. Laboratory confirmation may follow, **but advice is usually required right now.**

4.  Without adequate records, a reliable diagnosis may not be possible.

5.  Record and report accurately and fairly.

**Disease is a departure from a normal state of health, or production.** In intensively produced poultry, disease usually has its origin in the methods of management. Often, the causes of such problems involve many factors. For example, an infectious agent may express itself when factors such as those of nutrition and/or management are also at fault.

**The diagnosis of poultry problems in the field today is not a simple, straightforward business involving an infectious agent that it was in the early days of the industry.** It is not only the multi-factorial nature of the problems involving nutritional, managemental, environmental and genetic factors, but also the usually ill-defined nature of the complaints, that is so demanding and challenges the investigator. For example, the 5% or 10% drop in production, shell quality faults, drops in hatchability, leg weakness problems, or loss of performance. Such problems are more difficult and also tedious to cope with, than a classical disease involving diagnostic symptoms, mortality, and characteristic postmortem findings.

Basically, then, **there are two categories of problems that require investigation.**

(1)  The postmortem-based, laboratory-confirmed, **relatively easy and straightforward problems** for making a diagnosis of some disease conditions, and possibly prescribing specific treatment.

(2)  The 'in-depth' (very thorough) investigation to find out the underlying cause of an infectious disease, or to attempt to define a **more vague, possibly a multi-factorial condition and determine its origin and treatment.**

## History

The first step in any investigation is to obtain and record a **detailed history**. This needs time. While carrying out an on-farm or on-site investigation, the following guidelines may be observed.

**Start in the office.** Take a calculator. Collect all the history and write it down. Records of mortality, egg production, hatchability, etc. may be taken. Make sure you practise to **carry out quiet observations** when watching birds in a house. That is, not in the surroundings of talk, movement and noise.

**Do not be in a hurry.** Walk around the site or farm, and observe. Get to know the people involved, evaluate them and gain their confidence.

**Remember that common things occur commonly.** A drop in egg production may be caused by theft of eggs and increased feed consumption by poor feed conversion, or by theft of feed.

**Ask questions.** Important questions should be put on more than one occasion, but in different ways and to different staff during the course of investigation in order to get an overall idea. At the right place and time the observations and thoughts of all concerned may be of real value.

**It is essential to know the 'normal' before 'abnormal' can be appreciated.** Therefore, in addition to experience at the farm, **it is advisable to read the poultry periodicals and to be familiar with the technical books.**

**Postmortem examination forms only one part of any such investigation.**

## Problems

**Usually, the problems are of two types:**

1.  Mortality (deaths)/morbidity (sickness) in chicks, growers, or adult birds.

2.  Drop in production and/or quality of either growth (body weight, feed conversion ratio), or eggs.

**Investigation of disease involving mortality and morbidity**

The case history, a postmortem examination, and usually laboratory investigations are required. A visit to the farm/site may be helpful.

## History

**For a routine straightforward problem** involving sickness and deaths, investigations should include:

Type of bird

Age

Percentage sick

Number submitted for postmortem

Number in house

Mortality record for the last seven days

Symptoms of disease, duration, etc.

Postmortem findings

Laboratory findings

Tentative diagnosis and immediate recommendations

Final diagnosis and recommendations

However, solution of **a more difficult problem**, such as a drop in production and/or quality of either growth (body weight, feed conversion ratio, FCR) or eggs, **requires a more detailed investigation.** The following aspects may be considered.

Flock of origin

Strain of bird

Flock size, or total number of birds on site

Weight for age at various stages of growth or production

System of rearing

System of management (all-in, all-out, or multi-age)

## Building and Management

Size and type of building(s)

Management system

Stocking density

Type and condition of litter and number of times used

# Equipment

Brooders, heaters

Cage design, stocking

Feeders, drinkers

Space per bird

Cleanliness, efficiency

# Ventilation

Fans: number, type, condition, whether functioning

Temperature, air flow, spread of birds on the floor

Control system in use

Variation of ventilation/temperature within the house

# Lighting

Pattern

Intensity

Control system

# Nutrition

Supplier or home mix

Type of rations

Specification

Formulation

Raw materials

Quality, quality control

Premix/supplement

Minerals

Other conditions, e.g. medicines, growth promoters, enzymes

Feed and water systems: failures, size, space per bird, allowance per bird

Feeding system, feed consumption, feed wastage

Feed and water consumption records

Recent change of feed/system/method

Pellet quality

## Production Details

Broilers (weight and feed conversion ration, FCR)

Layers: weeks in lay, production percentage/bird/day (hen day production)/birds housed (hen housed average); egg size/egg mass

Records of previous flocks

## Disease

Vaccination details and record

Previous history of illness in the flock; results of previous investigation

Drug treatment record

Mortality and morbidity record for the duration of the flock

Presence of external parasites, worms, flies

## Symptoms of present problem and possible 'stress' factors

**External:** Feathering extent/quality, skin/eye/lesions, parasites

**Respiratory:** Coughing, snicking (making slight sharp noise), head shaking, swollen eyes, nasal discharge.

**Nervous:** Trembling, ataxia (muscular incoordination), falling, lying down, paralysis, circling, blindness

**Locomotor:** Crooked toes, enlarged hocks or other joints, slipped tendon, spread out legs, paralysis, leg trembling, leg weakness, posture, bone conformation

**Digestive:** Off-feed (disinclined to eat), droppings (**intestinal**: consistency, bloody, white, and green; **caecal**: consistency, colour, frothy)

**Recent stress factors:** For example, shifting, overcrowding, vaccination, drug treatment, weather extremes (hot and cold), overheating or chilling, lack of feed or water, change of feed or method, deworming, noise

**Body weight:** May be very important. A suitable spring balance and a loop of string may be used to do a flock sample weighing.

For postmortem examination, and for materials to be sent to the laboratory for disease diagnosis, refer to Chapter 14 and 15, respectively.

## Investigation of drop in egg production, quality, growth, body weight or feed conversion

Investigation involves enquiry into a potential (latent) disease, or a management or a nutrition fault. A detailed history is required along with a site investigation, as discussed earlier in this chapter.

## Drop in Egg Production - General

The investigator must have knowledge of disease and conditions that lead to production drop, and also of the management of layer flocks.

**Short falls** in production up to 6-8% may occur from quite small reasons, such as a reduction in feed consumption for 2 or 3 days. However, return to normal may take several days. The time of egg collections in relation to lighting patterns can be important. **Drops of 20-30%, taking a week or weeks to recover, are serious.** They may cause failure to peak, reduce bird's potential, or bring about a drop at the end of production.

It may be difficult, or impossible, to find out whether a 20% egg production loss is due to all birds producing 20% less, half the flock producing 40% less, or 20% of birds going out of production.

**If there are no symptoms,** for example, this sometimes happens in egg production drops, then it is necessary to find out the birds which are not laying. This can be very difficult. However, with birds in cages, each cage without eggs can be marked, for three successive mornings using pegs. Birds can then be selected from any of the cages, with three pegs. Similarly, when birds are to be weighed, cages thought to be representative may be marked with pegs. Bird weight is usually very important in egg production problems. Weighing may be done using a spring balance.

**When associated with infectious diseases,** especially those involving the oviduct, serious drops in production may last for months, and the flock may never regain full production. Drops in production are usually accompanied by a decline in egg quality (shell and internal faults).

If disease is suspected, it is important that any laboratory investigation carried out is relevant, economically justified and meaningful. Negative findings, for example in virus isolation; or results of tests of doubtful value, may not be of much help. Also, a diagnosis based on ambiguous (unclear) findings in one small set of blood samples, may be misleading and unwise. **On the other hand, serological investigation may be very helpful, particularly if it can be done sequentially in time.**

**While considering history,** discussed earlier, **special attention should be given to:**

1. **Diseases:** Such as Ranikhet disease (RD), infectious bronchitis (IB), infectious laryngotracheitis (ILT), egg drop syndrome (EDS), avian encephalomyelitis, avian influenza (AI), *Escherichia coli*, **Mycoplasma, Haemophilus, Pasteurella, Chlamydia.**

2. **Environment:** Ventilation, temperature, wind proofing, light pattern, intensity, light

proofing.

3.   **Housing or caging:** Design, size, stocking density.

4.   **Nutritional aspects:** Feed formulation, raw material ingredients, feed and water space allowance; feed consumption; do all birds get feed?; cleanliness; changes in feed; errors in mixing (for example, sodium chloride, calcium, vitamin A, anticoccidials); interrupted or inadequate feed or water supply. Mycotoxins have serious effects, but present diagnostic difficulty.

5.   **Stress:** Management, change of manager or personnel, presence of strangers, fright due to noise, vaccination, cannibalism (pecking), debeaking.

6.   **Birds:** Genetic strain, weight at the time of laying, body weight.

7.   **Eggs:** Quality, hatchability, fertility.

## Drop in Egg Production - Caged Layers

**Broadly speaking, management plays a greater part in egg production loss, than disease.** Alternate up and down production graphs usually indicate a managemental fault. Causes are often multifactorial (involving many factors), and can be very time-consuming to investigate.

A first visit to the farm is useful in investigating management and general aspects, and also in obtaining such samples as may be initially required for laboratory examination. But one should be careful in making a diagnosis based on findings on one set of blood samples.

Before examining birds in houses, while in office, define the problem and its duration in terms of production. Also, check records of bird numbers and body weights, mortality, egg numbers, size, bird feed intakes, vaccination, and house temperature.

## Regarding the feed, consider the following:

Distribution system: Uneven troughs; 'caked' feed, stale feed, mould growth; flow (e.g. feathers blocking the channel)

Inadequate feed

Timing, irregular feeding

Feed runs missed by staff (e.g. at the end of day), long feed runs

Over-restriction, inadequate calcium or phosphorus

Inadequate protein

Poor formulation, poor raw materials, poor mixing

## Regarding water, consider:

Temperature (**birds do not like very cold or warm water**); consumption; quality (*E. coli*, high saline, high metal ions)

Deprivation: caged layers

Nipples leaking, damp manure, flies, ammonia. Distribution from tank, sediment, blockage or air lock towards end of run

## Regarding temperature, consider:

High temperature: inefficient fans, reduced feed intake

High humidity, ammonia

Low temperature, high feed intake? Feed available?

## Regarding light, consider:

Distribution within the house (even or varying)

Poor maintenance of equipment and fittings (for example, bulbs, dimmers)

External light leakage

Repair work in house

## Regarding ventilation, consider:

Reduced to maintain temperature?

Distribution in house

Fans not working, inlets blocked

Fail-safe (foolproof) system, stand-by generator?

## Regarding pests and vermin, consider:

Rats and mice cause nervousness, consume and spoil feed, damage house and equipment, damage insulation (causing fires), contaminate eggs and may bite hens on nests.

Red mites etc. cause irritation to birds and staff, and 2-3% production loss.

Flies and moths cause irritation to birds and staff, and 2-3% production loss. Staff are reluctant to spend time in houses.

## Regarding management, consider:

Changes in daily routine, timing, excitement, different staff

Sudden noise, disturbance: trucks, lorries, dogs (white birds are more nervous and susceptible to stress), aircrafts or aeroplanes, drills

Basic feed, water and egg collection management: well-supervised?

Mechanical systems, inefficiency or breakdown: egg breaking; manure build-up

Regarding systems, timing must be similar from day to day (so also the egg collection times)

Manipulation of records

Does staff really know what to do?

Theft of eggs?

## Factors affecting egg quality

**Egg size – general:** Lighting patterns in rearing; lighting patterns in lay; nutrition, nutrient intake, linoleic acid, protein, amino acids; disease; water supply; moulting; house temperature (**heat stress reduces egg size**)

**Egg size – small:** Flock early in lay; inadequate nutrient intake, inadequate protein (methionine), energy, fatty acids (linoleic) in feed, inadequate water; high temperature; disease (Gumboro)

**Egg weight:** Storage temperature and humidity

**Shell weight:** Remains fairly constant as hen ages but egg weight increases, that is, decreased shell quality.

**Shell strength:** Nutrients that influence shell strength include calcium, phosphorus, magnesium, zinc, manganese, chlorine, potassium and vitamins; disease, especially respiratory system diseases.

**Shell quality:** High house temperatures; excess salinity (or other mineral salts) in water (e.g. from borehole); older flocks; collisions between eggs; damage by bird's feet; time of day egg laid (early in day larger eggs, weaker shells); disease.

The shell may show the following changes:

1. **Soft shell, shell-less:** Birds coming into lay; disease (Ranikhet disease, infectious bronchitis, egg drop syndrome); sulpha drugs.

2. **Misshapen (badly formed):** Genetic; disease (Ranikhet disease, infectious bronchitis); older birds higher incidence (inadequate oviduct muscle tone, insufficient protein in thick albumen); coming into lay.

3. **Thin, porous, or soft:** Mean thickness should be about 330 μm in chicken (measure by micrometer); nutrition, calcium or phosphorus deficiency or imbalance, zinc, manganese or vitamin D3 deficiency, separation of feed ingredients, feed intake inadequate; disease (Ranikhet disease, infectious bronchitis, egg drop syndrome);

excessive temperature; older birds; disturbance at night; sulpha drugs and other antimicrobials.

4.  **Rough:** Genetic; disease (Ranikhet disease, infectious bronchitis); sulpha drugs; excessive antibiotic; excessive calcium; young birds coming into lay; older birds (loss of oviduct muscle tone); stress (adrenaline release).

5.  **Mottled (i.e. marked with coloured spots/patches):** Genetic; humidity extremes; cage marks on freshly laid eggs.

6.  **Yellow:** High tetracycline level in feed.

7.  **Cracked:** High house temperature; high stocking density; cage design (cage floor, slope); collection method, handling staff; shell thickness or strength or weight per unit area.

8.  **Loss of colour:** Genetic; disease (Ranikhet disease, infectious bronchitis, egg drop syndrome); sulpha drugs; piperazine; high temperature, high production.

**The yolk and white of the egg may show the following changes:**

1.  **'Blood' spots:** Genetic; cold environment; marked temperature change; continuous light; older birds; low vitamin K level (especially with sulphaquinoxaline), low vitamin A level, following avian encephalomyelitis (for one month); mycotoxins; disease (Ranikhet disease, infectious bronchitis).

2.  **Abnormal yolk colour:** Pigment levels in feed (carotenoids, i.e. vitamin A/ xanthophylls); oxidative breakdown of natural and/or synthetic carotenoids.

3.  **Decreased yolk colour (with normal carotenoid levels in feed):** Flock disease; low feed consumption; intestinal parasites; mycotoxins (aflatoxin, ochratoxin, T-2); oxidative breakdown of natural or synthetic carotenoids.

4.  **Mottled or flecked (spotted) yolk:** (A very limited amount of mottling is normal). Causes include excessive dietary pigment, improper pigment ratios, poor mixing, oxidative breakdown of natural and/or synthetic carotenoids; excessive chilling; high storage temperature (yolks mottled, flaccid and fragile); genetic; ammonia; piperazine; phenothiazine.

5.  **Yolk taint (acquired before egg is laid):** Anticoccidial robenidine; unsaturated fatty acids (fish oils); moulds.

6.  **Yolk and albumen taint (acquired after egg is laid):** Unsuitable detergents; storage near strong odours, that is, as the egg cools and respires.

7.  **Watery white (when the albumen loses its viscosity, it is called 'watery white'):** Causes include genetic; disease (Ranikhet disease, infectious bronchitis); warm storage, prolonged storage in inadequate temperature; older birds; ammonia;

low protein in ration (also affects production and size). (Note: the thin white of a newly laid egg is watery, but the thick white is firm).

## Conclusion

To conclude, it can be easily seen that investigation of diseases, or other problems involving sickness and deaths, or drop in egg production, quality, growth, body weight, or feed conversion, requires **a three way approach.**

1.  **History**

2.  **Postmortem examination**, and

3.  **Laboratory investigations**

The history has already been dealt with in this chapter. The next chapter therefore discusses **postmortem examination** as a tool of disease diagnosis.

Chapter **14**

# Postmortem Examination

**P**ostmortem examination of poultry is essential to determine the cause of **death.** That is, to arrive at a correct diagnosis so that disease outbreaks, if any, can be effectively controlled. Postmortem examination is one of the most valuable diagnostic techniques available. However, before carrying out postmortem, the first most important aspect of diagnosis is the **compilation of a good history**, as discussed in the previous chapter. **Postmortem examination should be carried out as early as possible** because once putrefaction sets in, then it becomes difficult to identify the tissue changes (lesions) and isolate the organisms responsible for the disease.

## Selection of Birds

Selection of birds is very important. This is because a wrong conclusion of a situation may be arrived at from postmortem carried out on improperly selected birds, especially if the flock is not seen. Sometimes farm managers tend to pick out a few of the worst birds they can find, which may not be typical of the existing problem. Therefore, a few each of the dead, live ailing birds showing symptoms of a disease, and sometimes apparently normal birds may be examined to obtain a true picture.

## Killing of Birds

Several methods can be used to kill the birds. Each has certain advantages. **The objective is to kill the bird at once so that it does not suffer in the process.** Following are the commonly used methods.

### 1. Cervical Dislocation

Also known as **'breaking the neck'**, this is the quickest way to kill a small bird **(Fig. 26.** It is also considered to be a humane method of killing. That is, it causes as little pain as possible.

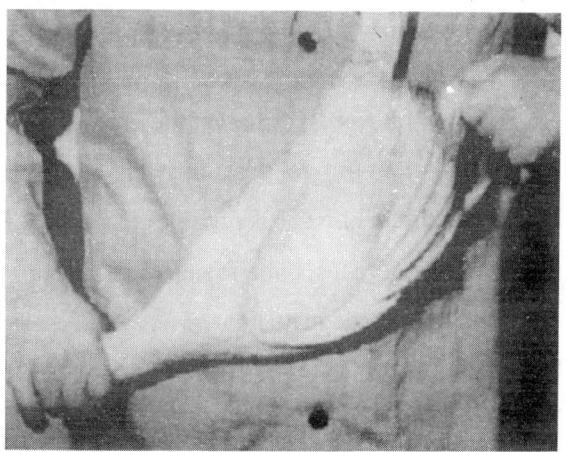

**Fig. 26.** Breaking the neck of a chicken (cervical dislocation)

The left hand holds the legs, while the right hand grasps the head with the palm. The head is then bent vertically upwards by the thumb under the beak, while at the same time the head is pulled firmly and steadily forward, stretching the neck, dislocating the skull from the neck and breaking the cord. Stretching must stop as separation is felt, otherwise the head will be pulled off the body. There will be violent reflex movement of the limbs for a while, during which time the base of the wings should be held firmly.

In very young birds, the neck can be broken easily by pressing it firmly with the thumb against a sharp table edge, or by pinching between thumb and index finger, or by placing the neck between the two shafts of the handle of a large pair of scissors which are then fully closed together.

## 2.  Inhalation Euthanasia

**Euthanasia is the act of killing painlessly.** For some conditions, cervical dislocation may not be the most useful means of destruction. **Chloroform inhalation** is then preferred.

**Birds are very susceptible to chloroform.** Chloroform can conveniently be placed on a thick cotton wool pad at the bottom of a narrow jar. The bird's head is then placed in the mouth of the jar. Care should be taken to allow air to enter the jar. That is, the bird is anaesthetized and not suffocated. Death soon follows anaesthesia.

## 3.  Injection Euthanasia

Pentobarbitone solution, or some other suitable anaesthetic agent, may be injected intravenously (i.e. within a vein - a blood vessel), or by the intracardiac (within the heart), intrathoracic (within the thoracic cavity), or intraperitoneal (within the body cavity) routes.

## Requirements for Postmortem Examination

1.  Disinfectant (dettol, savlon), or detergent solution in which to dip the entire bird (except the head), or to wet the body to control dust and feathers.

2.  Postmortem tray for easy, efficient clean-up.

3.  Postmortem gloves (disposable).

4.  Scissors, forceps, bone forceps and scalpels of different sizes.

5.  A table and adequate light.

6.  Balances for weighing.

7.  History sheets for recording results.

8.  Microscope, slides, swabs, containers, blood tubes, self-seal plastic bags, labels, felt pens, fixative, plastic waste bags, etc.

## Postmortem Technique

When birds are submitted live, note for any symptoms or behavioural abnormality. In addition, blood samples may be taken before killing. Body weights should be recorded, if necessary.

The dead bird is placed on its back and examined for any physical deformity, external parasites, discharges from nostrils and eyes, paleness of comb and wattles, dehydration, emaciation, etc.

The carcass should then be dipped in clean water having some 'dettol' or 'savalon', and kept on the postmortem table on its back. The angle of the jaw is cut through. With the blunt point of scissors inside the oesophagus, the cut is continued down the neck. This will expose the pharynx, oesophagus, and inside of the crop for examination. The trachea is cut down its length from the larynx and examined.

Each leg, in turn, is drawn outward away from the body, and the skin is cut between the leg and abdomen. Each leg is then held firmly in the area of the femur and pulled and twisted so that head of the femur is broken free from the hip attachment and the leg comes to lie flat on the table.

Then skin from the vent to the beak is cut. The cut edge is then forcibly reflected forward, cutting as necessary, until the entire vertical aspect of the body, including the neck, is exposed. Haemorrhages in the muscles, if present, can be detected at this stage.

**The next step is to expose the organs.** Strong scissors are used to cut through the abdominal walls transversely midway between keel and vent and then through breast muscles on each side. Bone scissors are used to cut the rib cage and then the coracoid and clavicle bones on both sides. With some care, this can be done without cutting the large blood vessels. The sternum and attached structures can now be removed from the body and placed on one side. The organs are now in full view and may be removed as they are examined. Lungs, airsacs, etc. should be examined in position. **At this stage of postmortem, microbiological samples are collected.**

The intestines are freed by cutting through the oesophagus and blood vessels of the liver just anterior to the proventriculus and liver. The intestines can be removed by gentle traction which breaks mesenteric and airsac attachments. The lungs, heart, and kidneys remain in the body cavity for later examination.

The tracheal cut previously made may now be extended left and right along the bronchi. This will show the inside of these passages for examination. After removal of the intestines, ovary and oviduct should be observed as also the organs beneath, such as kidneys.

The sciatic plexus beneath the kidney should be examined by removal of kidney tissue by blunt dissection. The bronchial plexus should be examined on either side near the thoracic inlet.

The softness or hardness of the ribs should be noted during cutting, and the degree of bend and snap (sound of breaking) in the bones should be assessed. **The nasal cavities and sinuses may be examined for the presence of exudate (inflammatory discharge)** by cutting through the upper beak at the appropriate level with sharp scissors.

The brain may be examined and removed for histopathological examination. After separating the head, reflect the skin over the skull and upper mandible. The skull may then be carefully cut in the midline with a sharp, firm scalpel and then transversely likewise. The four quarters may be reflected outwards from the middle by firmly holding with suitable forceps, **exposing the entire brain** which may then be removed with small scissors, cutting the nerve attachments carefully.

## Laboratory Examinations

## Impression Smears

If the above procedure has been carried out aseptically and the intestine is not cut, the internal organs will not be contaminated. Therefore, impression smears may be taken in the usual manner.

## Bacterial Cultures

If gross lesions indicate that bacterial cultures are needed, they can be made from unexposed surfaces of the organs without searing the surface. **If contamination has occurred, the surface of the organs should be seared (burnt) with a hot spatula before inserting a sterile culture loop.** Care must be taken not to sear and heat the tissue too much. It is better to transfer large tissue samples aseptically to a sterile Petri dish and take them to the microbiology laboratory for culture in cleaner surroundings.

## Respiratory Virus Isolation

If a respiratory disease is suspected and virus culture is to be carried out, the trachea should not be cut as described earlier, but an intact portion be taken from the lower trachea This should be placed along with a portion of the upper lung tissue, which should be removed aseptically, into antibiotic (penicillin and streptomycin) normal saline.

## Tissues for Histopathological Examination

Tissues for histopathological examination should be taken in slices, preferably not thicker than 3-5 mm or so, and placed in 10% formol-saline in a ratio of tissue to fixative of 1:15.

## Coccidia

The outer and inner surface of the intestine should be examined throughout its length for the presence of characteristic lesions of the various coccidial species in the freshly killed bird. Wet mount smears of mucosal scrapings from various segments of the intestine may be examined for the presence of oocysts and schizonts (see **'diagnosis of coccidiosis'**).

## Conclusion

**To conclude,** postmortem examination forms only one part of disease diagnosis. Laboratory examination is essential where examination of history and postmortem is not of sufficient help. The next chapter therefore discusses what materials should be sent to the laboratory for disease diagnosis.

## Note:

1.  The postmortem procedures described in this chapter should be taken only as guidelines, as there are several variations of the technique.

2.  Also when different organs and tissues are examined, always refer side by side to Chapter 17 **"Disease diagnosis on the basis of postmortem findings"** for an interpretation of the abnormal changes to arrive at correct diagnosis.

# Chapter 15

# Materials to be Sent to the Laboratory for Disease Diagnosis

**L**aboratory investigation is necessary in those cases where history and postmortem reports are of not much help in arriving at a diagnosis. It then becomes necessary to take help of the diagnostic laboratory. This chapter discusses what materials should be sent to the laboratory for disease diagnosis.

Having opened the carcass, the general appearance of organs and the presence of gross lesions (changes) should be noted. It is possible that at this stage a tentative (presumptive) diagnosis may be reached. Further detailed examination and tests may be undertaken to confirm the tentative diagnosis. The materials indicated against each disease should be sent to the laboratory to confirm diagnosis of that disease.

## (A) Viral Diseases

### Ranikhet Disease (Newcastle Disease)

(i)   Serum samples for serological tests (antibody detection).

(ii)  Intestine, intestinal contents and trachea, along with proventriculus and brain, for isolation and identification of the virus. Send samples in phosphate-buffered isotonic saline, containing antibiotics, or in 50% glycerine and saline.

### Gumboro Disease (Infectious Bursal Disease)

(i)   Bursa and spleen for isolation and identification of the virus in antibiotic-treated saline. However, bursa is the most commonly used.

(ii)  Macerated bursa and serum samples for serological tests.

(iii) Bursa and kidneys in 10% formalin for microscopic examination of tissue sections.

### Infectious Bronchitis

(i)   Trachea, lungs, airsacs, caecal tonsils, kidneys and oviduct in 50% glycerine saline for virus isolation and identification (only in the early stages of disease).

(ii)  Serum samples for serological tests.

332

## Infectious Laryngotracheitis

(i) Tracheal exudate to demonstrate the presence of virus by various methods, such as serological tests, examination of intranuclear inclusions, electron microscopy, inoculation into developing chick embryo and cell culture, and examination with DNA probes.

(ii) Trachea in 10% formalin for examination of intranuclear inclusion bodies.

(iii) Serum samples for serological tests.

## Fowl Pox

(i) Pieces from skin and other tissue lesions in 10% formalin for examination of intracytoplasmic eosinophilic inclusion bodies.

(ii) Smears prepared from lesions for detection of inclusion bodies.

(iii) Lesions of fowl pox in 50% glycerine saline for detection and identification of virus.

(iv) Serum samples for serological tests.

## Marek's Disease

(i) Nerve lesions (from sciatic and brachial nerve) and lymphoid tumours (from liver, spleen, ovary, lungs, kidney, proventriculus, heart) in 10% formalin for microscopic examination.

(ii) Feather tips in 50% glycerine saline for isolation and identification of the virus.

(iii) Serum samples for serological tests.

## Lymphoid Leukosis

(i) Pieces of liver, spleen, bursa, thymus, bone marrow, gonads (ovary, testes), sciatic and brachial nerves and any other tumour tissue in 10% formalin for microscopic examination.

(ii) Impression smears of fresh tumour tissue for cytological examination.

(iii) Tumour tissue, liver, serum and plasma for isolation and identification of the virus.

(iv) Serum or plasma for serological tests.

## Avian Encephalomyelitis

(i) Brain in 50% glycerine saline for isolation and identification of the virus.

(ii) Smears from the brain, or cryostat sections, for demonstration of the virus.

(iii) Serum samples for serological tests.

(iv) Brain, proventriculus and pancreas in 10% formalin for microscopic examination.

## Egg Drop Syndrome

(i) Affected eggs for isolation and identification of the virus.

(ii) Serum samples for serological tests.

## Avian Influenza

(i) Tracheal or cloacal swabs; faeces or intestinal contents and trachea for isolation and identification of the virus.

(ii) Serum samples for serological tests.

## Inclusion Body Hepatitis

(i) Liver in 50% glycerine saline, or a faeces suspension for isolation and identification of the virus.

(ii) Pieces of liver in 10% formalin for microscopic examination of intranuclear inclusion bodies.

(iii) Serum samples for serological tests.

## Leechi Disease

(i) Pieces of liver in 10% formalin for demonstration of intranuclear inclusion bodies.

(ii) Pieces of liver in 50% glycerine saline for isolation and identification of adenovirus.

## Reoviruses (viral arthritis, cloacal pasting, stunting syndrome)

(i) Faeces and spleen in 50% glycerine saline for isolation and identification of the virus. If arthritis is present, also include synovial fluid and synoviae from the tendon sheaths.

(ii) Serum samples for serological tests.

## Chicken Infectious Anaemia

(i) Serum samples for serological tests.

(ii) Liver impression smears and cryostat sections, fixed with acetone, for detection of antibodies.

(iii) Formalin-fixed, paraffin-embedded sections for detection of antibodies.

(iv) Thymus, bone marrow and liver from affected chicks in 50% glycerine saline for isolation and identification of the virus. **However, virus isolation is not recommended because it is a slow and expensive method.**

## Reticuloendotheliosis

(i)   Affected tissues (lymphoma), whole blood or plasma from affected birds for virus isolation and identification.

(ii)  Serum samples for serological tests.

## Avian Nephritis

(i)   Suspension of either the kidneys or the rectal contents for isolation and identification of the virus.

(ii)  Serum samples from recovered birds for serological tests.

## (B) Bacterial Diseases

## Colibacillosis

Heart, liver, and lungs for isolation and identification of the causative organism, *Escherichia coli.*

## Infectious Coryza

(i)   Swabs from infraorbital sinus, trachea and airsac from acutely diseased chicken for isolation and identification of the causative organism *Haemophilus paragallinarum.*

(ii)  Serum samples for serological tests.

## Salmonellosis

(i)   Liver, gallbladder, or yolk sac for isolation and identification of salmonellae from chicks dying of septicaemia. **In older birds, caeca is the most likely site for isolation.**

(ii)  Serum samples for serological tests.

## Fowl Cholera

(i)   Impression smears from the liver and lungs, or smears of the heart blood for demonstration of the causative organism *Pasteurella multocida.*

(ii)  Liver, bone marrow, heart blood for isolation and identification of the organism.

## Fowl Typhoid

(i)   Liver, spleen and caeca for isolation of the causative organism *Salmonella gallinarum.*

(ii)  Whole blood and serum for serological tests.

## Pullorum Disease

(i)   Liver, spleen and caeca for isolation of the causative organism *Salmonella pullorum.*

(ii)  Whole blood and serum for serological tests.

## Necrotic Enteritis

Intestinal contents, scrapings of intestinal wall, or haemorrhagic lymphoid nodules for isolation and identification of the causative organism *Clostridium perfringens.*

## Ulcerative Enteritis

Liver or spleen for isolation and identification of the causative organism, *Clostridium colinum.* The organism is present in the liver in pure form, rather than in the intestine.

## Gangrenous Dermatitis

Exudates of skin and subcutaneous tissue, or underlying muscle, for isolation and identification of the causative organisms, *Staphylococcus aureus* and *Clostridium perfringens.* However, isolation can be misleading since both the organisms are present on the skin of normal chickens.

## Staphylococcosis

Suspected clinical material, such as exudate from joints, yolk, and swabs from internal organs for isolation and identification of causative organism, *Staphylococcus aureus.*

## Streptococcosis

(i)   Blood smears or impression smears from liver, spleen, affected heart valves, or lesions from sick birds for demonstration of the causative organisms streptococci. However, this will provide only a presumptive diagnosis.

(ii)  To confirm diagnosis, isolation of streptococci from typical lesions is needed. This should be attempted without any faecal contamination, as these organisms are found in the faeces of normal poultry.

## Tuberculosis

(i)   Crushed lesions (from liver, spleen, or other organs) for demonstration of acid-fast tubercle bacilli for presumptive diagnosis. Even smears from infected liver and spleen are very helpful in diagnosis.

(ii)  Young lesions and bone marrow for isolation and identification of the causative organism *Mycobacterium avium.*

(iii) Whole blood for serological tests (rapid agglutination test and ELISA).

## Campylobacteriosis

(i) Caecal contents, even cloacal swabs or fresh faecal samples, for isolation and identification of the causative organisms **'campylobacters'**.

(ii) With systemic infection, the organism can also be recovered from liver, bile, and blood.

## (C) Mycoplasmal Diseases

## Mycoplasmosis

### *Mycoplasma gallisepticum* Infection (Chronic respiratory disease, CRD)

(i) Swabs from nasal cavity, airsacs, trachea and lungs as well as exudate aspirated from the infraorbital sinus and joints for isolation and identification of *Mycoplasma gallisepticum.*

(ii) Serum samples for serological tests.

### *Mycoplasma synoviae* Infection

(i) Trachea, lungs, airsacs and joint lesions for isolation and identification of *Mycoplasma synoviae.*

(ii) Serum samples for serological tests.

## (D) Fungal Diseases

## Aspergillosis (Brooder pneumonia)

(i) Smears from lesions (white caseous nodules in the lungs or airsacs) for demonstration of branched, septate **Aspergillus** hyphae.

(ii) Lesions (granulomas or plaques in the lung or airsacs) for cultural isolation and identification of the causative fungus.

## Candidiasis (Crop Mycosis, Thrush)

(i) Pieces of crop and oesophagus in 10% formalin for microscopic demonstration of the causative fungus *Candida albicans* in tissue sections.

(ii) Crop and oesophagus for cultural isolation and identification of *Candida albicans.*

## Mycotoxicosis

Samples (500g) of suspected feed, feed ingredients and mouldy clumps (compact masses) should be collected and submitted in separate containers for chemical analysis and screening of aflatoxin, ochratoxin, T-2, DON, and fumonisin. Isolation, identification, and quantification are done by various analytical chemical methods, as well as by feeding trials. Samples should be promptly submitted to a feed testing laboratory for analysis.

Mycotoxin formation may not be uniform, in a batch of feed or grain, and **multiple samples from different sites increase the chance of confirming a mycotoxin.** Samples should be collected and submitted in separate containers. Clean paper bags or polythene bags, properly labelled, are adequate.

## How to take a feed sample

While taking a sample of any kind of feedstuff for laboratory analysis, it is essential that samples are taken in a correct manner so that the sample used is truly representative of the feedstuff. **Failure to make this makes laboratory analysis meaningless.** Also, results could be misleading if unrepresentative samples are taken.

Samples should not be taken from feed troughs.

**The principle of taking a feed sample is that from the bulk at least four samples are taken from different places by a mug or a large cup, or by a grain probe if from a bag. These samples are then pooled to form an aggregate (combined) sample, from which the final sample (at least 500g or 1 lb) is taken for analysis.**

## (E) Chlamydial Disease

## Chlamydiosis

(i)   Impression smears from the surface of the liver or spleen; and cloacal, tracheal or conjuctival swabs for demonstration of the causative organism *Chlamydophila psittaci.*

(ii)  For isolation and identification of chlamydia, pieces of liver or spleen, exudate or faeces in a diluent containing antibiotics which reduce contaminants but have no adverse effect on chlamydia.

(iii) Serum samples for serological tests.

# Chapter 16

# Disease Diagnosis on the Basis of Symptoms

S ome diseases show certain characteristic symptoms. These are most helpful in arriving at an almost correct diagnosis. **This is particularly helpful in respect of nutritional diseases which show minimal gross changes.** A few typical symptoms that characterize certain diseases are presented below.

| **Symptoms** | **Disease** |
|---|---|
| 1. Paralysis of the legs and wings in birds 6 weeks or older. | Marek's disease |
| 2. Sudden deaths without any clinical signs, accompanied by marked bluish discoloration of comb, wattles, shanks (portion between hock joint and foot) and toes; severe head swelling; and eye discharges | Suggestive of avian influenza (bird flu) |
| 3. Swollen abdomen and congestion of abdominal skin. | Ascites |
| 4. Blood in droppings. | Coccidiosis |
| 5. Nasal discharge, facial oedema, conjunctivitis, and open-mouth breathing. | Infectious coryza |
| 6. Paralysis in laying hens in cages. The birds are unable to stand. | Cage layer fatigue |
| 7. Stunting and retarded development. | Infectious stunting syndrome Lysine deficiency |
| 8. Curled-toe paralysis. | Riboflavin deficiency |
| 9. Head swelling, puffy appearance of the face, and swelling around the eyes. | Swollen head syndrome |
| 10. Typical star-gazing pose. | Thiamine deficiency |

11. Thin-shelled, soft-shelled and shell-less eggs.     Egg drop syndrome

12. Thin-shelled, rough, and deformed eggs.     Infectious bronchitis

13. Healthy, fast-growing broilers dying on their back suddenly with a short, wing-beating convulsive attack.     Sudden death syndrome (Flip over)

14. Stunting, poor feathering, and short, thick, bowed legs typical of chondrodystrophy.     Choline deficiency

15. Facial oedema with haemorrhagic conjunctivitis.     Ranikhet disease

16. Falling forward with legs outstretched behind and lying paralyzed for several minutes.     Chloride deficiency

17. Difficult breathing with dried blood around nostril and along the lower beak.     Infectious laryngotracheitis

18. Stiff-legged gait and progressive lameness with a tendency to remain squatted.     Rickets

# Chapter 17

# Disease Diagnosis on the Basis of Postmortem Findings

T he symptoms in most poultry diseases tend to be similar, except in a few, and are therefore not of much diagnostic help. **On the other hand, postmortem findings (gross lesions/changes) can be very helpful, in several cases, in arriving at a correct diagnosis.** This is because such lesions are characteristic and typical of that disease (**pathognomonic lesions**), and indicate without doubt the correct cause of the disease. This is of great diagnostic value particularly under field conditions and also in a diagnostic laboratory where postmortem examination is usually the starting point of disease investigation. Also, it is most helpful in starting the treatment and controlling the disease in the face of mortality. As such, **this chapter discusses those postmortem findings that are of diagnostic importance.**

## Remember

1. Examine as many birds as possible to get a representative sample or a cross section of the lesions. This is because **lesions may differ considerably from bird to bird, even if the disease is the same.**

2. **Only fresh carcasses should be examined.** Do not examine the putrefied carcasses, because the decomposition that has set in will confuse the picture.

3. If available, birds with fully developed symptoms should be examined after sacrificing the sick ones.

4. Continue to examine the birds in cases of serious outbreaks. This is because birds dying in the early stages (e.g. in Ranikhet disease) may not show typical postmortem findings (lesions). Also, the subsequent examination gives a chance to partly evaluate the effectiveness of treatment.

The postmortem findings that follow are presented in the same order in which diseases have been described in the text under Section I.

## Typical Postmortem Findings in Various Diseases of Poultry

## (A) Viral Diseases

## Ranikhet Disease

Pinpoint haemorrhages on the tips of glands in proventriculus, haemorrhagic caecal tonsils, haemorrhagic changes in the intestinal wall, and white spots of dead tissue on the spleen.

## Gumboro Disease (Infectious Bursal Disease)

Greatly enlarged and swollen bursa, presence of cheesy mass within its lumen, small and large haemorrhages on its inner surface, and haemorrhages in the thigh and breast muscles.

## Infectious Bronchitis

Caseous plug in the lower trachea or bronchi, and airsacs. Lungs are congested and kidneys may contain urates and show gout.

## Infectious Laryngotracheitis

Trachea is inflamed red and contains blood. It may also contain cheesy inflammatory material.

## Fowl Pox

**Skin Form:** Severe fowl pox lesions on the comb and wattle.

**Diphtheritic Form:** Small white nodules or cheesy plaques in larynx and trachea.

## Avian Influenza (Bird Flu)

Marked bluish discoloration of comb, wattles, shanks (portion between hock joint and foot) and toes; severe head swelling and eye discharges; small haemorrhages on the heart and bigger haemorrhages in the muscles; severely congested trachea and lungs; and haemorrhages in the proventriculus. **All these changes are highly suggestive of avian influenza, but not confirmatory.**

## Marek's Disease

**Classical Form:** Marked enlargement of one or more nerves, mainly sciatic and brachial plexus.

**Acute Form:** Tumorous enlargement of the liver, spleen, kidneys, gonads (ovary, testes), proventriculus and heart.

## Lymphoid Leukosis

Greatly enlarged liver. Spleen, bursa of Fabricius, kidneys and ovaries are also usually enlarged due to formation of tumours.

## Avian Encephalomyelitis

No gross changes in the young or older birds.

## Avian Nephritis

Visceral gout

## Egg Drop Syndrome

Inactive ovaries and a decrease in the size of oviducts.

## Chicken Infectious Anaemia

Reduction in the size of thymus and bursa of Fabricius. Change of bone marrow from red colour to yellow or white colour.

## Inclusion Body Hepatitis

Liver pale, friable and swollen. Small and large haemorrhages in the liver and skeletal muscles.

## Leechi Disease

Presence of up to 10 ml of clear fluid in the pericardial sac (i.e. under the covering of heart.) Heart looks like a **peeled 'leechi' fruit.**

## (B) Bacterial Diseases

## Colibacillosis

Heart, liver, and airsacs covered by a layer of white inflammatory material.

## Infectious Coryza

Swelling of the face. Presence of mucus or pus with fibrin in nasal passages and infraorbital sinus.

## Necrotic Enteritis

Small intestine is greatly thickened and shows a loose to tightly attached yellow or green layer that is deeply cracked.

## Gangrenous Dermatitis

Affected area is very dark and moist. The underlying muscle is discoloured and oedematous. The tissue is dead and tends to slough.

## Ulcerative Enteritis

Severe haemorrhagic enteritis (inflammation of intestine). Ulceration in the caeca.

## Pullorum Disease

**In chicks:** Inflamed, unabsorbed yolk sac. Lungs congested and liver is dark. Foci of dead tissue found in the liver, lungs, and heart.

**In adult birds:** Ova are irregular, cystic, deformed, discoloured, and pedunculated.

## Fowl Typhoid

Liver swollen, friable, and dark red. Its surface has a characteristic coppery bronze shine.

## Salmonellosis

Lungs, liver, spleen, and kidneys swollen and congested. Unabsorbed yolk. White areas of dead tissue in the lungs, liver, and heart.

## Fowl Cholera

Pinpoint foci of dead tissue in liver. Liver is also enlarged and may show haemorrhages.

## Tuberculosis

Irregular, greyish yellow nodules in liver, spleen, intestine and bone marrow.

## (C) Mycoplasmal Diseases

### *Mycoplasma gallisepticum* Infection

Cheese-like inflammatory material in airsacs and some degree of pneumonia (inflammation of the lungs).

### *Mycoplasma synovie* Infection

Accumulation of fluid and thickening of the tissues surrounding joints.

## (D) Fungal Diseases

## Aspergillosis (Brooder pneumonia)

Nodules in the nasal passage, trachea, and airsac. Older nodules are green to black. Lungs may be greyish yellow with cheese-like inflammatory material.

## Thrush

Layer of white cheesy material in the crop.

## Aflatoxicosis

Enlargement of the liver, kidney, and spleen. Liver is greatly enlarged, is yellow and friable with small haemorrhages. Also, there is **'bloody thigh syndrome'.**

## (E) Helminthic Diseases

## Tapeworm Infection

Larger tapeworms may completely block the intestine.

## Ascaridia Infection

In severe infection, intestinal blockage can occur.

## (F) Protozoal Diseases

## Coccidiosis

**Caecal Coccidiosis:** Caeca greatly enlarged and distended with clotted blood.

**Intestinal Coccidiosis:** Middle portion of the small intestine distended to twice its normal size (ballooning) and the lumen is filled with blood.

## (G) Metabolic Diseases

## Gout

**Visceral Gout:** Kidney, heart, proventriculus and lungs show urate deposition. The deposits on the surface of the organs appear as white chalky coating.

**Articular Gout:** When joints are opened, tissues surrounding the joints are white due to urate deposition.

## Ascites

Presence of a large amount of fluid in the abdominal cavity. Heart is markedly enlarged. There is also accumulation of fluid under the covering of the heart. Liver is swollen and congested. Lungs are extremely congested and oedematous.

## Rickets

Bones are soft and rubbery. Keel bones are curved, ribs are 'beaded', and legs are bowed.

## Fatty Liver and Kidney Syndrome

Liver and kidneys are enlarged, pale, and fatty.

## Fatty Liver-Haemorrhagic Syndrome

Pools of blood, or large blood clots, in the abdomen. Liver is enlarged, fatty, very friable, and is of light greyish brown to yellow colour.

## Cage Layer Fatigue

Bones are easily broken. Fractures may be found in leg and wing bones, and in the thoracic spine. Sternum is often deformed.

## (H) Miscellaneous Diseases/Conditions

## Heat Stress

Carcass markedly dehydrated and congested. Breast muscles present a pale to white **'cooked meat appearance'**.

## Smothering

Congestion of trachea and lungs.

## Swollen Head Syndrome

Puffiness of the skin over the head.

## Egg-Bound Condition

Egg is found lodged in the cloaca.

## Egg Peritonitis

Scattered pieces of yolk, thickened yolk, cheesy semi-solid material, or milky fluid in the abdominal cavity. The cheesy mass gives a very offensive smell.

## Bumble Foot

Abscess in the foot pad.

# Section III

# DISEASE TREATMENT / PREVENTION

# Chapter **18**

# Introduction

After diagnosis, the next step is effective treatment of diseases. Actually, outbreaks of diseases indicate failures of management, nutrition, biosecurity, cleaning and disinfection, or vaccination programmes. Protective measures effectively control the disease but when they fail, medicines should be used to treat the disease and return the flock to its normal condition. **However, medicines should never be applied alone without correcting the management failures that caused the outbreak.**

Proper use of medicines can stop mortality and reduce the financial loss. Conversely, improper use of medicines can be costly, ineffective, and sometimes harmful. Therefore, no drug should be given until a diagnosis is obtained, or a veterinarian consulted. If a wrong drug is given, it may not only be a waste of money but can even be disastrous.

In most cases, administration in the drinking water is the best method of giving medicines. **This is because during a disease outbreak, birds may not eat but they still drink.** To be effective, a drug must reach the site of infection at curative level and must remain at that level for several days. Therefore, it is extremely important that doses and their schedules recommended by the manufacturers are followed carefully.

**Antibiotics are of no value against infections caused by viruses** (see 'viral diseases'). However, they are sometimes given in viral diseases to prevent secondary infection with bacterial agents like *Escherichia coli.* **Sulphonamides can be quite toxic for chickens and should be used with extreme caution,** and only under the guidance of a poultry veterinarian.

**When antibiotics are used over a long period, bacteria can become resistant, making antibiotics ineffective.** For this reason, antibiotics should be used only after diagnosis of the disease has been made. In recent years, an increasing number of bacteria have become resistant to several antibiotics. **A sensitivity test using bacteria isolated from the disease will determine which antibiotic should be used for maximum effectiveness.**

**To help the farmers,** the first chapter of this section presents the commercial medicines and vaccines currently available in the market for treating and controlling the poultry diseases. In addition, there are eight other chapters which deal with drugs/ chemicals that help either in the treatment, or in the prevention of diseases.

# Chapter 19

# Medicines and Vaccines

his chapter deals with commercial medicines and vaccines currently available in the market, along with their trade names, names of the manufacturers, indications and dosage.

All attempts have been made while compiling the list to make it as thorough as possible. However, despite the exhaustive search, it is by no means thorough or all-inclusive. This is because literature on some products was not available or accessible, mainly because the manufacturers of such products did not appear to trade in this region. It is advised that manufacturers whose products are not listed may bring them to the knowledge of the author, so that they could be included in the next edition of the book.

**The chapter is divided into two parts: (a) Medicines, and (b) Vaccines.** For easy reference, various categories of **medicines and vaccines have been listed alphabetically.** Also, all categories of medicines and vaccines can be readily traced from the index. Under medicines, the preparations to be given in drinking water are mentioned first, followed by premixes to be given in the feed. Regarding vaccines, live vaccines have been described first and then the killed vaccines.

**The various categories under which the medicines have been listed are:**

**The various categories under which vaccines have been listed are:**

**For the sake of convenience, the list of medicines and vaccines is presented at the end, on page 547.**

# Chapter 20

# Antibiotic Growth Promoters

## First, what is an antibiotic?

**An antibiotic is a substance that kills or stops the growth of bacteria.** There are hundreds of naturally occurring antibiotics, but only a few are useful in treating conditions in poultry.

Antibiotics are used to control bacterial diseases in chickens. They prevent bacterial growth, provided they are used at recommended levels and the organism is not resistant. **Antibiotics are of no use in diseases caused by viruses.** However, antibiotics are sometimes given in viral disease outbreaks to prevent secondary infection with bacterial agents like *Escherichia coli.*

## What are antibiotic growth promoters?

Also known as **'growth promotants'**, these substances, as the name indicates, are antibiotics that are used in feed continuously at a low level to improve growth and feed conversion. This supplementation is not to be confused with the therapeutic (curative) uses of antibiotics in which high levels are given to treat a specific disease problem. Therefore, **feed levels of antibiotic growth promoters should be those recommended by the manufacturer.** However, development of resistance by bacteria has been associated with their use and therefore this practice is not permitted in many countries.

## What are the benefits of using antibiotic growth promoters?

They improve bird's performance, health status, uniformity, and production efficiency.

## How do they work?

Antibiotic growth promoters (AGPs) act by modifying the intestinal microflora (bacterial population). On the basis of Gram's staining, bacteria are divided into two groups: **Gram-positive** and **Gram-negative**. Most AGPs act against Gram-positive organisms, which are associated with poorer health and performance of the bird.

Recent work has revealed that use of AGPs in germ-free birds has no benefit on the performance. This clearly indicates that their effect is due to antimicrobial (antibacterial) activity, rather than due to any direct interaction with the physiology of the bird.

## How do intestinal microflora (bacterial population) reduce bird's efficiency?

**They achieve this through the following mechanisms.**

1.  By competing with the host for nutrients in the intestinal tract. The bacteria use a significant amount of energy of the diet. This energy is then not available for the bird.

2.  In some circumstances, bacteria produce an immune response that causes appetite depression, and also breakdown of muscle protein to continue this response.

3.  By producing diseases, particularly **necrotic enteritis.**

4.  By reducing digestive efficiency of the bird, by destroying the digestive enzymes and reducing the absorptive surface area.

5.  By increasing the size of the intestinal tract through the production of certain compounds that stimulate its size, such as polyamines (i.e. compounds having more than one amino group, NH2) and volatile fatty acids. The net result is an increase in the energy required to maintain the intestine, thereby leaving less energy available for productive processes, such as muscle growth.

## Under what environmental conditions do AGPs provide best results?

The negative effects of the intestinal bacteria, outlined above, indicate that the best results depend on the microbial loading of the small intestine. For example, as already indicated, in germ-free birds use of AGPs in the feed has no beneficial effect on the performance of the bird. This means that the lack of a microbial challenge will limit the response to growth promoters. This challenge is made up of the background microflora present in the cage, pen, or shed, where the bird lives. The **environment** is particularly important in this context because the intestine of the chick is sterile (free from bacteria) before hatching. **The first bacteria to enter the intestinal tract are not at all challenged by others for space and nutrient. As a result, if they find the intestinal environment suitable, they rapidly become established.**

As more and more bacteria enter the intestinal tract, competition between the species increases, **and only the fittest survive.** Bacteria which become established and successfully colonize (grow) on day one, are not able to do so several days later, because the environment in the intestine becomes increasingly unfavourable to new comers (invaders) for reasons of space, the presence of toxins and the availability of nutrients. The growth of bacterial species that come to live in the intestine therefore depends on the bacteria present in the environment of the cage, pen or shed; and the order in which the birds are exposed to such organisms. **To conclude,** environment plays the main role in the response to AGPs, and **best results are obtained under conventional (routine) conditions of poultry farming, and not under germ-free conditions.**

## What influence does diet have on the microflora and therefore on the response to antibiotic growth promoters?

From the above, it is clear that for a particular bacterial species to become established in the intestine, it must not only be present **but must also find the correct nutrition and space in which to live.** The nutrition present in the intestine ultimately comes from the diet given to the chicken. It is now known that the diet can influence the microflora, and therefore the response to antibiotic growth promoters.

**It is important to remember that diet is a source of nutrient for the microflora as much as it is for the bird.** Poultry have a very rapid process of feed processing. Because of the very low pH in the gizzard/proventriculus, **feed entering the duodenum has very few bacteria.** They are largely destroyed by the acidic environment of the gizzard and proventriculus. The various digestive enzymes, the high oxygen tension, and the presence of high concentration of antimicrobial compounds (i.e. acting against bacteria), such as bile salts in the duodenum, further restrict the bacterial growth in this portion of the small intestine. However, **after duodenum, further down in the small intestine the environment changes and becomes more favourable for the bacterial growth** because of the low oxygen tension, somewhat alkaline pH, and the lower concentrations of enzymes and bile salts.

**When digestion is at its best,** the rate of nutrient digestion and extraction from the intestine is such that there is little material left that can be digested (e.g. starch and protein) by the native microflora of the small intestine. As a result, under ideal circumstances, best digestion and best absorption of nutrients restricts the bacterial population of the small intestine. The bacterial population is therefore kept to a minimum because nutrients are not available to the bacteria. Populations in the caeca are supported only by dietary fibre (see Chapter 23 on **'Enzymes'** for information on **'dietary fibre'**).

**However, when digestion is poor** (for whatever reason), more starch and protein reach the lower part of the small intestine and the restrictions on bacterial population are then removed to some degree. Also, there is a change in the type of food available, with more starch and protein than fibre. Therefore, not only population density but also species dominates change. High viscosity diets, or diets with poorly digestible starch and/or protein, produce such reactions.

## How does the bird respond to such a challenge?

**The bird responds to such a challenge through several mechanisms. These include:**

1. There is an increase in the rate of production of digestive enzymes.

2. There is an increase in the weight of pancreas.

3. The size of the intestine increases to deal with the unabsorbed nutrients. The increase

in size is brought about by bacterial by-products, such as **polyamines**. Polyamines are known to stimulate mucosal growth and enterocyte (lining intestinal epithelial cell) turnover. In other words, **they increase size of the intestine.** Thus, the bird tries to compensate for the reduction in the rate of nutrient absorption by increasing the digestive capacity.

## How effectively is the bird able to cope with diets having poorly digestible starch and/or protein?

Unfortunately, in an attempt to increase the size of the intestine, the lining epithelial cells (enterocytes) grow and move up the villi more rapidly. Such epithelial cells are immature and are less able to absorb nutrients efficiently. This is because they have a limited range and concentration of digestive and absorptive enzymes. Moreover, the surface glycoproteins in immature cells differ greatly from those of mature cells. As a result, a totally new environment is presented to the intestinal bacteria. Due to this, a rapid change in the species of bacteria and their distribution takes place. This usually results in intestinal disorders. **Thus, a simple change in the diet can have far-reaching consequences. Antibiotic growth promoters markedly reduce the damage caused by such dietary fluctuations by directly destroying the harmful bacteria. As a result, adverse effects of dietary changes are kept to a minimum.**

## What then is the overall conclusion regarding the use of antibiotic growth promoters in poultry?

Antibiotic growth promoters have undoubtedly improved performance and health status in poultry throughout the world, and are extremely helpful.

**Note:** For a list of commercial antibiotic growth promoters available at the market, refer to Chapter 19 under **"Antibiotic growth promoters"**.

# Chapter 21

# Probiotics

## What are probiotics?

The word **'probiotic'** is derived from Greek. **'Pro'** in Greek means **'for'** and **'bios'** means **'life'**. **Thus, a 'probiotic' is a substance that promotes life, and is the exact opposite of antibiotic which acts against life.** (Greek anti=against; bios=life).

The term **'probiotic'** was first introduced in 1965 to describe growth promoting factors produced by micro-organisms. **At present a 'probiotic' means a live microbial feed supplement** (i.e. consisting of micro-organisms) that improves the microbial environment of bird's intestinal tract to its advantage. In other words, **a probiotic is not a drug, but a mixed culture of living micro-organisms which helps the bird by improving the properties of its natural intestinal microflora (i.e. micro-organisms).** Recently it has been suggested that the term **'direct-feed microbial (DCM)'** be used, rather than **'probiotic'**, since the naturally occurring micro-organisms may also include fungi and yeast, besides bacteria. However, most scientists consider probiotics to be 'selected and concentrated live counts of lactic acid bacteria (i.e. **Lactobacillus, Streptococcus**).

**In future, probiotics will come to occupy a position of great importance in poultry industry.** This is because continued use of antibiotics in poultry feeds may result in the presence of antibiotic residues (remains) in chicken products, and the development of drug-resistant bacteria for humans. For this reason, **the use of antibiotics as routine feed additives has recently been banned in Europe, and probiotics have been introduced as an alternative to antibiotics.**

## What are the benefits of feeding probiotics?

Feeding poultry with either pure lactobacilli cultures, or mixtures of lactobacilli with other bacteria, produces positive results. **In broilers,** probiotics improve live weight gain and feed conversion rate, and markedly reduce mortality. **In layers,** supplementation of probiotics improves egg production and feed conversion. There is an increase in egg size, egg mass, egg weight, and improved albumen quality, reduced yolk cholesterol concentration, and an improved body weight gain.

## How does a probiotic work?

The different mechanisms by which a probiotic works are as follows:

## 1. By maintaining useful microflora in the digestive tract

Healthy birds have a well functioning intestinal tract. This is important for the efficient conversion of feed for maintenance and for growth or production. A most important feature of a well-functioning intestinal tract is the **proper balance of its bacterial population**. Lactic acid bacteria occur throughout the digestive tract, and in some places, are the main organisms. This situation is disturbed when the bird is subjected to stressful conditions, such as high temperature and humidity, change of feed, use of antibiotics, transportation, etc. **Continuous feeding of probiotics maintains the beneficial microflora in a healthy state, and this ensures proper functioning of the intestine.** The probiotics are able to achieve this in two ways.

## A. By antagonistic activity

It has been shown that lactic acid bacteria (**Lactobacillus** species) are able to inhibit the growth of pathogens (disease-producing organisms.) **Lactobacillus** species inhibits **Salmonella** species, **Staphylococcus** species, and *Escherichia coli*, which are very important pathogens of the intestinal tract in poultry. Lactic acid bacteria are able to do this because they produce several bactericidal substances that kill disease-producing micro-organisms (**competitive inhibition**). These substances include **bacteriocins, lactocidin, organic acids (lactic and acetic acid), hydrogen peroxide, lysozyme, lactoferrin, lactoperoxidase, acidolin,** and **acidophilin.** Lactic acid and acetic acid inhibit the growth of many organisms, including disease-producing Gram-negative bacteria. The activity of these acids depends on the pH. **Lower pH increases the level of acids in an undissociated form which is most bactericidal.** The inhibition of *E. coli* by *Lactobacillus acidophilus* is related to the strong germicidal action of lactic acid at low pH. It is now believed that the antibacterial action produced by *L. acidophilus* is due to a combination of factors which include acids, hydrogen peroxide, and bacteriocins. Yeast *Saccharomyces cerevisiae* releases metabolite **mannan-oligosaccharide (MOS)** which is antagonistic to disease-producing organisms (see **'mannan-oligosaccharides'** under Chapter 24 and also 22).

## B. By competitive exclusion

**Competitive exclusion (CE) is the competition between beneficial and harmful bacteria in occupying the attachment (adhesion) sites on the cells of the intestinal tract of the bird.** Attachment is necessary for proliferation (growth) of the organisms and for a reduction in the rate of their removal from specific sites in the digestive tract. Their expulsion is due to the movement of intestinal contents caused by normal waves of intestinal contractions (peristalsis). **This means that whosoever**

occupies the attachment site first will remove the other. For example, if there is only one chair and if Mr A occupies it first, then Mr B is excluded. Similarly, if the useful organisms present in the probiotic reach the intestine first, they will not allow the disease-producing organisms to occupy the attachment sites, and thus the occurrence of disease is prevented.

It has now been shown that lactobacilli compete with pathogens for sites of attachment on the intestinal surface. Maximum colonization of chick intestine by the organisms (i.e. settlement and growth) occurs between 48 and 72 hours after probiotic treatment. The colonization of the intestinal wall by a dense layer of microflora appears to play an important role in the initial protection of chick against such pathogens as **Salmonella**, *Escherichia coli*, *Clostridium perfringens* and *Campylobacter jejuni*. This indicates that direct competition for attachment sites is probably the primary mechanism for competitive exclusion.

## 2. By altering bacterial metabolism

### A. Digestive enzyme activity

**Enzymes** released from the microflora in the intestine are beneficial to the chicken because they increase the digestion of nutrients. **Lactobacillus** species produce enzymes which may enrich the concentration of intestinal digestive enzymes. **Lactobacillus** spp. secrete enzymes **alpha-amylase** (digests carbohydrate), **protease** (digests protein) and **lipase** (digests fat), and thus improves digestion.

### B. Ammonia production

Ammonia produced from the breakdown of urea in the intestine by the enzyme urease can cause significant damage to the lining cells. Suppression of ammonia production and urease activity can be beneficial in improving bird's health and growth. Probiotics, containing *Lactobacillus acidophilus,* *Streptococcus faecium* and *Bacillus subtilis*, reduce the concentration of ammonia in the excreta and litter of broilers. Feeding of probiotic containing *Lactobacillus casei* decreases urea activity in the small intestinal contents of broiler chicks during the first three weeks.

## 3. Other effects of probiotics

### A. Enterotoxin neutralization

Enterotoxin (a toxin that damages intestine) produced by harmful bacteria may be neutralized by a probiotic. For example, *Lactobacillus bulgaricus* produces a metabolite which has neutralizing effect on the enterotoxin released from *E. coli*.

### B. Stimulation of immune system

**Immunity**, which results from exposure of the intestine to disease-producing bacteria, is important in the defence of young chickens against intestinal infections.

**Lactobacilli,** present in probiotics, could be important in the development of immune competence (i.e. ability to fight an infectious disease). Recently it has been found that **Lactobacillus** supplementation in layers increases cellularity of Peyer's patches in the ileum (a portion of small intestine). This indicated a stimulation of the immune system of the intestine which responded to bacteria by secreting antibody **immunoglobulin A (IgA). IgA antibody is most important in protecting the intestinal lining against bacterial infection.** In addition, immunostimulation is also brought about by increasing the macrophage and lymphocyte activity. (Refer to Chapter 32 for more information on IgA and role of 'macrophage' and 'lymphocyte' in the production of immunity).

## Conclusion

**The addition of probiotics to the feed has been found to improve growth performance and feed conversion in broilers; and egg mass, egg weight and egg size in layers.** However, the probiotic preparations should be of adequate concentration and sufficiently stable both in storage and during administration to the birds.

**Note:** For a list of various commercial probiotic preparations available at the market and their indications and dosage, refer to Chapter 19 under **"Probiotics".**

Chapter **22**

# Mould Inhibitors and Toxin Binders

The problem of mycotoxin exists all over the world. **Mycotoxins are toxic fungal metabolites.** A fungal metabolite is a product of fungal metabolism. **Mycotoxins, in poultry, even at low concentrations, reduce feed intake, growth rate, feed conversion, egg production, immunity, and increase susceptibility to disease** (see Chapter 6, under **'Mycotoxicosis'**).

**Mycotoxins** occur in grains quite commonly and therefore their harmful effects must be controlled. They are formed in high concentrations in **conditions of high temperature and humidity.** Moreover, the level of contamination by fungus directly influences mycotoxin production. Therefore, it is most important to prevent growth of the fungus (mould) in the feed. But this is extremely difficult in a tropical country like ours, where both temperature and humidity are high. However, the mycotoxin problem is mostly seasonal and is generally seen in rainy and winter seasons.

**Usually, it is the last of the old season maize, because of storage, and the first of the new season maize, because of the moisture content, that create the most problem.** Actually, mycotoxins are always present in the feed, usually at levels too low to be detectable. Moreover, **the harmful effects of most mycotoxins are additive (synergistic)** (see 'Mycotoxicosis'). **This means that concentration of mycotoxins in feed, even at harmless levels, can be of great importance to bird's health and productivity.** Mycotoxins increase flock disease and reduce productivity. **The main impact of mycotoxins is on the immune system of the bird.** As discussed under 'mycotoxicosis' (Chapter 6), **mycotoxins are immunosuppressive,** that is, they suppress the production of immunity against an infectious agent, or following vaccination. **It is therefore wise to use a mould inhibitor and an effective toxin binder.** Their inclusion in the feed prevents immunosuppression, ensuring an effective immune response. Also, economic losses from reduced growth and poor vaccination response, are prevented.

## MOULD INHIBITORS (Antifungal Agents)

**Mould inhibitors added to feeds to prevent fungal growth have no effect on the toxin already formed.** Organic acids as mould inhibitors are effective, but their effectiveness may be reduced by particle size of feed ingredients and buffering by certain ingredients. **Organic acids** are corrosive (eat away by chemical action) and irritating to skin. Some have been modified to neutralize this action. Organic acids most commonly used are propionic acid, acetic acid, citric acid, sorbic acid, and benzoic acid. At times salts of propionic, acetic, 2, 4-hexadienoic acid, benzene carboxylic and isobutyric acid are used as mould inhibitors. Propionic acid acts as an antifungal agent, and is added to kill vegetative growth (mycelium). Propionic acid is also added to ensure that there is propionate in the feed throughout its storage period. This is because propionate prevents spore's germination and growth. Acetic acid prevents the calcium and sodium salts, present in layer and breeder feeds, from neutralizing the propionic acid. Hexadienoic acid is effective against yeasts and some of the bacterial spores found in feeds. Benzene carboxylic acid has antibacterial and antifungal properties. Isobutyric acid also has antibacterial and antifungal properties. **Lower pH in the intestine, induced by organic acids, helps in better feed digestibility.**

**Thus, organic acids provide double benefits.** Apart from antifungal activity, they help in acidification of the intestine. Acidification increases protein digestibility and amino acid utilization, and also keeps under control the load of *E. coli* and **Salmonella**. **However, as stated, they do not destroy any mycotoxins present in the feed.**

The other shortcomings are that **mould inhibitors only stop the growth of moulds. They do not kill them.** Also, the activity of mould inhibitors in feed is limited by several factors. For example, mould inhibitors are weakly acidic with a pH of about 5. Therefore, the pH of the feed determines the antifungal activity of the inhibitors. The average pH of maize is 6.5. Any variations in the pH of feed significantly affect the antifungal activity of organic acid mould inhibitors. Moreover, mould inhibitors tend to lose their ability to control fungi with continued use. It therefore becomes necessary to increase the amount of mould inhibitor used each year, to achieve the same degree of control. Mould inhibitors may also affect the nutrient quality of feeds. For example, it has been found that they can destroy vitamin E.

Other agents that reduce fungal growth or mycotoxin formation include phosphates (tetrasodium pyrophosphate and alkaline polyphosphate), ammonium hydroxide, essential oil extracts, potassium sorbate, silicon dioxide, propylene glycol, and 3-p cymenol. Gentian violet is effective but has now been replaced by better antifungal agents. **Copper sulphate is a poor mould inhibitor for poultry feeds.**

More recently, **oxine copper** has emerged as an effective antifungal agent. It acts against a wide range of fungi. Oxine copper reduces the fungal load in the feed, preserves its nutrients, and also acts as a growth promoter.

## TOXIN BINDERS

**Detoxification** (removal of toxin or its effect) is another approach for using mycotoxin-contaminated feeds, while not allowing the disease mycotoxicosis from occurring.

# 1. ZEOLYTES

**Zeolytes** are silicon-containing compounds. They are practical and economical feed additives that can reduce the effects of certain mycotoxins, especially aflatoxin. **Hydrated sodium calcium aluminosilicate (HSCAS) binds aflatoxin B1** in the digestive tract of chickens and reduces its absorption, and thus toxicity. **However, inactivation occurs mainly in the case of aflatoxin, as zeolytes are ineffective against ochratoxin and certain others.** This is because aflatoxins have polar functional groups. Therefore, aflatoxins are inactivated due to their specific fixation to the adsorbing (sticking) components of HSCAS. (Adsorption means adhesion or sticking of molecules to the surface.) Thus, when HSCAS comes in contact with mycotoxins, HSCAS attaches aflatoxin on its surface in the form of an extremely thin layer, and this binds and removes it. However, the quality as well as the quantity of HSCAS is important to have better effect. For example, pore size has to be exact to adsorb toxins. **Zeolytes bind toxins by virtue of their pore size.** Uniform pore size provides a selective and stable binding and an effective mechanism for inactivating mycotoxins. Uniform pore size of zeolytes also ensures that they do not bind nutrients in feed. HSCAS adsorbs and retains aflatoxin at the intestinal level, which is then excreted in faeces. When mycotoxin toxicity is eliminated or diminished, there is better absorption of nutrients. **However, it is emphasized that HSCAS does not prevent toxic effects of mycotoxins, other than aflatoxin.**

# 2. ACTIVATED CHARCOAL

Activated charcoal provides high porosity for toxin binding. **It is a multiple toxin binder,** and binds ochratoxin, T2, and particularly aflatoxin. **However, at high levels it can bind nutrients.** It has therefore to be used carefully for the desired toxin binding effect.

# 3. GLUCANS

More recently glucan has been found as an effective mycotoxin binder. Glucan is a natural complex carbohydrate, a polysaccharide (like cellulose), and is composed of the basic unit **glucose**. It is derived from the cell wall of the yeast *Saccharomyces cerevisiae*, but is inert. That is, without active chemical or other properties. It has therefore been modified to convert it into an effective mycotoxin binder. The modified glucan is known as 'esterified glucomannan (EGM)', which acts as an effective mycotoxin adsorbent. That is, when glucan comes in contact with mycotoxins, it attaches mycotoxin on its surface, and thus binds and removes the toxin.

Whereas HSCAS binds only aflatoxin, **glucan binds a wide range of toxins.** It can successfully bind aflatoxins and fusariotoxins, including T-2 toxin. Because glucan has high affinity for mycotoxins, it is included in the feed at low level, and therefore, it does not block the absorption of nutrients.

## 4. MANNAN-OLIGOSACCHARIDES

**Mannan-oligosaccharide (MOS),** a potent modifier of intestinal microflora and an immunity enhancer (see Chapter 24: 'Oligosaccharides'), **also acts as a toxin binder.** It is also derived from the cell wall of the yeast *Saccharomyces cerevisiae,* but is composed of sugar **mannose. It can bind a range of mycotoxins,** namely, aflatoxin, ochratoxin, T-2 toxin, fumonisin, citrinin and others, **with the lowest levels of inclusion in the feed. MOS provides an extremely high surface area for toxin binding.** Moreover, toxin binding by MOS is highly stable, and is unaffected by enzymes or by variations in the intestinal pH.

Advantages of using toxin binders containing esterified glucomannans (EGM)/ mannan-oligosaccharides (MOS)

1.  Both are **broad-spectrum toxin binders.** They bind a range of mycotoxins. Aluminosilicates (HSCAS), on the other hand, bind only aflatoxin.

2.  Both provide a **stable binding.** They bind the toxins strongly. As a result, toxins are not easily released.

3.  Compared to aluminosilicates, they are **effective at much lower inclusion levels.** This is because of their very vast surface area.

4.  **Their toxin binding ability is unaffected by the intestine's pH.** To be effective their binding capacity must remain intact, despite changes in the pH.

5.  **Their ability to bind toxin is also unaffected by the digestive enzymes.** During digestion, they are exposed to attack by the enzymes, but they retain their ability to keep mycotoxins in a bound state.

6.  Moreover, **their binding capacity is unaffected by the feed ingredients.** Binding sites on aluminosilicates are usually occupied by other feed constituents (vitamins, minerals, etc.). This reduces their binding capacity. EGM/MOS, on the other hand, retain their ability to bind mycotoxins when mixed with poultry feed.

7.  Both **promote bird's performance.**

8.  Both **enhance bird's immune response.**

9.  Higher levels of aflatoxin B1 in layer feed result in increased levels of toxin in liver. EGM, added to the diet, **reduces liver mycotoxin content,** by more than 50%.

10.  MOS provides mannose sugar, which binds bacteria that would otherwise attach to the intestinal wall. As a result, **MOS prevents attachment and growth of disease-producing bacteria, especially *E. coli* and Salmonella, in the intestine** (see Chapter 24).

## Benefits of mixing mould inhibitors and toxin binders in poultry feed

1. Better growth and production

2. Better FCR and weight gain

3. Enhanced immunity and improved resistance

4. Better response to vaccination

5. Reduced mortality

## Conclusions

1. Remember that, despite the best efforts, contamination of feed with mycotoxins is unavoidable.

2. **Mycotoxins are highly heat resistant,** and can be present in the grains after the fungi that produced them are dead.

3. It is uncommon to find only a single **mycotoxin** under field conditions. **Usually they occur in combination of two or more.**

4. Therefore, mycotoxins usually act in combination, and their combined effect is much more damaging than that of the individual toxin.

5. **Absence of one mycotoxin does not mean the absence of others.**

6. Sun drying is the best method to prevent mould growth. However, it does not destroy the mycotoxins.

7. Therefore, the most practical way to tackle the problem is to **use an effective mould inhibitor** and a scientifically tested broad-spectrum toxin binder.

8. Remember that mould inhibitors added to feeds to prevent fungal growth have no effect on toxins already formed. **Therefore, use a compound that contains both a mould inhibitor and a toxin binder.**

9. In selecting a toxin binder, **make sure that the binder used covers a range of mycotoxins, and not just aflatoxin.** Aluminosilicates (HSCAS) bind only aflatoxin, whereas esterified glucomannans (EGM) and mannan-oligosaccharides (MOS) also bind several others. **Therefore, use a toxin binder containing either EGM or MOS.**

10. After selecting the most effective toxin binder, **ensure its thorough mixing in the feed,** and then enjoy the lucrative results!

**Note:** For a list of various commercial preparations containing 'mould inhibitors and toxin binders', refer to Chapter 19 under **'Mould inhibitors and toxin binders'.**

# Chapter 23

# Enzymes

## Introduction

**Antibiotic resistance has become a major issue globally.** As a result, at the end of June 1999 the majority of **antibiotic growth promoters (AGPs)** were removed within the European Union. These products had been used for many years by the poultry industry and had proved effective in improving bird's health status, uniformity, and production efficiency. **But now they have been banned in animal feeds in Europe.** This is because hospital-acquired infections in humans are currently causing one-third of all deaths around the world. Since no new antibiotics have been introduced in past 10 years, does it mean that due to their continued use in feed soon all antibiotics in humans will be ineffective? Many believe so. Does this suggest that soon there could be a situation when there will be no antibiotics available to treat even the common bacterial infections?

**The question now faced is that if antibiotic growth promoters are on the way out, what do we have to replace them with?** The removal of a whole class of 'antibiotic growth promoters' from diets has posed a difficult problem in Europe, since antibiotic growth promoters have undoubtedly improved bird's performance and health status. After removal of antibiotic growth promoters what alternative products can help to solve the problem? There are many ways to influence the intestinal microflora once antibiotic growth promoters are removed. **It is now believed that enzymes will help in reducing the extent of the problem.**

**As enzymes have a significant impact on bird's health and are going to occupy an important role in future poultry industry,** this chapter discusses at some length various aspects of enzymes, including their benefits and applicability for poultry.

## Impact of Enzymes on Poultry

**Enzymes, as additives to feeds, are having a great impact on poultry industry.** Not only have they improved the utilization of feeds containing cereals, but they have also improved the quality of the environment by reducing the output of excreta and pollutants, such as phosphorus, nitrogen, and ammonia.

The main objectives of enzyme supplementation to poultry feeds are to destroy the anti-nutritive factors (discussed later) in feed ingredients, to increase the overall digestibility of feed, to make certain nutrients biologically more available, and to reduce pollutants from excreta.

**Enzymes are now being widely used in poultry feeds in an attempt to improve nutrient utilization, the health and welfare of the birds, products quality, and to reduce environmental pollution.** Enzyme supplementation is beneficial, but feed has to be formulated carefully to derive the maximum benefits.

The use of enzymes in poultry feeds has mainly centred on the hydrolysis (breakdown) of **fibre** or **non-starch polysaccharide fractions** (discussed later) in cereal grains and other **anti-nutritive factors** (discussed later) in feed ingredients. **The non-starch polysaccharides (NSPs) and anti-nutritive factors cannot be digested by bird's own enzymes and therefore produce harmful effects.**

Since enzymes as feed additives are so important, various aspects of digestive enzymes are discussed next. This would also include the nature of dietary fibres and non-starch polysaccharides and their anti-nutritive effects; and as to why the use of enzymes is necessary to derive the maximum benefits. **For convenience, the entire subject is split into two parts. Part I deals with 'enzymes other than phytase', whereas part II discusses 'phytase', at some length.**

## Part I    ENZYMES OTHER THAN 'PHYTASE'

### What is an enzyme?

An enzyme is a protein produced by living cells. It modifies and increases the rate of specific chemical reaction at body temperature. **The enzyme itself remains unchanged at the end of the reaction.**

The enzymes are of various kinds. Those involved in the digestion of food (carbohydrate, protein, fat) are known as **'digestive enzymes'**.

### What are the different types of digestion in birds?

**These are of two types:**

1.  In the first case, digestion is due to the action of enzymes that originate in the bird's body. It is called **'autoenzymatic digestion'** ('Auto' in Greek means 'self'. That is, digestion from enzymes of self origin).

2.  In the second case, digestion is due to the enzymes of some other source, mainly bacteria. This type of digestion is called **'alloenzymatic digestion'.** ('Allo' in Greek means 'other'). That is, digestion from enzymes of other sources than bird's body).

This second type of digestion usually occurs in the caeca, posterior part of the small intestine, and rectum. Because of the low oxygen tension in these areas (mainly caeca) digestion, which is actually fermentation (discussed later), is carried out through anaerobic microbial activity. Anaerobes are those microbes or micro-organisms which live in the absence of oxygen. Alloenzymatic digestion is therefore commonly known as **'fermentation'**. Fermentation is digestion of food through the action of enzymes (**ferments**) produced by the micro-organisms, namely, **bacteria, moulds, and yeasts.**

## Why do birds need two types of enzymes?

This is because birds can digest, from their own enzymes, only carbohydrate, protein, and fat. **They are unable to digest the 'dietary fibre' present in the feed.** Dietary fibre is that part of the food of plant origin which cannot be digested by bird's own enzymes. This is because birds are unable to produce those enzymes that digest dietary fibre. However, enzymes produced by the bacteria in the caeca, or enzymes added in the feed, can digest the dietary fibre. Therefore, the second type of enzymes for **'alloenzymatic digestion'** is also required.

## Where are dietary fibres present?

They are present in the carbohydrate, and not in protein or fat. **Carbohydrates can be divided into two groups:** those that can be digested by the bird and those that cannot be digested. These latter indigestible carbohydrates are known as **'dietary fibre'** (discussed later). In fact, dietary fibres consist of such glucose units, whose linkages (bonds) cannot be hydrolyzed (broken) by bird's enzymes. Digestion of such fibres therefore requires outside help from enzymes of the bacteria present in the caeca, and the major form of the usable energy produced for the bird is volatile fatty acids.

**Dietary fibre is mainly composed of non-starch polysaccharides (NSPs) and lignin.** Dietary fibre in most foods is found in the plant cell wall, but legumes store a large amount of NSPs within the cells of their seeds.

**Feed ingredients for diets have been estimated to form 70-80% of the total cost of rearing poultry.** The most commonly used plant ingredients are maize, soyabean meal, sunflower meal, or beans. **Soyabean remains the protein source of choice** because of its high protein and relatively low fibre content, and its balanced amino acid profile. These ingredients may constitute about 80% of the final formulated feed. However, all these ingredients have problem compounds that can have harmful effects on the performance of the bird **(Table 3).**

**Table 3.   Plant ingredients used in poultry feeds and their problem  compounds**

| Ingredient | Problem Compounds |
|---|---|
| Maize | Lectins, phytate, resistant starch |
| Soyabean meal | Oligosaccharides and NSPs, trypsin inhibitors, lectin |
| Rice | Phytate, arabinoxylans |
| Sunflower meal | Oligosaccharides, NSPs |
| Beans | Tannins, trypsin inhibitors, lectins, oligosaccharides, NSPs |

NSPs = Non-starch polysaccharides

# What are non-starch polysaccharides?

Non-starch polysaccharides consist of celluloses, hemicelluloses, pectins, and lignin. **Cellulose** is the main component of plant cell wall. It is a fibrillar polysaccharide made up of beta-glucose units with beta-1, 4 linkages. **Hemicellulose** is also a plant polysaccharide, but is less complex than cellulose and easily hydrolyzable to simple sugars. **Pectins** are various water-soluble substances that bind neighbouring cell walls in plant tissues and yield a gel which is the basis of fruit jellies.

Both **hemicelluloses** and **pectins** are present in the plant cell as matrix polysaccharides, that is, as intercellular (between cells) substances. In other words, they act as cementing substances and bind together two neighbouring plant cells. **Lignin** is an insoluble dietary fibre and not a true NSP. In structure, it is related to cellulose, and is mainly an encrusting (covering) substance. It provides rigidity to the cell wall, and together with cellulose, forms the woody cell wall of plants and the cementing material between them.

**While 90-95% of the starch is digested in the small intestine of poultry, NSPs pass through the bird's intestine largely untouched unless exposed to enzymes produced by the bacteria.** Even a low fibre ration (3.5% crude fibre) contains a minimum of 10-11% NSPs.

**Birds can produce enzymes that can hydrolyze starch, which is alpha-linked. In contrast, they do not secrete beta-linked carbohydrate specific enzymes that can break NSP into digestible nutrients.** When NSPs cannot be digested by the bird's enzymes, they are fermented into gases and volatile fatty acids by the bacterial enzymes, **mainly in the caeca.** But these are of no use to the bird. Very less energy is derived from them, and they also cause **digestive disturbances.**

Table 4 shows total NSP present in the common ingredients fed to poultry.

Non-starch polysaccharides are the major anti-nutritive factors found in cereals and a variety of feed ingredients.

# Why are birds unable to digest NSPs?

As already stated, **chickens cannot digest NSPs because they lack enzymes to digest them.** On the other hand, **bacteria,** mainly in the caeca and also to some extent in the rectum and posterior part of small intestine (ileum), produce the enzyme beta-(1, 4)-glycosidase which is necessary for the digestion of beta 1-4 glucose linkages (bonds) of cellulose. The bacteria also produce enzymes capable of at least partially digesting hemicellulose, pectin, lignin, gums, mucilages, and other complex molecules. However, the bacteria cannot oxidize the resulting sugars, due to a lack of oxygen in the lumen of the caeca and rectum. **Therefore, sugars are fermented to volatile fatty acids, namely, acetic, propionic and butyric.** Of these, acetic acid production

**Table 4.   Total NSP present in common ingredients fed to poultry**

| Feed Ingredient | Total NSP (g/kg) | Glucose Equivalent (g/kg) |
|---|---|---|
| Maize | 124 | 77.7 |
| Soya-meal | 234 | 102.8 |
| Wheat | 94 | 68.8 |
| Jowar | 99 | 65 |
| Bajra | 80 | 53.2 |
| Rice polish | 87 | 61.4 |
| Rice kanaki | 144 | 106 |
| DORB* | 271 | 202 |
| GNC** | 167 | 110.4 |
| GNC deoiled | 186 | 123 |
| Sunflower cake | 367 | 170.40 |
| Extract rapeseed | 362 | 192.80 |

*DORB  = Deoiled rice bran

** GNC  = Groundnut cake

predominates, but all three are readily absorbed from caeca and rectum. **However, in the chicken, caecal fermentation contributes only about 3-4% of the energy requirements of the bird**, and this amount does not change with the level of dietary fibre.

In the chicken, carbohydrates are the main source of energy. Glucose, disaccharides such as sucrose, and polysaccharides such as **amylose** and **amylopectin**, are the most common forms of dietary carbohydrates of plant origin that are digested by bird's own enzymes **(autoenzymatic digestion). Amylose** is a component of **starch** and is made up of **straight** chains of glucose units with alpha -1, 4 linkages (bonds). **Amylopectin** is also a component of starch, but has a **branched** structure and consists of alpha - 1, 6 - **linked** amylose units. Thus, **starch** is the chief form of carbohydrate in plants, and is made up of glucose units with **alpha-linkages**.

## What is the nature of bacterial population in caeca?

**In the chicken,** the main contribution of bacteria to the digestion occurs in the **caeca,** although some fermentation may occur in the posterior part of the small intestine. **The caeca contain a large and complex group of micro-organisms.** The main group is of those bacteria known as **'obligate anaerobes'**. These organisms live in the absence of oxygen. They occur in the lumen of the chicken caeca at a concentration of

$10^{11}$ per gram wet weight. **At least 38 different types of anaerobic Gram-negative and Gram-positive bacteria have been isolated from chicken caeca. The caecal mucosa (i.e. lining) of the chicken has a layer of Gram-negative bacteria about 200 cells deep.** These bacteria are attached to the mucus secreted by the lining cells of the caeca.

## What are soluble, insoluble and crude fibres?

Functionally, dietary fibre can be divided into **'soluble fibre'** (pectins, gums, beta-glucans, dextrins, pentosans, mannans, and some hemicelluloses), and **'insoluble fibre'** (lignin, cellulose, and some hemicelluloses) **(Table 5).**

**Table 5. Non-starch polysaccharides (NSPs)**
          **(Dietary fibre)**

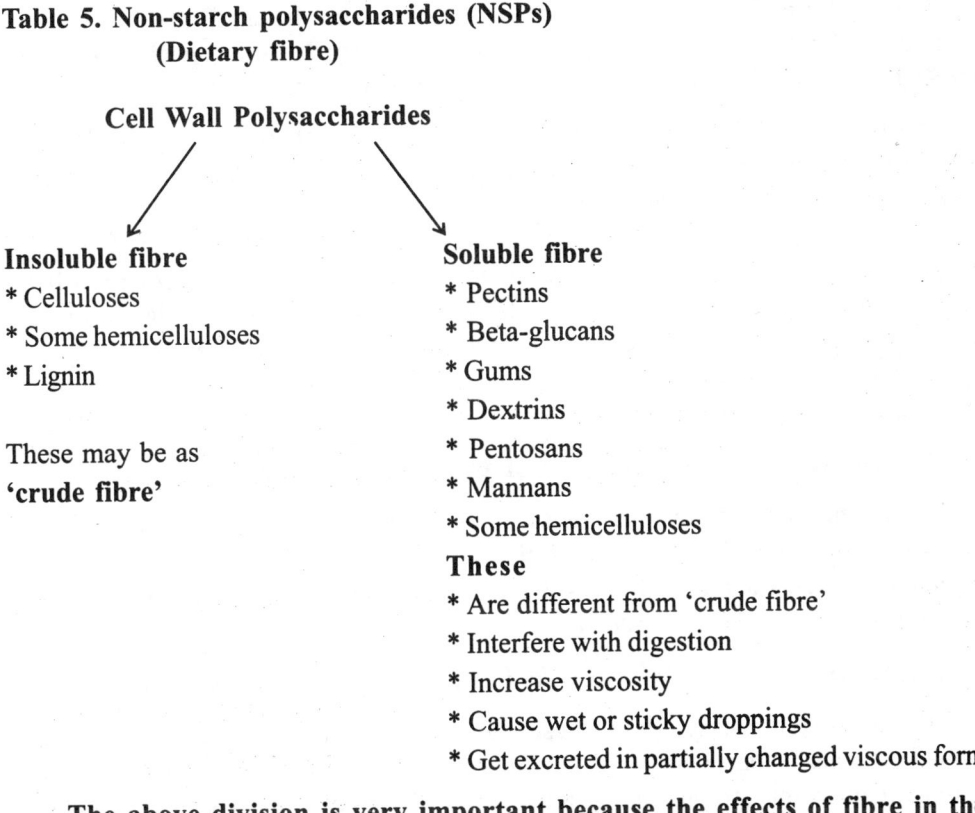

**Cell Wall Polysaccharides**

**Insoluble fibre**
* Celluloses
* Some hemicelluloses
* Lignin

These may be as
**'crude fibre'**

**Soluble fibre**
* Pectins
* Beta-glucans
* Gums
* Dextrins
* Pentosans
* Mannans
* Some hemicelluloses
**These**
* Are different from 'crude fibre'
* Interfere with digestion
* Increase viscosity
* Cause wet or sticky droppings
* Get excreted in partially changed viscous form

**The above division is very important because the effects of fibre in the intestine depend on its solubility. Beta-glucans** are polysaccharides (such as cellulose) which are made up of beta-glucose units. **Dextrins** are any of various water-soluble gummy polysaccharides obtained from starch, by the action of heat, acids, or enzymes. **Pentosans** are polysaccharides present in plant fibres that yield pentoses (arabinose and xylose) on hydrolysis. (A **pentose** is a monosaccharide that contains **five** carbon atoms in the molecule. A **hexose** is a monosaccharide, such as glucose, that contains **six** carbon atoms in the molecule.) **Gums** are colloidal polysaccharides of plant origin

371

that are gelatinous. **Mannans** are polysaccharides composed of sugar mannose. They occur especially in plant cell wall.

**'Crude fibre' is an old term** that refers to the remnants of plant material left after extraction with acid and alkali during proximate analysis (feed analysis). Crude fibre does not adequately estimate the amount of hemicellulose in feed and therefore underestimates the amount of dietary fibre. Moreover, it also fails to subdivide functionally different types of fibre. **As a result, its use in avian (bird's) nutrition has decreased.**

## What are the physiological effects of fibre?

Some birds can digest fibre in the caeca and obtain useful amounts of energy in the form of volatile fatty acids. It is the soluble components of the dietary fibre that are most susceptible to fermentation and provide most of the energy. **In some species, such as ostrich, but not in the chicken, cellulose can also be fermented.**

This is because the so-called **'large intestine' in the chicken** is very short. **It is only 4% of the total gastro-intestinal length and is therefore not referred to as 'large intestine', but as 'rectum' or 'colon'.** Interestingly, among the birds, **ostrich** is an exception. **Its rectum is the largest of any bird and makes 52% of the total length of the gastro-intestinal tract. Ostrich is therefore the most efficient bird at utilizing dietary fibre.** Fermentation in its rectum and caeca produces high levels of volatile fatty acids and may supply as much as 75% of the metabolizable energy as against only about 3-4% in the chicken. **In fact, dietary fibre digestibility in the ostrich approaches that in the horse.**

## What is the anti-nutritive feature of the dietary fibre?

When high levels of dietary fibre are eaten by the chicken, the anti-nutritive or negative character of the fibre acts against the energy obtained. **It is mostly the soluble components of the fibre that are involved in anti-nutritive activities. That is, in producing harmful effects on poultry.**

## What kind of an anti-nutritive effect is produced by the soluble fibre?

**Soluble fibre increases the viscosity of the intestinal contents.** That is, the intestinal contents become sticky and acquire a glutinous consistency (i.e. become like glue or gum; gelatinous, resembling gelatin or jelly). This increase in viscosity is highly correlated with the solubility of the fibre, and is not dependent on the amount of non-starch polysaccharides present. In other words, **viscosity is due to the soluble fibres, and not insoluble fibres.** Pectins, gums, beta-glucans, pentosans, and some hemicelluloses are soluble fibres and therefore they are the main viscous components, whereas lignin, cellulose, and some hemicelluloses are insoluble fibres and do not produce viscosity. **The soluble fibres absorb large amounts of water and this makes the intestinal contents viscous.**

## Why only soluble fibres enter the caeca and insoluble fibres are kept out?

The junction of small intestine, caeca, and rectum is surrounded by **three sphicters**. A sphicter is a circular muscle that can close an opening on contraction. These sphicters regulate the direction of intestinal contents when they leave the small intestine. The two sphicters, one for each caecum at the junction, control the two caecal openings. **Recently it has been shown that lining of the caecal sphincters has very long villi, that is, minute finger-shaped projections.** Contractions of the sphincters narrow the openings, which causes these finger-shaped projections to inter-digitate. That is, the villi become inter-locked like the fingers of folded hands, and then act like a filter. **The network formed permits entry of only liquid fraction of the intestinal contents containing soluble fibres into caeca, and keeps out the insoluble, indigestible solid fibrous portion. Thus, only soluble fibres are allowed to enter caeca.**

## What are the harmful effects of viscosity?

1. High intestinal viscosity interferes with the diffusion of substrates (i.e. substances on which enzymes act, namely, carbohydrates, proteins, fats) and also the digestive enzymes. As a result, the interaction between a substrate and the enzyme is prevented. **This leads to decreased digestion of food.** Moreover, the gel-forming components of fibre (gums and pectins) interact with the glycocalyx of the intestinal lining and increase the thickness of the unstirred water layer. This leads to poor absorption of the end products of digestion. **The net result is that NSPs are poorly digested and therefore reduce the metabolizable energy and nutrient contents of the feed.**

   Moreover, the increase in **viscosity interferes with the intestinal absorption of nutrients,** and can result in 'wet or sticky droppings', **vent pasting,** and **unhygienic litter conditions.** In order to help the digestive processes, water consumption increases that further enhances the production of **wet and sticky excreta.** In addition, increased retention time on contents in the intestine decreases oxygen tension. **This favours the bacterial colonization (growth) of anaerobic toxigenic (i.e. toxin-producing) micro-organisms.** That is, those disease-producing bacteria which thrive best in the absence of oxygen, such as **clostridia. All this may have harmful effects on the health of the bird. Therefore, enzymes (of microbial origin) are commonly added in the feeds to decrease the viscosity of grain-based diets.**

2. Some components of the fibre, such as **pectins,** have a high charge density and ionically interact with dietary cations, such as manganese (Mn), iron (Fe), zinc (Zn) and copper (Cu). **This interaction decreases the digestibility of these minerals.**

3. **Soluble fibres** (pectins, gums, beta-glucans and some hemicelluloses) have **very**

**high water-holding capacities.** If these components are not fermented, they also provide bulk to the faeces. Insoluble fibres can also absorb a large amount of water. But they do this without increasing the viscosity of the intestinal contents. However, some of the insoluble components of NSPs capture fat, starch and protein, making them unavailable to the birds. The insoluble fibres and the water absorbed by them also increase the bulk of the faeces. **The bulk caused by insoluble fibre reduces the residence (retention) time of the intestinal contents, and this may lead to lower feed digestibility.**

4.    NSPs bind salts, lipids and cholesterol, and thereby change the digestive and absorptive dynamics (processes, patterns) of the intestine.

**All the above interactions lead to poor assimilation (absorption), poor feed conversion, chronic deficiencies, and other health related problems in poultry.**

## What are anti-nutritive factors?

The non-starch polysaccharides, namely, pectins, beta-glucans, gums, celluloses, and some hemicelluloses, are also known as **'anti-nutritive factors'**. This is because they are not only poorly digested but also have harmful effects on poultry, as discussed above.

## Why are enzymes added in poultry feed?

Poultry feed contains ingredients of both plant and animal origin. Animal feedstuffs can be easily digested by chicken. However, plant material has certain residues which chickens are incapable of digesting by their own enzymes. These indigestible plant residues include NSPs, galactosides, phytates and other anti-nutritional factors like lectins, trypsin inhibitors, etc. Even a low fibre ration (having 3.5% crude fibre) contains minimum 10-11% NSPs.

**The use of NSP-degrading (breaking) enzymes as food additives is highly advantageous.** Most of the beneficial effect is because these enzymes prevent viscosity of the intestinal contents by leaching (removing) NSPs from the cell walls of grains. **As viscosity is greatest in the youngest bird and decreases with age, the value of adding enzymes for older birds is limited to secondary effects.** These include the release of nutrients trapped in the cereal grains of the feed.

**Galactosides** are carbohydrates found in legumes like soyabean. They yield sugar galactose on hydrolysis. Galactosides interfere with the gut function and may cause flatulence (too much gas formation) and poor assimilation (absorption) of nutrients. **Other anti-nutritional factors** interfere with the action of bird's enzymes. For example, they inhibit action of trypsin-like enzymes. The anti-nutritive effects of phytates will be discussed in Part II under the enzyme **'phytase'**.

NSPs, phytic acid or phytate (see under 'phytase'), and tannins are anti-nutrients (anti-nutritional factors). **Supplementation of diet with enzymes can reduce the** harmful effects of these compounds. Further, **cocktails of enzymes have a much better beneficial effect on the performance of growing chickens and laying hens.** Recently, enzyme supplementation has also been shown to influence the absorption of fats and fatty acids as well as fat-soluble micronutrients (trace elements) contained in the diet.

## Is there any significance of feed enzymes in older birds?

**Intestinal viscosity is highest in youngest birds and decreases with age.** Addition of enzymes results in decreased viscosity, improved feed intake and daily weight gain in **young broiler chicks.** Thereafter, benefits are seen as **improved feed conversion efficiency,** which means that viscosity reduction is playing a lesser role and that other effects become more important as the bird grows older.

## What is the effect of soluble NSPs on metabolizable energy?

Release of soluble NSPs from cereal grains within the digestive tract causes a decrease in the metabolizable energy (ME) of the diet **(Fig. 27).** This is because NSPs increase the size and stability of the unstirred water layer at the inner surface (mucosal surface) of the intestinal tract. This reduces the contact between the feed and the digestive enzymes and slows the absorption of released sugars, amino acids and lipids, resulting in defective digestibility (availability) of the major nutrients. Moreover, **increased viscosity of the intestinal contents promotes bacterial proliferation which is harmful to both overall digestive efficiency and bird health.**

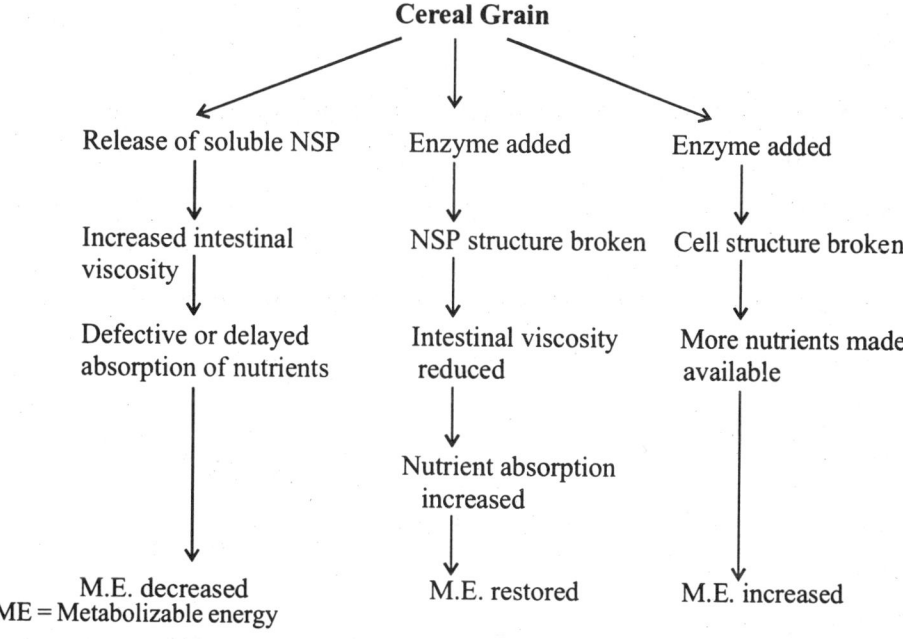

**Fig. 27. Effects of adding NSP-degrading enzymes on cereal-based poultry diets.**

**Following enzyme treatment, there is reduction in viscosity and an increase in the nutrient absorption.** However, this should be taken as restoration of normal or expected performance, which would be otherwise lost, rather than any added or extra advantage (Fig. 27). But when there is breakdown or disruption of cell structures in the grains of feed, brought about by enzymes, more nutrients become available to bird, and then there is a definite increase in the metabolizable energy for the bird **(Fig. 27). This certainly is an added advantage.**

## Which enzymes should be used?

The enzymes shown in **Table 6** may be mixed in the feed, depending on feed's composition, for **digestion of indigestible plant residues.**

**Table 6.   Enzymes used in poultry feeds**

| Enzymes | Substrates |
|---------|-----------|
| **Carbohydrases** | |
| Cellulases | Cellulose, hemicellulose |
| Hemicellulases | Hemicellulose |
| Pectinases (polygalacturonases) | Pectins |
| Alpha-galactosidases | Galactosides (short-chain carbohydrates) |
| Amylases | Starch |
| Beta-glucanases | Beta-glucans |
| Xylanases | Xylans (arabinoxylans) |
| Beta-glucosidases | Glucosides |
| Amyloglucosidases | Amyloglucosides |
| Arabinoxylanases | Arabinoxylans |
| **Proteases** | |
| Acid proteases | Proteins |
| Alkaline proteases | Proteins |
| **Others** | |
| Phytases | Phytic acid (phytate) |
| Lipases | Fats |
| Esterases | Fats |

**Note:** The importance of adding **'phytase'** is discussed later in this chapter.

## What are the different methods of adding enzyme to feed?

**Enzymes are available in various forms for adding to poultry feeds.** They may be supplied as **powders** and added to the diet before mixing and pelleting, or they can be added as **granules** before the feeds are mixed and pelleted. Both these procedures allow the enzymes to mix intimately with the dietary ingredients, and this permits them to react effectively with their substrates. Many enzymes, however, tend to be thermolabile (destroyed when heated), and therefore processing at high temperatures may reduce their activity.

A more recent development is to add enzymes as **liquid** after pelleting. This avoids the problem which occurs with pelleting at high temperatures, but has the disadvantage of enzyme getting coated onto the surface of the pellets. This does not allow the enzyme to have intimate contact with most of the components of the pellet. This may reduce the pre-ingestion (prior to eating) action of the enzyme compared to application of the enzyme before pellet formation. However, it is clear that enzymes applied as liquids to the surface of pellets usually have superior benefits on the nutritional value of the diet and on performance.

## What qualities should a good feed enzyme possess?

1.  **It should assist the bird's own digestive enzymes.** This is because poultry do not have all the necessary enzymes in their digestive tract to achieve the best utilization of feed. **The enzymes in feed must break the long-chain NSPs into smaller pieces so the nutrients can be absorbed and utilized.**

2.  It must be active in the environment of the gastro-intestinal tract, for example, temperature and pH.

3.  It must have **a wide range of activity** that may allow its use both in cereal and vegetable proteins.

4.  **It must be stable during storage, in premixes, and under normal feed manufacturing conditions.**

5.  It must be **safe and non-toxic** to those working with the product and to the poultry to which it is fed.

6.  It must not leave harmful residues in poultry products, or the environment. Of course, as enzyme is a protein, it will be digested once its function is over, but it must not contain any heavy metals. Otherwise, they may accumulate in carcass, or be present in the excreta and pose a threat to the consumer of the poultry product, or to the environment.

7.  It must show a consistent improvement in the bird's performance. That is, **it must be effective both in broilers and layers.**

8. It must be **economical** to the poultry farmers.

## What are the advantages of adding enzymes to the feed?

1. **Increased nutrient digestion.** This is particularly important in poultry because of the relatively fast digesta transit-time and limited scope for absorption of nutrients in the lower intestinal tract. Addition of enzymes, not produced by the bird, breaks down fibres, releases simple sugars, and by breaking open grain cells exposes otherwise undigested starch and protein to the action of bird's own enzymes.

2. **Enzymes hydrolyze the NSP contained in the feed, decrease gut (intestinal) viscosity, and thus improve nutrient absorption. This greatly reduces wet, sticky, or loose droppings.** Moreover, the energy level of the diet may be lowered without reducing the bird's performance.

3. The **reduction in wet droppings,** in turn, **brings a number of benefits to the broiler farmer.** These include:

   (i) Less wet litter problems.

   (ii) More hygienic litter conditions.

   (iii) **Reduced ammonia build-up in the poultry shed,** and therefore improved air quality and reduced stress on birds.

   (iv) Cleaner poultry shed.

4. **Enzymes modify intestinal environment.** Improved nutritional digestibility leads to better absorption and reduces the amount of undigested nutrients available for bacteria present in the lower intestine. **This reduces the overall bacterial population,** and when this is combined with a reduction in intestinal viscosity, indirectly **modifies the intestinal environment in favour of the growth of useful bacteria like Lactobacillus species at the cost of harmful bacteria like *Escherichia coli*, Salmonella species, and Campylobacter.**

5. **Faster growth** and improvement in body weight.

6. **Better feed conversion ratio (FCR).** This is because enzymes unlock metabolizable energy and proteins trapped in the soluble fibres.

7. **Better phosphorus and mineral assimilation** such as that of **calcium, magnesium,** and **zinc.**

8. Reduction or **removal of the anti-nutritional factors present in feed.** For example, proteases can improve the effects of lectins and trypsin inhibitors in soyabean meal.

9. **An increase in egg production.**

10. Improvement in bioavailability of metabolizable energy.

11. **Fat digestibility.** Many vegetable proteins contain high levels of oil following oil extraction. **Lipases** have positive effects on fat digestibility, especially on saturated fats. Fat has a high energy value and therefore only a small increase in its digestive efficiency is required.

12. Flexibility in feed formulation, making it most cost-effective without compromising on the quality.

13. Reduction in phosphorus deficiency related sickness.

14. **Phytase helps in reducing or removing DCP from the feed.**

15. **Improvement in eggshell quality.**

16. Less manure and nitrogen due to improved feed utilization. As a result, there is **less environmental pollution.**

## Conclusion

No physiologically harmful effects have been reported from enzyme addition to feed, and **enzyme treatment is now an accepted method of enhancing the nutritional value of poultry feed.** Several enzymes are 'cocktails' or combinations of enzymes that may also contain proteases to help the digestion of proteins.

**Note:** For a list of commercial preparations of various enzymes available at the market and their indications and dosage, refer to Chapter 19 under "**Enzymes**".

## PART II PHYTASE

## Introduction

Poultry feeds mainly consist of seeds (cereal grains) and products derived from seeds (oil seed meals, cereal by-products). **However, some nutrients in feeds are not digested and absorbed by poultry.** It is now known that the availability of nutrients can be affected by the presence of **natural complexing agents in the feeds.** This is particularly true for cereal grains, legume seeds and oil crops containing **phytic acid,** also known as **phytate.**

**Dietary phosphorus may be present in inorganic or organic form.** Inorganic phosphorus found in foods is readily absorbed from the diet. **However, the organic phosphorus in the seeds of plants is poorly utilized, because it is a component of phytic acid (Fig. 28).** Only a small part of the total plant phosphorus is present in the inorganic form, which is fully available to the birds. **The majority, some 60-80%, is in the phytic form.** This means that whereas phosphorus found in animal by-products is completely available, **plant phosphorus has low biological availability for poultry.**

Also known as phytate, phytic acid is an organic complex. It is the main form in which the phosphorus is stored in plants. Unfortunately, many grains, oil seed meals, and plant derived products contain high concentrations of phytic acid. As indicated **phytic acid contains 60-80% of the total phosphorus present.**

The phosphorus present in phytic acid (phytate) is not available to poultry because they lack the enzymes to hydrolyze (break down) phytic acid into inorganic phosphorus. To be nutritionally available, phytic acid must be broken down by enzymes known as **'phytases'. There is a lack of phytase in chicken intestine, especially in young chicks. The limited ability of poultry to utilize phytic acid presents two problems.**

1.	The first is about the feed formulation, to satisfy the bird's physiological requirements of phosphorus.

2.	The second involves the environmental impact of unused dietary phosphorus excreted in the faeces.

In order to meet the phosphorus requirements of the bird, poultry feeds have been traditionally supplemented with inorganic phosphorus sources, such as **dicalcium phosphate (DCP).** This is not only expensive, but also fails to deal with such problems as over-supplementation. This leads to potential environmental phosphorus pollution. Therefore, attempts were made to examine other ways to make phytate phosphorus available to birds. As a result of these efforts, there has been a renewed interest in the use of **enzyme phytase**. The purpose is to reduce the need for inorganic phosphorus supplementation and to improve the utilization of the phosphorus present in feedstuffs.

## What is phytic acid?

Also known as **'phytate'**, phytic acid is an organic complex. It was discovered in 1855 and purified in 1900. **Phytic acid has six phosphate groups (Fig. 28),** and is a naturally occurring component of many seeds. At neutral pH, the phosphate

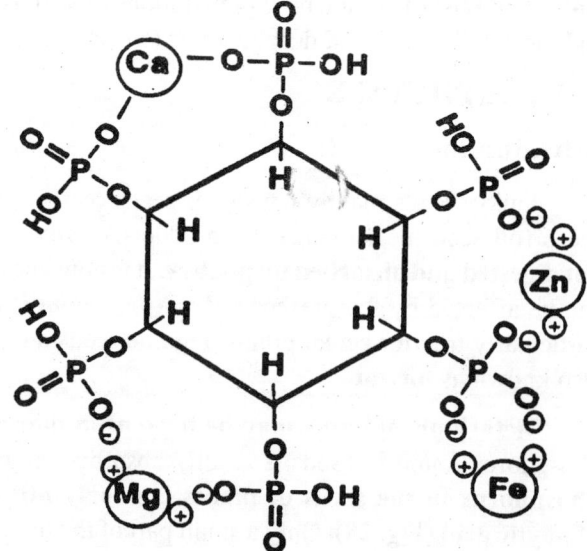

**Fig. 28. Structure of phytic acid.** Note chelation (binding) of positively charged calcium, zinc, iron and magnesium ions by the negatively charged oxygen atoms in the four phosphate groups.

groups in phytic acid have either one or two negatively charged oxygen atoms. Therefore, various cations (ions with positive charges) are able to **chelate** (bind) strongly between two phosphate groups, or weakly with a single phosphate group **(Fig. 28)**. (The word **'chelation'** means removal by binding. It comes from the Greek word 'chela' which means 'claws of a crab'. The meaning is to strongly bind like the crab's claw, and then remove it.) In the present case, **the negative charges of phosphate groups in phytic acid bind strongly with the positive charges of ions of calcium, magnesium, zinc, and iron (Fig. 28).** Thus, these important minerals are bound and removed from the diet, and **thus become unavailable to the birds.** Phytic acid also binds in a similar way with proteins, making them less soluble.

**Phytic acid is considered as a nutrient because it contains phosphorus.** On the other hand, it is also considered to be **toxic because it binds various essential elements and reduces their availability. Table 7** shows the amount of total phosphorus and phytate phosphorus in various feed ingredients of poultry. **Table 8** also presents similar findings from another study.

**Table 7.** Total phosphorus and phytate phosphorus in various feed ingredients of poultry

| Feed ingredient (%) | Total 'P' (%) | Phytate 'P' (%) |
|---|---|---|
| Maize | 0.49 | 0.22 |
| Soyabean meal | 0.65 | 0.39 |
| Rice polish | - | 1.2 |
| Sorghum | 0.31 | 0.22 |
| Wheat | 0.35 | 0.20 |
| Wheat bran | 1.23 | 0.99 |
| Cotton seed meal | 1.20 | 0.84 |
| Sunflower meal | 1.05 | 0.58 |

**Table 8.** Phytic acid and phytate phosphorus concentrations in cereals (from another study)

| Cereal | Sample | Phytic acid (%) | Phytate phosphorus (%) |
|---|---|---|---|
| Maize | Commercial hybrid | 0.89 | 0.25 |
| Maize | High lysine | 0.96 | 0.27 |
| Wheat | Soft | 1.14 | 0.32 |
| Rice | Brown | 0.89 | 0.25 |

**Phytate phosphorus** constitutes the major portion of the total phosphorus present in cereal seeds, grain legumes and oil-bearing plants. **About two-third of the total**

**phosphorus in these materials is present in this form.** The concentration of phytic phosphorus in feedstuffs depends largely on the part of the plant from which it is derived. In rice more than 80% of phytate is present in the outer bran. In contrast, phytate in soyabean appears to have no specific site of localization.

## Digestion of phytate and its bioavailability

In order that phytate phosphorus can be used by the bird, phytate must be hydrolyzed (broken down) to inorganic compounds containing phosphorus within the digestive tract. This is brought about by a family of enzymes called **'phytases'. Otherwise, phytate phosphorus is poorly utilized by poultry.** The hydrolysis can occur in the digestive tract of the bird, or in the feedstuff before its consumption. The breakdown of phytate in the digestive tract of poultry can occur from the action of **phytase from four possible sources.**

(i)     Intestinal **phytase** present **in digestive secretions,**

(ii)    Phytase originating **from microbes** living **in the intestinal tract,**

(iii)   Phytase present in some **feedstuffs,** or

(iv)    Phytase produced by **outside micro-organisms**

Recent work indicates that **phytase activity in the intestinal secretions of poultry is extremely low, at least in young birds.**

## What are the factors that influence phytate phosphorus utilization?

The hydrolysis and absorption of phytate phosphorus are complex processes, which are influenced by factors such as dietary calcium, inorganic phosphorus (available phosphorus), vitamin D3, age and type of birds, dietary ingredients, and feed processing.

## 1. Dietary calcium and phosphorus level

Utilization of phytate phosphorus in poultry is influenced by both dietary calcium and phosphorus concentrations. **The effect of dietary calcium is much greater.** At very high calcium concentrations phytate hydrolysis is completely prevented. That is, the availability of phytate phosphorus decreases with increasing calcium content. At high levels in layer feeds (about 4% calcium) and in feeds for very young chicks (about 1% calcium), **phytate phosphorus is considered virtually unavailable.**

A high calcium, or calcium:total phosphorus ratio of 2:1 impairs the digestion of phytate because of the formation of an insoluble calcium phytate complex in the intestine. Chicks fed on a diet with a calcium:total phosphorus ratio of 1:1 performed better than those fed on a diet where the ratio was 2:1.

## 2. Dietary vitamin D3 level

**Phytate phosphorus utilization decreases when diets are deficient in vitamin**

**D3. Addition of vitamin D3 greatly increases the amount of phytate phosphorus utilized by chickens.** This improved utilization of phytate phosphorus in response to vitamin D3 supplementation may be due to: (1) increased synthesis or activity of intestinal phytase, (2) increased phytate hydrolysis by stimulation of calcium absorption. This makes phytate more soluble and available for utilization, and (3) increased absorption of phosphorus.

## 3. Age of Birds

**Older birds hydrolyze phytate phosphorus to a greater extent than do chicks because** there is more phytase activity present in the digestive tract of older birds. **The ability of poultry to utilize phytate phosphorus increases with age.** For example, 21 day-old broilers utilize phytate phosphorus better than 14 and 7 day-old broilers. However, it has been observed that there is only a slight increase in phosphorus utilization by the older birds. Moreover, the ability of layers to utilize phytate phosphorus appears to decrease with advancing age. For example, retention of phytic phosphorus is high at 34 weeks of age, but decreases markedly at 50 and 72 weeks of age. A significant effect of sex has been reported, with males retaining more phytate phosphorus than females.

## 4. Type of dietary ingredients

The utilization of phytate phosphorus by poultry can be improved by dietary incorporation of plant-derived ingredients with known phytase activity. There are differences in the solubility of phytate from different sources. For example, phytate in soyabean meal is more soluble than that in sesame meal. Since soluble phytate is a better substrate for enzymatic action, variation in phytate solubility may be responsible for the differences in the extent of hydrolysis of phytate from different feedstuffs.

## 5. Genotype of birds

Limited evidence indicates that there may be breed and strain differences in the utilization of phytate phosphorus within poultry. Average retention of phytate phosphorus by Leghorn chickens is greater than that by meat-type broilers.

## Effects of phytate on bioavailability of other nutrients

## 1. Effect on bird

As already stated, phytate (phytic acid) has strong chelating potential. It forms a wide variety of insoluble salts with divalent and trivalent mineral cations, that is, carrying positive charge at neutral pH. This renders these elements unavailable for intestinal absorption. **Phytic acid in feeds derived from plants forms complexes with essential elements such as calcium, zinc, copper, iron, and magnesium, and makes them biologically unavailable to the bird.**

Although calcium has the lowest binding affinity, phytate has the greatest impact on the bioavailability of **calcium**, next to **phosphorus**. This means that if diets contained ingredients high in phytate, more calcium would be required to compensate for the portion that was unavailable as insoluble calcium phytate. **However, because of the greater cost of phosphorus, we are mostly concerned about the availability of phosphorus from phytate, rather than calcium.** **Zinc** may become a limiting (deficient) mineral in high phytate diets because it forms a highly insoluble salt at pH 6.0, the approximate pH of the upper intestine where most of the mineral absorption occurs. The effect of phytate on the availability of minerals, other than calcium and zinc, has received relatively little attention in poultry nutrition. However, high phytate diets also cause decreased **magnesium, copper** and **manganese** availability.

## 2. Effect on protein availability

The importance of phytate is further complicated by **protein-mineral-phytate interactions** and the inhibitory effects of phytate on proteolytic enzymes (i.e. which digest protein). The association between phytate and protein begins in seeds. Phytic acid-protein interaction reduces the availability of legume protein and the protein source is an important factor. It has been shown that **phytate-protein complexes** are more resistant to proteolytic digestion than protein alone. The interaction between phytic acid and proteins is thought to be ionic and dependent on pH. **Phytic acid can form complexes with protein at both acidic and alkaline pH.**

At low pH (about 2), phytate is strongly negatively charged while proteins are strongly positively charged. Therefore, phytate-protein complexes are formed. At high (alkaline) pH, both phytate and protein are negatively charged so that multivalent cations, such as calcium, are thought to mediate such **phytate-protein complexes. This interaction between phytic acid and protein leads to decreased protein solubility.** As a result, certain functional properties of the protein can be damaged because they depend on solubility.

**Phytate inhibits a number of digestive enzymes,** such as pepsin, alpha-amylase and trypsin. Inhibition may result from the chelation of calcium ions which are essential for the activity of trypsin and alpha-amylases. Protein digestion may also be inhibited **indirectly** because proteolytic enzymes in the digestive tract form complexes with phytate.

The main nutritional effect of **phytate-protein complex formation** is a **reduction in mineral availability.** Recent studies also indicate that phytate-protein interactions can interfere with protein and amino acid digestibility.

## 3. Effect on starch digestibility

The **enzyme alpha-amylase** requires calcium ions for its activity and to increase its stability. Phytate suppresses alpha-amylase activity by complexing with the calcium ions necessary for enzyme activity. **Inhibition of alpha-amylase may lead to low digestibility of starch and reduction in the availability of energy.**

## Characteristics of phytase

Phytase is an enzyme that hydrolyzes phytate to **inorganic phosphorus** and inositol. Phytases are present in most cereals, but their activity varies widely among cereals. For example, while wheat and barley are rich in phytase, maize, oats, sorghum and oilseeds are found to contain little or none of this enzyme. Phytase is also produced by fungi, bacteria, yeast, and some soil micro-organisms.

Phytase has been used as a commercial feed additive for more than 10 years. Commercial production of phytase for use as an enzyme supplement for diets is done by using microbial cultures. **Microbial phytases** have a broader pH activity range than plant phytases and are therefore more effective within the gastro-intestinal environment.

**Attempts are currently being made to insert foreign genes into the relevant plant DNA to enable it to synthesize enzymes, such as phytases. Phytases would then be present in the products, such as soybean meal.** Such genetic manipulations to introduce appropriate enzymes into the constituents of diets to allow them to be more efficiently used are exciting developments.

## Use of microbial phytase to increase nutrient availability

**Developments in genetic engineering** have resulted in the isolation of micro-organisms capable of producing large amounts of phytase. **It is now increasingly realized that phytase provides a cost-effective alternative to inorganic phosphorus supplementation.** In future, much attention may centre on the effects of phytase on nutrients other than phosphorus. This, in turn, may further increase the cost-effectiveness of the enzyme.

## Effects of microbial phytase on phytate phosphorus availability

**In broiler chickens**, microbial phytase supplementation of a low phosphorus maize-soyabean diet increased the availability of phosphorus to over 60%, and decreased the amount of phosphorus in droppings by 50%. The growth rate and feed conversion ratio (FCR) of the birds on the low phosphorus diet containing microbial phytase were even better than those obtained by birds fed on the control diet. **Thus, not only phosphorus availability increased and phosphorus excretion decreased, but the performance was also improved.** Several other studies have indicated that microbial phytase supplementation increases the availability of phytate phosphorus in broiler chickens. Improvements in phosphorus availability resulting from phytase supplementation are generally reported to be in the range of 20-40%. **Laying hens appear to benefit more from phytase addition**, 300 FTU / kg releasing the same amount of phosphorus as 500 FTU / kg in broilers. (FTU means 'phytase unit').

The amount of phytate phosphorus released by microbial phytase depends on the concentration and source of the added phytase and the dietary phytase, calcium and vitamin D3 contents, and the calcium: phosphorus ratio. **Microbial phytase**, unlike **plant phytase**, is active over a wider range of pH and is thus active within the proventriculus and gizzard. In poultry, phytate hydrolysis occurs mainly within the crop (pH 5-6), the proventriculus, and the gizzard (pH 2-4). This may explain the effectiveness and consistency of action of microbial phytase compared with that of plant origin.

## Effect of microbial phytase on the availability of minerals

As already discussed, phytate (phytic acid) has strong chelating potential and forms a variety of complexes with minerals and proteins, making these nutrients biologically unavailable. Theoretically, when phytate is hydrolyzed by microbial phytase, all minerals bound to it should be released. It is now known that microbial phytase supplementation improves the availability of **calcium** to broiler chickens.

**Zinc** availability is also affected by phytate in chicks. **Zinc is the mineral most prone to phytate binding.** Therefore, zinc deficiency is most likely to result from feeding a diet that includes phytate-containing plant protein diets. In fact it has been shown that in poultry phytate is an important factor in the origin of zinc deficiency. **Addition of phytase to the diet increases the absorption of zinc, magnesium, copper, and iron.**

## Effect of microbial phytase on the availability of protein and amino acids

Phytase supplementation appears to release phytate-bound protein for utilization. Recently it has been shown that phytase liberates a substantial amount of extra protein (amino acids) and energy for the bird. The effect of phytase on protein and amino acid utilization is of great practical importance.

## Effect of microbial phytase on the performance of broiler chickens

**Microbial phytase supplementation increases body weight gain and feed intake in broiler chickens.** The improvements in growth in chickens fed on a low phosphorus diet with phytase may result from:

1.  An increase in absorbed phosphorus

2.  The release of other minerals from the phytate-mineral complex

3.  An increase in digestibility, or

4.  Increased availability of amino acids

## Effect of dietary calcium and calcium: phosphorus ratio on the effectiveness of microbial phytase

Dietary calcium content and the calcium:phosphorus ratio are important factors that determine the extent of phytate hydrolysis (breakdown). Excess dietary calcium can gradually precipitate all the phytate by forming an insoluble calcium-phytate complex in the intestine. The result is that the phytate phosphorus as well as the calcium becomes largely unavailable for absorption. High contents of dietary calcium and magnesium are known to reduce intestinal phytase activity in chicks. There are only a few studies on the influence of calcium:phosphorus ratio on the efficacy of phytase in broiler diets. It has been shown that a diet high (0.9%) in dietary calcium and supplemented with microbial phytase resulted in reduced body weight gain, feed intake and phosphorus and calcium retention **compared with a diet containing low dietary calcium (0.6%) plus microbial phytase.**

## How does phosphorus from poultry faeces cause environmental pollution?

Figures are not available for our country, but in the United States 2, 60, 000 tonnes of phosphorus are excreted from poultry annually. Because of the contamination of lakes and streams, phosphorus is of great practical importance as it is the most limiting (deficient) nutrient for plants that grow or live in water (i.e. aquatic life).

When phosphorus comes in contact with soil, it binds tightly with soil particles. Phosphorus then does not leach from the soil. That is, it does not pass out, diffuse, or percolate through, but is rather adsorbed (gets adhered/coated) on the surface of soil particles. It then causes damage on erosion of the soil. As topsoil (surface soil), rich in phosphorus, erodes and passes into the streams and lakes, it can lead to good growth of algae, other aquatic plant life, and to significant **eutrophication**. Eutrophication is the process by which a body of water becomes enriched in dissolved nutrients, such as phosphorus. **Phosphorus then stimulates the growth of aquatic plant life.** (**'Eutrophication'** means **'good nourishment'.** In Greek **'eu'** = **good,** and **'trophe'** = **'nourishment'**). This process affects water quality as plants consume oxygen both during the 'dark cycle' and when the plant decays. **This results in the depletion of dissolved oxygen.** If this problem is allowed to continue unchecked, **it can ultimately lead to death of fishes on a large scale.** Eutrophication has therefore also been called as **'poisoning'** of the water source.

## Conclusions

1.  Phytate or phytic acid is a naturally occurring organic complex found in plants. **Phytate is a molecule rich in phosphorus. Phytate phosphorus** constitutes the major portion of the total phosphorus in the cereal seeds, grain legumes, and oil bearing plants.

2.  Typical poultry feeds contain 0.25-0.40% phytate phosphorus. **Only one-third of the total phosphorus is available to young chicks, and perhaps one-half is available to adult birds.** To compensate for the limited supply of available phosphorus, various inorganic phosphates, like dicalcium phosphate (DCP), are

usually included in the feed. DCP and bone meal are the two major phosphorus sources in the poultry feed.

3. **Phytate forms a wide variety of insoluble salts with minerals.** Phytic acid also complexes with proteins and starch and reduces their availability. Phytate also reduces the activity of enzymes pepsin, trypsin, and alpha-amylase. **It therefore has anti-nutritional properties.**

4. Because of a lack of enzyme phytase, which hydrolyzes phytate, **phytate phosphorus is biologically less available to poultry.** As a result, there is a high phosphorus concentration in the manure from birds fed on diets containing phytate, and this leads to **pollution of the environment.** About 70% of the phosphorus in the vegetable feed ingredients, along with valuable minerals, is excreted.

5. A number of factors influence phytate hydrolysis, such as dietary calcium content, inorganic phosphorus and vitamin D3, and the age and genotype of birds.

6. Cereal-based poultry diets supplemented with **microbial phytase** result in increased digestibility and availability of phytate bound phosphorus, calcium, zinc, copper, magnesium, manganese, and iron as well as amino acids. **Phosphorus availability of feeds is increased to 70%.** In general, an increase of 1-3% amino acid digestibility (availability) has been reported on addition of phytase to the feed. There is an effect on energy utilization as well. In other words, **phytase supplementation improves the digestibility of protein and amino acids** (perhaps lysine, methionine, arginine, histidine, threonine and tryptophan), **in addition to the positive effect on the phosphorus digestibility.** There is higher growth rate in broilers. In layers, addition of phytase prevents production drops and improves the shell thickness. In general, there is prevention of leg weakness and improvement of phosphorus related diseases.

7. Thus, excretion of phosphorus, calcium, copper and zinc, and perhaps, nitrogen to the environment can be reduced when the feeds are formulated with microbial phytase. **Therefore, instead of polluting the environment these nutrients benefit the poultry.** This helps to keep feed costs down as well as **helps to protect the environment.**

8. **Microbial phytase** supplementation also increases the intestinal digestibility of crude protein and amino acids in broiler chickens.

9. Supplementation of poultry feeds with microbial phytase results in clear benefits in terms of increased availability of phosphate-bound minerals and crude protein, and reduced environmental pollution through the lower levels of phosphorus and nitrogen excretion. **Phosphorus excretion in poultry can be reduced by 30% by including phytase in their feeds.**

10. Finally, **it is strongly recommended that phytase be added to poultry feeds.** Besides all the advantages narrated above, **it would also be economical and cost-effective, as dicalcium phosphate (DCP) may not be required to be added in the feed.** That is, addition of phytase improves the digestibility of phytate-phosphorus to the extent that phosphorus supplementation may become unnecessary.

**Note:** For a list of commercial preparations of the enzyme phytase available at the market, along with their indications and dosage, refer to Chapter 19 under **"Enzymes"**.

# Chapter 24

# Oligosaccharides

Oligosaccharides are coming up in a big way as an alternative to antibiotic growth promoters. This is because antibiotic resistance has become a major issue globally. Phosphorylated mannan-oligosaccharides (complex carbohydrates), derived from walls of certain yeast strains, appear as good as antibiotic growth promoters in their performance.

## What is an oligosaccharide?

'Oligo' is a Greek word which means 'few'. Thus, 'oligosaccharide' is a saccharide (i.e. a carbohydrate) that contains a known **small number** of monosaccharide units, such as mannose, fructose, or galactose.

Earlier, 'oligosaccharides' were classified as 'dietary fibre'. However, with the improvements in analytical techniques, 'oligosaccharides' are now grouped within the 'non-starch polysaccharide' moiety (i.e. component). This is because of the similarities in the response to the bird's intestinal enzymes. However, oligosaccharides are fermented by mainly beneficial intestinal micro-organisms. This explains the difference in bird's responses when oligosaccharides, rather than non-starch polysaccharides, are included in diets fed to birds. (For information on 'non-starch polysaccharides', refer to Chapter 23: "Enzymes").

## What are the different types of oligosaccharides?

These are of **two types:** (1) **Natural**, and (2) **Synthetic.** However, there are differences in the responses of the bird to natural and synthetic oligosaccharides. **Whereas natural oligosaccharides have harmful effects on bird's health and productivity, the synthetic oligosaccharides have beneficial effects.** These are due to the very low concentration at which the synthetic oligosaccharides are usually included in the feed.

## What are the sources of natural oligosaccharides?

Grain legumes are the most common natural sources of oligosaccharides. Concentrations of oligosaccharides are similar in soyabeans and legume seeds. In many grain legumes the most common oligosaccharide is stachyose (a sugar), followed by raffinose (a sugar) and verbascose (a sugar).

# What are the synthetic oligosaccharides?

**These are commercially manufactured oligosaccharides.** Production of **synthetic oligosaccharides** was started with the realization that, in contrast to natural oligosaccharides, many synthetic oligosaccharides possessed **beneficial effects** when present in feed. Some of the commonly used synthetic oligosaccharides are fructo-oligosaccharide, **mannan-oligosaccharide,** and galacto-oligosaccharide.

# What qualities do oligosaccharides possess?

Oligosaccharides possess several qualities. They have an ability to withstand high temperatures during feed pelleting. They also withstand the physical and chemical conditions of the gastro-intestinal tract.

Oligosaccharides are not digested by bird's enzymes. When fermented, they produce volatile fatty acids, which stimulate peristalsis (wave-like movements that force the intestinal contents forward) and decrease transit time through the intestine.

# What are the effects of oligosaccharides on bird's growth?

Mannan series of oligosaccharides, derived from oil palm kernels (seeds), increase muscle weight gain when fed to chickens. However, fructo- and galacto-oligosaccharides fed to broiler chicks do not increase any body weight gain. Variations in the effects of different classes of oligosaccharides depend on the age and species of bird and management conditions.

# What are the effects of oligosaccharides on bird's health?

Oligosaccharides do not have any direct effect on the feed. However, they indirectly influence productivity. **Their beneficial actions include:**

# 1. Prevention of intestinal colonization by disease-producing bacteria

**Mannan-oligosaccharide (MOS)** has a direct stabilizing effect on the normal intestinal microflora. In mannan-oligosaccharide, the monosaccharide units are sugar **mannose.** For most bacteria to colonize the gastro-intestinal tract (i.e. to establish themselves and grow), they must first attach to the intestine's lining epithelial cell's surface. They do this by their **lectins,** which recognize certain sugars (**mannose**) present on the intestinal epithelial cells **(Fig. 29).** Many disease-producing (pathogenic) bacteria which infect the intestine attach to these sugars through their type 1 fimbriae (fine thread-like structures) which recognize **mannose. Mannan-oligosaccharides occupy the lectin attachment sites on type 1 fimbriae and thus block the attachment of disease-producing bacteria to intestine (Fig. 29). As a result, bacteria are unable to establish themselves in the intestine and multiply (i.e. colonize).**

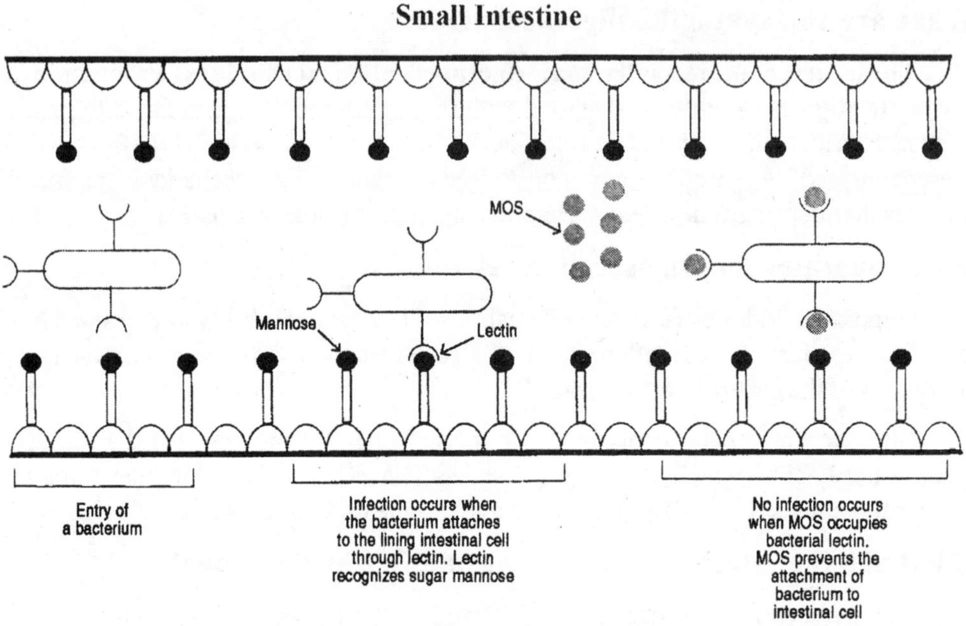

## Small Intestine

**Fig. 29.** MOS (mannan-oligosaccharide) blocking bacterial attachment.

Feeding of MOS has been found to significantly reduce the ability of *Escherichia coli* and *Salmonella typhimurium* to attach and establish infection in the caeca of chicken. Even some positive results have been observed with **clostridial organisms** (cause of necrotic enteritis), although they do not depend on mannose-sensitive lectins for intestinal attachment. Thus, by maintaining a stable gastro-intestinal environment, **MOS is able to reduce colonization by disease-producing bacteria. This, in turn, improves flock health and performance.**

When broiler chickens were fed **fructo-oligosaccharide (FOS)** and challenged with **Campylobacter** (intestinal bacteria that produce enteritis, i.e. inflammation of the intestine), only 8% of the chicks given FOS were colonized by the bacteria compared with 80% of chicks on the control feed. It was found that **gluco-oligosaccharide (GOS)** supported the proliferation (growth) of beneficial bacteria and not disease-producing species, such as **Clostridia** and **Salmonella**. For example, disease-producing bacteria cannot grow on fructo-oligosaccharide (FOS) and mannan-oligosaccharide (MOS). A low incidence of intestinal colonization with *Salmonella typhimurium* was observed in chickens fed on feeds supplemented with FOS than those fed on control diet. Chicks on the FOS-supplemented diet also grew faster than those on the control. Chickens treated with FOS had a fourfold reduction in the level of **Salmonella** in the caeca.

## 2. Direct inhibition of disease-producing bacteria

Oligosaccharides may directly prevent the growth of certain intestinal organisms, including the disease producing bacteria. They achieve this **by increasing the acidity through** an increase in the concentration of lactic acid in the lower intestine.

## 3. Increase disease resistance by improving the immune response of the bird

Phosphorylated mannan-oligosaccharides (MOS) have the capacity to modulate (regulate) the **immune system** and the intestinal microflora in the bird, and also to preserve the integrity of the intestinal absorptive surface. To understand how oligosaccharides improve the immune response, it is important to know the manner in which disease-producing organisms are dealt with in the body after their entry.

**For antibody (immunity) production, the antigen (a disease-producing organism) first has to be processed by antigen-processing (presenting) cells of the body** (see Chapter 32: "**The avian immune system**"). An antigen is any foreign substance that can induce an immune response. Bacteria, viruses, and other disease-producing organisms, are the most common antigens. On entry into the bird's body they are ingested by the antigen-processing cells **(Fig 30)**, broken down, processed and then presented to antibody-producing cells (see **Fig. 38**). **This step (processing of the antigen) is a must for induction of immunity.** The most important antigen-presenting cell in the chicken's body is a large phagocytic cell (i.e. capable of engulfing or eating an antigen) known as **'macrophage' (Fig. 30).** The macrophage is derived from a blood cell known as **'monocyte' (Fig. 30). The better the antigen processing by the macrophage, the better is the immune response.** Although resting macrophages can ingest the antigen, they are not as efficient to process the antigen as the activated cell. An **activated macrophage** is in a state of increased metabolic and functional activity. It therefore becomes a very effective antigen-processing cell.

**Chicken macrophages have mannose-binding receptors on their surface (Fig. 30).** MOS induces macrophage activation by occupying these

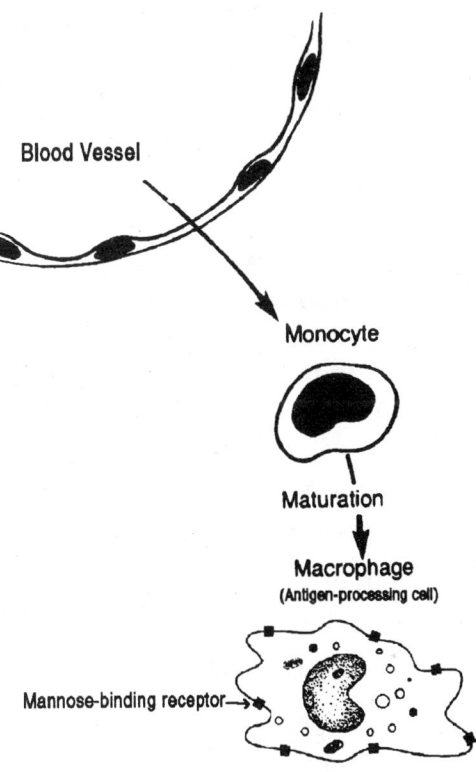

Fig. 30. Origin of macrophage in the chicken. Note the presence of mannose-binding receptors on the macrophage.

mannose-binding receptors. Once three or more of these receptors are occupied, a series of reactions are initiated which result in **macrophage activation**. The **activated macrophages** are more efficient in engulfing and destroying the disease-producing bacteria (i.e. antigens). On this account, adult macrophages are far more efficient in antigen processing and presentation to antibody producing cells. **MOS is thus able to initiate and induce a better immune response.** Moreover, it improves both the extent and uniformity of the response.

## 4. By increasing the body weight gain and FCR

With improvement in intestine's environment (see S. No. 1), **the efficiency of both digestion and absorption is improved.** As much as 50% of the dietary amino acids are used directly by the gastro-intestinal tract for repair and regeneration (replacement) of the lost cells. The lining epithelial cells of the gastro-intestinal tract are shed and replaced by new cells every 24 hours. Therefore, **by limiting the damage caused by disease-producing bacteria and their toxins, oligosaccharides make available more of the nutrients for conversion into muscle protein.** This is on account of both digestion and absorption. This has a positive effect on feed efficiency. As a result, there is an improvement in FCR of MOS-fed birds. It is now believed that **oligosaccharides, such as MOS, may provide a very useful substitute for antibiotic growth promoters.**

5. **Mannan-oligosaccharides also reduce the anti-nutritive or anti-nutritional properties of dietary lectins.**

6. **Toxin binding**

**MOS also acts as a toxin binder, and can bind a range of mycotoxins,** namely, aflatoxin, ochratoxin, T-2 toxin, fumonisin, citrinin and others, **with the lowest level of inclusion in the feed.** (See Chapter 22: **"Mould inhibitors and toxin binders"**). MOS provides an extremely high surface area for toxin binding. Moreover, toxin binding by MOS is highly stable and is unaffected either by intestinal enzymes or by variations in the intestinal pH.

## 7. Performance Enhancement

MOS, in poultry feed, has also a beneficial effect on bird's performance, namely, **FCR, weight gain, egg production, and liveability.**

## How do oligosaccharides differ from 'prebiotics'?

Oligosaccharides are in fact prebiotics. A prebiotic is an indigestible carbohydrate that selectively stimulates the growth and/or activity of one or a limited number of bacterial species already present in the large intestine of chickens. **Fructo-oligosaccharide (FOS) and mannan-oligosaccharide (MOS) are examples of prebiotics.**

## What is the relationship between oligosaccharides and 'synbiotics'?

**A synbiotic is a combination of probiotic and prebiotic** (i.e. an oligosaccharide). This combination improves the survival of the probiotic organism **because its specific substrate is available.** The chicken then gets the benefits of both, live micro-organisms of probiotic and the prebiotic as their substrate. The combination of fructo-oligosaccharide (FOS) and bifidobacteria is an example of synbiotic.

## What is the significance of having a uniform immune response? (Based on S. No. 3)

**Poorly immunized birds within the flock are prone to infectious diseases.** Once disease is established in these susceptible birds, the level of infection to which other birds in the flock are exposed is greatly increased as a result of organism's growth within the bird's body, and afterwards shedding. Vaccination failures and disease outbreaks are thus much more likely to occur in a flock with a non-uniform immune response. By improving the uniformity of the flock response to vaccination, it is possible to significantly reduce the risk and untoward effects of exposure to an infectious disease. **MOS enables to achieve this.**

## What are the negative effects, if any, of using oligosaccharides?

1. While there is plenty of evidence to show the benefit of including synthetic oligosaccharides in the diet, there is at the same time, **evidence of the negative effects of natural oligosaccharides to bird's health and productivity.** Therefore, various methods have been used to reduce or eliminate oligosaccharides from the feed, but the results are not entirely satisfactory. For example, ethanol extraction achieves only up to 90% reduction of the oligosaccharides present in soyabean meal. Enzymes (alpha-galactosidase and invertase) have often been employed to reduce the level of raffinose (a sugar) series oligosaccharides.

2. **The evidence of improved health status of the flock with inclusion of synthetic (commercial) oligosaccharides in the feed is convincing.** However, the response depends to some extent on the rearing environment. Flocks exposed to disease-producing organisms benefit more from oligosaccharide supplement than flocks raised under relatively hygienic environments. **Therefore, where disease risk is low, it would be better to reduce the level of oligosaccharide supplement in the feed.**

## What then is the overall conclusion?

1. Natural (raffinose series) oligosaccharides have negative effects on the growth of broiler chickens.

2. On the other hand, **synthetic oligosaccharides, such as mannan-oligosaccharide (MOS), have beneficial effects on the growth of the broiler chickens.** MOS

may provide a very effective method of improving flock health, uniformity and productivity, by:

(i) **Increasing disease resistance** by improving the extent and uniformity of vaccine response.

(ii) **Preventing intestinal colonization** with those bacteria that cause infection in the intestine.

(iii) **Indirectly improving intestine's health and integrity,** thus increasing nutrient digestion and absorption, and therefore FCR.

3. **Most of the current research favours the inclusion of various oligosaccharides in the feed on account of their beneficial effects.** In fact, phosphorylated mannan-oligosaccharides are now included as a standard ingredient in many poultry feeds around the world.

**Note:** For a list of various commercial (synthetic) oligosaccharides available at the market, and their indications and dosage, refer to Chapter 19 under **"Oligosaccharides".**

# Chapter 25

# Osmoregulators and Methyl Donors

## What is an osmoregulator?

An **'osmoregulator'** is a substance that helps in the maintenance of water and ion balance within the cell. This balance prevents cell's dehydration (water loss), and also maintains its function.

Birds maintain the concentration of water within the cell by **osmoregulation**. This is vital for the survival. Put simply, osmoregulation is the ability of a cell to maintain its structure and function by regulating movement of water in and out of the cell. And, any substance that regulates the water movement is known as an **'osmoregulator'**. An osmoregulator is also known by two other names, **'osmoprotectant'** and **'osmolyte'**.

## How does an osmoregulator act?

When the bird is subjected to stress, such as heat stress, or a disease like coccidiosis, the body cells come under **osmotic stress**. In such cases, water is drawn out of the cell because of a higher concentration of ions (salts/solutes) outside the cell. This loss of water **(dehydration)** causes the cell to shrink (become smaller), and if this water loss is not corrected, **the cell finally dies. An osmoregulator** (osmolyte) helps in maintaining water and ion balance within the cell, and thus **prevents its dehydration and also enables the cell to maintain its function.**

## How osmoregulation occurs in poultry?

**In poultry**, the kidney, large intestine, caeca and cloaca maintain body's osmoregulation. Body's water from drinking and eating, and also that formed from metabolism, must equal water lost by evaporation and through urine, faeces, and secretions from glands, in order for poultry to maintain osmoregulatory balance. **Electrolyte ingestion must also equal electrolyte excretion.**

## How diarrhoea disturbs osmotic balance in poultry?

**In diarrhoea**, following the water loss, amount of fluid outside the cell (i.e. extracellular or intercellular fluid) is reduced. As a result, osmotic pressure in this outside fluid increases since it now becomes hypertonic due to concentration of ions (salts/ solutes), following fluid loss. As a result, the osmotic pressure within the cell becomes comparatively low (hypotonic). **Thus, the osmotic balance is lost.** As per the rule of osmosis, fluid from a place of low osmotic pressure passes towards the site of high osmotic pressure. **Accordingly, following diarrhoea, water is pulled out of the cell.** This loss of water causes the cell to shrink, and if this water loss is not corrected, the **cell eventually dies.**

In an attempt to save itself, the cell then struggles to restore the water and ion balance, by using certain other mechanisms. But these other mechanisms put a high energy cost on the bird. The net result is that the amount of energy available to the bird for growth and reproduction is directed elsewhere. Here, **betaine (an osmoregulator)** helps in correcting the disturbed water and ion balance. **It accumulates within the cell and enables it to retain water. It thus prevents cell from dehydration and shrinkage, and its function is maintained.** The bird is therefore able to save energy, and then more energy becomes available for growth and reproduction.

Diarrhoea may result from coccidiosis, bacterial infection (*Escherichia coli, Clostridium perfringens, Pasteurella multocida,* and species of **Salmonella**), viruses (rotavirus) and fungi (*Candida albicans*). It may also occur from excessive consumption of water, sodium chloride, potassium, magnesium sulphate, and indigestible carbohydrates. **Diarrhoea in poultry is of great practical importance because it increases litter moisture,** and as a result, **increases atmospheric ammonia and foul-smell.** High litter moisture increases the susceptibility of a flock to infections (see '**Effects of ammonia**' and '**Litter management**').

## Do osmoregulators have a beneficial effect on diarrhoea?

Yes. **Osmoprotective substances prevent dehydration from the body cells and are therefore effective in stopping diarrhoea. Coccidiosis** in birds results in diarrhoea which may lead to dehydration. Osmoregulators protect the integrity and function of the cells. Osmoregulators may therefore also have beneficial effects in poultry under the influence of severe stresses, such as heat, high sodium intake, mycotoxin intake, and corticosterone. This aspect is being currently worked out.

## Which osmoregulators play a major role in osmoregulation?

**Organic osmoregulators.** These are the major modulators (regulators) of intracellular osmolarity. That is, the concentration of an osmotic solution within the cell. Of the different organic osmoregulators, **betaine** has emerged as the most important osmoprotective compound. It possesses beneficial osmolyte properties. As stated, **it accumulates within the cell and enables it to retain water.**

## What is betaine?

Betaine is a naturally occurring substance found in a wide variety of plant and animal species. For example, sugar beet molasses, a by-product of sugar production, is a major source of betaine.

In poultry, oxidation of **choline**, yields **betaine**. Betaine molecule possesses three methyl ($CH_3$) groups and acts as a methyl donor (i.e. giver of a methyl group). Betaine donates a **methyl group** to a substance called **homocysteine** to form **methionine** in the liver **(Fig. 31).**

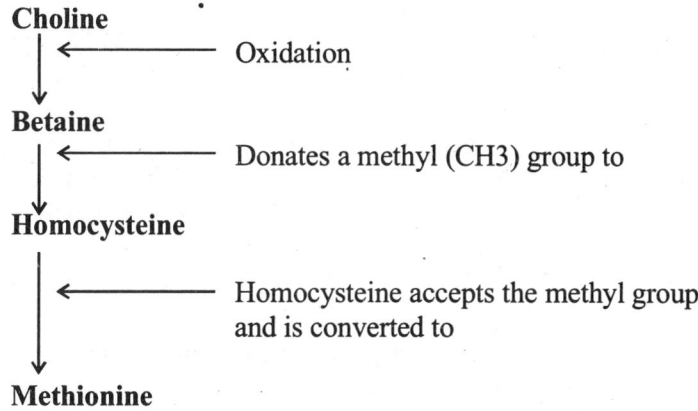

Fig. 31. Formation of methionine in the chicken.

## Is betaine being used in poultry?

Yes, because of its osmoprotective properties. Betaine has a beneficial effect in diarrhoeal diseases in poultry, and may also be helpful in poultry under the influence of severe stresses (stressors). **Betaine treatment has been reported to be effective in stopping diarrhoea.** It exerts protective effect on the integrity and functions of the intestinal lining epithelial cells and may be **an effective intracellular osmolyte in poultry.** For example, **in coccidiosis**, the presence of coccidia in the bird's intestine causes the water to flow out of the bird's intestinal epithelial cells into the content's of the intestine, **resulting in diarrhoea and dehydration.** The osmolyte function of betaine helps in removing the osmotic stress and intestinal changes caused by coccidia. **In the presence of some coccidiostats, betaine can improve bird's performance**

Betaine supplementation of feed, or in drinking water, may therefore be helpful in the control of dysfunctional osmoregulatory conditions, such as diarrhoea, diuresis (increased excretion of urine), and **ascites.** If the bird's total betaine requirement cannot be met through metabolism, a dietary source may be necessary. This is because, physiologically (functionally), betaine is one of several compounds used by body cells to regulate osmotic pressure.

## And, how does betaine act as a methyl donor?

As discussed, **choline** is first converted in poultry to betaine which then donates a methyl group ($CH_3$) to **homocysteine** to form **methionine** in the liver. Choline is transported from cytoplasm of the liver cell into the mitochondria (structures within the cell) where it is oxidized to betaine, and then betaine is transported back into the cytoplasm where it functions as a methyl donor to form methionine. **The growth responses obtained from betaine are due to its ability to provide methyl groups.**

For example, **during stress, the chicken needs more methionine.** This is because methionine generates a compound called 'S-adenosyl methionine' which donates methyl groups required in important chemical reactions in the body, such as DNA, RNA, and protein synthesis, **and the immune responses.** Betaine can reduce the amount of methionine required by providing the methyl groups needed for the regeneration of methionine from homocysteine in the transmethylation cycle. **This means that in the bird dietary methionine is spared.** Methionine can therefore be used for its other important function of protein synthesis, and thus growth and reproduction.

### As a methyl donor what then is the usefulness of betaine in poultry?

Methyl groups ($CH_3$) are fundamental for life. They are involved in hundreds of metabolic reactions. However, **methyl groups cannot be synthesized by the bird and so must be supplied in the diet.** The major dietary sources of methyl groups are methionine, choline, and betaine. **Betaine has three methyl groups, whereas methionine has only one.** Therefore, betaine is the more efficient methyl group donor. All animals require a constant supply of methyl groups. **In poultry, requirement for methyl groups increases during periods of high temperature, or stress, or in a diarrhoeic disease like coccidiosis.**

### Is commercial betaine available in the market?

Yes, some companies are preparing betaine and it is now available in the market.

### What then is the overall conclusion about the use of betaine in poultry, both as an osmoregulator and also as a methyl donor to save the cost of feeding choline and methionine?

**Betaine**, as a methyl donor, allows some methionine and choline to be spared from feed formulation. It can spare some added methionine and choline from broiler feed. By sparing supplementary methionine and/or choline in the diet, **betaine can reduce feed cost per tonne, while maintaining bird performance.**

However, recent work has revealed that poultry do not have a specific requirement for betaine provided they consume or synthesize sufficient choline. **But betaine does have an osmolyte function which helps the bird to maintain cell water balance under periods of stress.** It is therefore concluded that supplementation with betaine may be beneficial during certain challenging conditions, including the high metabolic demand of rapid growth, disease, and osmotic stress.

**Note:** For a list of various commercial osmoregulators and methyl donors available at the market, and their indications and dosage, refer to Chapter 19 under **"Osmoregulators and methyl donors".**

# Chapter 26

# Acidifiers

## What is an acidifier?

**Acidifiers are various organic acids** having an antimicrobial and pH regulating activity in the intestine. They include acetic acid, propionic acid, citric acid, phosphoric acid, formic acid, lactic acid, fumaric acid, etc. and their salts. In fact, they are a synthetic combination of organic acids and their salts.

## Why use an acidifier in poultry ration?

**An acidifier maintains gut health.** Health of the gut (intestine) is an important factor that governs the performance of birds, and therefore the farm economics. The health of the gut, in turn, depends on the population of its microflora (bacteria). The gut microflora consists of both Gram-positive and Gram-negative bacteria. **The Gram-positive bacteria are largely commensals (i.e. harmless or useful), while Gram-negative are disease-producing.** In general, there exists a delicate balance between the Gram-positive and Gram-negative populations of bacteria **at an ideal pH. A healthy gut has a greater number of Gram-positive bacteria.** This balance gets disturbed when there is a change in the pH due to the ingestion of certain toxic or chemotherapeutic agents (e.g. antibiotics, sulpha drugs), or an alteration in the feed composition. Disease occurs when the shift is towards bacteria that produce disease in the intestinal tract. **Thus, maintenance of the ideal pH for microbial balance is essential for keeping the gut healthy. It is here that the use of acidifiers is helpful in maintaining the microbial balance of the gut.**

## How do acidifiers work?

**Acidifiers effectively regulate the pH of the intestine.** They promote growth and health of the chicken by:

- **Decreasing the gastric (stomach) pH.** Common disease-producing bacteria, such as *Escherichia coli*, **Salmonella** sp., **Streptococcus** sp., **Staphylococcus** sp., and **Clostridium** sp. act within the range of 6 to 8 pH. **Their growth is inhibited when the pH falls and becomes acidic,** that is, outside their range of growth.

- In general, **the more acidic the pH of the medium, the greater is the antibacterial activity.** This is because acidic pH causes major damage to lipopolyssacharides of the outer membrane of Gram-negative bacteria. . Acidic pH also inactivates essential enzymes at the cell surface of bacteria.

- **At an alkaline pH,** the organic acids of the acidifiers are present mostly in a '**dissociated form**', whereas in the acidic pH they remain mostly '**un-dissociated**'. **It is in the un-dissociated form that they are able to enter into the bacteria through their cell membrane.** This is because, by partitioning into membrane lipid bilayers, un-dissociated organic acid molecules interfere with the activity of membrane protein/enzymes. **Thus, organic acids inhibit the growth of bacteria when concentration of the acid reaches a critical level.**

- **Once inside the bacteria** the more neutral environment within causes the organic acids to dissociate into H+ ions (hydrogen ions) and anions (negatively charged ions). The acid anions disrupt and interfere with DNA and protein synthesis, **causing bacterial death.**

## Why free acids are not used as such, instead of their salts or along with their salts?

This is because one of the major problems in their use as free acids is **corrosion**. That is, they destroy slowly by chemical action. Any liquid, including tap water, is to a certain degree corrosive. Therefore, free acid is combined with calcium, sodium, or ammonium. The advantage of salts over free acids is that they are easier to handle because they are no longer volatile (changing rapidly into gas). **Moreover, the strong corrosive effect which most free acids have on metals is greatly reduced.** Unfortunately, this neutralization of free acids into salts also has an effect on their efficiency. Their acidifying effect in the feed is reduced. Most of the acid in the salt is in dissolved form, making it less effective compared to free acids.

To overcome this problem, '**acid salts**' are prepared. In these products, the acid is only partly neutralized, giving the advantage of the free acid and the salt. **Such products are acidic without having the negative aspects of the free acids,** like corrosion and unpleasant smell. Therefore, the overall efficacy of **acid salts** is higher than that of the common salts, or the straight organic acids.

## How do acidifiers regulate pH and microbial balance of the gut?

After ingestion, the feed reaches the stomach of the chicken. Gastric acid (hydrochloric acid) is secreted in the proventriculus to lower the pH of the digesta. **A low pH in the stomach and upper intestine is important for the following reasons.**

1. **Pepsin,** the proteolytic enzyme (i.e. enzyme that digests protein) of the stomach, is activated from pepsinogen **only at low pH (2 to 4).** In other words, the low pH activates pepsinogen. This results in **better digestibility of proteins and absorption of amino acids.** If the stomach pH remains high, protein breakdown is

interfered with. This not only affects the digestibility and utilization of protein, **but also of minerals.**

Passage of digesta through the proventriculus coats food particles with hydrochloric acid and pepsin. The secretions of the proventriculus have a pH of about 2, but the digesta usually buffers some of the acid, resulting in slightly higher pH within proventriculus and gizzard.

2.  **Acidifiers decrease the gastric pH.** A low gastric pH is also essential to control the bacterial population in the stomach. **Proliferation (growth) of disease-producing bacteria, such as** *Escherichia coli,* **decreases in an acid environment, whereas beneficial Lactobacilli species are more tolerant to low pH values.**

3.  When using feeds with high **B-values** (B-value is discussed later), the pH in the upper digestive tract remains too high. Protein digestion then does not proceed normally. This leads to undigested protein reaching the lower digestive tract. Excessive protein fermentation may then occur, resulting in the **formation of toxic biogenic** (produced by living organisms) **amines.**

4.  **The low pH** does not allow less fermentable substrates to pass through, and therefore **prevents the fermentation that occurs in the lower intestine. It thus inhibits proliferation of harmful bacteria.**

## What then are the benefits of using acidifiers?

1.  Acidifiers **regulate pH and microbial balance of the gut.** Treatment with salts of propionic acid and formic acid can cause a significant drop in the caecal counts of *Salmonella typhimurium*. Synergistic acid blends also **reduce the counts of** *E. coli* and coliforms in the small intestine, caeca, and rectum, without affecting the lactobacilli counts.

2.  Acidifiers **promote digestion** by activating the digestive enzymes.

3.  Acidifiers **favour mineral absorption** by creating an ideal pH in the intestine.

4.  Acidifiers **promote palatability of feed.**

5.  Acidifiers **enhance nutrient utilization** by birds.

6.  By inhibiting the growth of disease-producing bacteria in the **feed or drinking water,** and also in the intestinal tract of the bird, but at the same time allowing growth of beneficial intestinal bacteria, **acidifiers can significantly improve bird's health and performance.**

7.  Organic acids in the feed reduce pathogenic (disease-causing) micro-organisms and as a result there is **less stimulation of the bird's immune system.**

8. **In poultry,** organic acids also play a role in the **bird's growth.** The acidic environment on the intestinal epithelial surface allows diffusion of the undissociated acids into the bacteria and enterocytes (intestinal epithelial cells) for their effect. The positive influence of fumaric acid, propionic acid, sorbic acid, and tartaric acid has been seen on **feed conversion ratio (FCR), or growth performance.**

## How do acidifiers bring about improved absorption of nutrients?

**Organic acids influence gut morphology, that is, intestinal structure.** They increase villus height, and therefore the absorptive capacity of the intestine. Villi (singular 'villus') are minute finger-shaped processes found on the mucous membrane (i.e. inner surface) of the small intestine. These are involved in the absorption of nutrients. **The increased absorptive capacity contributes to improved protein, energy, and mineral absorption.**

## Are there differences in the effects of different organic acid supplements?

Yes. Acetic acid and propionic acid show moderate effects on feed pH, while formic acid, lactic acid, fumaric acid, citric acid and phosphoric acid lower feed pH substantially. Furthermore, some organic acids also show antibacterial properties, as in formic, lactic, acetic, and propionic acids. Therefore, **to obtain the best results those acidifiers must be used that possess the strongest antibacterial properties.**

## What is the guideline on which acidifiers should be formulated and mixed in the ration? What is B-value?

This guideline is based on the **acid binding capacity of feed raw materials and ingredients.** Each feed ingredient has a particular acid binding capacity. This has to be taken into consideration while formulating poultry ration.

'B-value' indicates the amount of acid required to lower the pH of a feed to a certain value. Different methods are used to determine the **'buffering capacity' or 'B-value'.**

Protein ingredients (soyabean meal, fish meal) generally have relatively high buffering capacities, whereas cereals (maize, rice, wheat, barley) have low B-values. Premixes show high B-values mainly because calcium carbonate ($CaCO_3$) is used as a carrier.

## Is it possible to calculate the B-value of feed from the B-values of the feed components?

Yes. However, this is correct only when the B-value of the feed component is assessed using an end point pH of 5. When using a lower end point pH (3 or 4), B-values are no longer additive. Also, B-values of feed ingredients may vary between batches.

**Therefore, it is not easy to use ingredient B-values from tables to calculate the B-value of a finished feed.**

Formulating diets to reduce their acid binding capacity depends on the composition of the feed. One approach is to adjust the protein and mineral content of the diet. **Diets with high protein and mineral (calcium and phosphorus) content tend to have higher B-values.**

## Are there any problems in young birds?

High B-values may pose particular problems to the health of young birds, mainly because **young birds have limited capacity to secrete gastric acid (hydrochloric acid).** That is, young chicks may have difficulties in lowering their gastric (proventricular) pH. **In poultry, the main problem with high buffering capacity of feedstuffs is the proliferation of harmful bacteria in the digestive tract.**

## What then is the overall conclusion?

There is a movement toward antibiotic-free poultry farming and **acidifiers can be used as an alternative to antibiotics.** It is expected that acidifiers will gain widespread application as they benefit poultry industry.

**Note:** For a list of commercial acidifiers available in the market and their dosage, refer to Chapter 19 under **"Acidifiers"**.

# Chapter 27

# Biosurfactants

### What is a 'biosurfactant'?

A **'surfactant'** is a surface-active substance (<u>surf</u>ace–<u>act</u>ive+<u>ant</u>), such as a detergent. A detergent is a cleansing agent, such as soap. A **'biosurfactant'** acts on the living surfaces ('bio' in Greek means 'life'), that is, it acts on the internal surfaces of animals/ birds.

### Why use a biosurfactant in poultry ration?

A biosurfactant is used **to increase absorption of nutrients.**

### How does a biosurfactant increase absorption of nutrients?

A nutrient is of use to the bird only after it is absorbed from the intestine into the blood circulation. Under the present intensive poultry farming, where the birds are given high quality and density nutrition, and also because of the short length of the intestine, there is not enough time for complete absorption of the nutrients. **Thus, some nutrients are excreted unabsorbed. This results in poor performance of the flock.**

A nutrient is absorbed only when it is soluble in water, and then it is taken into the blood circulation. Thus, water soluble nutrients like sugars and certain amino acids are readily and completely absorbed. **The absorption of water insoluble nutrients like fatty acids, fat soluble vitamins and certain amino acids in the intestine is helped by 'biosurfactants'.** Biosurfactants form complexes with these nutrients, called **'micelles'**, which can then be easily absorbed. (**'Micelle'** is a Latin word and means **'an extremely small particle'**.) The rate of absorption of micelles is inversely proportional to their size. This means that if size of micelles is small, absorption is more, and if size is large, absorption is less. Phospholipids in bile are the natural biosurfactants produced by liver, which facilitate micelle formation. **Recent work has revealed that supplementation of biosurfactants helps in rapid and complete absorption of nutrients from the intestine.**

**Note:** For a list of commercial biosurfactant preparations and their dosage, refer to Chapter 19 under **"Biosurfactants".**

## Section IV

# DISEASE CONTROL

# Chapter **28**

# Introduction

The importance of disease control in poultry industry cannot be over-emphasized. This is because to achieve the best genetic potential in respect of egg and meat production, hatchability, liveability and growth, it is necessary to maintain healthy flocks. **It is more economical to pay proper attention to methods of disease prevention, rather than fight a losing battle afterward once a disease outbreak has occurred.**

Vaccination and to some extent medication, along with a regular programme of health monitoring, have helped in improving the health status of many flocks. **Hygiene and biosecurity are the key factors.** In fact, to achieve the best disease control, it is necessary to maintain good hygiene standards. Hygiene is concerned with preventing the entry of infectious organisms into the flock, in minimizing the spread of infection should it occur, and finally in eliminating infection from the farm. To achieve the best results from any disease control programme, attention has to be given to the ways in which disease-producing organisms can spread and to look closely at management to find out where and how this can be minimized. **All these aspects are discussed at some length in the first three chapters, namely, biosecurity, disinfection, and sanitization.**

The second part of the section deals with controlling diseases through **vaccination.** Vaccination builds protection against disease-producing organisms known as **'immunity'.** **Vaccination is an extremely important aspect of disease control.** But there are already so many vaccines in the market and new ones keep coming. As a result, a farmer often gets confused. Moreover, so much technical literature on vaccines and chicken's immune system keeps pouring all the time that the farmer may be totally lost. **Therefore, in the 5th chapter of this section (Chapter 32), the fundamentals and certain basic concepts of the avian (of the bird) immune system are discussed in some detail.** Then, the next chapter discusses the ways and means to boost bird's immune system to obtain the best protection. This is followed by a discussion on the nature of live and killed vaccines and the various vaccination schedules.

**It is only through the collective implementation of biosecurity, disinfection, sanitization and effective vaccination programme that diseases can be kept under control and the flock healthy.**

# Chapter 29

# Biosecurity

## What is biosecurity?

'**Bio**' in the word '**biosecurity**' is of Greek origin, and means '**life**'. Here, it implies '**living organisms**'. **Thus, biosecurity is security, or safety and protection of birds against disease-producing organisms. Biosecurity therefore includes all the measures that should be taken to prevent viruses, bacteria, fungi, protozoa, parasites, rodents, and wild birds from coming in contact with birds on the farm.**

**Biosecurity is the most efficient and cost-effective method of disease prevention. Disease management and eradication are difficult and expensive.** In fact, they are alternatives to a failed disease prevention programme. Effective implementation of biosecurity measures prevents many threats to poultry health. As the topic is of great practical importance, it is being dealt with at some length.

## The Nature of Disease-Producing Organisms

In all biosecurity programmes, it is most important first to consider the nature of various disease-producing organisms, **particularly in respect of their ability to survive in the environment.** This is because their capacity to survive away from the bird would influence their chances of infecting the birds. **This in turn will determine the extent to which biosecurity may have to be used.**

Mechanical spread occurs when the disease-producing organism is carried on the surface of people and their clothes, equipment, wild animals, or insects. They are then brought into physical contact with a susceptible chicken. **All-in, all-out management systems help in the removal of disease agents that do not survive well outside the chicken, such as mycoplasma, infectious coryza bacterium, avian influenza virus, and infectious laryngotracheitis virus. Providing at least two weeks of rest (downtime) to the poultry house between flocks** (i.e. keeping it vacant) will improve the effectiveness of disease management on the farm and reduce the time and money spent on vaccines and medicines. Traffic should follow from younger to older birds and from healthy to sick birds.

The risk of infection from a previous flock depends, in part, on the **nature of infectious agents.** For example, some infectious agents persist in the environment longer than others **(Table 9).** The infectious status of the previous flock should be considered when planning the placement of a new flock. **After a disease outbreak, period of rest given to the poultry house should take into consideration the shedding time of the agent and its survival time in the environment (Table 9).**

Table 9.   Survival time of disease-causing organisms

| Disease | Infectious agent | Life-span away from birds |
|---|---|---|
| Ranikhet disease | Virus | Days to weeks |
| Gumboro disease | Virus | Months |
| Infectious bronchitis | Virus | Weeks to months |
| Infectious laryngotracheitis | Virus | Weeks |
| Avian influenza | Virus | Weeks to months |
| Marek's disease | Virus | Months |
| Lymphoid leukosis | Virus | A few hours |
| Fowl pox | Virus | Months to years |
| Infectious coryza | Bacterium | Hours to days |
| Salmonellosis | Bacterium | Weeks |
| Fowl cholera | Bacterium | Weeks |
| Pullorum disease | Bacterium | Months |
| Fowl typhoid | Bacterium | Months |
| Staphylococcosis | Bacterium | Months |
| Avian tuberculosis | Bacterium | Years |
| Mycoplasmosis (MG, MS) | Mycoplasma | Hours to days |
| Coccidiosis | Protozoa | Months |

## I.   Sources of Infection

**Infections enter into a flock from various sources.** To understand why various biosecurity measures are important, it is necessary first to examine briefly the sources and routes of infection.

## 1.   Humans

**Because of their movements, duties, curiosity, ignorance, lack of concern, carelessness, or total concentration on profits, humans constitute one of the greatest potential causes of introduction of disease.** This is because they come in contact with infectious agents, use contaminated equipment, or manage their flocks in such a way that spread of disease is unavoidable.

Usually, **footwear** (shoes, 'chappals') is suspected as the means of transport of disease, but **hands** can become contaminated with infected material, such as exudates (inflammatory fluids) when lesions and discharges are examined. **Clothing** can also become contaminated with dust, feathers, and droppings. At least one disease-causing organism (Ranikhet disease virus) has been found to survive for several days on the mucous membrane (i.e. lining) of the human respiratory tract, and has been isolated from the sputum.

## 2. Neighbours

A common source of infection is a disease outbreak at a neighbouring farm. Visits among poultry farmers are a common way of spreading diseases. If a neighbour's flock is infected with a serious disease, **discuss it by telephone.** It is best to warn neighbours not to visit when disease is in progress, and certainly do not walk around on a neighbour's farm for any purpose.

## 3. Contract Workers/Labourers

Much of farm management requires periodic use of a group of workers for debeaking (beak trimming), vaccination, blood testing, weighing, and shifting birds from one place to another. The farm manager usually has difficulty in finding workers who are easily available and have sufficient knowledge of handling poultry. Therefore, people who work at many poultry farms are contacted and hired. Such workers travel around the poultry farms handling many flocks, and must therefore be regarded as a potential source of infection. **The farm manager should take strict precautions to safeguard the health of every flock with which they work.**

## 4. Visitors

**No casual visitors are to be permitted in or near the poultry premises.** Official visitors should always be taken to the flocks in increasing order of age, observing the precaution that they have not visited any other farm on that day. They should be provided with footwear and a clean outfit of clothing before visiting the flocks. **Visitor's vehicles should not be allowed inside the farm premises.**

Disease outbreaks on a farm have been known to follow the visit of a careless visitor. **If visitors do not enter premises or buildings, they cannot bring in or carry away diseases.**

The source of a new or dreaded disease like Gumboro is often puzzling. World trade and travel are becoming more commonplace. It is not uncommon for a person to leave one farm in the morning and be visiting another farm or place of business in another part of the country on the same day. **Some disease agents easily survive during** that period. All who travel should be aware of this, and must be careful against introducing the disease into their own flocks, or into the premises of friends, or fellow farmers when returning from a trip.

## 5.  Recovered Carriers

**Carrier birds are those which appear to have recovered from disease, but still retain the infectious organism in some part of the body.** While they appear healthy, the infectious organism continues to multiply (increase in number) in the body and to be shed into the environment. Like actively infected flocks, they can spread a disease on a farm and thus constitute a threat to other birds. **Many commonly occurring diseases are known to be transmitted by carriers.**

## 6.  Multiple Ages

**Multiple ages on premises constitute a serious disease threat, from both diseased bird and recovered carriers.** This is particularly important if birds of different age groups are closely associated through management practices, or nearness. Disease organisms from sick birds, or recovered carriers, are passed by various ways, including direct contact, to each new susceptible flock brought into the premises. Serious drops in production may occur in young laying flocks moved into laying premises where carrier birds from previous disease outbreaks had remained.

## 7.  Induced-Moulted Hens

Induced-moulting of laying hens (or breeders) is usually practised, particularly during times of economic stress to meet an emergency egg demand, or improve declining shell quality, or because it is considered economical at that time. One advantage of keeping induced-moulted hens, rather than rearing new replacement growers, is that old hens are not likely to suffer from a disease that normally occurs during the rearing age. If such flocks are moulted and kept in the same house, **then there is no risk of disease problems developing**. On the other hand, a farmer who collects spent hens for moulting from many poultry farms and mixes them on one premise at one time runs a serious risk. This is because any of the moulted groups may be carriers of a disease to which the others are susceptible.

## 8.  Poultry Show Birds

Birds exhibited at poultry shows may be exposed to **infected or symptomless carrier birds** of exhibitors from which they contract disease. The **contact-infected birds** may not develop symptoms until returned to the owner's farm, where they may then be a source of new infection. **A basic rule for show birds is that they should never be returned to the owner's farm.** If birds must be shown, such should be selected that can be sold after the exhibition. If the birds must be returned, they should be quarantined for several weeks.

## 9.  Mixed Species of Poultry

One species which is naturally very resistant to a disease may act as a carrier of that disease for another species that is very susceptible. For example, histomoniasis may cause mild death losses in chickens, but in turkeys, the losses can be extremely serious. Also, a silent mycoplasma infection in chickens may spread to mycoplasma-free turkeys and result in extremely serious sinusitis and airsac infection. **Therefore, two species should never be run together.**

Some diseases may be rather harmless in one species of chicken, but very serious in another. **Also keep meat and laying chickens separate, since the same disease may have different economic importance in the two types.**

## 10.  Hospital Pen

Sick birds from several pens collected into one hospital pen, or house, and later returned to their respective pens may carry back one or more **diseases contracted while in the hospital area.** Therefore, hospital pens are not recommended for routine segregation of sick birds **unless they are ultimately to be sent to the diagnostic laboratory, or burned.** If used for a special purpose (such as observation, injury, pecking), there should be a temporary arrangement within the house, **and it should hold birds from only one pen or house.**

## 11.  Backyard and Pet Fowl

Poultry kept as pets, or to supply household eggs or meat, are just as capable of carrying and transmitting diseases as are commercial flocks.

## 12.  Soiled Vehicles and Equipment

Diseases and parasites can be carried on vehicles and equipment. Vehicles and equipment usually have accumulations of litter and faeces that can be a threat to other farms and houses. **Soiled vehicles and equipment can carry disease organisms.** They should be washed free of litter and droppings, and also disinfected after each transport of live birds, before use in another farm area. **One gram of chicken faeces can contain enough virus particles to infect one million (ten lakhs) birds with avian influenza.**

**Fowl pox, Gumboro disease and Marek's disease viruses, coccidia, roundworm eggs, and other infectious material** can be carried on crates (large containers for carrying eggs and birds), footwear, and vehicles, particularly on the floor and foot control pedals of a vehicle.

**Artificial insemination equipment,** particularly reused inseminating tubes, offer an excellent method of transmitting disease.

Poultry transporting vehicles and equipment can spread infectious material through feathers, faeces, blood, exudates, and skin scabs (crusts) left in the crates, or picked up at the slaughter plant. **Transport equipment should be washed and disinfected after use before being taken to another farm.**

## 13. Laboratory exposure

A farmer, particularly a small flock owner, may like to take a bird home after a veterinarian has examined it at the laboratory. While in the laboratory, even for a short time, live birds have a good chance to contract some infectious agent. **Therefore, no bird should be returned from the laboratory to the farm,** because it could develop disease and be the source of a new infection on the home premises. **The bird should be sacrificed and subjected to postmortem.**

**A disease may be carried from laboratory to a farm by careless laboratory or service workers, or the farmers. Therefore, precautions against carrying disease from the laboratory to the farm should be taken by the farmer and service worker.**

## 14. Rodents

Rodents are a group of small animals with strong sharp front teeth, such as **rats, mice, squirrels** and beavers (see 'rodents'). **Rodents contaminate feed and litter with their faeces.** They are particularly important in the control of **Salmonella**, because they are frequently infected with these organisms and can maintain and spread the disease on a farm.

## 15. Household Pets

**Dogs** and **cats**, like rodents, are capable of harbouring enteric organisms (i.e. those infecting intestine) which are infectious to poultry. When these pets are not confined to the household area, but roam among the poultry in the pens and farms, they constitute a serious health hazard. **Such pets are just as capable of carrying contaminated material on their feet and in their hair, as people.**

## 16. Wild Birds

Wild birds are capable of carrying a number of diseases and parasites. Some cause illness in the wild birds themselves; for others, the birds act as mechanical carriers. Every effort should be made to prevent their nesting in the poultry farms. **Domestic pigeons can also be a source of dangerous strains of Ranikhet disease virus.**

## 17. Insects

**Many insects act as transmitters of disease.** Some are intermediate hosts for blood and intestinal parasites; others are mechanical carriers of disease through their biting parts. Still others, because of their feeding habits and hiding places, appear to be reservoirs of disease by means of which the infectious agent survives from one flock to the next.

## 18. Feed

**Some ingredients may contain infectious agents,** particularly **Salmonella**, from contamination at their source, or anywhere along the production line, or storage areas. Pelleting, if done properly, is a practical method of greatly reducing infectious agents because of the heat generated in the process. **Meat meal** and **bone meal** are the feed ingredients most likely to introduce **Salmonella** species. The risk can be avoided by using only vegetable protein ingredients, supplemented as necessary with synthetic amino acids.

## II. Management Factors in Disease Prevention

Good disease-prevention practices have been compared with a chain which is only as strong as its weakest link. Many sound principles may become worthless from failures to carry out one or two related ones, which are either ignored or not considered essential. **Although it may not always be possible to use all the practices, the more are followed, the greater are the chances of avoiding disease outbreaks.**

## 1. Isolation

It is very important that the **poultry farm** has an **isolated location. This will avoid most disease problems.** No exact minimum distance from other poultry farms can be stated because this is influenced by prevailing winds, climate, type of houses, and other factors. **The greater the distance from other poultry farms, the less chances of contracting disease from them. Isolation** can be achieved by taking advantage of natural or artificial barriers, such as rivers, creeks, hills, cities, towns, or forests.

Not all farmers follow the same disease control practices. A close neighbour may ignore them and is then burdened with diseases until forced out of business by economic pressures. In the meanwhile, disease organisms present on his farm may be spread by air, or carried by various vectors (i.e. organisms, such as insects that transmit disease) and fomites (inanimate substances that mechanically spread disease-producing organisms) to neighbouring farms. **Thus a disease sometimes may enter into even well-managed farms.** Until a disease has been eradicated, it serves as a reservoir and potential source of infection for future flocks on the same premises and also those on the neighbouring premises. The closer the houses of one premises to those of another, the more likely is the spread of infection to healthy birds on a neighbouring farm. **Farmers who do not minimize losses go out of business.** Many left out poultry farms are purchased or leased by other poultry farmers.

## 2. Birds of One Age at One Farm

**From disease prevention point of view, it is always better to have birds of**

**only one age at one farm, rather than having birds of different ages.** When birds of one age are maintained, houses become vacant each time growers are moved to the layer premises, or each time the broilers are sold, or each time the old layers are sent to market. The premises are then cleaned, washed, and disinfected, and left vacant for as long as possible, **but at least for two weeks before healthy stock is introduced.**

**Keeping premises vacant is most effective in controlling disease organisms which do not survive for long outside the bird.** This applies to most respiratory infections (mycoplasma infection, infectious coryza, laryngotracheitis). However, it is not much effective in controlling disease agents that are more resistant and survive long periods in nature (coccidia, clostridia). **In general, the longer poultry house remains vacant, the lower the number of surviving disease-producing organisms.**

Moreover, in birds of one age at one farm, should a disease occur, the flock can be treated and handled in the best way possible until its disposal. **All this is not possible when birds of different ages exist on a farm.**

The best way to prevent infection from carrier birds is to remove the entire flock from the farm before any new replacements are added, and **to rear young stock in complete isolation from older recovered birds on a separate segment of the farm, or preferably on another farm and in an isolated area.**

## 3. Functional Units

For certain economic reasons, it is not always possible to limit the entire farm to a single age of poultry. In such cases, it should be divided into separate units, or areas for different groups of birds. **Each area is then periodically kept vacant, cleaned, and disinfected.** Much stricter security procedures for personnel, bird and equipment movements are necessary for this type of operation. There is no definite formula for minimum distances between houses or units. The most important factor in dividing the farm into isolated units is to provide units that can be quarantined (kept in isolation) to prevent spread and facilitate elimination of disease, should it occur.

## 4. Building Construction

The first rule in poultry house construction is to prevent flying wild birds and insects from entering. This is because many carry mites and harbour them on their nests (see **'mites'**). Also, many species of **wild birds** have been found susceptible to some common viral and bacterial diseases of poultry, and thus **could act as carriers. Bird-proofing can be done in open-type houses in hot climates.**

## (a) Entrances

An area (a slope or ramp) of concrete at the entrance of poultry house helps in preventing entry of disease into the unit. Rain and sunshine keep the area clean and sterilized. **A water tap, boot brush, and covered metal container of disinfectant** should be made available on the slope for disinfecting footwear (shoes, 'chappals', etc.) This further helps in keeping litter and soil-borne diseases out of the house. **Shoes must be thoroughly cleaned before the person steps into the container of disinfectant. Failure to remove organic matter will prevent even the strongest of disinfectants from destroying disease-producing organisms**. Moreover, the disinfectant is ineffective unless replaced frequently to ensure a potent solution at all times.

### (b) Ventilation

Poultry buildings should be constructed to provide protection against violent or severe weather conditions, yet not create stress conditions such as **excess dust**, insufficient ventilation with **ammonia build-up** (a gradual increase), or **wet litter.**

There are many advantages of windowless and temperature-controlled (i.e. environmentally controlled) houses, but one serious drawback is the development, in some cases, of extremely dry and dusty litter. **Colibacillosis outbreaks are usually associated with inhalation of excessive dust.** Coccidial oocysts require moisture to develop into the infective stage. Extremely dry litter prevents their development. On the other hand, **improper ventilation can lead to excessively wet litter, which favours the survival and development of coccidia and other parasites.**

**Ammonia fumes develop in wet litter.** If ventilation is poor and fumes accumulate, they may reach high concentration to prevent growth and performance of birds, cause kerato-conjunctivitis, and aggravate respiratory infections.

Litter will dry better if it can be stirred (mixed up) frequently. However, in spite of all efforts, it may remain wet in winter or in humid climates. **If wetness and excess ammonia concentration persist, litter should be replaced and ventilation improved.**

### (c) Floors and Cages

All surfaces inside the building should be of impervious material (i.e. not allowing water to pass through), such as concrete, so that it can be thoroughly washed and disinfected.

Raised slatted floors have been used successfully for years for laying chickens, both for adults and rearing birds. Such floors have alternate wooden pieces and spaces, each about ¾ inch wide, to allow droppings to fall through the open spaces and be out of reach of the birds. **This prevents recycling of infection and thus helps in the control of intestinal diseases and parasites.** Coccidial infection is thus avoided or greatly reduced. Broilers are likely to develop leg problems and breast blisters if raised on completely slatted or wire floors.

Keeping laying hens in cages has become an accepted practice in both closed and open-type houses in hot climates. Cages and wire floors are widely used also to rear growers, destined for cages as adults. The system is so successful in preventing intestinal diseases that birds have no chance to develop immunity to them. **Coccidiosis occurs if chickens reared in cages are transferred to litter floors.** Drugs can be used successfully to control coccidiosis in these birds.

## (d) Feeders and Drinkers

**Rats, mice** and other rodents should be out of feed because they may introduce and **spread salmonella,** or other disease organisms, which can be the source of an outbreak in the poultry flock.

Feed spilled in litter increases intake of litter and litter-borne disease agents. For example, more coccidial oocysts and less coccidostat are ingested, and a clinical disease may occur. **If poultry are allowed to eat litter,** mortality and depression can occur from impaction of the gizzard, and litter fragments may cause enteritis by mechanical irritation.

**Feed troughs** should have some type of guard to keep poultry out, and should not be overfilled to avoid spilling of feed into litter. Feeders without guards allow defaecation into feed, which results in the spread of infectious agents shed in faeces. Wet feed in litter attracts wild birds and rodents and provides a good medium for growth of **fungus and moulds,** which can cause liver, kidney, immune system disorder, or other damage to poultry.

**Drinkers** are usually set or hung over the litter area. In such a case, drinkers should be so managed **that the spillage of water on the litter is minimum.** Drinkers are basically of two types: (1) those which provide a constant reservoir of water, such as troughs (i.e. channels) and hanging plastic bells, and (2) nipple drinkers, which supply water on demand when activated by a bird.

**Drinkers which provide an open reservoir of water must be cleaned and disinfected regularly to prevent the build-up of potentially disease-causing organisms in the water supply.** These drinkers are also more prone to spillage and may cause problems of wet litter. The advantages of nipple drinkers are that they provide water free of organisms which are commonly present in the poultry houses, and also there is a decreased water spillage. **The dry litter conditions provided by nipple drinkers result in decreased growth or maturation of coccidia, bacteria, and fungi in the litter.**

## (e) Feed and Water Medication

**In spite of all precautions, birds may become sick.** When birds are grouped in large numbers in one big pen, separation and treatment of individuals is not possible; mass medication and vaccination are then necessary if any treatment is to be given.

Feed medication is not the best method of treatment for sick birds because of the loss of appetite (desire for food) and their inability to compete for feed. **Water medication is better because the sick birds usually drink when they will not eat.** Mass medication keeps the disease in check until the bird can respond with a successful immune response. Mass vaccination through drinking water is an accepted and successful labour-saving practice. **If drinking water is chlorinated or otherwise treated, the sanitizing agent may destroy the vaccine.** Therefore, use untreated or distilled water for mixing and administering water vaccine.

Several methods are used to reduce, remove, or neutralize chlorine in chlorinated water supplies. **The best practical method is to add protein to the water when mixing vaccines.** A common practice is to add 1 lb of non-fat dried milk to 50 gallon water, in tanks.

If a building is constructed with a big water tank, the tank should be of plastic, or lined with some non-reactive protective substance, and should be easy to reach for cleaning and for mixing of medicines. A metering device to measure feed and water consumption is useful to keep track of the health of the flock. **Use of a watering system with nipple drinkers for individual cage units helps in preventing spread of disease.**

## III. Personnel Control

### 1. Company and Farm Workers

Managers, supervisors, and owners are sometimes the worst people to break the sanitation rules. These people usually visit many different types of poultry farms, farm units, poultry industries, and spread disease organisms. **They should set a good example for the workers.** One of the most important aspects of disease control is **awareness on the part of everyone, that is, managers, supervisors, owners, workers, feed and supply delivery people; egg, bird and litter transporters; and all those who visit or work on poultry farms, that each has an important role in the disease-prevention programme.**

### 2. Visitors

Visitors can cause only minimum harm if they cooperate fully with strict sanitary rules. When they enter the poultry premises (houses, sheds) it is important that they wear disinfected rubber overshoes (gumboots) and other footwear. Also, they should wear protective clothes such as clean aprons. Disposable plastic boots may become punctured when used on gravel (mixture of small stones and coarse sand), or other sharp surfaces. Therefore, only heavy plastic disposable boots should be used. **These sanitary precautions are particularly essential when entering brooding and rearing houses, but will be helpful in keeping disease out of any house or pen.**

## IV. Sanitary Environments

## (A) Grounds around the Buildings

## 1. Rodent Control

Heaps of rubbish and unused equipment are good hiding and breeding places for **rats, mice and ground squirrels (see 'rodents')**. These may **serve as reservoirs of disease and contaminate troughs (water channels) with their faeces.** Rodents are reluctant to travel over open spaces which do not provide protective cover. A 20-metre strip (belt) of shortly cut grass, or gravel, discourages the migration of rodents into the poultry building from surrounding areas. It is more difficult to get rid of rodents once the premises are infected, than to keep them out from the beginning.

## 2. Insect Control

Many parasites and disease agents are: (1) harboured from one generation to another in insects, e.g., Marek's disease, or (2) require an insect for an intermediate stage of development, e.g., tapeworms, or (3) are simply carried from bird to bird mechanically or by biting, e.g., fowl pox virus. Control measures against insects are part of the sanitary environment and clean-up.

**Spraying the area around building with an insecticide prevents insect build-up.** A good practice during cleaning is to spray the grounds, litter, and buildings with an insecticide immediately after removal of the birds. Then allow a few days for effective insect killing before removing litter for cleaning and disinfection. After cleaning, the building should be sprayed again with an insecticide to prevent re-infestation.

## (B) Disposal of Dead Birds

**Dead bird disposal has become a major problem in poultry industry.** This is because farms have become larger and some of the older methods of disposal are no longer environmentally acceptable. **Following precautions must be observed in the disposal of dead birds.**

1.  Dead birds must be removed from the cages and the poultry house daily.

2.  Keep the containers having dead birds covered at all times to prevent contact with flies and other insects, dogs, cats, and free-flying birds.

3.  After dead birds are handled, wash your hands, and disinfect the house and its equipment.

4.  Don't allow trucks or people picking up dead birds to visit any area on the farm.

5.  **The disposal pits should be in an isolated area of the farm.**

## Foci of Infection

**When birds die from infectious diseases, carcasses remain a source of infection for other birds on the same or other farms.** Also, sick birds discharge infectious material into the environment and should be removed from the flock and killed in a manner that will not allow the discharge of blood or exudates. Whatever the cause, all carcasses should be disposed of by one of the following methods to prevent spread of disease.

## 1. Burning

**Burning is the most reliable way of destroying infectious material.** Many smokeless, odourless incinerators for disposal of animal carcasses are available commercially.

## 2. Burying

Where environmental regulations allow, **a deep pit may be dug** and the carcasses buried so that animals cannot get at them. The best and easiest way is to use a backhoe (an excavating machine) and dig a deep narrow trench (a long narrow channel, a ditch). Each day's collection of dead birds can be deposited and covered until the trench is filled.

## 3. Pit or Tank Disposal

For small losses, **a decomposition pit** can be used. Precautions should be taken to ensure that: (1) it is not located where it will contaminate drinking water supplies, (2) that walls will not collapse, (3) that animals will not dig into it, (4) that flies and other insects cannot get into it, and above all, (5) **that children cannot fall into it.** The pit cover should be sealed with tar paper or plastic, and be strong enough to hold a foot of soil on it.

## 4. Cooking

Freshly dead birds can be rendered (i.e. treated to convert) into fertilizer or other products. The rendering temperature should be adequate for sterilization. It should be remembered that commercial or contract transporters of dead carcasses can introduce another disease from some other outbreak, unless strict precautions are taken.

## 5. Composting

Composting is the process by which a mixture of decayed organic matter is converted into fertilizer. Composting of poultry carcasses is an important method of disposal. Compost mixtures of straw, whole poultry carcasses, manure, and water in the proportions of 1:1:1.5:0.5, respectively (one-third of water added to each layer), decompose rapidly and odourlessly. Composts heat rapidly, reach temperatures of between $145^\circ$ and $165^\circ$ F, and reduce soft tissues completely within 14 days. **The process is biologically reliable.** *Escherichia coli*, **Salmonella-like bacteria, and Gumboro virus get destroyed.**

## (C)  Buildings and Runs

### 1.  Clean Buildings

A clean hygienic environment is good protection against disease outbreaks.

### 2.  Litter Removal

When all the birds from a house are disposed of and the house falls vacant, the litter or droppings should be removed before cleaning. **With very big poultry farms, proper and economical disposal of litter and poultry manure has become a serious problem.** There is no clear-cut answer. Generally, it is removed far away from the buildings so that insects do not crawl or fly back into houses; and to dry it, compost it, or spread it onto fields and work it into the soil. If cleaning is done while chickens are still present, remember that hired people, trucks and equipment may recently have been on another farm where a disease may have occurred.

**For most disease agents, composting of litter or droppings is sufficient, because of the heat generated.** However, one must remember that wherever litter is spilled or piled, it remains as a disease reservoir for varying lengths of time.

### 3.  Washing and Disinfection

**Once the litter or cage droppings have been removed, drinkers, egg collecting and other equipment, walls, floors, cages, outside concrete runs, and entries to buildings should be washed thoroughly and disinfected.** If the supply of water is limited and washing is not possible, **dry cleaning** may be sufficient if it is thorough, and includes scraping and sweeping or vacuuming surfaces, corners, ledges, nests, and feeders. The amount of disinfectant used on dry-clean surfaces must be increased over that required for washed surfaces.

If possible, it is better to clean the house without removing equipment. If not, all portable equipment should be removed, soaked with water, then thoroughly washed and dried. A high-pressure water hose is effective. Equipment that cannot be removed should be washed in place, and then the entire inside building surface washed clean.

**After washing, disinfection should be done** (see Chapter 30: **'Disinfection'**). There are many good disinfectants sold under different trade names. Follow the manufacturer's recommendations. **The important thing is that the surfaces be clean before application. Disinfectants applied on dirt-covered surfaces are ineffective and wasted.** Not only are they inactivated by organic material in the dirt, but they never reach the infectious organisms below it. Thorough washing removes most infectious agents from the house and equipment, and leaves a clean surface, so the disinfectant can reach those that remain. **Two or four weeks of vacancy (resting) before a new flock is moved in,** is additional protection against carrying over of diseases. However, the **vacancy period (downtime)** should be taken only as an additional measure, and not as a substitute for thorough cleaning, washing, and disinfection.

## 4. Built-up Litter and Uncleaned Buildings

Farmers demand chicks that are free of infectious agents acquired through egg transmission, or from unsanitary hatchery or delivery environments. To maintain this standard, these healthy new flocks should be placed in cleaned and disinfected buildings, with fresh clean litter. To provide these ideal conditions is expensive because of labour and litter costs. Also, suitable litter materials are becoming less available. To reduce production costs and cope with shortages, rearing of several successive flocks on the same (**built-up**) litter has become an economically acceptable practice with broilers, where the life-span is very short and birds of one age group in each farm permit their complete removal at the end of each lot.

In developed countries, this trend has become common with the use of litter-processing machinery, which can break up caked litter and produce a litter that is acceptable. **However, the continual re-use of such built-up litter will result in an increase in the numbers of infectious organisms and parasites within the litter.**

**The practice of re-using litter is not advisable for rearing layer flocks,** where the life-span is usually more than 18 months. In any case, **those who re-use litter should be fully aware of the possible risks involved, and should follow other sound disease control practices to minimize the dangers.**

If old litter must be re-used, remove any caked or excessively dirty litter, accumulated feathers, and decomposed carcasses. A layer of fresh clean litter should then be placed under the heating brooders and over the area where the young will be confined, or will spend most of their time (i.e. the first few weeks of their life). One disadvantage of multiple brooding on the same litter is the excessive **dust** that accumulates. **Inhalation of the dust provides a means of entry into the respiratory tract for bacteria and fungal spores.**

# Chapter **30**

# Disinfection

A disinfectant is a chemical that destroys disease-producing organisms on contact. **To disinfect** is to free from disease-producing organisms (bacteria, viruses, fungi, etc.), or to make them inactive; and **disinfection** is the act of destroying infectious agents. (**To sanitize** is to reduce the number of bacteria present and also to prevent them from multiplying).

Disinfectants and disinfection procedures have been widely used for many years in the poultry industry. Natural disinfection agents, such as sunlight, heat, or just simply resting poultry houses, are considered to be of limited use. Increasing evidence of the prolonged survival time of a number of important chicken pathogens (disease-producing organisms) outside the body of the birds (see **'biosecurity'**), together with an ever-increasing economic pressure for quicker re-stocking of units, **has led to a greater dependence on chemical disinfectants.**

## Properties of a Disinfectant

The lethal action (i.e. causing death) of a disinfectant depends on the chemical composition of the disinfectant and the type of organism. **An ideal disinfectant should have all, or most of the following properties.**

1.  It **must be cost-effective** and produce benefit to the farmer in terms of improved production. That is, reduced mortality, increased live weight gain, and feed conversion.

2.  It **must be effective against all the infectious agents** (viruses, bacteria, fungi). That is, it must have a broad-spectrum activity. It must be effective under farm conditions, organic soiling, hard water and low temperatures.

3.  It must be **safe for humans and animals.**

4.  It must be soluble in water.

5.  It must be readily available.

6.  It must be safe to the environment.

7.   It must not corrode the utensils, fabrics, equipment or fittings.

8.   It must be stable when exposed to air.

9.   It should be free from any objectionable or lingering odour.

10.   There should be no residual toxicity.

11.   There should be **no harmful accumulation of any portion of the disinfectant in meat or eggs.**

**No disinfectant works immediately. All require a certain amount of contact time to be effective.** Use of disinfectants at the recommended concentration is important for their effectiveness. All disinfectants are less effective in the presence of organic matter, e.g., faeces, soil, etc. **Organic matter interferes with the action of disinfectants by coating the disease-producing organisms and preventing their contact with the disinfectant.**

Therefore, for any disinfectant to be effective, **it must be applied to surfaces that have been first freed from debris and organic matter by thorough scraping, scrubbing, brushing, and dusting, and washing with soap or detergent solutions.** Many disinfectants are highly efficient, but only when first these basic cleaning requirements have been met.

## Types

**There are a variety of disinfectants available nowadays.** Many disinfectants of similar composition are sold under different trade names. Before buying a product with an unfamiliar name, compare types and values with a well-known product. Directions for dilutions given by the manufacturers should be closely followed. Continuous use of certain chemicals, particularly at inadequate concentrations, may produce a population of micro-organisms resistant to that chemical.

A brief description of some of the commonly used disinfectants follows.

## 1.  Aldehydes

**Glutaraldehyde** and **formaldehyde** are the most commonly used disinfectant in this group. Glutaraldehyde is much stronger and more effective disinfectant than formaldehyde. **It has a very wide range of activity and is a potent bactericidal, virucidal, fungicidal, and sporicidal compound. It is also effective against both enveloped and non-enveloped viruses.** It also has a fair residual activity and is **effective in the presence of organic matter.**

## 2.  Formaldehyde

Formaldehyde is a gas. It is sold commercially in a 40% solution with water, under the name of **formalin. Formalin is a very effective disinfectant, also cheap and**

**easily available.** It is used for fumigation of poultry house, brooder, and hatchery with potassium permanganate. Formaldehyde is usually generated by adding formalin to potassium permanganate in an earthen pot, or metal container. Because of the heat generated by the chemical reaction, glass containers should not be used. Take also steps to avoid risk of fire. The container should be deep and have a volume several times that of the combined chemicals, because a lot of bubbling takes place. Therefore, not more than 1 litre of formalin should be used per container. The container is placed in the room meant for disinfection. The ratio of formalin is about twice the amount of potassium permanganate, that is, 2 ml formalin to 1 g of potassium permanganate. **Potassium permanganate is poisonous. Therefore, both the compounds must be kept in accident-proof containers in a safe place.**

About 60-70 g of potassium permanganate mixed with 120-150 ml of formalin is sufficient for disinfecting 100 cubic feet of space. Gas should be allowed to remain for 20-30 minutes in the rooms, incubators, brooders, etc. **Solution of formalin (5-10%) can be used for spraying as disinfectant for most bacteria and viruses.** Usually a 4% solution is used. Formalin vapour is very good to disinfect incubators, eggs, rooms, utensils, and is not very harmful except for its irritant action on eyes, nose, and skin.

**Though formaldehyde is a powerful disinfectant, it has many disadvantages.** It is extremely irritating to the conjunctiva and mucous membranes, and **some people are very sensitive to it.** Therefore, precautions must be taken to prevent its escape into areas where people work. Operator should wear rubber gloves when handling formalin. Its chief advantage is that formaldehyde can be used as a gas or vapour for **fumigation of hatching eggs** to destroy potential harmful shell contaminants, such as salmonella. **It is a good disinfectant in the presence of some organic matter,** and it does not injure equipment with which it comes in contact. Formaldehyde is also used to fumigate the inside of incubators and hatchers and their contents. **Fumigation of incubators and eggs has been an established practice in the industry.** The higher the humidity and temperature, the more effective is fumigation. Fumigation should not be done in incubators with eggs inside because of the danger of injuring embryos. 15 to 20 ml of pure formalin can disinfect about 100 cubic feet of a box or incubator.

Now the traditional method of formaldehyde fumigation is getting replaced by safer chemicals.

## 3. Phenols

Phenols are effective against bacteria, especially Gram-positive bacteria and enveloped viruses. They are bacteriostatic at lower concentration (i.e. stop the growth of bacteria but do not kill them) and bactericidal and fungicidal at higher concentration. Phenols are not effective against non-enveloped viruses and spores. Some commercial disinfectants have residual activity persisting after they have dried, giving continued suppression of bacterial and viral populations on sprayed surfaces. Therefore, they are effective in the presence of organic matter.

## 4. Chlorine compounds

Chlorine is bactericidal, virucidal, and fungicidal. However, it is relatively ineffective against spores. Its activity is reduced in the presence of organic matter, such as faeces and soil. Chlorine has poor residual activity.

## 5. Chlorinated Lime (Bleaching powder)

Chlorinated lime or bleaching powder, prepared by saturating slaked lime (i.e. lime treated with water) with chlorine gas, is one of the earliest recognized disinfectants. It has corrosive effect on metals and skin, and therefore should be used cautiously after proper cleaning of floor. A 20% solution is used for disinfecting floor and utensils for feed and water. **For water sanitization, use bleaching powder at the rate of 6 g per 1000 litres of water.**

However, chlorinated lime has now been largely replaced by **hypochlorites.** If used according to directions, **hypochlorites are highly efficient.** Their main use is for egg washing and sanitizing, and for disinfecting incubators, incubator and hatcher trays, small brooders, and water and feed containers. They can also be used on cement surfaces. All surfaces to be disinfected with hypochlorite solutions must first be thoroughly cleaned to ensure the greatest efficiency.

## 6. Organic Iodine Combinations

**Iodine has long been recognized as an effective disinfectant.** To overcome many of the disadvantages of the earlier products, 'iodophors' have been prepared. The term **'iodophor'** refers to a combination of iodine with a solubilizing agent that slowly liberates free iodine when diluted with water.

A group of iodophors have been developed and are marketed for a wide variety of disinfectant uses. Some of these products have a built-in indicator of disinfectant activity. As the solution is used up, the normal amber (brownish-yellow) colour fades. When the solution is colourless, it is no longer effective. The product can be mixed in cold and hard water. They have a wide variety of uses. They can be applied safely to all surfaces, and are useful for disinfecting hatchery and incubator surfaces, incubator and hatchery trays, feeders, footwear, and poultry buildings. **Iodophors are good disinfectants, but do not work well in the presence of organic matter.** Like all other disinfectants, these compounds are **most effective on clean surfaces.** Iodophor has a broad disinfecting range which includes bacteria, viruses, fungi and even coccidia and ova of parasites.

## 7. Quaternary Ammonium Surface Disinfectants

Quaternary ammonium products (quats) can be regarded as ammonium ($NH4$) compounds. Commercial products often contain various forms of ammonium chloride, or a combination of different ammonium compounds. Quaternary ammonium disinfectants are effective against bacteria, enveloped viruses, and some fungi. They are not effective against non-enveloped viruses and bacterial spores. However, they are moderately active in the presence of organic matter.

## 8. Chlorhexidine

Although it is bactericidal, virucidal and fungicidal, it is less effective against these agents than many other disinfectants. It is ineffective against non-enveloped viruses and spores.

## 9. Copper Sulphate

**Copper sulphate is toxic to fungi.** A 0.5% solution is generally used for destroying fungi on feed, hoppers, utensils, water fountains, and surrounding areas associated with outbreaks of fungal disease.

## 10. Lime

Lime is commonly used as a disinfectant for litter, floor, and **poultry carcasses.** It is mainly used in areas that are damp and cannot be exposed to the sun, as well as for disinfection of drains and faecal matter, and whitewashes. The action of lime depends on liberation of heat and oxygen when the chemical comes in contact with water. **Heat destroys bacteria and parasitic eggs and even coccidia, and keeps fungi under control.** It should be applied liberally using at least 4-7 kg/100 feet$^2$. For disinfection of poultry manure, lime should be added at the rate of 90 kg / tonne of manure. It also disinfects wall and crevices, if a solution containing 38 parts lime and 15 parts sodium chloride is used for washing the wall. **This combination acts as a good disinfectant.** As lime has a caustic action, birds should be kept away from it, until it has become thoroughly dry.

## 11. Hot Water

Hot water adds to the efficiency of most disinfectants. If applied in the form of boiling water, it is effective without addition of any chemical.

## 12. Dry Heat

Dry heat in the form of a **flame** is effective, if the flame comes in contact with the infective agent to be killed. All methods involving direct flame are fire hazards, and not recommended except possibly on cement surfaces.

## 13. Commercial Disinfectants

Various commercial disinfectants are available under different trade names.

## Among them, how to select a good disinfectant?

Selection of the most effective disinfectant is the key to a successful disinfection programme. **Select a disinfectant that has a broad-spectrum of activity, is effective against both forms of viruses (enveloped and non-enveloped), bacteria, bacterial spores, fungi, etc. and offers antimicrobial action for a long time. Besides, it should be effective in the presence of organic matter.**

A **disinfectant** that destroys viruses is called a **'virucide'**, bacteria as **'bactericide'**, fungi as **'fungicide'**, and bacterial spores as **'sporicide'**. A **'spore'**, also known as **'endospore'**, is the resting stage of certain bacteria. Under adverse conditions, bacteria enclose themselves within a **tough protective coat** called **'spore'**. Spore allows bacteria to survive under unfavourable conditions. On return of favourable conditions, the spore changes back to its vegetative or infective form. As an example, *Clostridium perfringens*, cause of necrotic enteritis in poultry, is **a spore-forming organism**. In the vegetative form, these organisms are susceptible to environmental changes and disinfectants, but their spores are extremely resistant to environmental influences like drying and heat, **and also to disinfectants.** These spores survive for years and thus increase organism's ability to spread. **Most disinfectants may be virucidal, bactericidal, fungicidal, but very few are sporicidal.** Among the disinfectants available, those with **glutaraldehyde** possess moderate sporicidal activity, whereas iodine compounds, oxidizing agents, and chlorine have only mild activity. **Other disinfectants appear ineffective against spores.**

## It is stated that a disinfectant should be effective against both enveloped and non-enveloped viruses. What does this mean?

Each **virus particle** (**virion**) has a central core of either **DNA** (deoxyribonucleic acid) or **RNA** (ribonucleic acid), but not both. The nucleic acid is surrounded by a **protein coat** called **capsid**. In some viruses, the nucleic acid core and capsid are surrounded by a **lipoprotein layer** (i.e. composed of **fat** and protein) called an **envelope**. Viruses having an envelope are called **enveloped viruses**. Those that lack envelope are called **non-enveloped** (or **naked**) **viruses.** In enveloped viruses, the disinfectant acts on the lipoprotein layer, whereas in non-enveloped viruses on the protein coat (capsid). Those disinfectants that have an affinity (**chemical attraction**) for lipids (lipophilic) are effective against viruses having a lipid layer, that is, **enveloped viruses.** For example, Ranikhet disease, avian influenza (bird flu), and lymphoid leukosis viruses are enveloped viruses and contain about 20-25%, 20%, and 30-35% lipid, respectively, in their envelope. These viruses are therefore easily killed by lipophilic disinfectants, **but they are unable to eliminate non-enveloped viruses,** such as those of Gumboro disease, avian encephalomyelitis, chicken infectious anaemia, and others. This is because, being non-enveloped viruses, they lack the lipid layer. The disinfectants then are required to act on the protein coat. **Therefore, it is more difficult to destroy non-enveloped viruses** than enveloped viruses, and some disinfectants fail to act on them. **Following is the list of common enveloped and non-enveloped viruses of poultry.**

| Enveloped Viruses | Non-Enveloped Viruse |
|---|---|
| Ranikhet disease | Gumboro disease (Infectious bursal disease) |
| Infectious bronchitis | Avian encephalomyelitis |
| Fowl pox | Egg drop syndrome |
| Avian influenza | Reovirus |
| Infectious laryngotracheitis | Rotavirus |
| Marek's disease | Chicken infectious anaemia |
| Lymphoid leucosis | Leechi disease |
| | Inclusion body hepatitis |

## Which disinfectants act only on enveloped viruses and which on both?

**Broad-spectrum disinfectants** are effective against both enveloped and non-enveloped viruses, bacteria, fungi, and even bacterial spores, such as those of *C. perfringens.* These include disinfectants such as glutaraldehyde, iodine compounds, oxidizing agents, and chlorine. **However, glutaraldehyde is the most potent member of the group.** It acts against both enveloped and non-enveloped viruse, bacteria, fungi, spores and is also effective in the presence of organic matter. Along with polymethyl urea derivatives and dihydroxy diohexane (formaldehyde liberators) it can provide prolonged disinfection. The higher the concentration of these two ingredients, the greater is the residual activity.

**Among the other disinfectants,** chlorhexidine, quaternary ammonium compounds and phenols are effective against only enveloped viruses. They do not appear to eliminate non-enveloped viruses. Also, they are ineffective against bacterial spores.

## Terminal Disinfection of Poultry Houses

Infectious agents present on the surfaces in poultry houses can transfer diseases from one flock to the next. The survival time of many disease-producing organisms on inadequately disinfected surfaces can run into months. Rodents (rats, mice) and insect vectors (transmitters) are often responsible for the transfer of both viral and bacterial infections. Such a situation can be dealt with by a process generally known as **'terminal disinfection'.** Apart from the selection of an effective disinfectant, the success of any **'terminal disinfection programme'** depends on careful attention to every step given below. Failure to appreciate the importance of the steps involved may not bring the expected results.

**431**

One should follow all, or as many as possible, of the following basic steps.

# 1. Dry clean

This involves the removal of any residual food from the feeders. Portable equipment for cleaning and sanitizing should be placed outside the house or pen. Litter should be completely removed from the house and transported to a safe area away from the store. After removal of the litter, dust from ceilings, water pipes, etc. should be blown down and then all loose debris from the floor blown out.

# 2. Sanitize the drinking water system

This procedure is sometimes neglected, or improperly carried out, but it is essential in order to avoid the transport of infections from one lot to another through the drinking system. The header tank should be drained and checked to ensure that it is free of debris. The tank should then be filled with required quantity of water, and the disinfectant added to achieve the required dilution. The solution should be allowed to fill the drinking system, and left to stand for an hour. After this, the system should be drained and filled with fresh water, and covers replaced on the tanks.

# 3. Pre-clean the house and equipment

Use a detergent sanitizer to properly clean surfaces to minimize organic matter and reduce the bacterial load prior to disinfection. All surfaces should be sprayed with the solution at low pressure, ensuring thorough wetting. This must include coverage of pipe lines, feeders, and drinkers. After the detergent application, cleaning should be completed with high pressure water until all the areas are visibly clean.

# 4. Disinfection of the house and equipment

This involves a thorough application by spraying of the selected broad-spectrum disinfectant to all surfaces and equipment in the house, strictly following the required dilution rate, application rate, and contact time. Application can be with any suitable spraying equipment. **Select the dilution at which the disinfectant is most effective against disease organisms.** Always select the highest concentration necessary to eliminate the most resistant disease organisms. Effective disinfection requires surfaces to be thoroughly wet. An application rate of 250-300 ml m$^2$ is the minimum required for any disinfectant. A higher rate is required on rough or very absorbent surfaces. **All disinfectants must remain in contact with the disease organisms for 'a minimum contact time'. In practice, at least 30 minutes contact time is generally required for effective disinfection.**

# 5. Setting up the house

All equipment removed from the house, after being cleaned and disinfected, are now replaced and litter spread.

## 6. Fumigation or fogging

After setting up the house **this is a final security measure.** In many cases the traditional method of formaldehyde fumigation has been replaced by safer chemicals either applied with fogging machines, or as a fine spray.

Ensure the house is closed as soon as these steps are completed to prevent the re-entry of disease organisms.

**Effective control of insects,** particularly litter beetle, is essential. They are known vectors (transmitters) of disease, e.g. Gumboro. **Rodent control (rats, mice)** is also highly important (see 'rodents'). **Rats and mice are a source of salmonella,** and are attracted to poultry houses by a large amount of easily available food. Mice are important vectors of *Salmonella enteritidis.* They become infected during the period a flock is kept, move outside the house when flock is gone, then re-enter and infect the next flock of chickens. Strict attention should be paid to control and, if possible, eradicate such vermin (rodents, insects) from poultry sites. **Domestic flies and beetles** are both capable of transmitting salmonella, and infection can persist through the contamination of their eggs and larvae.

**Note:** For a list of various commercial disinfectants available at the market and their usage, refer to Chapter 19 under **"Disinfectants".**

# Chapter 31

# Sanitization

A sanitizer is an agent which reduces the number of bacteria present and also prevents them from multiplying. These agents are used to sanitize drinking water.

**Drinking water can act as a very important source of infection for a number of diseases.** Utmost care should therefore be taken to ensure that drinking water does not become contaminated through wild birds, rats, and mice.

If the water supply is thought to be contaminated, or in the case of serious disease problems which could be spread through the drinking water, **treat the water continually with a sanitizer**. Chlorination may be desirable. **The drinking water given to birds can be a potential source of disease-producing organisms, viruses, bacteria, or fungi.** However, this fact is sometimes overlooked. (Sanitization of the 'drinking water system' has been discussed under 'terminal disinfection of poultry houses' in Chapter 30.)

**There are two other areas that must be considered. First** is quality of the water that is supplied and its regular sanitization when necessary. **Secondly,** prevention of the spread of disease organisms through the drinking water at the time of high risk. In certain areas, poultry units have to rely on water supplies of doubtful quality. Analysis of some supplies has demonstrated exceptionally high bacterial counts which often include *Escherichia coli* and **Salmonella** species. In these situations it is usually found that, despite every effort with management and hygiene, good results are not achieved. **Continuous water sanitization is the answer.** In the event of some disease problems, **the drinking water is the major means by which infectious agent is spread from bird to bird within the house.**

**Note:** For a list of various commercial sanitizers available at the market and their usage, refer to Chapter 19 under **"Water sanitizers"**.

# Chapter 32

# The Avian Immune System

## Introduction

During the process of development, nature provides a defensive mechanism to all living creatures, **the immune system**, which protects them against various microbiological and environmental attacks. **Poultry farming is profitable only when there is no morbidity (sickness) or mortality (losses) from infectious diseases.** This, in turn, depends on the immunocompetence of the birds. That is, on their ability to resist infectious diseases by mounting an effective immune response.

The ability of poultry to resist infectious diseases, caused by bacteria, viruses, protozoa, or other infectious agents, depends on the integrity of the immune system. **The immune system can be considered like the 'Ministry of Defence'. Its function is to defend the body against foreign invaders.** Without it, that is, without proper defence, the very survival of the bird would be threatened. For example, antibodies are the bird's best defence against infection, but when their production is hit in a disease like Gumboro, the bird succumbs to infection. Likewise, when the cell-mediated immune mechanisms of defence are destroyed as is the case in a disease like chicken infectious anaemia, the bird dies.

**So, how does such a vital system work?** What are the antibody and cell-mediated mechanisms of defence, and how do they impart protection to the bird? What are the different types of antibodies, what is their role, how does the day-old chick acquire them from the hen, and how do they protect the bird? How is the immunity produced following vaccination, and how do infectious agents attack the immune mechanisms?

As poultry producers, we are constantly manipulating the immune system and the immune response of the birds. **In its lifetime, a bird is faced with a variety of natural and man-made challenges, that is, infections and vaccinations.** To overcome these challenges, bird requires a competent immune response. But what do we, as poultry professionals, really know about the avian immune system, and how can we help the response to effectively meet these challenges.

**The purpose of this chapter** is to briefly discuss what is immunity and its different types, outline the basics of the avian immune response, and to discuss what measures can we adopt to boost up bird's immunity. An understanding of the avian immune system is also essential in monitoring various vaccination and serological programmes.

## What is immunity?

The word 'immunity' is derived from the Latin word **'immunis'**, which means **protection,** or **freedom from the disease.** In other words, **immunity is the ability of a bird to resist infection.** But before we proceed any further, as to how this occurs, it would be most helpful if first we consider a few important features of the immune response in general.

## THE IMMUNE RESPONSE

When we consider the immune response, the most important component is **protein.** Protein is nothing more than an assembly of 20 basic building units called **amino acids.** Even in a small protein composed of 10 amino acids, the variety of ways these amino acids can be assembled is almost limitless. The assembly of the amino acids is directed by the genetic code of the individual, and the sequence in which the amino acids are assembled governs the way protein folds and functions in the body. (Genetic code is the system by which genetic information is stored within the cell.)

When we talk about the immune response, and the various vaccination programmes and protection from infectious diseases, we are in fact talking about the protection of the bird from the protein present in the bacteria and viruses, **because this protein is foreign to the bird.** Foreign proteins, and not carbohydrates and lipids, make the best antigens. **An antigen** is a substance (usually protein) capable of stimulating an immune response. Proteins, because of their unique properties, produce the best immune response.

**Fundamental to the understanding of the immune response is the concept of what is foreign and what is self.** During the embryonic development, when proteins that make up the newly hatched chick are being formed, a process known as **tolerance** occurs. Explained simply, this process enables the chick's immune system to recognize the extremely large number of proteins that form the newly hatched chick as **self, that is, its own,** and to be tolerant to these proteins. In other words, chick should not develop an immune response against its own proteins. Without this awareness of self, the immune system would not be able to fulfill its role in the body, namely, **recognition and elimination of foreign proteins associated with infectious agents like bacteria and viruses.**

## What then are the components of an immune system?

What was first believed to be a simple response to a foreign invader has turned out to be an extremely complex phenomenon (event). The immune response depends on a carefully orchestrated and coordinated chain of events (discussed later), **which ultimately result in the destruction and elimination of the foreign protein (i.e. infectious**

**agents).** An effective immune response depends on the cooperation of several types of cells, all interacting through specialized chemical messengers (**cytokines**) to bring about swift and specific actions against foreign invaders.

**The immune system has two components: 1. Innate, and 2. Acquired or Adaptive**

## 1. Innate Immune System

Innate immunity is not acquired after birth. **It is present in an individual from birth itself. 'Innate'** is derived from the Latin word 'innatus' which means 'to be born with', that is, **'inborn or inherent'. Innate immunity** is therefore already present within, and becomes functional as soon the chick is hatched. **Birds have well-developed innate defence mechanisms.** However, these are relatively slow, non-specific, and to a certain extent inefficient.

## If innate immunity is relatively inefficient then why should the bird have it? And what does it consist of?

The bird needs **innate immunity** because this system **constitutes the very first line of defence** against foreign invaders (bacteria, viruses, etc.). **Innate immunity has three components:**

(i)  Barriers to physical attack,

(ii)  Chemical defence system, and

(iii)  Cellular components

**Intact skin,** and the **thick mucus layer** which covers the inner surfaces of the respiratory and digestive tracts, are the body's important barriers to physical attack. **They simply do not allow the infectious agents to gain entry into the body.** Further, the respiratory tract has cilia (minute hair-like processes) which constantly beat and sweep (remove) the infectious agents out of the body. In the digestive system movement is through peristalsis, which moves the infectious agents out of the gastro-intestinal tract without allowing them to attach and gain entry into the body.

**If the physical barriers are broken,** then the **second line** of the innate system comes into operation. This defence mechanism is present in the blood of normal birds and is known as the **'complement system'.** In the blood are various proteins which circulate along with the blood cells. The complement system consists of **a group of blood proteins.** These proteins, and the proteolytic enzymes (i.e. which digest protein) of certain blood cells, together act on the infectious agents and destroy them. However, the complement system is relatively slow and inefficient, but can be extremely effective when helped by antibodies of the acquired immune system. **Its purpose is to destroy those infectious agents that have defeated the physical barriers and entered into the bird's body.**

437

The **last two components** of the innate immune system in birds are two types of cells: (1) **natural killer (NK) cells**, and (2) **macrophages**. Here, again the purpose is to destroy those infectious agents that have overcome the physical barriers and entered into the bird's body. NK cells are large lymphocytes, and are different from T-lymphocytes and B-lymphocytes. That is, they are non-T, non-B lymphoid cells. **In chickens**, they are found in thymus, bursa, spleen, blood, and intestinal epithelium. **These cells** are present in normal birds and **can destroy virus-infected and tumour cells, without prior sensitization.** That is, they are not required to be produced in the body by immunization. These cells are therefore called 'natural killer cells' and are also the **first line of defence.**

. . The other cell is the **'macrophage'** It is derived from the blood cell called **'monocyte'** (see Fig. 30). **Macrophages** act as the scavenger system of the body. That is, **they search, find out, and dispose of waste materials of the body.** Macrophages possess a large stock of enzymes, which enables them to destroy various materials rapidly. These cells first engulf (eat) foreign invaders (infectious organisms) by a process called **'phagocytosis'**, and then kill and digest them through their powerful enzymes by a process called **'lysis'**. However, like the complement system, action of macrophages can be slow and inefficient **unless they work in association with the components of the acquired immune system, such as antibodies.**

**Under normal circumstances, the innate immune system works quite effectively.** That is, when the physical barriers are intact and only a few infectious agents are able to enter into the body. These few organisms are then easily handled by the complement components and cells of the innate system. **However, in cases of major attack** innate immunity is either overpowered (defeated), or it acts so slowly that a great damage is done to the bird before the infectious agent is adequately dealt with. **It is on this account that the acquired immune system has evolved.**

## 2. Acquired (or Adaptive) Immune System

Infectious agents that cross the physical barriers and are not controlled by innate defence mechanisms, initiate a specific immune response called **'acquired or adaptive immunity'. The purpose of acquired immunity is to destroy the infectious agents that could not be killed by innate immunity.** Acquired immunity is highly specific to the agent that stimulates its development, whereas innate immunity is non-specific.

In contrast to the innate immune system, acquired immune system is **characterized**, as we shall see, **by specificity, heterogeneity, and memory.** However, like the innate immune system, it is composed of both non-cellular and a cellular component. The **non-cellular component** is made up of **antibody** and the **cellular component** of a blood cell called **lymphocyte.**

## THE AVIAN IMMUNE RESPONSE

**The primary and most important function of the immune system is to provide the bird with the ability to resist the entry and harmful effects of the infectious agents.** The common belief about immunity in birds is that protection against infectious agents is entirely because of **antibodies.** However, this is only half-truth. We are largely unaware that **protection to birds against infection is also brought about through cells,** the most important being **lymphocyte,** a type of white cell present in the chicken blood. The protection given to the bird through the cells is known as **'cell-mediated immunity'**, and as we shall see later, it is equally important like that of antibody. Protection imparted to the bird through the antibodies is called **'antibody-mediated immunity'.** Thus, **antibody-mediated immune response** and **cell-mediated immune response** are the **two arms of the acquired immune system.**

### Why does the bird need two different mechanisms? Why can't it manage with just one?

In the antibody-mediated response, protection comes from the development of **antibody.** The antibodies neutralize, inactivate and weaken the infectious agents, which are then engulfed (eaten) by body's phagocytic cells (heterophils, macrophages) and destroyed. In this way, the innate and acquired immune systems work together. **However, in this manner, only those infectious agents can be destroyed by the antibodies that are outside the cells** (extracellular). If they are within the cells (intracellular), then antibodies are unable to harm them as they cannot be reached. How does then the bird get rid of the intracellular enemies? If they are left unattacked, they could comfortably grow within; destroy the cells, and eventually the bird. **This is where the second mechanism, the cell-mediated immune response, comes to bird's rescue.** Its basic purpose is to destroy the very cell that harbours the infectious agent, and thereby destroy the cluster of infectious organisms flourishing within it, and thus protect the bird. **This cannot be achieved with the antibody-mediated immune response. Hence the need for the cell-mediated immune response for the bird's very existence.**

**Infectious agents are like terrorists and the immune system like the army.** If the terrorists are out on the street, they can be shot dead with bullets, but if they are hiding inside a building, it needs a bomb to be thrown that would destroy not only the building but also the terrorists hiding within. **Bullets can be compared with antibodies (antibody-mediated immune response) and bombs with cells (cell-mediated immune response).**

**Let us take an example to understand this very basic difference between antibody- and cell-mediated protections (immunity).** The best example is that of diseases caused by viruses, such as Ranikhet disease and several others, or those bacterial diseases in which bacteria grow within the cells, such as avian tuberculosis. In the virus-infected cells and in diseases like avian tuberculosis (TB), however, both mechanisms operate. When the viruses or TB bacteria are outside the cells, antibodies are formed to protect the bird, but **if they are confined within the cell, the cell-mediated mechanism comes into operation.** In this mechanism, a type of white cell present in the chicken blood, known as a **'lymphocyte'**, kills the virus-infected cell by direct action (cytotoxicity).

**Lymphocyte**, in recent years, **has emerged as a remarkable cell. Both antibody-mediated and cell-mediated immune responses are brought about by this cell.** Since lymphocyte is the most important cell of the immune system, let us first examine what this cell is, where does it originate in the bird, and how does it produce both antibody- and cell-mediated immune responses. The subject is highly complex, but would be explained as simply as possible.

## ANTIBODY-MEDIATED IMMUNE RESPONSE

The chicken blood has two types of cells: red cells and white cells. **Lymphocytes are one type of white cells.** They are normally about 60% of the total number of white blood cells (range 45-70%). **In birds,** lymphocytes originate in the bone marrow (soft tissue within the bones) from a cell that has the potentiality (capacity) to develop into several types of blood cell. This cell is known as the **'pluripotent stem cell' (Fig. 32).** (A **'stem cell'** is an undifferentiated cell that produces all the specialized cells). Pluripotent stem cell, in turn, gives rise to another cell called **'lymphoid stem cell' (Fig. 32),** which gives rise to different types of **lymphocytes.**

During incubation of the egg, in the developing chick, the lymphoid stem cells migrate into two different directions through the bloodstream. **One set (B-cell precursors) goes to the bursa of Fabricius between 8-15 days of incubation (Fig. 32).** Bursa is a round sac located just above the cloaca **(Fig. 33).** In fact, it is a sac-like extension of the rectum (large intestine). This organ grows rapidly up to 4 weeks, then there is a plateau period for the next 5 or 6 weeks, and thereafter gradually disappears before sexual maturity (i.e. 16-20 weeks). **Another set of cells (T-cell precursors) goes to thymus (Fig. 32).** This organ consists of seven lobes present in the neck of the chicken **(Fig. 33).** These lobes lie on each side of the trachea. Thymus attains its maximum size around 16 weeks (i.e. at puberty) and disappears soon after sexual maturity. Unlike the bursa, the lymphoid stem cells enter the thymus in three waves: between 6 and 8 days; 12 and 14 days; and 18 and 20 days after incubation.

**Bursa and thymus are called 'primary lymphoid organs" (Fig. 33) because they regulate the production and differentiation of lymphocytes.** Mature lymphocytes of the chicken blood fall into two major populations, **B-lymphocytes or B-cells and T-lymphocytes or T-cells.** B-cells mature in the bursa, whereas T-cells mature in the thymus (Fig. 32 & 33). After maturation, the B- and T-cells populate

## Origin of B- and T-Lymphocytes in the chicken

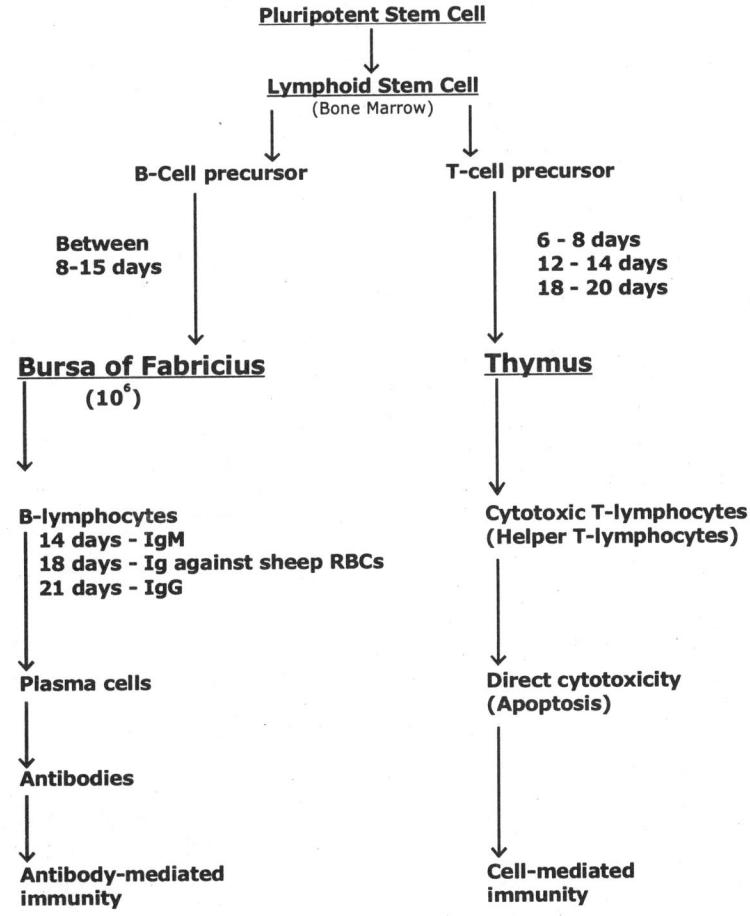

Fig. 32. Origin of B- and T-lymphocytes in the chicken.

(migrate to) the **'secondary lymphoid organs'** (discussed later).

## What happens after the lymphoid stem cells enter the bursa?

After lymphoid stem cells enter bursa, they undergo a period of processing and then differentiate into a type of mature lymphocytes called **'bursa-derived lymphocytes'** or **'B-lymphocytes'** or simply as **'B-cells"**. (**'B' stands for bursa**). The processing (maturation) within the bursa transforms them into **antibody-producing cells**. That is, they are assigned the job of producing antibody.

**By the time bursa disappears around sexual maturity, these antibody-producing B-cells populate the secondary lymphoid organs (Fig. 33)**. In the chicken these include spleen, bone marrow, Harderian gland (located near the eye), conjuctival-associated lymphoid tissue **(CALT)**, bronchial-associated lymphoid tissue **(BALT)**, and

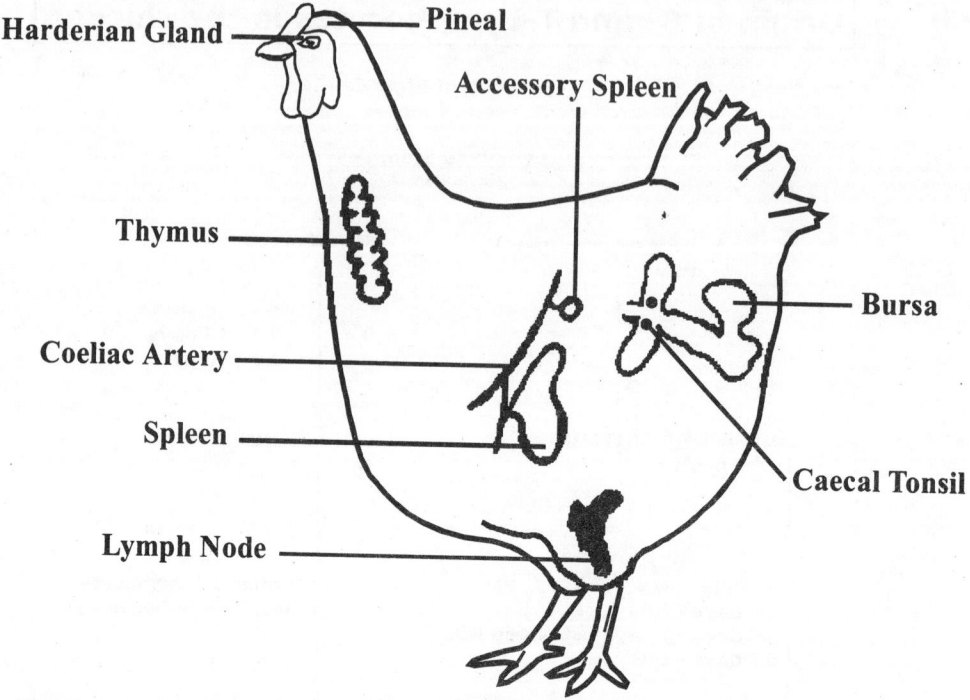

**Fig. 33.** Primary lymphoid organs, thymus and bursa of Fabricius, and secondary lymphoid organs, pineal, Harderian gland, accessory spleen, spleen, lymph node, and caecal tonsils.

gut-associated lymphoid tissue **(GALT),** such as caecal tonsils, Peyer's patches, Meckel's diverticulum (present in the small intestine at the junction of jejunum and ileum), and intestinal lymphocytes **(Fig. 33).** The purpose of the above exercise is to make the bird immunocompetent throughout its life. That is, to enable the bird to effectively produce antibodies to fight infections, **even after the bursa and thymus have disappeared.**

**Chickens lack lymph nodes** found in mammals but have **lymphoid nodules** along the course of the lymphatics.

## How do B-cells produce antibodies?

Following antigenic stimulation, that is, on contact with the infectious agent (viruses, bacteria, etc), B-cells do not themselves produce antibodies, but enlarge, divide repeatedly, and differentiate into another type of cell which is especially designed to synthesize and secrete large amounts of antibody. These cells are called 'plasma cells'. **Antibodies are technically known as 'immunoglobulins (Ig)',** and are **proteins** made up of amino acids. As already stated antibodies destroy infectious agents and protect the bird. To fight enemies, they are required in large numbers. **Plasma cells can make up to a million (ten lakhs) molecules of antibody per hour, that is, nearly 300 molecules per second; and these are secreted soon after they are formed.**

### In case B-cell starts producing antibody against bird's own protein, then would not that be fatal to the bird?

**Certainly in that case survival of the bird would be impossible.** To ensure that B-cells do not produce antibodies against bird's own proteins, bursa takes adequate precautions. Each B-cell is first thoroughly screened by the bursa for its loyalty to body, as if with a metal detector. Bursa then selectively destroys such B-cells that react against the body's own components (self antigens). This mechanism is known as **'negative selection'** or **'clonal deletion'**. Up to 99% of the B-cells are thus eliminated (destroyed) through a process known as **'apoptosis'** or **'physiological cell death'**. Those B-cells that are loyal to the body, that is, they act only against foreign invaders (infectious agents) and not against body constituents, are preserved, stimulated to multiply, and are **finally sent to secondary lymphoid organs for antibody production.**

### Apart from the infectious agents, there are thousands of different antigens in the environment. Does this mean that there are also thousands of different types of B-cells in the bird's body to deal with them?

Yes. One very important event that occurs in the bursa during the process of maturation and differentiation of lymphoid stem cells is that they develop what is known as **'antibody diversity'.** This means that during maturation and differentiation of the millions of B-cells in the bursa, **each B-cell is earmarked (set aside) to recognize one type of antigen/infectious agent.** In other words, if there are one million (ten lakhs) antigens in the environment that the bird may face during its lifetime, then there are also one million types of different B-cells, **each meant for one specific antigen/ infectious agent.** It is now known that **chicken B-cells are able to recognize as many as $10^6$ different antigens** (i.e. ten lakhs).

It would be wrong to presume that once mature (differentiated) B-cells are formed, they can produce antibodies against all types of infectious agents. The fact is that **one specific type of B-cell produces antibodies only against one particular infectious agent.** That is, for producing antibodies against Ranikhet disease virus, Gumboro disease virus, Marek's disease virus, or salmonella organisms, different types of B-cells must be activated to produce antibodies.

### How is this possible? How does it all work out?

**The process is extremely complex.** Explained simply, if you want to have a jacket, there are two options. Either you go to a tailor and get it stitched as per your requirements, or go to a departmental store and buy a ready-made jacket of your size and choice, from the hundreds available. **It is this latter mechanism that operates in nature, when it comes to antibody production against any particular infectious**

**agent**. It is now believed that B-cells carry tiny ready-made antibodies on their surface against each infectious agent/antigen present in nature. These antibodies (immunoglobulins) act as receptors for infectious agents, and are known as **'B-cell receptors (BCRs)'**. That is, when bound to B-cell surface, this antibody molecule acts as an antigen receptor. When released by the B-cell and free in the circulation, it acts as an antibody. In other words, **antibodies are simply soluble forms of B-cell receptors secreted by B-cells into body fluids.** Each B-cell is covered with about 2, 00, 000 to 5, 00, 000 antigen receptors. These antigen receptors are all identical. **Because they are all exactly the same, one B-cell will bind and respond to only a single (i.e. of one type) antigen/infectious agent.**

When an infectious agent enters the body, it starts looking for the B-cell meant for it. **The phenomenon (process) works on a lock and key basis.** In searching the specific B-cell meant for it, the infectious agent identifies the corresponding antibody present on its surface, which acts as a receptor for it. Thus, the infectious agent picks up that particular B-lymphocyte from among the countless present in bird's body. The organism then attaches itself to the specific antibody molecule (i.e. receptor) present on the B-cell. This means that from among the millions of B-cells, only one specific B-cell is picked up to produce antibodies against Ranikhet disease virus, another specific type B-cell for Gumboro disease virus, and so on. In other words, **antibodies against one infectious agent are derived from only one type of B-cell,** which then gives rise to a specific set of plasma cells.

## Once an antibody has been formed, how does it react against the infectious agent?

The antibody molecule is made up in such a way that if we look at it under a high power microscope, it would look like the letter **'Y'** (see **Fig. 35**). On the arms of the **'Y'** are the areas which recognize the foreign invader (infectious agent). **The situation is much like a lock and key,** where a portion of the invader (key) matches with a portion on the antibody (lock). When the matching is perfect like a lock and key, the two attach, and an immune response begins.

## How does a B-cell come to know that a foreign invader is present in the body, and that antibodies have to be produced to destroy it?

Earlier, under **"Innate Immune System",** it was discussed that the cell **'macrophage'** can engulf infectious agents and destroys them through its powerful enzymes. Cells, like macrophages, that can ingest, process, and present an infectious agent (antigens) to B- cells, are called **'antigen-processing (presenting) cells'** (see **Fig. 38 & 30**). During the processing, small fragments (broken pieces) of the infectious agent are left on the surface of the macrophage. In addition, the macrophage sends out chemical messages/signals (**cytokines,** see **Fig. 38**) which say to body cells **'come**

**and look',** here is the enemy. Various cells, including the B-cells, then come to the site. B-cells have on their surface tiny ready-made antibodies (receptors). As the B-cell examines what is on the surface of the macrophage, it tries lock and key method. If there is a matching, a signal is sent inside the B-cell saying that there is an invader (enemy) and that something should be done. **That something is the production of antibodies against that infectious agent.**

## How do antibodies destroy the disease-producing organisms?

They achieve this by **three mechanisms: (i) Neutralization:** Antibodies bind to specific disease-producing organisms and neutralize them. That is, they block the activity of that organism by coating its surface. This occurs particularly with **viruses. Neutralized viruses (i.e. coated with antibodies) are unable to attach to surface receptors of body cells and are therefore prevented from replication (i.e. multiplication, growth).** As a result, they are unable to produce disease. **(ii) Opsonization: If bacteria are coated with antibodies (opsonization),** they are more easily taken inside and destroyed by phagocytes of he body, (**Phagocyte** is a cell that is able to engulf/eat and digest bacteria. They include **heterophils** of blood and **macrophages** of tissues.) **(iii) Complement activation:** Antibodies bound to the surface of disease-producing bacteria can activate complement (described earlier) and produce new complement proteins. These complement proteins attach to receptors on phagocytes. **This makes phagocytosis and destruction of disease-producing bacteria easier for phagocytes.** (Phagocytosis is engulfment of bacteria by a phagocyte.)

## What are the different types of antibodies produced in the chicken against infectious agents, and what is their role?

Three main types of **antibodies (immunoglobulins)** are produced in the chicken. These are designated as **IgM, IgG, and IgA** ('Ig' means **immunoglobulin**). **Each has a specific purpose. Also, each antibody is specific for the bacterium or virus that initiated its production.**

### IgM

During the course of an immune response, **the first antibody produced in the chicken is IgM (Fig. 34).** That is, following infection, first IgM appears. Therefore, this is the antibody seen earlier in infection.

**IgM is actually five of the IgGs (or IgYs)** joined at the tails in a circular fashion **(Fig. 34).** (In the chicken IgG is also called IgY.) **The function of IgM is mainly to arrest the infectious agent.** When the lock and key matching occurs between IgM and the infectious agent, the antibody attaches itself tightly. As many of these antibodies attach or hang on, a framework (structure, lattice) of antibody is built around the infectious agent. This prevents the infectious agent from spreading and doing any damage.

Technically, this process is called **'agglutination'**.

Although produced in small amounts following infection, because of its very large size, IgM is much more efficient than IgG against infectious agents in preventing the damage. **However, also because of their very large size, IgM antibodies are usually confined to the bloodstream. Therefore, IgM antibodies are of no use in preventing damage caused by the spread of infectious agents in tissue fluids or body secretions, even at sites of acute inflammation. In other words, their protective actions are limited to the bloodstream only.**

## IgG

As the immune response progresses, the IgM-producing cells (B-cells) stop IgM production and start the production of IgG or IgA. This phenomenon is called **'class switch'**. Cytokines interleukin-4, transforming growth factor-beta, and gamma-interferon stimulate the class switch. **IgG consists of only one 'Y' (Fig. 35) which means that it is five times smaller than IgM.**

A typical immune response in the chicken

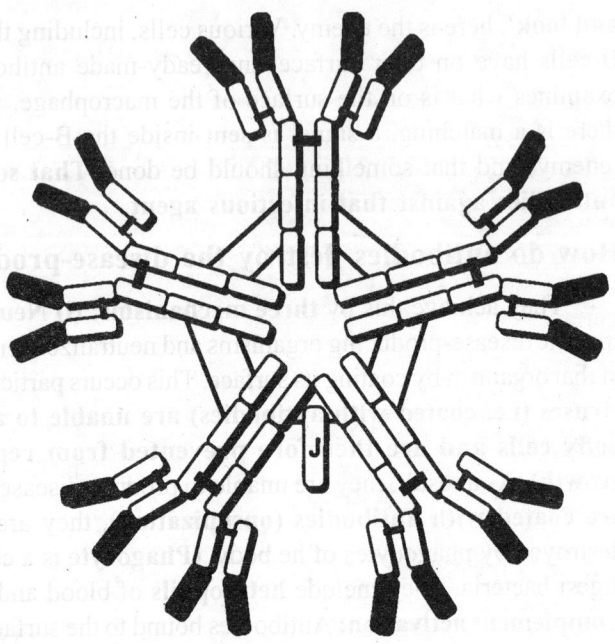

**Fig. 34.** Structure of **immunoglobulin M (IgM)**. IgM consists of five IgGs.

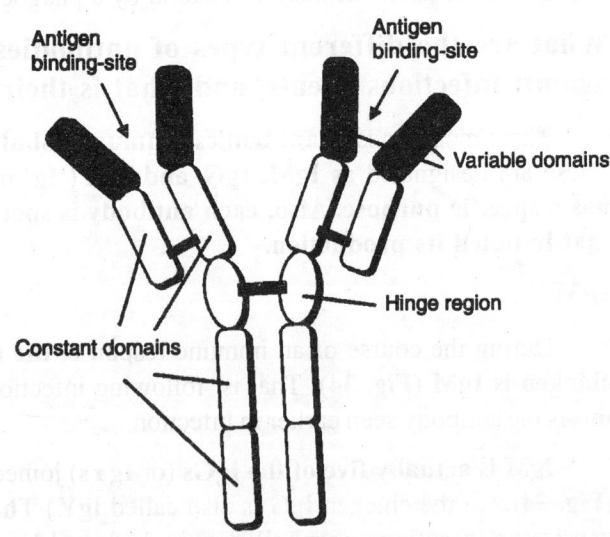

**Fig. 35.** Structure of **immunoglobulin G (IgG)**. Note IgG looks like the letter 'Y'. It contains only one 'Y'. Compare it with IgM (Fig. 34) which consists of five such 'Ys'.

begins with **IgM production**. After some time, IgM production switches over to **IgG production. IgG** is also the main antibody produced after secondary immunization (i.e. booster vaccination) and is the **predominant Ig class in chicken blood. Because avian IgG is larger than its mammalian counterpart, the chicken IgG is often called IgY.** Molecular cloning data suggest that IgY may be the ancestral precursor of mammalian IgG.

It is IgG which is measured with **enzyme-linked immunosorbent (ELISA) test.** As the lock and key match occurs between this antibody and the infectious agent, certain areas on the 'Y' are exposed. These areas activate the **complement system** and help **macrophages**, and make them much more efficient in quickly disposing of the infectious agents. IgGs cause clumping of the infectious agents (**agglutination**) and coat their surfaces. This facilitates **phagocytosis (engulfment and destruction)** of the infectious agent by macrophages.

**IgG is found in highest concentration in blood,** and for this reason, **it plays the major role in antibody-mediated defence mechanisms.** Because it is the smallest of the three antibodies, **unlike IgM, IgG can escape from the blood vessels.** This is extremely important, since **it permits IgG to participate in the protection of tissue fluid and body surfaces during inflammation, which IgM is unable to do.**

## IgA

The third important class of antibody in the chicken is IgA (Fig. 36). This antibody is manufactured by B-cells present in tissues immediately under the body surfaces, such as in the **walls of the respiratory and intestinal tract.** IgA produced in the body surfaces either passes through epithelial cells into **mucosal secretions**, or diffuses into the bloodstream. (**Mucosa** is the inner lining of the respiratory and intestinal tracts.) Thus, most of the IgA made in the intestinal wall is carried into the intestinal fluid. **Its blood concentration is usually lower than that of IgM.**

**IgA is the most important antibody in the mucosal secretions,** and is therefore the most important immunoglobulin involved in mucosal immunity. As such, **it is of critical importance in protecting the respiratory, intestinal, and urogenital tracts, and also the eyes against infectious agents.** In other words, in infections that are mainly localized on the surfaces of the respiratory and intestinal tract, IgA antibodies are the main line of defence in preventing the infectious agent from gaining entry into the body. IgA combines with a **secretory component** present on the surface of the mucosal epithelial cells. This combination with secretory component protects IgA from proteolytic digestion in the intestine. **In the chicken,** it is present in significant amounts in the intestinal fluid, tracheal secretions and secretions on the urogenital tract, saliva, tears, and urine. It is most concentrated on mucosal surfaces, although small quantities may be found in the circulation. **Bile** is also a rich reservoir of IgA in birds. IgA protects mucosal surfaces against disease-producing organisms, particularly **viruses by neutralizing and**

preventing their attachment to mucosal cells. IgA has been evolved mainly to protect body surfaces.

IgA does not activate the complement system and it cannot coat infectious agents for phagocytosis like IgG. It can, however, clump (agglutinate) infectious agents and neutralize viruses. **Its most important function is to prevent the adherence (sticking, binding) of infectious agents (bacteria, viruses) to the mucosal surfaces, the process being known as 'immune elimination or exclusion'.** If bacteria or viruses cannot bind to the intestinal lining epithelial cells, they will then simply move forward along with the intestinal contents, and would be expelled without doing any harm.

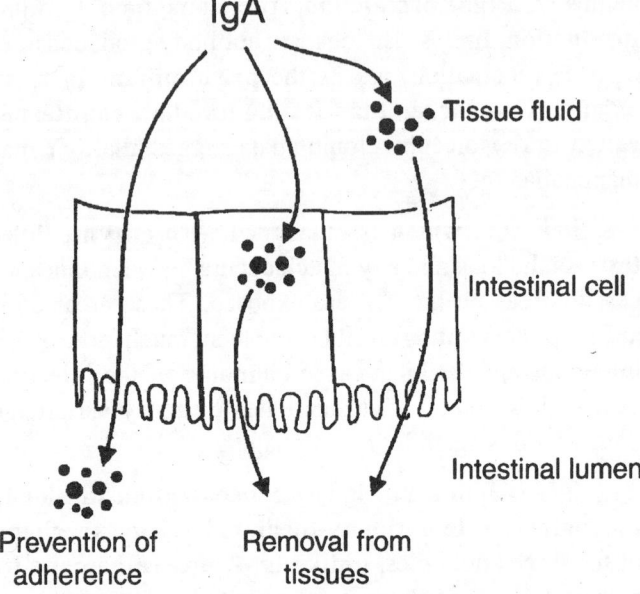

**Fig. 36. Immunoglobulin A (IgA) is unique in that it acts at three places.** It can bind infectious agent in tissue fluid, within the intestinal cell, and also in the intestinal lumen. The bound infectious agent in tissue fluid or intestinal cell is carried to the intestinal lumen.

Because IgA is transported through intestinal epithelial cells, **it can also act inside these cells**. Thus, IgA can bind to viruses present inside the epithelial cells and stop their growth. **This is a unique example of an antibody which can act inside the cells.** Another unique function of IgA is to remove the infectious agents. IgA can bind to infectious agents that penetrate into the submucosa. (Submucosa is the loose tissue that lies below the mucosa of the intestine.) Once bound, the **IgA-infectious agent** complex is actively transported across the lining epithelial cells into the intestinal lumen. **IgA can therefore act at three different levels to keep infectious agents out: (1) within the submucosa (tissue fluid), (2) within the lining intestinal cells, and (3) within the intestinal lumen (Fig. 36). This is a unique feature of IgA. With current technology, it is not practical to routinely measure IgA. This is unfortunate, because in infections with viruses such as those of Ranikhet and Gumboro disease, measurement of circulating IgG alone may not be the best index to judge whether the bird is protected or not.**

An interesting feature in the chicken is that between 30 and 75% of the IgA produced within the intestinal wall diffuses into the blood circulation and is carried to the liver. It is then released into the bile. **Bile is therefore extremely rich in IgA** and is a major route by which IgA reaches the intestine in the chicken. **By this route infectious agents in the chicken, bound to circulating IgA, are removed from the body.** The situation in the domestic animals is different. Less than 5% of IgA enters the bile in dogs, ruminants (cattle, sheep, goats), and pigs.

**Earlier it was mentioned that one of the characteristics of the acquired immune system is memory. What is memory, and what is its significance in the immune response of the chicken?**

Besides being stimulated to produce antibodies, following lock and key match with the infectious agent, **B-cell is stimulated to undergo 'clonal expansion'.** This means that B-cell reproduces itself so that there are more cells of this type available to keep a careful watch (surveillance). Why? This is because, basically, the body is saying that we have seen this infectious agent once and we must be on the alert in case it attacks again. Should it attack again, these B-cells immediately recognize it and start producing antibodies against it without delay, to destroy it. This immediate increase in the number of B-cells on future recognitions, specific against that infectious agent, **is the memory - a characteristic feature of the acquired immune system. Memory cells have a great longevity and 'remember'** their encounter with the infectious agent even after the infectious agent has been cleared from the body and the immune response has subsided. Memory cells respond to the subsequent exposure to the same infectious agent by initiating a rapid and highly effective immune response. **Booster vaccinations, used routinely in poultry, take advantage of this memory response. An example is the greater response** to the second vaccination against Ranikhet disease compared to the lower level of response to the first.

## How does the newly hatched chick acquire antibodies from the hen?

**A day-old chick has an inadequately developed immune system and therefore has to depend on the immunity obtained from the mother.** Newly hatched chick emerges from the sterile (bacteria free) environment of the egg and as such requires temporary immunological protection until it is able to produce antibodies. Antibodies are therefore transferred from the hen's blood to the yolk, while the egg is still in the ovary **(Fig. 37). IgG in yolk is therefore found at levels equal to those in hen's blood.** The transfer of IgG from the yolk sac begins during the first week of incubation, but it mainly occurs during the last 3 days before hatching and continues after hatch. **Peak levels of maternal IgG in the circulation of the newly hatched chick are reached around 2-3 days of age.** Maternally derived antibodies decrease thereafter and become undetectable after 2-5 weeks. In addition, as the egg passes down the oviduct, **IgM and IgA from oviduct secretions are acquired with the albumen (Fig. 37).**

As the chick embryo develops, it absorbs some of the yolk's IgG, which then appears in its circulation. **The maternal (obtained from hen) IgM and IgA from the albumen diffuse into the amniotic fluid and the developing embryo (developing chick) swallows IgM- and IgA-containing amniotic fluid. Therefore, when the chick hatches, it possesses IgG in its blood and IgM and IgA in its intestine (Fig. 37).** The newly hatched chick does not absorb its all yolk sac antibody until about 24 hours after hatching. These maternal antibodies effectively prevent successful vaccinations between 10 and 20 days after hatching.

**The function of maternal antibodies is to prevent pathogenic (disease-causing) organisms from producing disease in young chicks.**

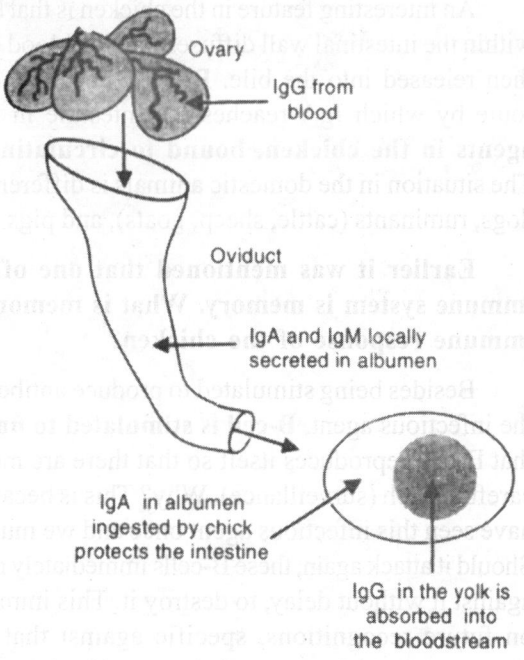

**Fig. 37.** The passive transfer of maternal antibodies from hen to the chicken.

Chicks usually receive up to 3 weeks of protection from maternal antibodies. This allows their immune system to develop to a level capable of producing an effective immune response when exposed to harmful viruses or bacteria. However, high levels of maternal antibodies can interfere with vaccination in many diseases. It is therefore important to know the level as well as the uniformity of maternal antibodies when planning the vaccination programme. **Strains of some vaccines are available that are strong enough to overcome maternal antibodies.**

## CELL-MEDIATED IMMUNE RESPONSE

### What happens after the lymphoid stem cells enter the thymus?

Lymphoid stem cells undergo a period of processing in the thymus (see **Fig. 32**) and differentiate into mature lymphocytes. The differentiated mature cells are called **'thymus-derived lymphocytes'**, or **'T-lymphocytes'**, or simply as **'T-cells'**. (**'T'** stands for thymus). The processing (maturation) and differentiation transform them into **'cytotoxic T-cells' (Fig. 38). That is, they acquire the ability to kill the cells that harbour the infectious agents.**

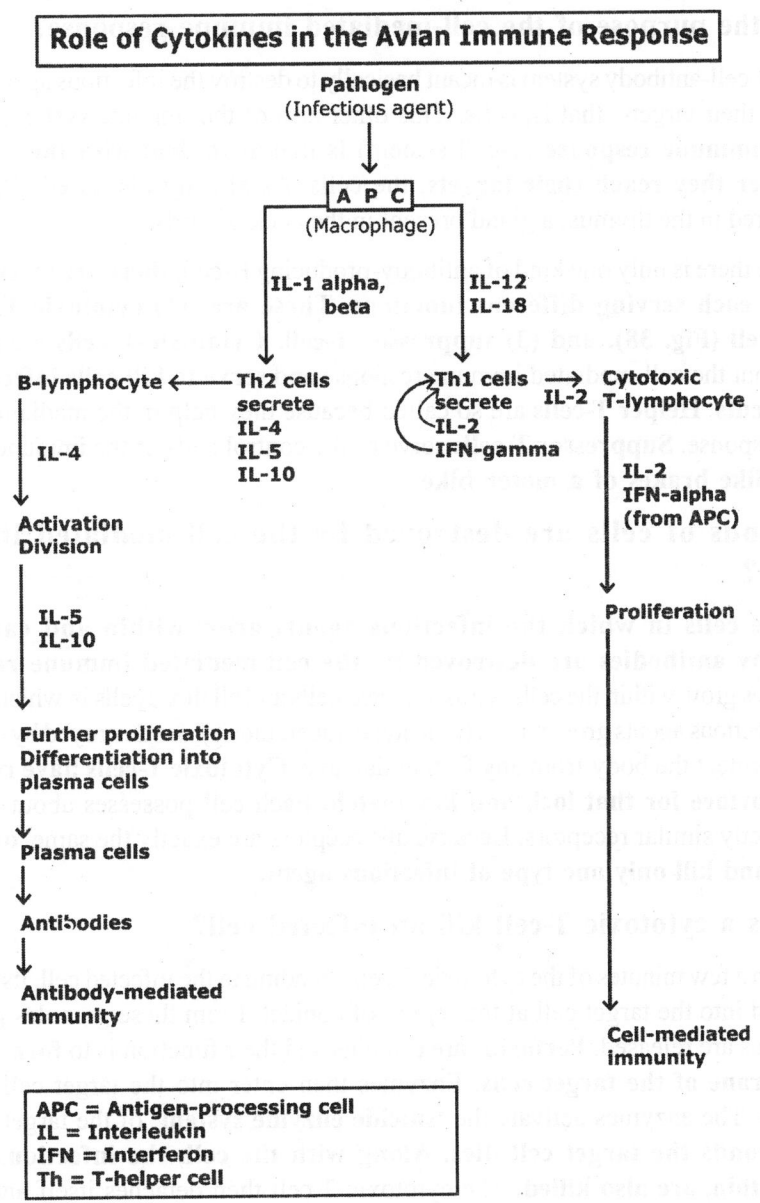

**Fig. 38.** Role of cytokines in the avian immune response.

By the time thymus disappears, which is soon after sexual maturity, **T-cells populate various secondary lymphoid organs.** These have been described earlier under 'antibody-mediated immune response'.

## What is the purpose of the cell-mediated immune response?

The B-cell-antibody system is meant basically to destroy the infectious agents **before** they reach their targets, that is, cells. This other arm of the immune system, the **cell-mediated immune response** (T-cell system) **is meant to deal with the infectious agents after they reach their targets,** the cells. As already discussed, T-cells are manufactured in the thymus, a gland present in the neck of birds.

While there is only one kind of antibody-producing B-cell, **there are several kinds of T-cells, each serving different functions. These are: (1) cytotoxic T-cell, (2) helper T-cell (Fig. 38), and (3) suppressor T-cell. Cytotoxic-T cells** are the ones that carry out the cell-mediated immune response and **serve to kill cells infected with disease agents. Helper T-cells** are so called because they help in the mediation of the immune response. **Suppressor T-cells** serve as the control cells of the immune system. **They are like brakes of a motor bike.**

## What kinds of cells are destroyed by the cell-mediated immune response?

**Those cells in which the infectious agents grow within and cannot be attacked by antibodies are destroyed by the cell-mediated immune response.** Since viruses grow within the cells, virus-infected cells and all those cells in which bacteria or other infectious agents grow within (as in avian tuberculosis), are destroyed by cytotoxic T-cells to protect the body from any further damage. **Cytotoxic T-cells have receptors on their surface for that lock and key match.** Each cell possesses about 10,000 - 20,000 exactly similar receptors. Because all receptors are exactly the same, **one T-cell will bind and kill only one type of infectious agent.**

## How does a cytotoxic T-cell kill an infected cell?

Within a few minutes of the cytotoxic T-cell's binding to the infected cell, its granules are released into the target cell at the region of contact. From these granules perforins and enzymes are released. **Perforins** are proteins and their function is to **form holes in the membrane of the target cells.** Enzymes then enter into the target cell through these holes. The enzymes activate the 'suicide enzyme system' of the target cell and **within seconds the target cell dies. Along with the cell, the infectious agents present within, are also killed.** The cytotoxic T-cell then detaches itself and moves on to find another target (i.e. another infected cell), and deals with it likewise.

## What then is the role of helper T-cell in an immune response?

It is now well established that neither the cytotoxic T-cells which kill the infected cells, nor the B-cells which produce protective antibodies (see **Fig. 32**), **can function without the signals (instructions) received from 'helper T-cells'.** Helper T-cells secrete certain chemical substances (cytokines) which act as messenger molecules (**Fig.**

**38)**. These molecules help both B-cells and T-cells in the mediation of antibody- and cell-mediated immune responses, hence the name 'helper T-cell'. In other words, these cells regulate the immune responses. **Helper T-cell is like the conductor of a musical orchestra. It commands the entire show.**

## What then is the role of macrophages in an immune response?

The immune response is very complex. The B-cells and T-cells do not themselves pick up (engulf, phagocytose) the infectious agents (bacteria, viruses, or whatever). **The infectious agents are first engulfed by a 'macrophage'** (already discussed earlier), which is derived from a blood cell known as '**monocyte**' (see **Fig. 30**). For antibody production, **the infectious agent has to be processed first. This is done by the macrophage.** After ingestion (engulfment) by the macrophages, the infectious agents are broken down, processed and then presented to B- and T-cells. This step, processing of the infectious agent, is a must for induction of immunity. **Macrophages act as 'antigen-processing' or 'antigen-presenting cell'** (already discussed earlier) **(Fig. 38)**.

## Do innate, antibody and cellular arms of the immune system act separately or together in the production of antibody?

The process is extremely complicated, **but they all work toward the common cause of protecting the bird against the infectious agent.** For example, the production of antibody actually depends on a specific interaction between the macrophage (the innate system), specific B-cell (the antibody system), and helper T-cell (the cellular system). All the three arms must communicate with each other through chemical messengers (cytokines) to produce a measured (accurate) and specific response against an infectious agent.

## Finally, what can we do to protect chickens against infectious agents and improve their immune responses?

1.  As can be seen, the immune response is a tremendously complex chain of events. As with life insurance, it is most effective if it is not called on for use. The very basis of any programme to ensure that birds are protected **is an effective and well implemented biosecurity programme** (see 'biosecurity'). **Even the best vaccine administered by the best methods is ineffective, if the birds are challenged by new and different invaders.**

2.  When we talk about the innate immune system, the single most important step that we can take to protect our birds **is to ensure best management.** One very important component of innate immunity is **an intact and effectively functional barrier to invasion.** The management factors that can damage this barrier and expose the bird to infection are many. Overcrowding can lead to scratching and

picking, which can disrupt the skin barrier and cause infections. Each time we give an injection to a bird, we break this barrier, and if our equipment is not clean and sterile, we can actually inject the infectious agent into the bird.

3. We often talk about **air quality** and its effect on litter and heating and cooling costs. But we often forget about the **effect of poor ventilation on immunity. When birds are forced to breathe poor quality air high in ammonia and dust, the defence barrier breaks down** (refer to 'effects of ammonia'). The bird is then unable to effectively eliminate infectious agents **because the immune system is overpowered.**

4. **The same is true for feed and feed quality.** When birds are given feed ingredients of poor quality, or if feed contains **mycotoxins,** the **local defence mechanisms again break down, making the bird prone to intestinal infections.** In addition, in intestinal disease the bird is less capable of absorbing or manufacturing nutrients that are important in the immune response.

# Chapter 33

# Impact of Nutrients on Avian Immunity

**T**he ability of birds to resist infectious diseases depends on the integrity of their immune system (see Chapter 32: 'The avian immune system'). Efficient function of the immune system, in turn, depends on the availability of certain nutrients (i.e. nourishing substances) which mediate cell functions required for the bird's defence. It is now being increasingly realized that **nutrition plays a significant role in the functioning of the bird's immune system.** There are extremely important interactions between nutrition and immunity, among cells, that greatly affect productivity of poultry. Proteins, certain vitamins and trace elements are important for these interactions. As such, **nutrition can significantly influence the immunocompetence of the birds.** That is, their ability to mount an effective immune response against infectious agents, and thus increase bird's natural resistance.

**A major objective of poultry industry is to minimize the losses and obtain good flock liveability.** To achieve this, farmers continuously strive to improve the environmental conditions and management at their farms. However, commercial poultry environments contain ubiquitous organisms (i.e. present everywhere) that continuously challenge the bird's immune system. This makes them more susceptible to disease.

In recent years there has been much research on the role of nutrients that improve bird's health through **'immunomodulation'.** That is, by improving the working of their immune system. Some nutrients have been shown to enhance certain cell functions important for disease resistance, when added to the diet of poultry. **The purpose of this chapter is to highlight how best disease losses can be prevented in poultry by tuning their immune responses through nutrition.**

However, before we proceed any further, it would be helpful if we first understand certain unique features of the avian immune system. In other words, how does the bird's immune system differ from that of the mammal?

## Differences between avian and mammalian immune system

1.   **A unique feature of the immune system in birds is that it consists of rapidly dividing cells.** This is not so in mammals. A 100 g broiler chick doubles its weight

to 200 g in less than 5 days, whereas a fast-growing laboratory animal like rat takes nearly 10 days to double its weight from 50 g to 100 g. Moreover, **during the first several weeks, bursa and thymus grow at a rate much faster than the rest of the body.** B-cells proliferate rapidly in bursa, with more than 5% of bursal lymphocytes dividing per hour. Bursa and thymus are the primary immune organs, as they play a central role in the production of immunity (see Chapter 32). **This very fast growth of the immune organs and the extremely rapid division of their cells soon after hatching, unlike in mammals, continuously for several weeks, makes the avian immune system particularly prone to damage.** As a result, any nutritional deficiencies in the life of chick, especially of those nutrients that influence the immune organs, would greatly harm both bursa and thymus. **This would result in a poor immune response and increased susceptibility to infectious diseases.**

2.  The developing embryo (chick) in the incubating egg has no connection with the hen, whereas the needs of a mammalian embryo are fulfilled through placenta connected to mother. This means that the **chick embryo depends entirely on the supply of nutrients present in the egg,** and any deficiency thereafter cannot be corrected once the egg is laid.

3.  In addition, **if deficient, the newly hatched chick cannot go to the hen for further requirements of antibodies, or other protective substances. In humans and animals,** these antibodies are obtained through colostrum (the first milk secreted after parturition) from breast-feeding and suckling, respectively. Colostrum is rich in antibodies and other defensive substances. **Therefore, deficiency of a nutrient** that has an impact on the immune system, **such as vitamin A, will harm birds faster and more seriously, than mammals.**

4.  In the newly hatched chick, the immune system undergoes a period of development and maturation, and becomes functionally competent only by about three weeks of age. At a young age, the immune system is not sufficiently developed to produce a response adequate enough to destroy the infectious agents. **Therefore, any deficiency of nutrients, especially during the early weeks, is particularly harmful and makes the bird immuno-compromised.** That is, the bird loses its capacity to mount an effective immune response throughout its life.

5.  **Vaccination failure(s):** Many factors can cause vaccination failures (see 'vaccination failure", under Chapter 34) in poultry. In the present case, **vaccination may fail to produce immunity because birds were deprived of necessary nutrients required for the proper growth and development of the bursa and thymus.**

Having discussed the unique features that characterize the avian immune system, let us now examine the nutrients that play an important role in the production of immunity in poultry.

# PROTEINS

Right from the time a chick is hatched, a number of vaccinations are carried out. What do they mean in terms of the immune response? Each vaccination stimulates only one type of B-cells, which then divide and differentiate into **plasma cells**, and plasma cells produce antibodies against that particular infectious agent present in the vaccine (see Chapter 32).Vaccination against another disease produces another set of plasma cells, and a third vaccination yet another, and so on. With so many different vaccinations as many different sets of plasma cells are produced (see Chapter 32). **Each plasma cell is capable of producing nearly 300 molecules of antibodies per second.** As **antibodies are protein,** made up of amino acids, with millions of plasma cells continuously producing billions of antibody molecules, **protein requirements of the growing bird during vaccinations, can be enormous.** Moreover, plasma cells die after 3-6 days, and are then replaced by a fresh lot. Production of new plasma cells again requires protein.

Antibodies being protein, importance of adequate protein supply cannot be over-emphasized while the bird is producing antibodies. **Any deficiency of protein during the growing stage, when various vaccinations are carried out, will lead to poor antibody production.** This would result in a poor protection of the bird against infectious diseases, and an increased susceptibility to infections.

# AMINO ACIDS

**Methionine** is the **first limiting** (i.e. in short supply) **amino acid for growth of poultry,** and is **also the first limiting amino acid in most commercial feeds.** Methionine is essential for the functioning of immune system. Antibodies (immunoglobulins) show a significant improvement with dietary increases of methionine. **The methionine deficiency depresses immune responsiveness.** The level of methionine required for obtaining best body weight is adequate to obtain best antibody response. **Requirement of methionine for obtaining maximal antibody- and cell-mediated immune response is greater than that for growth. Lymphocytes** appear to have specific methionine requirements. This is because lymphocytes, which play such a vital role in the production of immunity (see Chapter 32), are unable to form methionine from its precursor homocysteine (see **Fig. 31**). Other cells are able to do this. **Therefore, in the deficiency of methionine, unless lymphocytes have an access to available body reserves (pools), even a very small deficiency would first affect lymphocytes before affecting other cells.** As such it is very important to increase the level of dietary methionine beyond that required for obtaining best growth.

The amino acid **threonine is found in high concentrations in chicken antibodies.** Because antibodies depend on amino acid sequences to form the variable regions for binding an infectious agent and in providing structural support, **threonine deficiency may suppress antibody activity.** Work on Newcastle disease (Ranikhet disease) revealed that birds achieved maximum growth with 0.7% threonine in the diet, **but higher amounts were required to obtain best antibody production.**

Recent work has revealed that **avian macrophages are unable to synthesize amino acid arginine,** whereas mammalian macrophages can do so. Therefore, birds require arginine in the feed. In macrophages, arginine is converted to reactive nitrogen intermediate **'nitric oxide (NO)'.** Nitric oxide is a free radical and can kill ingested bacteria and intracellular parasites, and is also antiviral. **Better nitric oxide production** will result in better processing of an infectious agent and in **better immune response** (see Chapter 32).

# VITAMIN A

**Low dietary vitamin A, in the chicken, causes reduced antibody production in response to infections and following vaccinations.** In addition, cytotoxic T-cell responses are defective; there is reduced antigen-specific T-cell proliferation, defective phagocytosis, and **reduced resistance to infection.** Vitamin A deficient birds also have reduced absolute and relative weight of bursa.

## Why should vitamin A deficiency result in the above changes?

Vitamin A is an essential nutrient that has a great impact on the development and function of the immune system. **Its deficiency causes lymphocyte depletion both from bursa and thymus and results in reduced weights of these organs. Vitamin A deficiency increases susceptibility to infectious diseases. This results from a defective immune response.**

**Vitamin A (retinoids) controls differentiation and development of B-cells in the bursa.** Retinol and retinoic acid (forms of vitamin A) bind and interact with their cytoplasmic and nuclear receptors on cells and induce expression of genes that regulate cell proliferation and differentiation. **Recently,** a retinoic acid receptor has been identified in the chicken lymphocytes, and it has been found that expression of this receptor is clearly regulated by dietary vitamin A. Therefore, **in the absence of vitamin A, development and proliferation of not only B-cells, but also that of T-cells, are affected** and this leads to the changes discussed above. The deficiency also affects activity of macrophages and results in **defective phagocytosis and antigen processing.**

In addition, in the absence of vitamin A, the basal cells of bursa change into keratinized squamous epithelial cells. This change is known as **'squamous metaplasia'.** In the absence of vitamin A, the normal differentiation of basal epithelial cells into cuboidal and columnar cells is lost. The resulting keratinization (i.e. formation of dead horny tissue) of basal cells destroys the functional capacity of bursa and results in poor differentiation of B-cells. **This leads to inadequate antibody production. Responses of T-cells are also affected. Deficient chicks are very susceptible to infections and deaths may occur.** For example, vitamin A deficiency increases mortality from Ranikhet disease and *Escherichia coli* infection as well as **Mycoplasma** and coccidial infections.

Good immune responses are obtained with dosages of 5-10 mg vitamin A/kg feed. Further, it has been found that antibody production in the immune response is increased by large single doses of vitamin A (10 mg). This is a useful way to increase the immune response following infection. However, it must be remembered that excessive dietary vitamin A levels, that is, exceeding 10 μg / kg diet damage immune responsiveness in poultry. This means that both low and very high vitamin A intakes result in defective immune response.

## ZINC

In virus-infected cells, and those bacterial diseases in which the organisms live within the cells, such as in avian tuberculosis, **the infectious agents are destroyed by cytotoxic T-cells** (see Chapter 32).

**Dietary zinc deficiency results in poor development of thymus, depletion of T-cells within thymus, decreased helper T-cell functions, and poor cell-mediated immune responses.** Chickens are unable to produce antibodies against T-cell dependent infectious agents **even though B-cells are capable of immunoglobulin production.**

**Zinc is among the metabolically most active of the trace minerals.** It is an activator or a cofactor of more than 200 enzymes and has a very large number of functions. In growing chicks zinc stores last for only about few days. Bone stores last a few days longer, **but a zinc deficiency soon develops.** Thus, of all the trace minerals, storage pools of zinc are the smallest compared to the requirement, and dietary deficiencies are not well compensated for by the body.

## Why should zinc deficiency cause the changes described above?

1. The above changes are due to **a decrease in zinc-containing hormone** (a secretion) produced by thymus (a gland in the neck of birds) known as **'thymulin'.** Thymulin is necessary for T-cell development. In addition, there are **two zinc-containing enzymes,** namely, **DNA and RNA polymerase, and one zinc-dependent enzyme deoxythymidine kinase.** All these enzymes are necessary for T-cell growth and multiplication. Inadequate lymphocyte proliferation may be due to defective nucleic acid synthesis. **The functions of all these enzymes and thymulin hormone are destroyed in the absence of zinc.**

2. Under Chapter 32 ('The avian immune system') it was stated that for antibody production B-cells require help (stimulation) from helper T-cells through chemical

messengers known as 'cytokines' (interleukin 4, 5 and 10) **(Fig. 38)**. For the production of antibodies against most of the infectious agents, except **pneumococcal polysaccharide** and **Brucella organisms**, chickens depend on helper T-cells for help. Therefore, these infectious agents are known as **'T-cell dependent antigens'. Since in the absence of zinc, helper T-cells are unable to function, B-cells cannot produce antibodies against most infectious agents even though they are capable of antibody production.**

3.  Likewise, **cytotoxic T-cells**, which kill virus-infected cells, **also require stimulation from helper T-cells** for their activity. This help comes in the form of a chemical messenger (a cytokine), known as **interleukin-2**, produced by helper T-cells **(Fig. 38)**. In zinc deficiency, there is defective production of inteleukin-2 by helper T-cells. **Due to inadequate production of interleukin-2, and therefore insufficient stimulation, cytotoxic T-cells are unable to destroy virus-infected cells.**

4.  More recently, it has been revealed that zinc is also necessary for **macrophage function**, that is, **in phagocytosis**. Macrophages in bird are the first line of defence against infectious agents, once physical barriers are broken. It was discussed under Chapter 32 that the infectious agent has first to be processed by **'antigen-processing cells'** and then presented to cells of the immune system for antibody production. **Macrophage is the most important antigen-processing cell in the chicken's body.** An infectious agent cannot be processed unless it is engulfed, that is, phagocytosed. **In zinc deficiency, this function of the macrophage is seriously damaged.** Therefore, in zinc deficiency, there will be poor processing of the infectious agent, **resulting in poor antibody production and increased susceptibility to infectious diseases.**

**To conclude, most antibody responses in poultry are thymus dependent. That is, they require co-operation between B-cells, T-cells and macrophages for the production of immunity. Since zinc deficiency severely damages the activity of all these immune cells, zinc must be added in adequate amounts to poultry feed.**

## NUTRIENTS AS PROTECTORS OF TISSUE DAMAGE (Vitamin E, Selenium, Vitamin C, Vitamin A, Manganese, Copper, Zinc)

When the immune system reacts against infectious agents, several harmful substances are formed. **One of the most important is free radical. A free radical** is an atom, or a group of atoms, that has one or more **unpaired electrons** in the outer orbit. In such a state, the free radical is **extremely reactive and unstable**. It then enters into reactions and severely damages the cells. In the body, **they are mostly derived from oxygen and nitrogen.** Those derived **from oxygen are superoxide, hydroxyl radical, hydrogen peroxide, and singlet oxygen;** and that from nitrogen **is nitric oxide (NO).**

The rapidly proliferating cells of the stimulated immune system are particularly prone to damage by free radicals (i.e. **oxidative damage**). **Free radicals can harm all types of biological molecules, and it is only the presence of natural antioxidants in the body that enables cell's survival.** Free radicals act on the double bonds of the unsaturated fatty acids present in the lipids of the cell membrane. This leads to **peroxidation** (a form of oxidation) of the cell membrane, which eventually results in extensive damage of both cell membrane and also the cell. **If the integrity and stability of the cell membrane of the immune cells (B- and T-cells) is threatened, they cannot produce immune responses effectively.** (**Peroxidation** is oxidation to the greatest possible extent resulting in the formation of **peroxides. Peroxide** is a compound, such as hydrogen peroxide, in which oxygen is joined to oxygen.)

**Free radicals have an electrical charge** and try to get an electron from any molecule or substances in the neighbourhood. Once, they get an electron, the unpaired electron in the free radical gets paired. As a result, free radicals are neutralized, that is, inactivated. In other words, they now become stable and do not cause damage. On the other hand, **if free radicals are not neutralized, they produce more free radicals and these cause serious damage** to the cell membrane, vessel wall, proteins, fats, and even to the DNA of the cell. This damage is called as **'oxidative stress'**.

It is here that the body's **antioxidants** come to bird's rescue. **An antioxidant is a substance that has the ability to give an electron to a free radical and balance out the unpaired electron. This neutralizes the free radical.** As mentioned, the free radical then becomes stable and does not cause the damage. The **antioxidants** are so named because they inhibit oxidation or reactions produced by oxygen free radicals.

**Some of the antioxidants are produced in the bird's body.** These are mainly enzymes, such as **superoxide dismutase, catalase,** and **glutathione peroxidase**. However, the bird does not produce all the antioxidants that it needs. **The rest it gets from feed.** As long as adequate amounts of antioxidants are available for the amount of free radicals produced, **no damage is caused to the body.** But when more radicals are produced than there are antioxidants available, **such as under stress, oxidative damage occurs.**

**The most common antioxidants are vitamin E, vitamin C, vitamin A and selenium, which bird must get through the feed. Each has a specific role.** For example, vitamin E is fat-soluble and is best antioxidant within the cell membrane. **Vitamin C is water-soluble and is therefore best antioxidant to destroy free radicals in the blood. Glutathione** is the best antioxidant inside the cell, that is, in the cytosol. **Vitamin C** has the ability to regenerate vitamin E and glutathione, so that they can be used again.

## Vitamin E

**Vitamin E is a very effective natural antioxidant.** It is present in all the cell membranes to prevent oxidation of their unsaturated fatty acids. In the membrane, it captures the free radicals and inactivates them. Vitamin E is unique among all antioxidants in that, being fat-soluble, it preferentially accumulates in the cell membranes, and not in the fluid portion of the cell - cytosol. **It works in close association with selenium** (discussed next).

## Selenium

**Selenium is a component of the antioxidant enzyme glutathione peroxidase.** This enzyme removes active peroxides (free radicals) from the cells, before they could damage (oxidize) unsaturated fatty acids. Vitamin E and selenium together prevent cell damage caused by free radicals. Vitamin E prevents peroxide formation in the cell membranes. In case this could not be prevented and peroxides diffuse into the fluid portion of the cell (cytosol), then selenium through the enzyme glutathione peroxide removes peroxides from the cytosol. **Thus, vitamin E and selenium work together, to protect cells from oxidative stress of free radicals.**

## Vitamin C and A

**Vitamin C and A also possess significant antioxidant activity.** Vitamin C being water-soluble can inactivate free radicals directly within the cell (cytosol), and also indirectly by regenerating the antioxidant form of vitamin E. **Thus, vitamin E and C also work together.** In addition, enzymes **superoxide dismutases** also destroy free radicals. This group of enzymes, localized inside the cells, includes **manganese-containing superoxide dismutase** present in mitochondria and **copper- and zinc-containing superoxide dismutase** found in the cytosol. Dismutases convert free radical superoxide to **hydrogen peroxide ($H_2O_2$)**, and thus protect the cells of the immune system from **oxidative damage (oxidative stress).**

It has been observed that **deficiency of vitamin E and selenium depresses weight of bursa, reduces total number of lymphocytes both in bursa and thymus as well as in the spleen, and causes very damaging structural alterations within these organs. Dietary copper and zinc deficiencies** cause reduced superoxide dismutase activity in poultry. **The amounts of vitamin E, copper, zinc and manganese in tissues are directly affected by their dietary levels.**

## Organic Selenium

As stated, body requires **selenium** on account of its incorporation in the **antioxidant enzyme glutathione peroxidase.** This enzyme destroys toxic peroxides so that immune cells can function efficiently, **producing the best immune response.** However, in the inorganic form (sodium selenite), selenium is poorly absorbed from the intestinal tract, and has also limited biological activity. In contrast, in the organic form, selenium is actively and efficiently absorbed, is biologically more available, and is also very active. It is therefore most advantageous to feed selenium to poultry in the organic form.

Organic selenium is produced in the yeast in the form of **seleno-amino acids,** that is, amino acids containing selenium. Selenium is incorporated in the place of sulphur atoms in the sulphur-containing amino acid **methionine.** Thus, organic selenium is obtained from **seleno-amino acids** that possess special properties. **Firstly,** selenium-containing amino acids are efficiently absorbed through amino acid transport mechanisms. **Secondly,** they are able to move via blood throughout the body. **Thirdly,** instead of being largely excreted through urine like inorganic selenium, seleno-amino acids (organic selenium) are converted into biologically active seleno-proteins and structural tissue protein. Seleno-amino acids can be used by any tissue taking up methionine. **Incorporation of organic selenium into tissue protein is very important because it increases selenium retention in body (mainly muscles). As a result, selenium content of tissue protein is increased.**

**At the cellular level,** body protein is continuously recycled. That is, it is broken down and re-synthesized. **Selenium-containing protein thus serves as an excellent source of selenium for seleno-protein synthesis.** It is now known that selenium forms an integral part of 14 biologically active seleno-proteins in the body, **six of which play a central role in the bird's antioxidant defence system.** For example, the **antioxidant enzyme glutathione peroxidase, a seleno-protein, is composed entirely of seleno-amino acids.** It is therefore most important that seleno-amino acids be part of the muscle amino acids **so that a reserve is available during periods of stress.**

**Thus, by replacing dietary inorganic selenium with organic selenium, we can increase both selenium absorption and its biological availability and activity.** We therefore derive the maximum benefit from the limited levels allowed in the diet. The selenium-dependent antioxidant pathway is crucial to bird's health, and hence productivity. **Disease, either from infectious agent, or due to physical stress arising from environmental mismanagement, results in over-production of free radicals and tissue damage.**

**Nutritional stress, that is, either a deficiency of selenium, vitamin E, zinc or manganese, or an excess of polyunsaturated fatty acids, iron or vitamin A and the presence of toxins and toxic compounds, is most important.** This is because on the one hand it reduces antioxidants and on the other it increases pro-oxidants, that is, substances that damage cell membranes by bringing about their lipid peroxidation. **By ensuring adequate supply of organic selenium** (i.e. biologically active selenium), **it is possible to improve the antioxidant defence system of the bird, and thus improve flock health and productivity.**

## Organic Zinc

Similarly, **organic zinc (zinc-methionine) is more bioavailable to the bird than its two inorganic forms** - zinc sulphate and zinc oxide. Also, inorganic zinc is poorly available in maize-soya diets due to phytic acid chelation (see 'phytic acid' under Chapter 23: 'Enzymes'). **Increased absorption of zinc from the organic form of zinc-methionine creates a larger zinc pool in the body.** This, in turn, boosts functions of those cells of the immune system that require zinc, such as the various types of T-cell in the thymus. **Zinc-methionine, when added to the diet, improves the immune system of poultry and increases their disease resistance. This is because zinc is very essential for normal development, maintenance and function of the avian immune system.**

**To conclude, for getting better results, it is recommended to include both selenium and zinc in the feed in the organic form rather than the inorganic form.**

**Note:** For a list of various commercially available preparations **containing organic selenium,** and their indications and dosage, refer to Chapter 19 under **"Minerals".** It is not known whether preparations containing organic zinc are currently available.

## ACUTE PHASE PROTEINS

Following infection, within a few hours, body synthesizes what are known as **'acute phase proteins'. Acute phase proteins appear earlier than antibodies.** These are non-antibody proteins. The purpose is **to ensure immediate protection for the bird,** since protection from antibodies takes a few days. Acute phase proteins impart **protection** and **resistance** to birds against infectious agents **within a few hours** and then subside (by 24-48 hours). Afterwards, the immune response takes over and does the job. **Explained simply, acute phase proteins are like the 'border security force' which promptly checks the invader, and antibodies like the 'army' meant for a major fight with the enemy.**

During the acute phase of an immune response, or following an infectious disease, the greatest nutritional need is for the synthesis and release of various **'acute phase proteins'.** Under the influence of certain cytokines (i.e. chemical messengers like interleukin-1, interleukin-6, and tumour necrosis factor-alpha) released from macrophages following infection, **liver cells increase protein synthesis and secretion. Synthesis of acute phase proteins requires about 10 times more energy and amino acids than are needed by lymphocytes producing an immune response.** Moreover, their synthesis is more sensitive to deficiencies of several nutrients, including amino acids methionine and cysteine.

One of the important acute phase proteins, **in the chicken,** is copper-containing **ceruloplasmin.** Most of the blood copper in the chicken is found as a component of ceruloplasmin. **Ceruloplamin,** in poultry, plays an important role in the acute phase of the immune response. **It reduces the formation of free radicals.** Also, ceruloplasmin protects the bird against excesses of the immune response by its antihistamine activity and by removing oxygen derived free radicals produced during phagocytosis.

**Ceruloplasmin is greatly increased within 24 hours following** *Escherichia coli* **infection.** Similarly, ceruloplasmin increases in *Eimeria tenella* infection, that is, in caecal coccidiosis. Its increases in other infectious diseases of poultry are currently being investigated. Thus, the need to synthesize ceruloplasmin during an infection **increases the copper requirement.** Ceruloplasmin activity is influenced by the levels of copper in the diet of chickens undergoing an acute phase response. Feeding more dietary copper increases the level of ceruloplasmin, the major transporter of copper in the blood.

## Conclusion

An adequate supply of good quality protein containing essential amino acids like methionine, and also certain vitamins, minerals, and trace elements, is a must to ensure protection of poultry against infectious diseases through successful operation of the immune mechanisms. This would ensure effective immunity. Demand for these essential nutrients is greatly increased while the immunity is being produced following infections and vaccinations. **Therefore, dietary supplementation of essential amino acids and necessary vitamins and trace elements should be recommended at higher levels for poultry to maintain a high level of immune protection in the face of stress and the considerable infectious pressure which may occur in modern poultry production practices.**

## PREVENTION OF EARLY CHICK MORTALITY

It is suggested that the following measures, if properly implemented, would greatly help in the prevention of early chick mortality by boosting up the immune resistance, both in broilers and layers.

**(A)** On arrival of the day-old chicks, give a **probiotic** in the very first drinking water, even though a probiotic has been added to the feed. This is because the intestine of the newly hatched chick is sterile, that is, free from bacteria (see Chapter 20: 'Antibiotic growth promoters'), and the first bacteria to enter are *Escherichia coli*. Therefore, if the beneficial bacteria of probiotic are introduced into the intestine first, they occupy the attachment sites and exclude the disease-producing bacteria through **'competitive exclusion'** (see Chapter 21: 'Probiotics'). Remember that probiotic only through the feed does not serve the purpose. Probiotic must also be given along with in the drinking water in proper dosage for at least 5-7 days.

**The probiotic also boosts the immune system.**

**Note:** For a list of commercial probiotic preparations available in the market and their indications and dosage, refer to Chapter 19 under **'Probiotics'.**

**(B) Then, in the same drinking water, administer the following vitamins and minerals also for 5-7 days. Their suggested dosages are:**

1. Vitamin A - 10,000 IU / litre of drinking water

2. Zinc - 60 mg / litre of drinking water

3. Vitamin E - 250 IU / litre of drinking water

4. Selenium - 600 ppm / litre of drinking water

5. Vitamin C - 400 mg / litre of drinking water

6. Copper 6 mg/litre of drinking water

## Feed Supplementation

**The above formula is no replacement for the feed supplementation.** The feed must also contain the above nutrients in the dosages suggested below.

1. Vitamin A - 10,000 IU / kg of feed

2. Vitamin E - 200-240 IU / kg of feed

3. Vitamin C - 150 - 200 IU / kg of feed

4. Zinc 60 mg / kg of feed (inorganic)

5. Selenium 0.4 mg/kg of feed (inorganic)

6. Copper - 6-8 mg / kg of feed

It is advised that **inorganic selenium and zinc should be replaced by organic selenium and zinc,** if available.

## Benefits of the Formula

1. The above measures **will prevent the early deaths in chicks** significantly.

2. Since these measures boost the immune system, **there will be no vaccination failures** in the later part of the bird's life.

3. As these measures build up bird's resistance, there will be an increase in flock liveability. That is, **much less morbidity (sickness) and mortality (deaths);** and, it will all add up to **profitable poultry farming.**

# Chapter 34

# Vaccines and Vaccination

**Disease prevention and control depend on:**

1. Proper management

2. Proper nutrition

3. Proper sanitation

4. Proper disinfection

5. Proper biosecurity

6. Proper disease diagnosis and treatment, and

7. **Proper vaccination**

**Vaccination is the most practical method of protecting the birds against viral diseases, since there is no treatment for a viral disease.** Therefore, birds must be protected from common viral diseases by means of correct and timely vaccinations. Remember: **'Prevention is always better than cure'.**

Although vaccination is carried out mainly against viral diseases, vaccines against bacterial diseases are also produced, under specific circumstances.

**There are a large number of vaccines available for poultry,** and their number is ever increasing with the emergence of new diseases. For example, we now have a vaccine against leechi disease and inclusion body hepatitis. Disease control by vaccination is more effective for some diseases than others. **Vaccines work best under conditions of good biosecurity and hygiene.**

## What is a vaccine?

**A vaccine** is a preparation which contains either killed micro-organisms, or live attenuated organisms (i.e. organisms whose disease-producing power has been weakened), or live fully virulent organisms (i.e. organisms with full disease-producing power). The preparation is administered to produce immunity (resistance) against a particular disease.

## What are the different types of vaccines?

**Vaccines for poultry are of two types:  (1) live (viable), or (2) killed (inactivated).** Each type has specific advantages and uses. Vaccines against different diseases are usually combined to give protection against a number of viral and bacterial diseases.

## What are the differences between a live and a killed vaccine?

**The differences are:**

1.  **Live vaccines:** Usually they **contain only antigen.** An antigen is a substance which, when introduced into the body, induces the formation of antibodies. **The antigen is either a virus or a bacterium.** ('Bacterium' is singular of 'bacteria'). The antigen may either be a disease-producing organism which has been deliberately attenuated, that is, made much less harmful, for example H120 strain of infectious bronchitis virus; or it may be a naturally occurring mild strain of the organism such as B1 strain of Ranikhet disease virus.

    **Killed vaccines, on the other hand, consist of concentrated antigen combined with an oil emulsion or aluminium hydroxide adjuvant.** (An **adjuvant** is any substance, which when given with an antigen, increases the immune response of the antigen.) Antigens against two or three different disease-producing organisms can be included in one vaccine.

2.  A **live vaccine** may be administered by spray (aerosol), intranasal route (through the nose), drinking water, or eye drop. An exception is Marek's disease vaccine, which must be injected. **A killed vaccine, on the other hand, must always be injected.**

3.  **A smaller amount of antigen is required in live vaccine** because the virus multiplies rapidly in the target organ(s). This organ is the respiratory tract for viruses such as Ranikhet disease (RD) and infectious bronchitis (IB), or the intestine for Gumboro disease and avian encephalomyelitis (AE, epidemic tremor). **The live vaccine may stimulate the production of local or mucosal immunity as well as general immunity.**

    **Multiplication of vaccine virus in the vaccinated birds is important and excretion may be helpful in producing good flock immunity.** For example, cycling of vaccine virus is essential in achieving good flock immunity against Ranikhet disease, Gumboro disease, and infectious bronchitis. Lateral spread of vaccine virus can be very undesirable on multi-age sites. For example, if avian encephalomyelitis and infectious bronchitis H52 strain spread into older, unvaccinated group of layer birds, **then the vaccine itself may produce disease.** It is quite common for birds to show a reaction after the administration of live vaccines. Examples include mild coughing or 'snicking' (producing a slight sharp sound) after Ranikhet disease, or infectious bronchitis vaccination. **A killed vaccine, on the other hand, requires a large amount of antigen. This is because no multiplication occurs after administration.**

4. **The immunity produced by live vaccines is usually short-lived,** particularly after first exposure. However, there are some exceptions, such as Marek's disease, fowl pox, and infectious laryngotracheitis. Repeated vaccinations, with increasingly virulent (powerful) vaccines may be necessary to provide long-term immunity with some agents. **Care must be taken with live vaccines that both appropriate vaccine and the correct dosage are used.** Severe vaccine reactions can result in unnecessary morbidity (sickness) and mortality (deaths) if too virulent (powerful) vaccine strain is used in young birds, or if the dose administered is too high.

   **Killed vaccines** (called **'bacterins'** in the case of bacteria), **usually produce long-term immunity.** Killed vaccines are usually virus preparations or whole bacteria combined with an **adjuvant** that are designed for subcutaneous or intramuscular injection. When used after **'priming'**, that is, **first vaccinating** with a live virus vaccine, oil emulsion killed vaccines can provide long-lasting high levels of immunity. This should be considered as an alternative to repeated live virus vaccinations during the laying cycle. **The vaccines must be given by subcutaneous** (beneath the skin) **or intramuscular** (inside the muscle) **injection.** In some cases, they are the final vaccinations after one or more **'priming'** vaccinations with live vaccines. The **labour and vaccine costs** associated with killed vaccines make them more practical for use in **layer and breeder flocks** in which long-term protection against disease and/or decreased egg production is desired.

   **To prime** means to satisfy **first** an essential requirement of killed vaccine for inducing a long-term immunity. The requirement is that a killed vaccine produces such immunity only when the bird is **first** vaccinated, that is, **primed**, with a live vaccine. The word **prime** is derived from the Latin word **'primus'** which means **first.**

5. With **live vaccines**, the onset of immunity is rapid, whereas with **killed vaccines**, the onset is generally slower.

6. **Live vaccines** are susceptible to existing antibody present in bird. **Killed vaccines** are more capable of producing an immune response in the face of existing antibody.

7. **Live vaccines** stimulate local immunity in trachea or intestine. **Killed vaccines** may re-stimulate local immunity if used as a booster. However, local immunity is poor, if it is not a secondary response.

8. With **live vaccines**, there is danger of contamination, for example, with egg drop syndrome or reticuloendotheliosis virus. With **killed vaccines**, there is no danger of vaccine contamination.

9. With **live vaccines**, tissue reactions (vaccine reactions) are possible. With **killed vaccines,** since there is no multiplication of the organism being dead, there is no tissue reaction, except that which is adjuvant dependent.

10. With **live vaccines**, there are relatively limited combinations. This is due to the interference of several organisms given at the same time, for example, infectious bronchitis virus, Ranikhet disease virus, and infectious laryngotracheitis virus. With **killed vaccine**, combinations are less likely to interfere.

**Liquid nitrogen freezing of live vaccines** preserves and prolongs cell culture viability. This is essential for cell-associated vaccines, such as **Marek's disease vaccines.**

## What is the primary purpose of vaccination?

**The primary purpose of a vaccination programme is to prevent disease,** and also to improve decreased productivity associated with infectious diseases. **In broiler flocks,** a vaccination programme is designed to protect against the infectious agents that are a significant threat to the productivity of a flock in a specific geographical area. **A universally effective vaccination programme cannot be designed, due to differences in the prevalence of diseases.** The purpose of a **vaccination programme for layers** is to prevent disease and provide long-term protection against decreased egg production and egg quality. The **vaccination of breeder flocks** in addition must also ensure that antibody levels against selected viruses are high enough to provide progeny with a uniform protective immunity during the first week of life in the form of maternally derived antibodies (i.e. antibodies derived from the hen through the egg).

### In designing a vaccination programme, what factors should be considered?

1. The general health of the flock and the local pattern of disease.

2. Vaccine must not be given to sick birds.

3. The cost-benefit of vaccination against potential loss.

4. The short or long-term protection required.

5. The genetic type and function of the bird.

6. Assessment of the vaccinations, or diseases that occurred in the previous generation, because they influence maternal antibody status. **Maternal antibody** may have a very significant effect on the design of a vaccination programme. For example, in the case of Gumboro disease, it is impossible to vaccinate in the face of high maternal antibody.

## What are the conditions when birds should not be vaccinated?

1. When birds are 'off feed'.

2.   During periods of extremely hot weather.

3.   When birds have some other disease, such as coccidiosis.

4.   When birds have been recently shifted.

5.   When birds are in a stage of recovery from another vaccination.

6.   When birds are being medicated, or are diseased.

7.   Following debeaking (beak trimming).

8.   When young birds are chilled.

9.   When maternal antibody titres are high.

10.  During the first few weeks of an induced moult.

## What are the different methods of administering a live vaccine?

**Live vaccines are usually supplied in vials in freeze-dried form.** That is, they are dried in a frozen state under high vacuum, especially for preservation. Marek's disease vaccine may also be supplied 'wet', frozen, and stored in liquid nitrogen. They should be kept at $4^0$ - $8^0$ C and transported in an insulated container to protect them from heat and light. **The different methods of administration are:**

### 1. Eye Drop and Nasal Drop

Of all the methods of administration of live vaccines, the **eye drop or nasal drop** (i.e. into the nose) **route is probably the most effective**, although time-consuming and labour-intensive. Accuracy is important and the vaccine must disappear after a blink in the case of eye drop, or inhalation in the case of nasal drop, before the bird is released.

**Vaccines should be procured from laboratories having a good reputation.** They should be transported in insulated, cooled and secured packing, and stored under conditions specified by the manufacturer.

### Procedure

1.   Store diluent bottles overnight in a refrigerator.

2.   With a sterile needle and syringe withdraw 5 ml of the chilled diluent and transfer it to vaccine vial.

3.   Dissolve the vaccine pellet by shaking the vial gently.

4.   Transfer reconstituted vaccine back to the diluent bottle and rinse the vaccine vial at least 2 times and transfer it to diluent bottle.

5.   Mix the final vaccine by gently turning the bottle upside down several times.

6.   Store the reconstituted diluent bottle throughout the entire procedure on ice, in a

flask, or a thermocol box.

## Administration

Using a clean dropper, administer one drop from a height of a few cms into the eye, or nostril. Hold the bird in the same position until the vaccine has been taken into the nostril, or has spread over the eye. Vaccine from the eye flows through the lachrymal duct into the respiratory tract.

## Precautions

1.  Do not use unclean and contaminated droppers, syringes, needles, etc. Sterilize them by boiling in water.

2.  Do not use any chemical for sterilization, such as dettol, savlon, soap, etc.

3.  Always keep vaccine vial plus diluent bottles on ice during transport.

4.  Keep also the prepared (reconstituted) vaccine on ice. Remove small quantities for use, frequently. Do not remove the entire vaccine, once diluted for vaccination.

5.  Do not mix all the vaccine vials at the same time. Reconstitute (prepare) one vial at a time.

6.  Use the entire quantity, once a vial is opened.

7.  Destroy the leftover vaccine, vaccine vials, etc. in a disinfectant solution.

## 2. Spray

**This is a method of mass administration of live vaccine.** It involves **application by spray or aerosol.** Generally an aerosol contains particles less than 5 μm in diameter, but this is not desirable as they can penetrate deep into the respiratory tract. This may initiate a severe vaccine reaction with bacteria, such as secondary *Escherichia coli*, resulting in **septicaemia.** (Septicaemia is invasion of the blood circulation by disease-producing bacteria from a local seat of infection). **Therefore, a coarser spray with particles greater than 10 μm is usually preferred to an aerosol,** and is less likely to cause a harmful reaction.

Vaccine should be reconstituted in distilled water, **and not tap water.** The tap water contains dissolved solids and salts which concentrate rapidly as spray droplets evaporate, and this is harmful to the virus particles. The volume of water is determined by trial and error with each type of vaccine. In general, 500 ml of distilled water per 10,000 - 15,000 doses is adequate. **Spray vaccine is generally more effective in a controlled environment than in open-sided houses.** In closed houses, fans should be turned off, all inlets and outlets closed, the lights dimmed, and the birds allowed to settle quietly before starting spraying.

## 3. Oral Drop Method

In this case, using a clean dropper, administer one drop of vaccine into the mouth, and not in the eye or nose.

## 4. Through Drinking Water

**This is an excellent method of mass administration of live vaccine.** Vaccines should be reconstituted in clean cold water in which **skimmed milk powder** has been dissolved at the rate of 5 g per litre. The milk powder should be mixed with the water 20-30 minutes before adding the vaccine to give time for neutralization of any damaging components in the water, such as chlorine or metallic ions.

Vaccine solution should not be put into metal storage tanks. It is very important that the entire drinking system is clean and does not contain any debris, such as rust or dirt. **Also ensure that there are no residues of any sanitizer, which might inactivate (destroy) the vaccine viruses.** Plastic header tanks are therefore preferred as they can be thoroughly cleaned.

## Procedure

1.  Remove all drinkers, or withdraw water for 1-2 hours before vaccination, to thirst the birds.

2.  Clean and rinse all drinkers, and also water channels, using plain water.

3.  **Stop adding sanitizer to water, such as bleaching powder, liquid chlorine or others, 24 hours before and also after vaccination. Also stop any antibiotic treatment to birds at least 24 hours before and after vaccination.**

4.  Add skimmed milk powder to the required quantity of water to be given, at the rate of 5-6 g per litre of water.

5.  Add ice to chill the water.

6.  Take small quantity of this water, mix vaccine vial thoroughly and make initial solution.

7.  Add this vaccine solution gently to the total quantity of water prepared earlier. Keep the water chilled.

8.  Provide this vaccine water to birds.

9.  Ensure that the entire water is consumed within an hour. The reconstituted vaccine should be diluted in required amount of water that will be consumed in one hour.

10. Make sure that all the birds have consumed the vaccine water.

## Water Requirements for Drinking Water Vaccination

| Age (weeks) | Water (Litres/1000 doses) |
|---|---|
| 4-5 | 15 |
| 15-16 | 20-25 |
| Adults | 30-50 |

## Precautions

1. **Use fresh cool water, free of water sanitizer.** Stop using routine water sanitizer 24 hours before vaccination. It has been found that as low as 1 part per million (ppm) of a sanitizer can inactivate a vaccine. Adding **skimmed milk powder** to the drinking water overcomes the inactivation caused by residues of the sanitizing agents. The mild proteins neutralize the small amounts of sanitizer that may be present in the water. **Besides, the virus remains alive and potent much longer when the milk proteins are present.**

2. Make sure to **thirst the birds** for at least 1-2 hours, to ensure proper intake of vaccine.

3. Use **skimmed milk powder** only, or fat free (non-fat) milk. **Do not use ordinary milk.**

4. **Vaccinate during cooler part of the day,** especially during early morning hours.

5. Prepare your own ice from bore water. Ensure that the ice is made from bore well water free of chemicals and sanitizer.

6. Vaccinate only healthy flocks.

## General Tips

The vaccine should be used as soon as possible after reconstition, and **certainly within two hours.** The procedure of administration is very important, as uptake of vaccine (i.e. taking in) by the individual bird is essential. **Most effective uptake of vaccine can be obtained as follows:**

1. The day before vaccine is to be given, the water meter should be read hourly to determine the pattern of drinking, especially in relation to the timing of the feeders. This will give an idea of the best time to vaccinate the birds and also the volume of water required. The drinkers should be cleaned.

2. On the day of vaccination, the drinkers should be raised 1½ hours before the feeders are used. The vaccine should be mixed in the calculated volume of water plus the volume of water within the lines. (The drinker lines in a shed may contain as much as 250 litres of water). The ball cock should be tied up. The drinkers should be

clean.

3. Once the vaccine is mixed, each drinker line should have the bung (stopper) removed and the water drained until the milk-stained water is visible.

4. When all the lines have been emptied, the drinker lines should be lowered to coincide with the feeders coming into use.

5. Walk along the side of the shed to stimulate bird movement.

6. Ensure the ball cock (stop cock) is released just before the tank runs dry.

5. **Injection**

   **All the killed vaccines and R2B live, Marek's disease live, and fowl-pox live vaccine are injected into the bird by either intramuscular or subcutaneous route.** Prepare the lyophilized vaccine (i.e. freeze-dried) **in physiological saline.**

## Procedure

1. The reconstituted vaccine should be injected subcutaneously or intramuscularly by using an automatic syringe having a 20-22 gauge needle.

2. Shake the reconstituted vaccine frequently during vaccination. Also, keep the reconstituted vaccine on ice during the entire procedure of vaccination.

3. **When injecting oil emulsion killed vaccines, subcutaneous route is recommended. This will reduce the risk of aseptic nodules left in the muscles** which cause loss or downgrading of the birds when dressed.

4. Birds should be **dewormed** before R2B vaccination. Ensure that the body weights are above750 g at the time of R2B vaccination.

5. Birds to be vaccinated should be healthy and free from diseases.

6. **Ensure to sterilize the needles frequently to prevent contamination.**

## General Precautions during Vaccination

1. Check quality of vaccine and source.

2. Ensure to maintain the cold chain of the vaccine.

3. Note down the batch/lot number, and the date of production and expiry.

4. Vaccinate during cool hours of the day, either early in the morning or at late night.

5. **Use only the trained personnel for vaccination.**

6. **Ensure to provide anti-stress vitamin medication before and after vaccination to reduce stress of vaccination.**

7. Destroy or burn the leftover vaccine and the used vaccine vials.

8. **Keep a minimum of 5 days between two vaccinations.**

9. Remember it takes a few days before adequate immunity is obtained. Therefore, **maintain good hygiene and cleanliness in the shed and the farm.**

10. **A profile of antibody level should be monitored at regular intervals** throughout the growing and laying period. For this, the blood samples from at least 1% of the flock should be collected, and sent to the laboratory. Titres will indicate the quantitative profile of antibodies and will also point to whether the vaccination was effective for diseases in which antibody formation is important. The monitoring is also useful in determining exposure of the virus, whether from vaccine or from field. Analysis should reveal the level and uniformity of antibody titres.

## Precautions to be observed by vaccinators

1. Wear clean clothes. Insist on separate footwear (shoes, etc.) at the farm.

2. Before vaccinating, observe the flock. Do not vaccinate, if you find that the flock is sick or diseased.

3. Check the flock's body weight and uniformity.

4. Check the flock for signs of coccidiosis, or other diseases, that may interfere with vaccination.

5. Check and note down the medications presently being given in the feed and water.

6. Handle the birds gently. **Remember vaccination produces severe stress and may interfere with the future production of the birds.**

7. Vaccinate no more birds from a vial than the directions recommend.

8. **Follow the manufacturer's procedures for vaccination.**

9. When using water-type vaccines, **be sure there are no sanitizers in the water.** (Neutralize the water with non-fat milk powder.)

10. Handle birds carefully for individually applied vaccines.

11. Lastly, vaccination is an important procedure. You are playing a vital role in prevention of diseases, and in maintaining a good health status of the birds at the farm. **Therefore, never be in a hurry and do a good job.**

**Live vaccines** may have to be administered by injection as in the case of Marek's disease and reovirus (cause of viral arthritis) vaccines. **For killed vaccines,** injection is the only method used, given either by intramuscular or by subcutaneous route. Automatic syringes are used to a pre-set (adjusted in advance) dosage. It is important that the equipment is regularly checked to ensure that the dosage is correct, and also that the needles are changed regularly (after about 200 birds) to minimize the spread of contaminants. Injection may be given subcutaneously in the back of the neck, or more commonly intramuscularly into the breast or leg. Accuracy is important because incorrect placing of needle can result in head swelling, granuloma formation, liver punctures or lameness, depending on the injection site. The most suitable needles are 12.5 mm (half an inch) 19 gauge in size.

## 6. Wing Web

Vaccination through the wing web is the main method of administration of **fowl pox vaccine.** Avian encephalomyelitis vaccine is compatible and sometimes the two products are combined. It is important to use a two-prong applicator. This provides twice the area inoculated and results in better protection. Care should be taken to avoid the vaccine coming into contact with the bird's eyes or mouth. The application site on the wing web should be examined 7-14 days after vaccination to ensure a **'take'.** A **'take'** is a local reaction which indicates that vaccination has been successful, and should appear as a slightly raised and swollen area.

## Vaccination Failure(s)

1.  **Many factors can cause vaccination failure.** One of the most common causes is the **inappropriate administration of the vaccine.** For example, virus in certain live vaccines, such as Marek's disease, is easily killed. Therefore, failure to follow the manufacturer's recommended handling precautions will result in the inactivation (destruction) of the virus before administration. Likewise, live vaccines administered in the drinking water can be destroyed before they reach the bird if they are mishandled, **or if sanitizers have not been removed from the water before addition of the vaccine.** Vaccines that are administered by intramuscular or subcutaneous route can also fail, if vaccinators do not deliver the vaccine to the proper vaccination site.

2.  Although the most common cause of vaccine failure is **an error in vaccine delivery,** there are a large number of cases where vaccines simply do not provide adequate protection. In some cases, the **field strain** of an organism is of very high virulence (very powerful) and the **vaccine strain** is highly attenuated (very weak). In such a situation, the flock may have been effectively vaccinated, but the immunity is insufficient to protect against disease completely. Many infectious agents have several different serotypes. Vaccine failure may be the result of the antigens in the vaccine serotype being different and not providing protection against the particular serotype of the agent causing the field challenge. For example, it is not uncommon for a vaccine break to occur with **infectious bronchitis virus** when the field challenge is of serotype different from that of the vaccine used.

3.  **Management conditions** also play an important role in the prevention of

vaccination failures. If **infectious agents** are allowed to build up on a farm over long periods without proper cleaning and disinfection, it is possible that the natural challenging dose of a particular infectious agent may defeat the normally effective vaccination programme.

4. **The immune status of the breeder flock** also can be involved in a vaccination failure. If the breeder flock provides progeny with high levels of maternal antibodies, vaccination during the first 2 weeks of life may result in the vaccine being neutralized. Therefore, the timing of the vaccination of young poultry with live vaccines must always take into consideration the presence or absence of maternal antibodies.

5. **Certain infectious agents and mycotoxins are immunosuppressive** (i.e. they suppress the development of immunity) and may result in vaccination failure. **Gumboro virus, Marek's disease virus, and chicken infectious anaemia virus** are examples of agents that may cause severe immunosuppression in chickens. One mycotoxin, known as **aflatoxin**, has been shown to be immunosuppressive and is involved in decreased resistance to disease (see **'mycotoxicosis'**).

Also, the flock in which vaccination is to be carried out has birds suffering from diseases that particularly affect the organs which produce immunity (bursa and thymus), **then such birds will fail to develop immunity.** Viral diseases, such as **Gumboro disease, lymphoid leukosis, Marek's disease**, and **chicken infectious anaemia** specifically affect either bursa or thymus; or, at times, even **reticuloendotheliosis** causes reduction of the thymus and bursa. Bursa and thymus are called primary immune organs, since without them immunity cannot be produced (see Chapter 32: "**The avian immune system**"). Therefore, the presence of above diseases in a flock would lead to **vaccination failure**. Gumboro disease virus severely affects bursa, B-lymphocyte being the target cell; lymphoid leukosis virus affects both bursa and thymus, B-lymphocyte is the target cell; Marek's disease virus also affects both bursa and thymus, T-lymphocyte being the target cell; and chicken infectious anaemia virus severely affects thymus, T-lymphocyte is the target cell.

6. Besides viral diseases, **aflatoxicosis** has emerged as an important cause of vaccination failure. **Aflatoxicosis causes reduction of both bursa and thymus.** It is particularly **toxic for B-lymphocytes** (see **'Aflatoxicosis'**).

For a detailed description of the role of bursa and thymus, and also that of B and T-lymphocytes, refer to Chapter 32: "**The Avian Immune System**".

**Note:**

1. For a list of various commercial poultry vaccines currently available in the market, and their dosage and route of administration, refer to Chapter 19 under '**Vaccines**'.

2. **Purchase vaccines from a reliable company that will stand behind its products,** and supply the service necessary to achieve the best vaccination.

# Chapter 35

# Vaccination Schedules

**V**accination schedules may differ from area to area and country to country, according to the local pattern of disease. This is particularly important in the case of viral diseases for which there is no treatment. Therefore, timely vaccinations with reliable vaccines are of prime importance. Vaccinations also reduce secondary bacterial complications. For these reasons all vaccinations must be taken seriously and carried out with utmost care. **The following precautions must be observed for successful vaccination and production of best immunity.**

1. Purchase vaccines from reputed manufacturers and their authorized distributors. Vaccines can also be obtained directly from the manufacturer and stored in a refrigerator, or better still in a deep freeze.

2. Make sure that the vaccine is well within the expiry date.

3. Follow strictly manufacturer's instructions, supplied along with the vaccines.

4. **Carry out vaccinations, preferably in the cool hours of morning or evening.** Keep the vaccine container in an ice box, and do not expose it to sunlight.

5. For vaccination through drinking water, keep the birds thirsty for few hours before giving vaccine. Also keep many water containers at a time, so that every bird gets the vaccine.

6. Use cold water, free from chlorine, offensive smell, or any drug, in which vaccine is to be dissolved.

7. Use vaccine within the prescribed time-limit after its preparation. This varies from vaccine to vaccine. **Generally, use of vaccine within an hour is safe.** Automatic syringes reduce time and labour.

8. If considered necessary, blood (serum) of some of the vaccinated birds may be tested to find out the development of sufficient immunity against that disease. This may be done 2-3 weeks after vaccination, and is particularly recommended in the case of Ranikhet disease.

9. Maternal antibodies (i.e. antibodies derived from the hen for the newly hatched chick through the yolk) can interfere with the production of circulating antibodies. It

is therefore important to design the vaccination schedule taking this aspect into consideration.

10. Use of a sanitizer in drinking water may be harmful to the vaccine. Sanitizers reduce the efficacy of the vaccine, sometimes making it completely ineffective. **Therefore, do not add vaccine to any drinking water containing a sanitizer.** First, flush the water system several times until it is free of any sanitizer. Then provide clean water to which the vaccine has been added.

   If unsanitized water is not available, the sanitizer may be neutralized by adding **dried skim milk** in the drinking water. Add 1 part of dried skim milk to 400 parts of water. Add the vaccine to the milk-water solution and mix thoroughly.

11. Dispose of all empty vaccine vials after vaccination is completed. Put them in a solution containing disinfectant, or burn them.

## VACCINATION SCHEDULE FOR BROILERS

As broilers are killed any time between 35 and 60 days of age, vaccine requirements may differ depending on slaughter age.

The virulent (harmful) strain of Gumboro virus is present in certain areas and **two doses of intermediate strain vaccine are usually required.** These are given at about 17 and 24 days, depending on levels of maternal antibody. Alternatively, one dose of 'hot' strain vaccine may be given on farms where there is a history of high mortality. This vaccine is given in the drinking water at about 14 days of age, **but should not be given to birds without maternal antibody.** The timing of Gumboro vaccination can be more accurately determined after measurement of maternal antibody in 20 one-day-old chicks from each flock.

The Ranikhet vaccine should not be given to day-old birds, if there is a possibility that they are infected with *Mycoplasma gallisepticum* **(CRD).** The first vaccination should be carried out using a mild strain (F1 of B1) by the eye drop or the nasal (the nose) route, one day one. This is usually followed by a stronger RD vaccine, such as LaSota, given in drinking water, around 10 and 25 days. Severe challenge conditions may demand the use of **killed vaccine** given by injection between 0 and 5 days of age. Marek's disease vaccine is given routinely by injection at day old in countries with a high challenge, or where birds are to be kept up to 55 days of age or more.

As a general rule, live vaccines should be given at the same time, **or separated by at least seven days to avoid the phenomenon of interference.**

A general schedule of vaccination for broilers is given below (Table 10).

**Table 10. Suggested Broiler Vaccination Schedule**

| Days | Vaccine | Route |
|------|---------|-------|
| 6-7 | Ranikhet disease (F1 or B1) | Eye drop or nasal drop |
| 10-12 | Gumboro (intermediate) | Drinking water |
| 18-21 | LaSota vaccine | Drinking water |
| 24-30 | Gumboro disease (intermediate) | Drinking water |

## VACCINATION SCHEDULE FOR LAYERS

The schedule of vaccination for layers may differ from area to area according to the local pattern of the disease.

**All layers receive Marek's disease vaccine at day old.** Generally the cell-associated 'wet' vaccine is considered the most effective, and it may be either attenuated (weakened) Marek's disease virus or turkey herpesvirus. Rispens (serotype 1) is regarded as a very effective vaccine, but in some countries SB1 (serotype 2) or various combinations of two or three serotypes are used. Sometimes a second dose of vaccine is given at two weeks of age, and is an effective means of preventing disease in areas of high challenge infection.

**Layers are always vaccinated for infectious bronchitis and Ranikhet disease (RD).** Live vaccine administered has two advantages. **First,** it gives protection from disease during the rearing period, and **secondly,** it also acts as a primer (first stimulation) for inactivated (killed) vaccine given afterwards. For Ranikhet disease, B1 or F1 vaccine is usually given first around first week, and this may be followed by one or more doses of B1, LaSota, or other strains, depending on the local level of infection. **Killed RD vaccine is given around 16-18 weeks of age to provide protection through the laying period.**

The first dose of **infectious bronchitis (IB) vaccine** (H120) is usually given at 3 weeks of age. An alternative to killed IB vaccine is to use live H52 vaccine at 16 weeks. Further doses of H120 vaccine may be given during laying if infection is high. There are a number of variant strains of IB vaccine available in different countries, and these may be used if permitted by the authorities. RD, IB and Gumboro killed vaccines are normally included in one injection at 18 weeks.

**Gumboro vaccine is required in areas of high challenge.** Young birds of layers are very susceptible to the virulent (extremely harmful) forms of Gumboro infection. Thus, up to three doses of intermediate strain may be given at 14, 21 and 28 days through drinking water. If the level of infection is very high, a single dose of killed vaccine at 4-7 days has been shown to give protection.

**Egg drop syndrome (EDS) vaccine** may be required and is given by injection at 16 weeks of age as a single dose. EDS immunity is unusual in that it requires only one dose of killed vaccine, and no live primer (first vaccine) is required. **Live infectious laryngotracheitis (ILT) vaccine** is given by eye drop in areas where ILT is present.

In some areas **live or killed** *Mycoplasma gallisepticum* and/or *M. synoviae* vaccines are used, where these diseases continue to pose a problem.

**Fowl pox vaccine** is used in endemic areas (i.e. in areas where the disease is regularly found).

A common plan of vaccination for layers is given below (Table 11).

**Table 11. Suggested Layer Vaccination Schedule**

| Days | Vaccine | Route |
| --- | --- | --- |
| 1-3 | Gumboro (intermediate) vaccine | Eye drop |
| 7 | LaSota vaccine | Eye drop |
| 14 | Gumboro (intermediate) vaccine (repeat) | Eye drop |
| 18 | Marek's disease vaccine | 0.2 ml by intramuscular or subcutaneous injection |
| 21-23 | Infectious bronchitis vaccine + LaSota as combined vaccine | Drinking water |
| 28-30 | Gumboro (intermediate) vaccine (Repeat) | Drinking water |
| 42 | Fowl pox vaccine | Wing web prick (stab) |
| Week 8 | LaSota vaccine (Repeat) Infectious coryza (bacterin) (only in endemic areas) | Drinking water Intramuscular injection |
| Week 11-12 | Infectious bronchitis + LaSota as combined vaccine (Repeat) | Drinking water |
| Week 13 | Ranikhet disease vaccine (R2B) | Intramuscular injection |
| Week 14 | Fowl pox vaccine (Repeat), if necessary | Wing web prick |
| Week 18 | Ranikhet disease vaccine (killed) | Subcutaneous injection |

**Note:** (1) **During the entire laying cycle, repeat LaSota 8 weeks from the date of R2B vaccination.** In case RD killed vaccine was administered on the 18th week, then LaSota vaccine may be given from 35 week onward.

(2) Infectious coryza killed vaccine (bacterin) is recommended in areas where the problem is endemic.

(3) A list of various poultry vaccines currently available in the market, along with their dosage and route of administration, is given in **Chapter 19 under "Vaccines".**

## Section V

# TIPS ON REARING AND MANAGEMENT

# Chapter 36

# Introduction

The purpose of writing this section is to highlight the fact that, apart from diseases, errors of rearing and management can be equally responsible for losses in poultry, thus upsetting farmer's economy. Anything discussed under this section therefore has either a direct or an indirect bearing on bird's health.

It is now abundantly clear that the **origin of more than 80% of the health problems in poultry lies in poor management.** In fact proper management forms the very basis in preventing losses, and yet it costs so little. **What is needed is awareness of its benefits, which many fail to appreciate, and in turn, pay the penalty.**

**A number of examples can be cited in support of the above statement.** Just to give a few, if proper care of chicks is not taken on their arrival; many may die on the very first day. The first 2 to 3 weeks are crucial in the life of chicks. For example, if water is not available in adequate quantity during this period, or if the number of drinkers is less, this could lead to an outbreak of **gout**, resulting in heavy losses. Then again, if the brooding is inadequate and the area remains cold, the chicks would crowd together and may get suffocated from **piling** (see 'smothering', 'piling'). Also, improper brooding and errors of ventilation, in broilers, can lead to **ascites** in future.

Inadequate space, from that recommended can result in increased mortality and reduced rate of growth. Likewise, proper management of water, feed, light and litter is equally important. For example, any lapses or shortcomings of litter management will cause several problems. **Wet litter will lead to production of ammonia. Ammonia, in turn, will invite respiratory tract infections, such as colibacillosis and infectious coryza; whereas wet litter will predispose to diseases like coccidiosis. Similarly, inadequate ventilation can lead to wet litter and ammonia formation.**

**Perhaps the most important managemental factor responsible for losses in poultry farming is overcrowding.** Yet it is surprising that most farmers fail to realize this basic fact in their zeal to earn more. They tend to put unreasonably large numbers of birds within a limited space. This proves counter-productive and exposes birds to a number of health problems. For example, overcrowding can cause dehydration, smothering, piling, cannibalism, and several other conditions. Besides, it makes birds more susceptible to respiratory tract infections. **The net result: poor growth, poor performance, more sickness, more deaths.**

**To conclude**, you can't make a profitable poultry farming without proper management, just as you can't make an omelette without breaking an egg. **This fact is being highlighted in the chapters that follow.**

# Chapter 37

# Preparations Before Chicks' Arrival

**The following preparations should be completed in advance, before receiving the chicks.**

1.  As soon as the birds at the farm are sold, or otherwise disposed of and the sheds fall vacant, remove all the litter, manure, feathers, dirt, dust, cobwebs, etc. from the floors, ceilings, walls and equipment as early as possible. Then sweep and scrub the shed by rubbing with a hard brush and water. The floors must be scraped visibly clean. Floors should be soaked with saturated washing soda for 24 hours. Then water is drained out completely. Afterwards flush with clean water.

2.  No litter should be kept at the farm. Insects, vermin, rodents (rats, mice), and wild birds should be eliminated or controlled.

    The poultry farmer must know what proper cleaning is, why it is necessary and how it is to be done. **Most disease-producing organisms are killed by disinfectants only after thorough cleaning.**

3.  Remove all weeds and rubbish from the area outside the house, burn feathers, cut the grass, and make any necessary road repairs.

4.  Now, wash the entire shed thoroughly with water, if possible, by pressure sprayer, or a car washer. The water supply should be very clean.

5.  Air-dry the building. That is, allow it to dry thoroughly by exposure to air.

6.  Now, wash the shed with a detergent solution, such as that of soap, thoroughly, and then rinse it with plain water.

7.  Complete all repair of wire mesh, walls, floors, electrical, plumbing, etc.

8.  **Using a flame gun,** burn the side walls, wire mesh, crevices, cracks, cages, floor, etc.

9.  **Spray the entire shed with a suitable disinfectant solution.** (For a list of various disinfectants, see **Chapter 19,** under **'Disinfectants';** and also refer to **Chapter 30: 'Disinfection'**). Wet the wall, roof, ceiling, side mesh, cages, floor, etc. thoroughly. Use the most powerful concentration of the disinfectant, as recommended on the label.

10.  Allow the building to dry.

11.  Test all the equipment like heating devices, thermostat, water valves, switches, feeders, drinkers (waterers), motors, etc. and make sure that everything is in order.

12.  **Assemble all the brooding equipment.** Wash brooders, feeders and drinkers with a detergent solution. Then dip or spray them with a suitable disinfectant solution. Allow them to dry completely. **Place brooder, brooder guards, feeders, and drinkers at the appropriate places.**

13.  **Ensure the availability of water and feed in enough quantity, and also the feeders and drinkers in adequate numbers.**

14.  **Two days before the arrival of chicks,** spread the new litter evenly 3 to 4 inches, or a minimum of 2 inches deep on the floor. Keep the curtains open to prevent dust problem. The litter should be new and fresh, and properly sieved. **Do not reuse old litter.** Make sure litter is in sufficient quantity at the brooding site. Spread newspaper on the litter in the brooding area. It is advisable to test the litter for any bacterial and fungal load, before spreading. **Special care may be taken during the rainy season that litter is dry.**

15.  **Switch the lights on to obtain the required brooding temperature, well in advance.** The old wire and bulbs should be cleaned by a cloth, before use.

16.  Also, before use with the new batch of chicks, the side curtains must be thoroughly cleaned and disinfected. Preferably use plastic curtains. **Avoid using the gunnybag (gunnysack) curtains.** Gunny curtains, or preferably fresh jute curtains, may be used during the summer for cooling the sheds. **Side curtains should have a gap of 6 to 12 inches on top to allow used stale air gases to escape.**

17.  **Allow a time period of at least 10 days for resting the sheds, after the above preparations**. Disinfection and fumigation kill most of the disease-producing organisms, whereas **an empty house breaks the life-cycle of most of those still remaining.**

18.  In case of any emergency, if the chicks have to be reared immediately, **fumigation** of the shed using formalin and potassium permanganate is essential to further increase the efficacy of disinfection (see Chapter 30: **"Disinfection"**).

# Chapter **38**

# Care of Chicks on Arrival

Chicks should arrive at the farm, preferably early in the morning. In that case, they will have the entire day to learn to drink and eat, and would also be under close supervision. **In case they arrive in the evening,** then allow them to remain in the boxes and take them out in the morning, if they are coming from a local hatchery. However, during summer they should be taken out immediately on their arrival, otherwise they may suffer from **severe dehydration.** Also, if they have travelled a long distance from a distant hatchery, then take them out immediately.

1. Before chicks arrive, fill the drinkers (waterers) and feeders. **Chicks should be fed and watered within 24 hours after hatching. Sooner is even better.** In hot weather, dip the beak of the chicks into drinker, after being placed from the boxes into the brooders.

2. Do not withhold the chicks in boxes for a long time.

3. **Chicks can become overheated during transport** from hatchery to the farm, particularly while waiting for unloading after reaching the farm. **Overheating** can cause **serious dehydration, heat stress,** and affect the **disease resistance** of the chicks. It is therefore important that chicks be **unloaded** from the transport vehicle and distributed in the house immediately upon arrival at the farm. Arrangement should be made beforehand for rapid unloading when the chicks arrive at the farm. **Make sure unloading of the chicks is rapid, but gentle.**

4. Count the chicks, before placing them in the brooder.

5. Observe behaviour of the chicks closely for the first week. **Much can be learnt about their comfort by watching and listening.**

   **Some advance preparations include:**

1. Keep maize grit ready.

2. Check all the medications required, namely:

   Sugar solution

   Electrolytes

   Vitamins

Probiotics

Acidifiers

Initial antibiotic to be given

3.  A few hours before the arrival of chicks, prepare sugar, electrolyte, vitamin, acidifier, and probiotic solutions **to be given in the first drinking water.**

4.  Ensure that the **drinking water** is suitably **sanitized** (see Chapter 31: **Sanitization**).

5.  In case of power failure, an alternate source of heat, such as 'bukharis', generator, petromax, lanterns will be required.

**An account of seven days care is given below, day-wise.**

# Day 1

1.  **The brooder temperature should be between 90⁰ - 95⁰ F.** On arrival, place the chicks in the brooder gently. Note the condition of the chicks and check the transit mortality. Gently teach the chicks to drink the medicated water by dipping the beaks of a few chicks into the water. **Make sure that all the chicks are drinking.**

2.  **Feed maize grit (chick-maize) at the rate of 10-15 kg per 1000 chicks for 24 hours.** If crumbs are available, they can be given right from the beginning. The first feed is given by sprinkling, or spreading it on a newspaper or feeder trays. **Ensure that all the chicks are eating.** It is advisable to keep the papers for at least six days to keep chicks away from eating litter. **The first two days are critical in the chick's life** and it is absolutely essential that all chicks learn to drink and eat as soon as possible.

3.  Check chick's comfort and behaviour. If a **vaccination** has to be carried out on arrival, complete it at the time of placing the chicks in the brooder.

4.  **Monitor the water consumption.** Twenty-four hours monitoring is essential from a responsible person. **Drinkers should be cleaned daily and disinfected weekly.**

# Day 2

**Start chick feed.** Ensure chick comfort. Awaken chicks frequently to ensure adequate water and feed intake. Check brooder and room temperature at different periods.

# Day 3

1.  Routine antibiotic course with vitamins be started. (For a suitable antibiotic, see Chapter 19 under **'Antibiotics'**).

2.  Ensure chick comfort.

3.  Check feed and water intake.

4.  Introduce chick feeders filled with feed. Keep the grill open.

5.  Gradually stop feeding on the paper, so that chicks learn to eat from the trays and feeders.

## Day 4

1.  **Remove the soiled newspaper.** Replace it with a new paper to avoid the dust inhalation that may lead to respiratory problem.

2.  **Increase the brooder area.** If possible, combine the two brooder units to a single larger one.

3.  Ensure chick comfort.

4.  Monitor feed and water intake. Is it increasing?

5.  Are chicks healthy?

6.  **Remove weak, small and dull chicks to a separate brooder.**

## Day 5

Increase the brooder height, and check whether the temperature is being maintained correctly. However, this will depend on the weather conditions.

## Day 6

1.  **Remove the newspaper.**

2.  **Put feed in the feeders only.**

3.  Gradually increase the floor space.

4.  **Stop sanitizer in the drinking water and the antibiotic course.**

## Day 7

1.  Check the body weight and monitor growth.

2.  Check total feed intake.

3.  **Vaccinate chicks with F1 or LaSota strain against Ranikhet disease by nasal or eye drop method.**

4.  Brooder guards may now be put at a distance to cover a bigger area.

## General Tips

1.  **Visitors from other poultry farms should be prevented because of the possible disease threat.**

2.  Soles of shoes should be disinfected by stepping on a pad.

3.  **Chicks of only one age group should be kept together.**

4.  **Twenty-four hours before and after vaccination no antibiotic or water sanitizer should be given.**

# Chapter 39

# Brooding Management

Brooding can be defined as the care and management of day-old chicks up to 4 - 6 weeks of age. For the first few weeks, chicks require heat until they are well feathered.

Newly hatched chicks are unable to regulate their body temperature fully. Then, gradually they pick up heat regulation. **The chick is not able to maintain a constant body temperature until sometime between 1 and 2 weeks of age.** This is where it needs brooding and proper brooding temperatures. Brooding also affects the body weight and feed conversion of broilers.

**Brooding is the most critical period in the life of chick, and has an impact on its future growth and performance.** Efficient brooding will lead to the production of healthy birds with less mortality and good weight gains. This will result in the full expression of their genetic potential. As a result, it is **an important procedure in poultry management.**

## Brooder Unit

**The brooder unit consists of:**

1.  **A brooder with a heating source (Fig. 39).** Usually it is a bamboo basket with bulbs as heat source. The height of the brooder should be about 6 inches in the first week.

2.  **Brooder guard:** A cardboard or a metal sheet of about 18-24 inches height, placed around the brooders to prevent the chicks from moving away from the heat source (brooder), feed, or water **(Fig. 39). In winter**, guard should be 25 to 30 inches away from the edge of the hover (equipment for

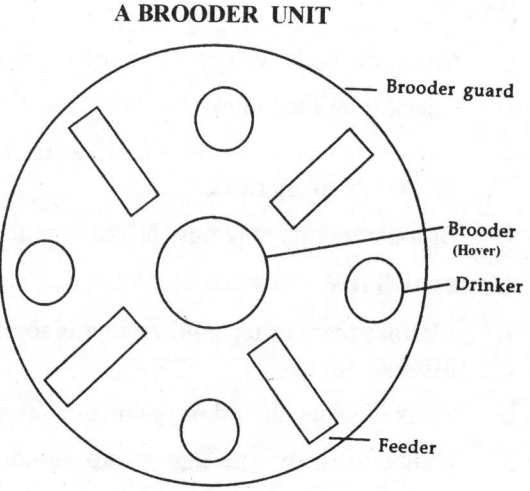

**A BROODER UNIT**

Brooder guard

Brooder
(Hover)

Drinker

Feeder

**Fig. 39.** A brooder unit.

keeping chicks warm), and **in summer** 36 inches. After the first few days enlarge the circle of the guards gradually, and **after 10 to 14 days remove them completely.** In warm weather, the guards may be made of wire network.

Usually a brooder fitted with 4 bulbs of 60-watt and a brooder guard of 5 feet radius may have 250-300 chicks comfortably. However, watt may be increased in winter, when one chick should get 3-4 watt's heat. If **gas brooders** are being used, adjust the temperature accordingly.

3.  **Drinkers and feeders (Fig. 39):** Four baby chick drinkers and four brand new egg trays, on which feed could be given, are sufficient for 250 chicks. Later, these would be required to be increased gradually.

All the equipment should be in place, with **brooders operating at least 24 hours before arrival of the chicks.**

## Brooding Requirements

## 1. Temperature

Best results are obtained when the temperature for the **first 7 days** is maintained around $35^0$ C (between $90^0 - 95^0$ F), and then as the chicks grow older the temperature may be reduced at the rate of $2.8^0$ C ($5^0$ F) on every successive week, until the room temperature of $21^0$ C ($65^0 - 70^0$ F) is reached, or chicks are 4-5 weeks old and fully feathered. **A thermometer, however, is a poor tool for measuring chick's comfort.** This is because thermometers often do not work correctly, and may register a few degrees high or low. **Therefore, the chicks themselves should be taken as the best guide, as they will indicate by their actions whether they are comfortable or not.** Fig. 40 illustrates how chicks could be the best indicator for the correct brooding temperature.

Since the temperature in our country varies a great deal, it is advisable to adjust the comfortable temperature for the chicks accordingly.

**Temperature Guidelines for Brooding**

| Age | $^0$F | $^0$C |
| --- | --- | --- |
| Week 1 | $90^0 - 95^0$ | $35^0$ |
| Week 2 | $85^0 - 90^0$ | $32^0$ |
| Week 3 | $80^0 - 85^0$ | $30^0$ |
| Week 4 | $75^0 - 80^0$ | $27^0$ |
| Week 5 | $70^0 - 75^0$ | $24^0$ |
| Week 6 | $65^0 - 70^0$ | $21^0$ |

Evenly distributed chicks around the hover with a contented peep (a short weak high sound) indicate they are comfortable **(Fig. 40A)**. When the chicks chirp (make a short, sharp, high-pitched sound) and squeeze themselves into a narrow space behind the hover, there is a draft (flow of cold air) **(Fig. 40B)**. If too cold, the chicks will chirp and pile under the hover **(Fig. 40C)**. If the chicks move away from the heat source and feel sleepy, they are too warm **(Fig. 40D). At low temperature** chicks will tend to huddle (crowd together) and may get suffocated; or this may lead to lowered weight gains due to reduced water/feed intake. **At high temperature,** chicks will get dehydrated, and this may lead to poor weight gain and increased mortality. In the case of broiler chicks, high brooding temperature should be avoided.

**Brooding Management**

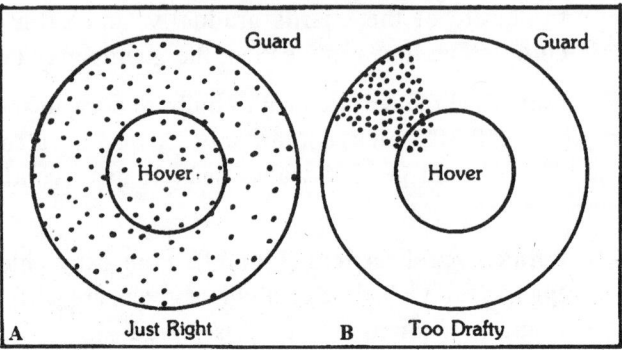

A. Evenly distributed chicks around the hover indicate that they are comfortable.

B. When chicks squeeze themselves into a narrow space behind the hover there is a draft.

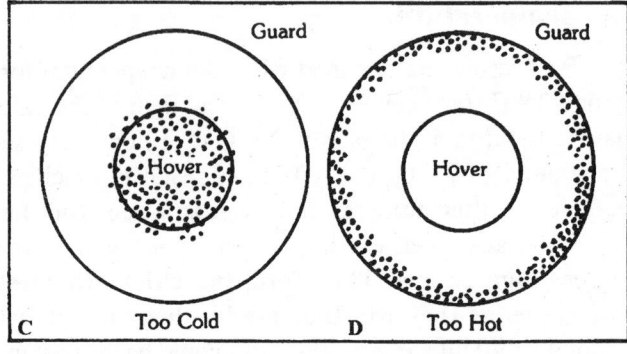

C. If too cold, the chicks will pile up under the hover.

D. If chicks move away from the heat source and feel sleepy, they are too cold.

**Fig. 40.** Brooding management.

The brooder house temperature should be kept at about $70^0$ F to $75^0$ F during the first 4 or 5 days. Thereafter, it should be lowered between $65^0$ to $75^0$ F.

## 2. Ventilation

Fresh air is very important for the health of chicks. It should be available continuously without chilling the chicks. Any errors in ventilation may later result in ascites in broilers (see **'ascites'**).

## 3. Space

Three to four square inches of space (hover space) per chick is the minimum required under the brooder. Not more than 500 chicks should be placed under one brooder, regardless of the size.

## 4. Feeders and Drinkers (Waterers)

Feed should be spread on paper, or given on chick box top or brand new egg trays. Regular feeders should be introduced after 3-4 days. **One tray for 100 chicks should be sufficient. Baby chick drinkers should be provided four per 250 chicks.**

Check the brooder temperature and room temperature with the brooders on. Make additional arrangements, if necessary.

## Effects of Crowding

Chickens should be given adequate floor space during the brooding period. This is very important. **They should not be crowded. Inadequate space from that recommended means an increase in mortality and reduced rate of growth.**

## Losses during Brooding

**Increased mortality,** mainly due to an increased incidence of **ascites**, also occurs in broilers brooded at low temperatures. **Cold weather and low brooding temperatures increase the susceptibility of broilers to ascites.** Low temperatures cause increased feed intake and higher oxygen demand. The increased need of oxygen for broilers at low temperatures, associated with the requirement to metabolize increased quantities of feed consumed to maintain body temperature, **set up an ideal situation for ascites to become a problem.**

Normally, chick mortality (deaths) during the first week is greater than in any week thereafter, **but it should not be over 1%.** Losses in the second week should be slightly less. From the third week, deaths should be at a relatively low level and thereafter run rather uniformly until the end of the growing period. **Most layer chickens are successfully reared with less than 5% loss to point of lay.**

# Chapter 40

# Water, Feed, Light and Litter Management

## WATER MANAGEMENT

1.  **Chicks must learn quickly to drink and eat.** Although they can get along without water and feed for up to 3 days after hatching, such a delay will be very harmful. Any delay only dehydrates and weakens them, and week chicks do not learn to drink and eat as rapidly. For best results, **chicks should be given water within 24 hours after they are hatched.** Remember, chickens of all ages consume about two times more water by weight than they eat feed.

2.  **Provide at least four drinkers for every 250 chicks.** The drinkers should be placed outside the edge of the hover and on the litter so that the water level is convenient for the chicks.

3.  Minimum water space per bird is 1 inch up to 4 weeks and 2 inches after 4 weeks. After 4 weeks one round drinker (automatic) should be provided for 50 birds. Water space should be increased by about 50% in hot weather. **No bird should have to walk more than 5 feet for a drinker.**

4.  **Adjust and raise height of the drinkers as the chicks grow.** As the broilers grow, the height of the drinkers should be maintained at their crop level. Birds consume more water when drinkers are maintained at the higher level. Also, water spillage is kept to a minimum when drinkers are maintained at 'correct height' resulting in better litter management. **Spillage of water in the litter should be avoided.**

5.  The water temperature should be somewhere between $55^0$ F and $65^0$ F. **Fill the drinkers 4 hours before the chicks arrival.** This allows time for the brooder to heat and warm the water. Do not use stale water. **Water must be fresh and clean.** Drinkers should be cleaned and washed daily with a scrubbing-brush. A disinfectant must be added to the water used for cleaning to destroy the micro-organisms and to prevent mould growth.

    Compared to mammals, chickens have only 250 to 350 taste buds in the mouth. Humans have about 9000. Thus, though **chickens** have poor taste judgment, they **can** differentiate as little as $3^0$ C ($5^0$ F) temperature differences between drinking water. Chickens will refuse to drink water at temperatures above $38^0$ C ($110^0$ F). It is therefore important to cool drinking water during summer. Chickens will not drink hot water, and as a result feed consumption will decrease and performance will suffer.

## 6. Water Consumption

As a rule of thumb, that is, as a rough practical method, one can determine the approximate consumption of water by multiplying the age of birds in weeks by two. The answer will be the litres of water per 100 chicks in those weeks. For example, 8 weeks x 2 = 16 litres of water per 100 chicks at 8 weeks. The following table gives the approximate water consumption of 100 chicks per day (**Table 12**).

**Table 12. Water Consumption of 100 Broiler Chicks per Day**

| Weeks | Days | Litres | Gallons |
|-------|------|--------|---------|
| 1 | 7 | 1.88 | 0.5 |
| 2 | 14 | 3.76 | 1.0 |
| 3 | 21 | 5.68 | 1.5 |
| 4 | 28 | 7.57 | 2.0 |
| 5 | 35 | 9.46 | 2.5 |
| 6 | 42 | 11.35 | 3.0 |
| 7 | 49 | 13.24 | 3.5 |
| 8 | 56 | 15.14 | 4.0 |

**In cool weather,** a broiler drinks 2-3 litres of water for every kg of feed it consumes. Water intake increases by 2-3 times **during summer months.** Thus, in hot weather, the ratio may increase to as much as 4 litres of water for one kg of feed.

**Table 13. Water Consumption of 100 Layer Chicks per Day**

| Weeks | Litres | Weeks | Litres |
|-------|--------|-------|--------|
| 1 | 1.75 | 11 | 12.72 |
| 2 | 3.50 | 12 | 13.65 |
| 3 | 5.45 | 13 | 13.65 |
| 4 | 5.90 | 14 | 14.00 |
| 5 | 7.25 | 15 | 14.10 |
| 6 | 8.65 | 16 | 15.00 |
| 7 | 10.00 | 17 | 15.45 |
| 8 | 10.90 | 18 | 15.90 |
| 9 | 11.80 | 19 | 17.25 |
| 10 | 12.25 | 20 | 18.20 |

7.  **Sugar Solution**

    **Addition of sugar solution to the first drinking water has been shown to reduce mortality.** An 8% sugar solution containing 1% sodium chloride is usually given for the first 15 hours after the chicks are placed in the brooder.

8.  **Vitamins and Electrolytes**

    Since chicks are under stress when they arrive at the farm, vitamins and electrolytes must be added to the drinking water for the first 3 or 4 days.

9.  **Use of a sanitizer in drinking water may be harmful to the vaccines.** Sanitizers reduce the efficacy of the vaccine, sometimes making it completely ineffective. Remember many vaccines are administered in the drinking water. Therefore, **do not use sanitizers 24 hours before and 24 hours after vaccination.**

10. **Give water before feed.** It is better that chicks drink before they eat because this procedure reduces dehydration.

11. Finally, it is emphasized that water constitutes as much as 78.8% of the body of the newly hatched chick. That is, **in a newly hatched chick more than 3/4th of the body weight is water.** Hence it is essential that clean fresh water is amply available by providing adequate number of drinkers. **Remember water is consumed twice the rate of feed. Even sick 'off feed' birds continue to drink.**

## FEED MANAGEMENT

1.  Ensure that the feed is supplied clean, and in amounts adequate to meet the nutritional requirements of the birds.

2.  **Give the first feed about 3 hours after the chicks arrive at the farm. Sprinkle it over** the entire area of the feeder lid or container. Feed should be fresh. Feed in small amounts and at short intervals during the first few days.

3.  **During the six weeks brooding period, chicks need feed at all times.** For the first few days of their life, it is important that the feed is made easily available. For this, large, flat containers make the most suitable feeders. Inverted chick-box lids, or similar trays, should be used. Supply one such feeder for every 100 chicks. Some use clean egg trays. Provide two of these for every 100 chicks.

4.  All chicks must eat. **Make sure that each chick is eating from the start.** Provide plenty of light on the feed to make it easier for the young chicks to see. Keep the brooder heat high enough so that chicks are not required to stay under the hover, that is, away from the feed, to keep warm.

5.  Some chicks have difficulty in learning to eat. This results in what are known as **'starve-outs'.** Examine some of the apparently shy or timid chicks on the first day to see if their crops are full. After a few hours on feed, a chick should have a well-

filled, distended crop. **If the chicks are not eating, find out where the trouble lies, and correct it.**

# LIGHT MANAGEMENT

**It is advisable to provide 23 hours of continuous light in the buildings** for broilers. A 23-hour programme is better than 24 hours, because it makes the flock aware of periodic darkness. Power failures can frighten a flock not used to total darkness.

Usually a high intensity of light is given during the first few weeks to help the chicks to get started on feed and water. This is done by using 60-watt per 100 sq. ft. of floor space. After two weeks, the lights can be dimmed to reduce the activity of the birds. Thus, the weight gain is higher. Low intensity light has a subduing (calming) effect on the activity of broilers. Therefore, they get more time in resting and converting feed for additional weight gain. **Also, they are less prone to pecking and cannibalism.** By 21 days, birds may be put on a low intensity light of 60-watt per 200 sq. ft.

# LITTER MANAGEMENT

The bedding material that covers the surface of the floor in a poultry house is called **litter. Litter serves a number of important functions. It absorbs moisture and promotes drying** by increasing the surface area of the floor. It also **dilutes faecal material,** thus reducing contact between birds and faeces. Further, it insulates chicks from the cooling effects of the ground and provides a protective cushion between the birds and the floor.

1. **There are many types of litter.** A good litter is absorbent (that can absorb) and not dusty. It should be fresh, dry and free from moulds and toxic substances. Do not use a litter that has been treated with an insecticide, herbicide, preservative, or other chemicals.

2. The most commonly used litters are **sawdust**, rice husk, and wood shavings. The particles should be large enough not to pass a 1/4 inch sieve.

3. **The litter should neither be too dusty nor too wet.** During the first 3 weeks of the chick's life, the litter should be only slightly moist. After that it should contain about 25% moisture. The litter that has correct moisture (20-25%) adheres slightly and breaks up when dropped from the hand. When litter contains an excess of moisture, it will ball up (i.e. form into a ball) in the hand when squeezed, and when dry it will not adhere. When moisture is below 20%, dust becomes a problem and when it is over 25%, the litter becomes wet and gets caked. That is, it hardens into a solid mass. **Wet litter can have serious consequences (see "Effects of ammonia").**

4. **Addition of chemicals to inhibit release of ammonia from used litter** during brooding is becoming more of an accepted practice. **Most litter treatments inhibit**

**ammonia release by decreasing the pH of the litter** to a level that stops the activity of bacteria that break down the uric acid in the litter to ammonia gas. **At a pH of 7.0 or lower, litter releases very little ammonia,**

5. Start the brooder one day before the chicks are to arrive, otherwise this tends to dry the litter too much. When chicks are placed on an extremely dry litter, this might increase their dehydration. After the chicks arrive, the droppings add moisture to the litter. **If the litter becomes too wet, increase the amount of air moving through the house.** If this does not dry the litter, more litter should be added, mixing the new with the old. But one has to be careful. Usually moulds grow under the wet litter, and stirring or turning only exposes more mouldy material for chicks. **Remove caked or wet litter before adding more.**

6. Cover the floor with three to four inches, or at least two inches, of litter. It is advisable that before spreading litter, a thin layer of sand is spread on the cement floor. Wet or caked litter may be due to less than two inches of litter. **Lack of ventilation, air movement and crowding worsen the conditions.** Turn the litter every now and then, especially in wet seasons. **Keep the litter always dry.**

7. **Avoid spillage of water.** It will lead to wet litter problem. To avoid excessive moisture, good management must be practised. Ventilation must be proper and adequate. Drinkers must be kept adjusted to avoid spillage and in good working condition to avoid leaks.

8. At least twice weekly, rake the litter up gently and remove moist lumps, cakes, etc. Stirring damp litter prevents caking. Apply hydrated lime powder at the rate of 1/2 kg per 10 sq. ft. during raking to keep the litter dry and free from unpleasant smell. **Do not use unhydrated lime powder, as it is an irritant. Also, do not stir the dry litter as it will lead to dust problem causing respiratory diseases.**

9. Finally, **it is emphasized that any lapses or shortcomings of litter management will lead to several problems,** and also invite diseases like coccidiosis and respiratory tract infections (see **"Effects of ammonia"**), such as colibacillosis and infectious coryza. These are serious diseases and may cause heavy losses. **These losses can be readily prevented through proper litter management.**

# Chapter 41

# Broiler Management

**B**roilers are those chickens that are raised purely for meat purposes. They achieve marketable weights very early, by 6-7 weeks (42-49 days). This is on account of their fast growth, high feed conversion efficiency, good body conformation, and early feathering.

Because of the extremely fast growth rate of today's high performing broiler, its proper management has become critical. The modern broiler is much less forgiving to errors of management than the bird of the past, making broiler management more challenging than ever before.

The chicks should be purchased from a reputable hatchery that provides pullorum-typhoid clean chicks. **The qualities of good broiler chicks are:**

1. Fast growth
2. Good liveability
3. Good fleshing
4. Fast feathering
5. Uniformity, and
6. Ability to convert feed into meat efficiently. **That is, good feed conversion ratio (FCR)**

## Systems of Rearing

(a) All-in, all-out system

(b) Multiple age groups system

## 1. All-in, all-out system

**This system means that all chicks of similar age are placed in the house at the same time, reared, and then disposed of also at the same time.** This programme is therefore called 'all-in, all-out', and **is much more successful.** This is because chicks of other groups are not placed in the house until all the older birds are moved out. All the premises are then thoroughly cleaned, disinfected and rested. **This provides a period when there are no chicks in the shed. This breaks any disease cycle at the farm.**

501

## 2. Multiple Age Group System

In this system, chicks of different age groups are reared at the same farm. This system of rearing is difficult to manage and disease outbreaks are difficult to control.

## Preparation of the broiler house

1. The shed should be thoroughly cleaned, disinfected and rested before chicks are placed.

2. Two days before the arrival of chicks, **litter** (sawdust, padding husk) should be spread evenly on the floor, 2-4 inches thick.

3. Place newspaper on the litter in the brooding area.

4. Place brooder and brooder guards, as discussed under 'Brooding management'.

5. Place properly cleaned and disinfected feeders and drinkers.

6. Make all electrical connections and **check on the functioning of brooders.** Check also if **correct temperature** is being obtained under the brooder.

7. Brooding unit should consist of four 60-watt bulbs suspended 6 inches above the floor, and a brooder guard of 5 feet radius along with 4 drinkers and 4 trays for feeding. This unit is meant for 250-300 chicks (see **'Brooding management')**.

8. After all the work is completed; **the entire shed should be disinfected using fine spray of a good disinfectant.**

9. The night before the chicks arrive, brooders can be switched on to obtain the correct temperature.

10. **A few hours before the chicks arrive; sugar, electrolyte, vitamin, acidifier, and probiotic solutions may be prepared for giving in the very first drinking water.**

## Management of the day-old broiler chicks

1. As soon as chicks arrive, check their condition.

2. **Place chicks in the brooder gently. Place all weak chicks in a separate brooder.**

   Chicks should receive fresh water only, and no feed, for several hours when first placed in the brooder. Adding sugar (sucrose) to the first water improves growth and liveability. If chicks are under stress when delivered to the farm, **water soluble vitamins plus electrolytes** may also be added to the water.

3. **Ensure that the chicks are drinking the sugar and electrolyte solution.** Teach a few chicks to drink water, by dipping their beaks.

4. **Check chick comfort.** Are they spread out evenly? Is it too warm? Is it too cold? Are they huddling together? Correct the problem immediately.

5. **Temperature requirements for chicks are as follows:**

   | | | |
   |---|---|---|
   | Week I | Day 1 | $33^0$ - $35^0$ C |
   | | Day 2 | $32^0$ - $33^0$ C |
   | | Rest of the week | $30^0$ - $32^0$ C |
   | Week II | - | $28^0$ - $30^0$ C |
   | Week III | - | $26^0$ - $28^0$ C |
   | Week IV | - | $24^0$ - $26^0$ C |

   **These are only the guidelines. The chick's behaviour is very important in determining the temperature.**

6. **Also, fresh air is equally important.** Make small gaps (at least 6 inches) in the side curtains on the upper side, but ensure that there is no direct wind or draft that will chill the chicks.

7. **Three hours after** placing the chicks in the brooder, when most of them have had water, **sprinkle the maize grit (chick maize) on the newspaper** and also keep it on the paper trays. **Ensure that the chicks are eating.**

8. **Constant 24-hour monitoring is very essential for the first few days.**

9. Usually the broiler starter feed/crumbs is given from 2nd day onward, or may be given from the first day itself, soon after maize feeding.

10. **On the 4th day, increase the brooder area** and also height of the brooders.

11. The **floor space requirements** of broilers are:

    | | |
    |---|---|
    | 1-10 days | 3 chicks / sq. ft. |
    | 11-20 days | 2 birds / sq. ft. |
    | 21-32 days | 1 bird / sq. ft. |

   Allow one square foot of floor space per broiler, if you intend to raise the birds up to 5 weeks (or up to 1 kg weight). **Floor space must be increased if you plan to keep the birds for a longer period of time after 1 kg of weight.** When birds are heavy, provide about 2 sq. ft. per bird.

   **Crowding the birds usually results** in more culls, uneven growth, a lower average body weight, poor feed conversion, more feather picking and cannibalism, decreased market value, more diseases, and higher mortality.

12. **Prevent overcrowding and dusty environments. This will lead to respiratory diseases.**

13. **On the 6th day papers can be removed,** and feed be given in the egg tray feeders. Keep the feeder grill open so that chicks can learn to eat from the feeder.

14. **On the 7th day, the brooder guard can be removed and the area is enlarged to provide more floor space.** Increase the height of brooders to about 1-1½ feet from the floor level. However, this will depend on weather conditions.

15. **Introduce more chick feeders** (3-4 per 100 birds) and **also additional drinkers** (3-4 per 100 birds).

16. **Brooders can be removed by about 3rd week in winter** when the feathering is complete. **In summer,** they can be removed **much earlier** (within one week).

17. **Take the body weights** at the end of first and second week to assess the flock performance. The average body weights should be 150g and 300g, respectively.

18. **Prevent feed wastage.** Feed at least 6 times per day at the beginning to stimulate feed intake. Afterwards, feeding can be reduced to four times a day.

19. **Check bird's activity and behaviour daily.** Is the appetite normal? Are they growing uniformly? Are they overcrowded?

20. **Remove weak, underweight birds to a separate pen.** Provide additional vitamins and growth promoters to these birds. Grading of birds can be done between 10-14 days.

21. **As the birds grow older, ventilation becomes very important.** Keep the curtains open throughout the day. Put curtains, only if necessary, but never full. If the air current or flow is strong, put curtains up to 4 feet from the side wall.

22. **Starter mash** should be given up to 21 days (550-600 g body weight). After this, **finisher mash** is given till marketing.

23. Remember always to **keep the water fresh and cool. Clean drinkers daily.**

## Water, Feed, Light and Litter Management

Refer to these points already discussed under Chapter 40. However, for ready reference, some important aspects are presented again. **Broilers drink a lot of water.**

## Water Management

1. **Provide at least 30 drinkers per 1000 birds.**

2. **Minimum water space per bird should be:**

   1 inch up to 4 weeks

2 inches after 4 weeks, and

One round drinker (automatic) for 50 birds

3. **Usually a bird drinks 2-3 litres of water for each kg of feed it consumes. However, this depends on the weather conditions.** It is therefore very important that fresh clean water is always available by providing adequate number of drinkers. **Water intake increases by 2-3 times during summer months.**

## Feed Management

**Growth rate of broilers** increases rapidly during the first few weeks, is highest between 6-7 weeks, and then decreases as birds grow older.

1. Feeds formulated only for broilers should be used.

2. **The broilers should be given full feed continuously to attain early market weights.**

3. Give broiler starter up to 21 days (550-600 g body weight).

4. Give broiler finisher feed from 22 days of age till marketing.

5. Broiler starter feed contains 22-24% protein with 2900 kcal/kg of energy.

6. Broiler finisher feed contains 20-21% protein and has slightly higher energy of 3100 kcal/kg.

7. Feeding 250 g of a pre-starter usually gets off to a good start. Pre-starter diet containing additional proteins and vitamins is more beneficial to the chicks.

8. Feeder space required is:

   Between 0-14 days       1 inch per bird

   Between 15-42 days     2-2.5 inches per bird

9. Remember, **methionine** is the most limiting (restricted) amino acid in the broiler diet. Therefore, **make sure that methionine in the diet is in adequate amounts.**

## Light Management

Light adjustment is used in the broiler house to increase growth, improve feed efficiency, decrease mortality, and reduce electricity costs.

1. It is advisable to provide continuous light (23 hours light: 1 hour dark per day) during the entire cycle.

2. After two weeks, the lights can be dimmed to reduce the activity of the birds. Thus the weight gain is higher.

## Litter Management

1.  The most commonly used litters are **sawdust,** rice husk, and wood shavings. **Litter should be fresh, dry, and free from moulds.**

2.  In well-managed farms, the **litter** is **neither too dusty nor too wet.** The litter that has correct moisture (20-25%) adheres slightly and breaks up when dropped from the hand. When litter contains an excess of moisture, it balls up (i.e. forms into a ball) in the hand when squeezed, and when dry it does not adhere.

3.  **Avoid spillage of water.** It will cause wet litter problem. At least twice weekly, rake the litter up gently and remove moist lumps, cakes, etc.

4.  **Apply hydrated lime powder** at the rate of 1/2 kg per 10 sq. ft. area during the raking **to keep the litter dry and odour free.** Do not use unhydrated lime powder, as it is an irritant. Also, do not rake the dry litter, as this will lead to dust problem that may predispose to respiratory diseases.

## Ventilation

1.  **Proper ventilation of poultry houses is extremely important.** It meets oxygen requirements of the birds, removes carbon dioxide and other harmful gases, controls moisture in the house, regulates the temperature, and helps in the control of diseases.

2.  **Draft-free ventilation is very important** to provide fresh air, carry away ammonia fumes, and to keep litter dry. **Poor ventilation increases the chances of respiratory diseases** and ultimately results in poor performance. The chicks may be chilled if there is too much ventilation.

3.  Ventilation in the broiler house requires constant attention, especially during winter and spring months. Changes in the weather require immediate adjustments. **With inadequate ventilation, ammonia may build up.** The production of **ammonia** depends upon the amount of feed in the litter, aeration (exposure to air), and possibly, porosity of the litter.

4.  During cold weather and during the brooding period, **the main function of the ventilation is to remove ammonia and moisture from the broiler house.** The key to **control ammonia** problem and provide good air quality is to control moisture in the poultry house. **Proper ventilation** removes moisture and reduces humidity levels, and is the most effective method to ensure good air quality.

5.  Ventilation must be increased as broilers increase in age and weight.

6.  **The major ventilation problem in summer is keeping the house cool.** Whitewashing or painting the roof helps in heat reflection. **Water sprinklers** on the roof will reduce the temperature and therefore radiation of the heat from the roof

7.   A house with wet litter, ammonia fumes and thick cobwebs tells that it is not properly ventilated.

## Debeaking

**Debeaking in broilers is not necessary.** However, if done for better conversion of feed, it is usually carried out between 9-10 days of age. When debeaked between 9-10 days of age, do not remove more than 1/3rd of the beak, or else growth will be depressed. **Debeaked birds show better feed conversion. For more information, refer to 'debeaking' under Chapter 42: "Layer management".**

## Disposal of Dead Birds

**The immediate burning or burying of dead birds is an important part of a good disease control programme.** Never leave birds in the pen or cage, feed rooms, or around the poultry house. **Also, never throw them in the field and never feed them to animals like dogs, cats, etc.**

**Dead birds act as a source of disease** that can be spread by rats, mice, dogs, cats, flies, free flying birds, etc. **There are two methods for the disposal of dead birds.**

1.   Burning them in an incinerator, or

2.   Burying them deep in a disposal pit

## How to determine broiler performance?

1.   Efficiency of broiler performance is calculated by using what is known as **'feed conversion ratio'**, or **'FCR'** in short. Feed conversion, or the amount of feed required to produce a unit of live broiler weight, is of great economical importance to a broiler farmer. **It is calculated as follows:**

$$\frac{\text{Total feed consumed (kg)}}{\text{Total live weight (kg)}} = \text{FCR}$$

**Feed conversion ratio of 2.0 and less is good. Any FCR above 2.0 is poor and uneconomical.**

2.   **Males are better feed converters than females.** Usually, **the fastest growing birds have the best feed conversion.**

3.   The broiler farmer should take proper care in feeding. Some of the **factors that have an important bearing on feed conversion and may cause poor FCR are:**

## 1. Feed Wastage

(i)  When feeders are filled full, 30% of the feed is wasted.

(ii)  When feeders are 2/3rd full, 10% of the feed is wasted.

(iii)  When feeders are 1/2 full, 3% of the feed is wasted, and

(iv)  When feeders are 1/3rd full, **only 1% of the feed is wasted.**

**Remember, the feed in the litter does not produce meat.** Therefore, frequent shallow fillings, not more than 1/4th and preferably 1/3rd full stimulates consumption and reduces feed wastage. **Put feed in the feeders four times a day.**

2.  **Poor quality feed** and **incorrect formulation.**

3.  Poor feed and water management. That is, **less numbers of feeders and drinkers.**

4.  **Overcrowding.**

5.  **Errors in brooding.**

6.  **Aflatoxin (mycotoxin) problem in feed.**

7.  **Litter management** can indirectly influence feed conversion. Slightly damp (wet) and wet litter can indirectly influence feed conversion. **Damp and wet litter is an excellent medium for coccidial, fungal, and bacterial development.**

8.  **Ammonia fumes** in the poultry house.

9.  **Ventilation**: Both over ventilation and under ventilation can increase feed conversion ratio.

10.  Duration and intensity of light.

11.  Floor space for bird.

12.  Moderate temperatures give the best performance.

13.  Nutritional diseases, such as **vitamin deficiencies** or their absence (avitaminosis), will lead to poor feed conversion.

14.  However, in spite of the above factors being fully under control, if the feed conversion drops, **then be careful of a disease problem. Diseases,** particularly those affecting the intestinal tract, such as coccidiosis; enteritis from bacterial and viral infections; worms; diseases like Ranikhet, Gumboro, and Marek's; toxins; and nutritional deficiencies, **are responsible for poor feed conversion.**

In many cases of **coccidiosis**, broilers look apparently normal, but their intestinal tract is severely damaged. **This intestinal damage interferes with food absorption.**

15. Finally, **increased mortality**, from whatever causes, will lead to poor FCR.

**Table 14.   Broiler Performance Standards**

| Age weeks | Average weight (g) | Feed per week (g) | Feed cumulative (g) | Feed conversion |
|-----------|--------------------|--------------------|----------------------|-----------------|
| 1 | 145 | 160 | 160 | 1.10 |
| 2 | 385 | 320 | 480 | 1.25 |
| 3 | 705 | 510 | 990 | 1.40 |
| 4 | 1065 | 655 | 1645 | 1.54 |
| 5 | 1445 | 785 | 1430 | 1.86 |
| 6 | 1835 | 930 | 3360 | 1.83 |
| 7 | 2240 | 1075 | 4435 | 1.98 |

## Vaccinations

**The immune system of the chick is not fully mature at hatching.** Therefore, the bird's ability to immunologically respond to an infectious agent is limited. The chick does receive some passive immunity against diseases from its mother in the form of maternal antibodies. However, maternal antibodies do not protect the chick very long. They decrease as the chick's own immunological system develops. Therefore, broilers are routinely vaccinated to provide protection from infectious diseases.

However, **vaccinations should be carried out keeping in view the diseases prevalent in that area.** The chicks must be vaccinated against Ranikhet disease with F1 strain or LaSota within the first week. It is generally not necessary to vaccinate against fowl pox unless the disease is prevailing in the area.

**Table 15.   Suggested Broiler Vaccination schedule**

| Days | Vaccine | Route |
|------|---------|-------|
| 6-7 | Ranikhet disease (F1 or B1) | Eye drop or nasal drop |
| 10-12 | Gumboro intermediate | Drinking water |
| 18-21 | LaSota | Drinking water |
| 24-30 | Gumboro intermediate | Drinking water |

**Table 16. Suggested Broiler Medication Schedule**

| | | |
|---|---|---|
| Days 1-2 | Electrolytes | 1-2 g / litre of water |
| Days 1-10 | Vitamin AD3CE | 3 ml / 100 chicks |
| | Vitamin B complex | 7 ml / 100 chicks |
| | Growth promoters | 7 ml / 100 chicks |
| | | **All given once daily for 10 days** |
| Days 3-5 | Antibiotic course | 1/2 g / litre of water |
| Days 8-10 | Probiotic course | 1 g / litre of water |
| Days 11-13 | Calcium supplements | 15-20 ml / 100 birds once daily |
| Days 15-20 | Liver tonics | 10 ml / 100 birds |
| Days 15-20 | Immunostimulants | 5 g / 100 birds |

## Mortality

High mortality during the first 7 days is usually related to a hatchery or breeder flock problem. High mortality after 7 days is usually related to disease or management problem. **A typical mortality pattern** begins with **1% in the first week,** decreasing to 0.5% the second week, followed by relatively low mortality during 3rd and 4th week, **and then a gradual increase from 5 weeks** to market. In many cases, **early mortality is associated with dehydration, starve-outs, and infections introduced at hatchery,** whereas much of the **late mortality** is caused by growth related factors such as **leg problems, ascites,** and **sudden death syndrome.**

**Note:** For a list of various commercial preparations containing electrolytes, vitamins, acidifiers, growth promoters, antibiotics, probiotics, calcium supplements, liver tonics, immunostimulants, etc., refer to Chapter 19: **"Medicines and vaccines",** under the appropriate sub-head.

# Chapter 42

# Layer Management

Layers are those chickens that are reared only for egg production. These are light weight birds developed from White Leghorn breed of chicken. **The present layer bird is capable of laying more than 300 eggs per year.**

There are three stages in layer farming:

1. Chick stage **(chicks)**          1-8 weeks

2. Growing stage **(growers)**        9-18 weeks

3. Layer stage **(layers)**           19 weeks onward, usually up to 72 weeks

## 1.   Chick stage

This stage can also be called as **'brooding stage'**, and birds during this period are called **'chicks'**. The brood shed is cleaned, thoroughly disinfected and kept ready in advance for receipt of day-old chicks, as discussed earlier for broilers.

During brooding, the chicks are fed with **chick starter feed (chick mash)**, containing around 2750 kcal/kg of energy, 21% protein, 1% calcium and 0.45% available phosphorus. The chick feed is continued until the time the body weights are around 580 g (i.e. by 7th week of age).

## 2.   Growing stage

The period, after brooding up to sexual maturity, is called as **'growing period'** and birds during this stage are referred to as **'growers'**.

Both chick and the growing stage are of great importance for the future performance of the layer bird. It is during these two phases that the correct body weight and uniformity are obtained, which shape the future performance of the adult bird. During this stage, chickens are given **grower feed (grower mash)** containing 2500 kcal/kg of energy, 17% protein, 1% calcium and 0.40% available phosphorus. The grower feed should be fed from the time flock reaches an average body weight of 580 g until the flock completes 15 weeks of age (body weight of 1000 g). As the production commences the birds are switched onto pre-layer diet containing 2500 kcal/kg of energy, 17% protein, 2.5% calcium and 0.40% available phosphorus.

A total of about 7 kg of feed is consumed between 1st and 20th week.

## 3.   Laying stage

This period is from the onset of production (5% at around 19 weeks) to the end of laying cycle (about 72 weeks). The birds at this stage are called **'layers'**. During this period the hen is provided **'layer diet'** containing 2500 kcal/kg of energy, 18% protein, 3.8% calcium and 0.46% available phosphorus. During this period the production should be as follows.

### For  BV  300  Breed

| Week | Production |
|------|------------|
| 20 | 15% |
| 26 | 97% (peak production) |
| 40 | 95% |
| 50 | 92% |
| 60 | 88% |
| 72 | 81% |

During the entire laying stage, a total of about 42 kg of feed is consumed per bird.

## Schedule of Week-Wise Management

For details, refer to the appropriate chapter. The body weights refer mainly to BV 300 breed.

## Week 1

1.   The **brooder temperature** should be between $90^0$ and $95^0$ F. Adjust temperature by carefully watching and monitoring the birds.

2.   Provide **sugar and electrolyte solution** in the first water, followed by an **antibiotic course with vitamins.**

3.   **Three hours later, feed maize grit (chick maize)** by spreading it on the paper and feeder trays.

4.   Introduce chick **feeders.**

5.   Ensure chick comfort.

6.   Body weights should be around 70 g on the 7th day. **Remove weak, dull chicks to a separate brooder.** Provide light on the first day for 22 hours, and by the 6th day gradually bring it down to 18 hours. A twenty-four hour monitoring be done by a responsible person.

## Suggested vaccinations

(i)    Gumboro intermediate vaccine by eye drop on arrival or by 3rd day.

(ii)   F1/LaSota vaccination on the 7th day by eye drop, or nasal route.

## Week 2

1.   The **brooder temperature** should be between $85^0$ and $90^0$ F.

2.   **Avoid overcrowding.** Expand brooder area by shifting the brooder guards.

3.   **Put more drinkers.** There should be a minimum of 25 for 1000 birds.

4.   **The first touch-up of debeaking should be done by the 10th day.** Provide **anti-stress vitamins** for 3-5 days following debeaking.

5.   Check whether chicks are growing uniformly.

6.   Provide light for 16 hours.

7.   Record body weights on 14th day. They should be around 120 g.

8.   **Suggested vaccination:** Gumboro intermediate or Gumboro invasive vaccine by mouth, or in the drinking water.

## Week 3

1.   The **brooder temperature** should be between $80^0$ and $85^0$ F.

2.   **Increase brooder area.** In summer, the entire house may be kept open. Avoid overcrowding.

3.   **Check water and feed intake.** Check also chick's behaviour, activity, and flock uniformity.

4.   Provide light for 14 hours.

5.   The body weights should be around 170 g.

6.   **Check droppings and bird's behaviour for coccidiosis.** Preventive anti-coccidiosis medication may be required (see 'coccidiosis').

7.   **Suggested vaccination**: On 21st day infectious bronchitis vaccine may be given by the eye drop route (only in areas where the disease is regularly found).

## Week 4

1.   The **brooder temperature** should be between $75^0$ and $80^0$ F.

2.   **Brooders can be removed fully, as feathering is complete by now.**

3.   Provide floor space of 1/2 sq. ft. per bird. The body weights should be around 230 g.

4. **Put more drinkers and feeders.**

5. Check feeding. Do not allow the feed to be wasted. Keep the feed at quarter inch depth and mix it frequently. Keep feeders clean.

6. Provide light for 12 hours.

7. Check water management. Clean drinkers regularly.

8. Check litter condition. Add fresh litter, if required.

9. **Vaccination**: Gumboro vaccine (between 28 and 30 day) by mouth.

## Week 5

1. Body weights should be around 310 g.

2. Check water, feed, and litter management.

3. Provide light for 10-12 hours. That is, normal day length only.

4. **Suggested vaccination:** LaSota vaccine between 20-25 days through drinking water.

5. **Remove all weak, underweight birds to a separate pen**, and feed them a diet containing higher protein.

## Week 6

1. Body weights should be around 410 g.

2. Switch over from starter mash (chick mash) to grower mash, if body weights are normal.

3. Provide light for 11-12 hours.

4. **Suggested vaccination:** Fowl pox vaccine by intramuscular route.

## Week 7

1. Body weights should be around 490 g.

2. Shift the birds to grower house (i.e. in cages).

   Grower cage dimensions should be:

   | | |
   |---|---|
   | Length (front) | 16 inches |
   | Width (depth) | 12 inches |
   | Height | 12 inches |

   **Keep 4 birds per cage =   48 sq. inches cage space per bird**

   | | | |
   |---|---|---|
   | Feeder space | = | 4 inches |
   | Water space | = | 4 inches |

3. Provide light for 11-12 hours.

4. **Watch out for gangrenous dermatitis (wing rot) problem at this stage,** and take immediate action, if noticed (see **'gangrenous dermatitis'**).

5. Do not overcrowd the birds.

6. **Provide anti-stress and anticoccidial medication soon after shifting.**

## Week 8

1. Body weights should be around 580 g.

2. Provide light for 11-12 hours.

3. For the isolated underweight weak birds kept apart, continue the feed containing high protein.

4. **Vaccination**: LaSota vaccination between 54-56 days through drinking water.

## Week 9

1. Body weights should be around 660 g.

2. Provide light for 11-12 hours.

## Week 10

1. Body weights should be around 740 g.

2. Provide light for 11-12 hours.

3. Grading of the flock may be done during this week.

## Week 11

1. Body weights should be around 820 g.

2. Provide light for 11- 12 hours.

3. **Vaccination:** Infectious bronchitis (IB) (repeat), and LaSota vaccine through drinking water.

## Week 12

1. Body weights should be around 900 g.

2. Provide light for 11-12 hours.

3. **Deworm the flock.**

4. **Preventive anticoccidial medication** may be given, if the birds have been shifted from deep litter to grower house at this stage.

## Week 13

1. Body weights should be around 970 g.

2. Provide light for 11 - 12 hours.

3. **Vaccination:** R2B vaccine to be given by the intramuscular route.

4. Give anti-stress medication.

## Week 14

1. Body weights should be around 1030 g.

2. Provide light for 11 - 12 hours.

3. Check uniformity of the flock, following grading.

4. Provide additional vitamins and growth promoting factors to underweight birds.

5. **Prepare the flock for final debeaking.**

## Week 15

1. Body weights should be around 1070 g.

2. Provide light for 11-12 hours.

3. **Check bird activity. Is the growth normal and uniform? Are they healthy? Is feed intake normal?**

4. **Suggested vaccination:** Repeat fowl pox vaccine by intramuscular route, if necessary.

## Week 16

1. Body weights should be around 1110 g

2. Provide light for 11 - 12 hours.

3. **Final debeaking may be done.** Conduct this operation gently and slowly. Remember that **this is the biggest stress in the life of a layer bird. At this stage one can 'make or break' the flock. Hence one has to be very careful.**

4. **After debeaking, provide anti-stress medication, such as electrolytes, vitamins, liquid protein and mineral supplements.**

## Week 17

1. Body weights should be around 1160 g.

2. Provide light for 11 - 12 hours.

3. **Shift the flock to layer cages during this week.** Final grading of the flock is done. Isolate weak underweight birds to a separate row. Cull very weak and lame birds.

4. First egg may be laid during this week.

5. Change over to pre-layer diet containing 2.5% calcium (i.e. more calcium) to prepare the birds for laying.

6. Layer cage dimensions should be:

| | |
|---|---|
| Length (front) | 15 inches |
| Width (depth) | 12 inches |
| Height | 18 inches |

**Keep 3 birds per cage**

| | |
|---|---|
| Feeder space | 5 inches |
| Water space | 5 inches |

## Week 18

1. Body weights should be around 1200 g.

2. Provide light for 11-12 hours (normal day light).

3. Continue pre-layer diet.

4. **Deworm the flock.**

5. **Suggested vaccination:** Ranikhet disease killed vaccine be given by intramuscular or subcutaneous (under the skin) route.

## Week 19

1. Body weights should be around 1280 g.

2. Provide light for 11 - 12 hours (normal day light).

3. Continue pre-layer diet.

4. Egg production gradually increases now.

5. Feed *ad lib*. That is, without restriction, but do not allow the feed to be wasted.

   Feed at least 2 - 3 times daily.

## Week 20

1. Body weights should be around 1360 g.

2. Provide light for 11 - 12 hours with an hour increase at 5% production.

3.  Change over to layer diet at 5% production.

4.  **Start anti-stress medication (vitamins, growth promoters) on a weekly basis.**

## Week 21

1.  Provide light for 12 hours.

2.  Feed *ad lib*. Feed intake increases now. Do not underfeed.

3.  Do not forget daily works, such as cleaning of feeders, water channels, interior of shed, etc.

4.  **Collect eggs frequently.**

5.  **Prevent fly problem** by keeping the shed and farm premises clean.

6.  **Suggested vaccination: LaSota vaccine to be given between every 6-8 weeks in the drinking water.** In case RD killed vaccine was administered on the 18th week, then LaSota vaccine may be given from 35th week onward.

## Week 22

Provide light for 12½ hours.

## Week 23

Provide light for 13 hours.

Between 23 and 28 weeks, increase the light by 30 minutes per week until a maximum of 16 hours is reached. The lighting programme given above is only for lighting the shed, and not for the warmth of the chicks.

The lighting programme indicated above is designed to have the flock lay the first egg by 19 weeks of age, reach 10% of production at 20 weeks, and peak production between 26-27 weeks. The average body weights at 20 weeks should be about 1360 g at the time of increasing the light. Do not increase the day length until the average body weight of the flock reaches 1360 g.

## Feed Management

1.  The nutrients must be supplied in proper proportion and in a form nutritionally available to the birds. That is, **birds should be given balanced feed.**

2.  **Feed at least three times in a day.** Take special care that the feed is spread uniformly.

3.  Texture, colour, and taste of the feed must be acceptable to the bird.

4.  Keep an accurate row-wise and pen-wise record of feed consumption.

5.  To avoid wastage due to spillage while feeding, use mugs or scoops. These days

feeder trolleys are being used to avoid feed wastage.

6.   Level of feed at the time of feeding should not exceed 1/3rd the height of feeder.

7.   Do not throw feed from one end of feeder to the other. This results in loss of essential minerals (trace elements) in the form of dust.

8.   Feed should not be dusty. It must be free from contamination by disease-producing organisms like **Salmonella** and harmful chemicals and toxins. Animal by-products like fish meal, meat meal, liver meal, and blood meal are widely used. **They should be completely free from any contamination.**

9.   The stock of prepared feed at the farm should not exceed the requirements of more than 3 to 4 days. **Always provide fresh feed.**

10.  Calcium should be added to the feed in the form of oyster shell with a particle size of 3-5 mm. If calcium is added in the form of limestone, 2/3rd should be used in the form of large particles (3-5 mm), and only 1/3rd in the form of powder.

11.  **Contamination of the feed during storage, delivery and transport must be avoided.** Wild birds and rodents can contaminate the feed at any of the above stage.

12.  **Formulate your own feed** according to the season, age, and body weight of the birds. The formulations should be based on each feed ingredient being accurately valued, before they are all mixed together.

13.  Formulation of the feed should be based on maximum profitability, naturally on a least cost. However, the least cost feeds are only sometimes and not always profitable.

14.  Summer season makes the birds eat less. Therefore, efforts should be made to cool the house and also to increase the nutritional intensity.

15.  **Check the following causes for any feed wastage.**
     Spillage outside bags
     Spillage while feeding
     Filling too high in feed buckets
     Filling too high in feeders
     Faulty design or damages in feeders
     Use of old, torn bags
     Bad storage
     Rat problem
     Pilferage (i.e. small thefts)
     Poor debeaking

## Storage of Feed

1. **Keep feed bags away from dampness,** as well as from sunlight. Leaky roofs should be repaired to prevent the feed getting wet.

2. Feed bags should be stacked on wooden or stone beams 6 inches away from the floors and walls.

3. **Contamination during storage as well as during delivery must be avoided, particularly in the rainy season.** Wild birds and rodents also contaminate stored feed.

4. **Feed should always be stored and used in the sequence of its arrival.** That is, on a first in, first out basis.

5. **Discard any bag of feed that has lumps in it, or has got wet in transit.**

## Water Management

1. The quantity of water given to the bird, and the way it is given, has a great influence on the performance of chicks. Some interesting facts are:

    (i) Water content of the newly hatched chicks is nearly 80%. In a grown up bird it is 55%.

    (ii) 70% of the weight of an egg is water.

    (iii) A bird can lose 50% of its protein and still survive. It can lose 40% of the body weight and carry on living. **But if it loses 20% of its body fluids, the bird dies.**

    (iv) A bird deprived of water for 25 hours requires about 25 days to return to its normal condition.

2. **Pure, clean and fresh water must be available at all times.**

3. Water should be **sanitized** using **bleaching powder** at the rate of **6 g per 1000 litres of water**.

4. All drinkers and water channels should be cleaned daily.

## Light Management

Sexual maturity is controlled by the lighting programme during the rearing period. Number of hours of light per day and its intensity are the important factors to be considered.

**Management of light is a valuable tool for improving egg production and growth of poultry.** Light can influence behaviour, metabolism, physical activity, and reproductive system. It influences both egg production and growth. **Light is commonly used to stimulate birds into egg production and maintain reproductive efficiency**

**over a long period of time.** There are specific requirements for period of light that must be met for poultry to become sexually mature (day length, already indicated).

**The following lighting programme is designed to have the flock lay the first egg by 19 weeks of age, reach 15% of production at 20 weeks, and peak production between 25-26 weeks.** At the time of increasing the light the average body weight of birds should be 1360 g and the age 20 weeks.

| Age | Light per Day |
| --- | --- |
| 1-2 days | 22 hours |
| 3-4 days | 20 hours |
| 5-6 days | 18 hours |
| 7-14 days | 16 hours |
| 15-21 days | 14 hours |
| 22-28 days | 12 hours |
| 29-133 days | 10-12 hours |
| 20 weeks | 11½ hours |
| 21 weeks | 12 hours |
| 22 weeks | 12½ hours |
| 23 weeks | 13 hours |
| Between 23-28 weeks | Increase half an hour every week to a maximum of 16 hours |

**This lighting programme is only for lighting the shed, and not for warmth of the chicks.**

## Body Weights

Information on gains in body weight indicates the growth of a bird. A sample of 100 birds will provide inadequate record. Therefore, the sample should be a minimum of 2% of the flock at 4, 8, 12, 16 and 20 weeks of age.

For birds in cages, they should be selected at cage level on a uniform basis. As early as possible, the birds should be weighed. **The underweight birds suggest excessive crowding, lack of sufficient feeder or drinker space, disease conditions, heat stress and feed problems, among others**. The information on body weights points to flock uniformity.

## Flock Uniformity

Flock of ready-to-lay growers has the most uniform weights. **Only uniform flocks produce more eggs.** Flocks show a wide range of variation in weight. The following figures indicate the uniformity rating.

| Percentage of growers within 10% of average flock weight | Uniformity rating |
| --- | --- |
| 85% and above | Excellent |
| 80-85% | Very good |
| 70-75% | Fair |
| Less than 70% | Not satisfactory |

## Disinfection and Biosecurity

### 1. All-in, all-out system

**This system is strongly recommended** for maximum extraction of the genetic potential of the birds.

**In this system, all the birds in the shed are of the same age, and preferably of the same strain and source of supply.** All the layers are culled after completing the cycle, preferably in one operation, or at least in one week. House should be completely depopulated (i.e. free of birds), disinfected and given enough rest (**downtime**) before the next flock is reared.

### 2. Cleaning and Disinfection between Two Flocks

1.  Remove all the dead or live birds from the premises.

2.  Eliminate or control all rodents and wild birds.

3.  Remove all manure, litter, litter feathers, dust, and clean the fan's wire nettings and water tanks.

4.  Floors should be soaked with washing soda for 24 hours. Then water is leaked out completely. Again wash the floors with an effective disinfectant.

    Fumigation and other methods are also used for disinfection of poultry sheds (see Chapter 30: **Disinfection**).

    After fumigation, close the sheds for 24 hours. Then curtains be opened.

### 3. Restriction on Visitors

1.  Salesmen, egg buyers, servicemen and visitors should not be allowed to enter into the farm. Workers should not be allowed to go from one shed to another, or else

they should take a shower bath and change clothes before entering into another shed.

2. The feed mill should be outside the premises of the farm, or else should be at least 200 feet away. The trucks delivering the grains should not be allowed to come near the sheds.

3. Cars should be halted on the roads outside the premises.

**Table 17. Suggested Layer Vaccination Schedule**

This has already been given in **Chapter 35: "Vaccination schedules"**. However, it is presented here again for ready reference.

| | |
|---|---|
| Day 1-3 | Gumboro intermediate vaccine (eye drop) |
| Day 7 | LaSota vaccine (eye drop) |
| Day 10 | Debeaking touch-up |
| Day 14 | Gumboro intermediate vaccine (Repeat, eye drop) |
| Day 18 | Marek's disease vaccine (0.2 ml by intramuscular injection) |
| Day 21-23 | Infectious bronchitis + LaSota, as combined vaccine through drinking water |
| Day 28-30 | Gumboro intermediate vaccine (Repeat, drinking water) |
| Day 42 | Fowl pox vaccine (wing web prick/stab) |
| Week 8 | LaSota vaccine (Repeat, drinking water) |
| Week 11-12 | Infectious bronchitis + LaSota (Repeat), as combined vaccine through drinking water |
| Week 12 | Deworming |
| Week 13 | R2B vaccine (by intramuscular injection) |
| Week 14 | Fowl pox vaccine (wing web prick/stab), if necessary |
| Week 15-16 | Final debeaking |
| Week 18 | Ranikhet disease vaccine (killed, subcutaneous injection) |

**Note: During the entire laying cycle, repeat LaSota vaccine every 8 weeks from the date of R2B vaccine.** In case RD killed vaccine was administered on the 18th week, then LaSota vaccine may be given from 35 week onward.

## Debeaking (Beak-trimming)

Eating of the flesh of one bird by another bird is known as **'cannibalism'**.

**Cannibalism is most common among chickens.** Chickens of all ages have a tendency to eat the flesh of another chicken (see **'cannibalism'**). Therefore, some methods of preventing this vice (abnormal behaviour) must be used. The common method used is to trim (cut) their beaks. The operation is known as **'debeaking'** or **'beak-trimming'**. But the age at which this is best done is controversial. All the same, **the operation should be completed at any age before the onset of egg production.**

It has been suggested that the term 'beak-trimming' be preferred over 'debeaking'. This is because beak-trimming accurately describes the operation, in that beaks are not removed; they are only cut (trimmed).

Debeaking is a standard practice in layer flocks. It reduces feed wastage and also losses from cannibalism. There are two basic requirements for good debeaking.

1.  Create as little stress to the bird as possible, and

2.  The beak should not grow again

Sometimes debeaking is done carelessly. It then creates more stress.

**Examples:** When the beak is cut too short, or by not removing enough. This allows the beak to grow, and it eventually reaches to an almost normal length. Too little (incomplete) debeaking may lead to pecking (vent pecking and cannibalism), especially in caged layers leading to considerable losses. Moreover, 'over' debeaking (too much) leads to poor performance of the flock as a result of inadequate feed intake, formation of culls, etc. (Culls mean rejected, inferior, worthless birds.)

## Timings

The beaks are cut at two different stages.

## 1.  Chick stage

The first debeaking is done in chicks between 6-10 days (**usually 10 days**) of age, or latest by 3-4 weeks of age.

## 2.  Grower stage

Growers may again be finally debeaked between 15-16 weeks (**usually 16**), using method and equipment suitable for that age.

## Methods

There are several methods by which beaks can be effectively cut. Usually the age determines the method selected.

## 1.  At chick stage

This procedure is sensitive and requires extreme refinement. It is therefore termed as **'precision' debeaking**.

It is also the most stressful procedure. It **may 'make or break' the flock.** Using a red-hot blade, both the beaks are cut and cauterized in one step. One-third of the beak should be removed and care should be taken to minimize the bleeding. The lower beak should be slightly longer than the upper beak. This is done by tilting the chick's head downward at the time of cut. Gentle pressure on the bird's throat will pull back the tongue and prevent it from burning. The cut beak should be in contact with the blade for about two seconds. If held longer, the beak may be burnt and permanently damaged. If held shorter, the beak may grow again.

## At this stage remember:

(i)   That the tongue and soft tissues of the beak (upper and lower palate) may be burnt too much, if held for longer than two seconds.

(ii)  That lower block of the debeaking machine may be hot, if the blade is in contact with the block for too long (by applying pressure from the foot lever). This may also damage the soft tissues of the lower beak.

## 2.   At grower stage

Remember that, **at this stage, debeaking is more stressful and bleeding could be severe** if not cauterized properly. **You may 'make or break' the flock once again.**

## Procedure

1.   The blade should be red-hot.

2.   Both the beaks are to be cut separately.

3.   Cut about 0.45 cm in front of the nostril. Cut the lower beak slightly longer than upper beak.

4.   Cut one beak at a time. Cauterize the area and round the corners of the beak, so as to give the 'V' cut.

## At this stage, again remember:

(i)   **That debeaking is the biggest stress in the life of a layer bird.** Therefore, anti-stress medication should be given. Vitamin K is included in the water the day before and also on the day of debeaking to protect against excessive bleeding.

(ii)  **Touch-up debeaking:** If the early debeaking has not been done properly, beaks partially grow back by the time the pullets are 8 weeks of age, or older, and will need to be touched up. This procedure is usually done on a bird-to-bird basis.

## Advantages of Debeaking

**Advantages are far greater than disadvantages.** Cannibalism in a flock, either through feather pulling, vent pecking, toe picking, or fighting, sometimes leads to deaths and heavy mortality. The vice tends to be habit-forming. A few cannibalistic birds pass on the character to others and soon the entire flock is affected. **The advantages of debeaking are:**

1.  It reduces mortality from pecking.

2.  There is less stress, less fearfulness and less nervousness in the flock.

3.  Feed efficiency is improved as a result of less wastage.

4.  Liveability is better, with fewer culls.

5.  There is more uniformity of the birds in the flock.

6.  Better feather condition.

7.  Debeaking reduces injurious and subnormal performance.

## Disadvantages of Debeaking

1.  Birds loose weight for 1-2 weeks after debeaking.

2.  Growth rate is reduced for a long period. It takes from 10-20 weeks for a bird to attain the weight of a similar non-beaked bird.

3.  Debeaking may delay slightly sexual maturity, reduce body weight at sexual maturity, reduce egg production, and may also reduce egg size.

## Precautions

1.  Flock should be healthy and conform to standard body weight.

2.  Do not debeak sick birds.

3.  Never be in a hurry. Debeak not more than 5-6 chicks and 2-3 growers per minute.

4.  Use new blades and change them for every 2000 chicks and 1000 growers.

5.  Remember to heat the blade to 'red-hot stage' to ensure correct cauterization and prevent bleeding. Do not over-cauterize. Remember the contact time of two seconds.

6.  Do not burn the tongue, or sear the eyes of the bird.

7.  Debeak only during cooler hours of the day. Early morning and night hours are preferred.

8.  **Do not trim beaks when chickens are under stress.** For example, never combine debeaking while shifting the birds or while vaccinating. Both shifting and vaccination are stress factors. Also, if possible, do not subject the birds to stressful conditions, such as handling, shifting, vaccination, etc. for two weeks after debeaking.

9.  **Do not delay the debeaking for more than 16 weeks.** Being the single most severe stress in bird's life, if done later than 16 weeks, it can lower body weights,

reduce egg production, and may reduce egg size. Even the growth may be reduced for 10-14 days after beak trimming.

10. Faulty technique, low temperature of debeaker and carelessness often result in insufficient cauterization of the beak. **This may result in excessive bleeding**, especially in birds deficient in vitamin K. **Any blood lost this way is swallowed by the chicken and is found in the crop on postmortem.** Digested blood also causes pasty vents.

11. Incorrectly debeaked chicks are usually slow to eat and drink because of the raw exposed surface of the beak. If the wound becomes infected, it can result in septicaemia (blood infection) and death of the bird.

12. Following stress of debeaking, major viral and bacterial diseases could come into the flock. Therefore, review the vaccine schedule and check for shortcomings.

13. About two days before and 2-3 days after debeaking, **vitamin K** (5 mg/litre of drinking water) and, if possible, **vitamin C** (20 mg/litre) should be added to the water to facilitate blood clotting and to reduce stress and dehydration. **Electrolytes** may also be given in the drinking water.

14. **Debeaking machines can be a source of infection.** Debeaking machines must be cleaned and disinfected regularly to prevent cross-contamination among chicks; otherwise mortality in the chicks may be increased about 10-12 days later. This is particularly true when debeaking is done in day-old chicks.

15. **When birds are more than 10 days old,** do not debeak during vaccination period, supply feed immediately, increase the level of both feed and water until the beaks are healed, add vitamin K to the feed during the hot weather, catch a number of birds at a time, and do not shift the birds to other sheds.

16. To minimize weight loss, birds can be fed a pre-starter, starter, or high-density stress diet for about one week after debeaking.

17. All the people carrying out debeaking must be carefully monitored. **Debeaking is a very tedious and responsible job and all steps must be followed properly.** Blades must be sharp and maintained at proper temperature. The amount of beak removed must always be the same from bird to bird. Growers should be monitored constantly during the operation and afterwards in the layer shed.

18. Lastly, remember that, while handling, you yourself can cause considerable stress to the birds. Thus, you could also be responsible for the future performance of the flock. **Therefore, do debeaking gently, steadily, and carefully.**

## General Point

Therapeutic beak trimming (i.e. for treatment purpose) is recommended at any age, if an outbreak of cannibalism occurs.

# Chapter 43

# Nutrition and Feed Basics

For profitable poultry farming, the broiler or layer bird must perform to its complete genetic potential. Nutrition, or feeding, plays an extremely important role in achieving this goal.

**Feed constitutes about 70 - 80% of the recurring expenditure in poultry farming.** It is the single most important input which determines as to how the broiler or layer bird is going to perform in terms of profitability.

**Commercial poultry rations today are known as complete rations.** That is, they contain all the essential ingredients for the bird to do the best job, whether in respect of growth or egg production, or the production of meat. Since the bird remains totally confined to its houses during its lifetime, it has no other source of food. Therefore, whatever it requires must come from the feed it is given each day.

## What are nutrients?

**Nutrients** are certain basic vital nutritional components, or nutritive (nutritious, nourishing) substances, that are required by every living being to sustain life. Nutrition is the process of supplying these nutrients. It involves ingestion (eating), digestion, absorption, and transportation of the absorbed foodstuffs to body cells, where they are metabolized and used.

**Metabolism** refers to those chemical changes in food components that occur after digestion and absorption. The various components of food (carbohydrate, fat, protein) are broken into simpler units and converted in forms that could be absorbed. Thereafter, further chemical reactions take place, so that tissues of the body are able to utilize the simpler compounds carried to them by the blood. By these additional processes **energy is released, fat is stored, heat is liberated, and many end products not of value to the bird are eliminated through the kidneys.**

**Birds require the following basic nutrients to be able to live, grow, and reproduce.**

Water

Carbohydrate

Fat

Protein

Vitamins

Minerals

## Water

**Water forms the major portion, around 55-85%, in the body of the chicken. Thus, 3/4th of the body weight is water.** It performs several vital functions. It is the major component of blood and tissue fluids, it transports nutrients or removes waste products from all cells of the body, and it helps in heat regulation. Water helps to cool the bird by evaporation through the lungs and airsacs. It helps in softening the feed in the crop and in the digestive processes. About 70% of the egg contents is water.

**Chickens of all ages consume two times more water by weight, than they eat feed.** This may vary depending on bird age and environmental temperature. Unlike animals, chickens must have a continuous water supply, since they drink only small amounts at a time. **An insufficient amount results in decreased growth and egg production.**

## Carbohydrates

**Carbohydrates are the major source of energy and heat for the body.** They are required for the maintenance of body temperature, growth, bird activity and production of eggs. **Excess of carbohydrate in the body is converted into fat.**

The major ingredients that contribute carbohydrates in poultry feed are the cereals, and grains such as **maize,** wheat, jowar, rice, etc.

## Fats

**Fats are another potential major source of energy.** They supply **essential fatty acids** like **linoleic acid** and **arachidonic acid.** Fats are the most concentrated source of energy that a bird can consume. **They have a gross energy value of 9.45 kcal compared to only 4.1 kcal for a typical carbohydrate.** They are digested and metabolized with high efficiency. Fats are the only component which is deposited intact into tissues with little or no modification. Because of their high energy content, relatively large amounts of fats or oils are added to some poultry rations, **particularly in broiler diets.**

Fats are an important component of the vital lipid known as **'phospholipid'.** Phospholipids are found in all living cells and in the cell (plasma) membrane. Both linoleic acid and arachidonic acid are important constituents of phospholipids. **Linoleic acid cannot be synthesized in the chicken body, but can be converted to arachidonic acid.** Essential fatty acid deficiency in laying hens results in low egg production, egg size, and hatchability. Most commercial feed ingredients are low in linoleic acid. **Linoleic acid is required for maintaining satisfactory egg size and weight.**

529

The fat content of the nervous tissue is also high. Fat also serves as an insulating material in the subcutaneous tissue of the skin and around certain organs.

## Proteins

Proteins were so named because these substances are of **primary importance** to the body as they perform innumerable vital functions. (The word **'protein'** is of Greek origin. **'Protos'** in Greek means **first** or **primary**.) **Enzymes, hormones, and antibodies (technically known as 'immunoglobulins') are all proteins.**

**Proteins** are first broken down to their basic units **'amino acids'** in the digestive tract by the enzymes, and then absorbed. In the chicken body, proteins are the major constituents of the structural and protective tissues, such as skin, feathers, bones, muscles, ligaments and organs. They are also important for growth and egg production.

**The absolutely essential amino acids for chicken include** arginine, histidine, isoleucine, leucine, lysine, methionine, phenylalanine, threonine, tryptophan, and valine. Of these, **methionine** and **lysine** are the most critical amino acids that should be taken into account while formulating ration for poultry. For example, in feeds composed of maize and soyabean as source of protein, **methionine** supplementation is usually necessary. **Lysine** may be slightly deficient in such diets unless alternate lysine-rich protein sources, or feed-grade lysine are included.

**Protein deficiency** (mainly that of essential amino acids) **will result in reduced growth, reduced feed consumption, decreased egg production and size, and loss of body weight in adults.** This would lead to **poor profitability.**

Energy can also be obtained from proteins as a last resort, but this is not desirable, as it is expensive and produces strain on the body.

Both **plant sources of protein** (soyabean meal, groundnut extract, sunflower meal), and **animal sources of protein** (fish meal, meat meal, bone meal) are used in poultry feed. Broiler chickens are more efficient in the utilization of dietary protein (64%) than layer birds (55%).

## Vitamins

**Vitamins are a group of organic substances that are essential in minute quantities for normal growth of the bird, maintenance, and egg production.** Since they are vital for life and all contain the **amino group (NH$_2$)** in their structure, they are called **'vitamin'**. (In Latin **'vita'** = life. Vita + amine = vital amine, or 'vitamin'). Vitamins are neither sources of energy nor do they serve as building blocks. But they are absolutely essential for normal function and maintenance of health. They are effective in minute quantities. They act mainly as regulators of metabolic processes and play a role in energy transformations, usually acting as co-enzymes in enzymatic systems.

Vitamins exist in most foods in minute amounts in their natural state. **All vitamins, except vitamin C, are essential for poultry.** Although the amounts of vitamins required in poultry diets range from parts per million (ppm) to parts per billion (ppb), **each is required for normal metabolism and health.** A marked deficiency of a single vitamin in the diet of chick leads to breakdown of the metabolic process in which that particular vitamin is involved. This results in a vitamin-deficiency disease.

**There are 13 vitamins necessary for the chicken.** They occur in foodstuffs in varying quantities and in different combinations. All foodstuffs do not have all vitamins, and some contain a greater quantity of certain vitamins than others. Some vitamins are produced by micro-organisms of the intestinal tract; one (vitamin D) by irradiation (action of ultraviolet light) on the bird's skin, while others are manufactured synthetically. Since vitamins are definite chemical compounds, commercially produced vitamins are as valuable as those found in the natural foodstuffs.

**Vitamins are classified into two groups:**

1. **Fat-soluble vitamins**       -       **Vitamins A, D, E, and K**

2. **Water-soluble vitamins**       -       **Vitamin B group and Vitamin C**

**No single foodstuff contains all vitamins in correct proportions.** Therefore, different ingredients must be considered and supplemented properly to meet the requirements of poultry. Poultry feeds are usually formulated to contain more than adequate amounts of all vitamins. They provide margin of safety to compensate for possible losses during feed processing, transportation, and storage, and variations in feed composition and environmental conditions.

# Minerals

Besides carbohydrates, fats, proteins, and vitamins, many other elements form a part of the bird's nutritional requirements. These are essential **'mineral elements'.** **Minerals are as important as amino acids and vitamins in the maintenance of life, well-being, and production in poultry.** They enter into composition of bones and give the skeletal the rigidity and strength needed to support the soft tissues. Minerals combine with proteins, lipids, and other substances that make up the soft tissues. They take part in the maintenance of osmotic pressure and acid-base balance (pH). Minerals are also necessary for activation of many enzymes of the body. In most cases, **the necessary quantity required for each is very small.**

**At least 13 minerals are required for the best health and productivity of birds.** Minerals that perform structural or osmotic function are required in relatively large amounts in the diet, and are referred to as **'macro-minerals'. These include:**

Calcium

Phosphorus

Sodium

Potassium

Chlorine

Magnesium

Minerals that are required in relatively low amounts in the diet are referred to as **'micro-minerals', 'trace minerals' or 'trace elements'. These include:**

Copper

Iodine

Iron

Manganese

Selenium

Zinc

**All the above macro-minerals and trace minerals are essential for the well-being of birds.** Fluorine in small amounts is a constant constituent of several tissues, particularly bones. Analysis of each mineral in the body of chicken has revealed that major portions of calcium, phosphorus, magnesium, and zinc are present in bones. Other essential elements are distributed largely in muscles, other soft tissues, and body fluids.

## Poultry Rations

Birds must get the above discussed nutrients, namely, carbohydrate, fat, protein, vitamins, and minerals from the food they eat daily. No single or individual feed ingredient can supply the entire requirement. **A combination of ingredients and other feed additives, such as mineral mixtures and vitamins, are formulated, balanced, mixed properly, and then fed in the form of:**

**Mash** (i.e. in ground form)

**Crumbles:** When pellets are coarsely ground, a type of product midway between mash and pellets is formed.

**Pellet (mash compressed to form pellets** of various sizes)

In our country, feed in the mash form is the most popular for feeding birds. **Various feed ingredients used to formulate and balance poultry diets include:**

1. Energy sources
2. Proteins of plant origin
3. Proteins of animal origin
4. Mill by-products
5. Mineral supplements
6. Vitamin supplements

7.    Other supplements. These include additives, such as **antibiotics, enzymes, probiotics, amino acids, antioxidants, toxin binders, immune stimulants,** and other useful **performance/growth promoters/enhancers.**

## 1. Energy Sources

## Maize

**Maize is the most common energy source in poultry feed.** It is easily available and highly digestible. It contains around 9% protein and has 3300 kcal/kg of metabolizable (usable) energy (ME). It has less fibre (2-3%). It can be used up to a level of 60% in the feed. Yellow maize is abundant in **carotenoid pigments** called **'xanthophylls'.** Carotenoids impart yellow colour to the fat deposits of chickens and to egg yolk. **Yellow maize** is a fair source of **vitamin A,** but storage tends to reduce its content by as much as 30%. **White maize** is similar to yellow maize except that it contains no xanthophyll and has virtually no vitamin A activity. **Maize is a good source of linoleic acid, an essential fatty acid.**

## Rice

Poor quality rice, unfit for human consumption (broken rice, or *'kanki'*), can be used in poultry feed. It contains around 8% protein and 2600 kcal/kg of metabolizable energy.

## Wheat

Wheat is an important human food. It is used only when there is a shortage of maize. It contains about 10% protein and 3000 kcal/kg of metabolizable energy.

## Fats and Oils

**Fats are solid, while oils are liquid.** They are excellent sources of energy. They give around 7000 kcal/kg of metabolizable energy. They are added at levels of 2-3% in feed to increase energy, especially in broiler rations.

It has long been known that when the vegetable oil content of the feed is increased, **egg size increases,** even when the total calories in the ration remain the same. Most of the effect is due to the increases of readily absorbable fatty acids, including **linoleic and oleic acid** in the vegetable oil. Most commercial feed ingredients are low in linoleic acid. **Therefore, fats and oils, such as certain vegetable oils, should be added to rations in order to prevent a deficiency of linoleic acid, which has a requirement of about 1.0% of the ration.**

## 2. Vegetable Protein

## Soyabean meal

**Soyabean meal has a high nutritional value.** It contains between 43-50% protein and around 2400 kcal/kg of metabolizable energy. When combined with maize, **methionine**

(an essential amino acid) is the only limiting factor. **At present, soyabean meal is very popular in poultry feed.** It can be used up to 30-40% level in the feed.

**Soyabean meal can be supplemented with some animal or fish protein to make up its deficiencies of certain amino acids, such as methionine.** Synthetic amino acids also can be used. Raw soyabeans should not be fed. They contain a trypsin inhibitor that must be destroyed by heat or other methods.

## De-oiled Groundnut Cake (Groundnut Extract)

This is another important vegetable protein source in our country. It contains 40-45% protein and 2300 kcal/kg of metabolizable energy. It can be used up to 10-20% in poultry feed.

## Full-fat Soyabean Meal

Full-fat soyabean meal is excellent for broilers, and helps in incorporating high levels of fat in feed. It has 37% protein and high metabolizable energy of around 3800 kcal/kg.

## Sunflower Meal

Sunflower meal contains around 35-40% protein, but is low in amino acid lysine. Because of its high fibre content (20%), it is usually not used in chick feed, and its use in layer feed is limited to a maximum level of 7% in diet. Higher additions will lead to diarrhoea, loose droppings and poor performance.

Other vegetable protein sources can also be considered, such as cottonseed cake, mustard oil cake, and sesame meal.

## 3. Animal Protein

## Fish Meal/Whole Fish

**This is the most important animal protein source in our country.** There are two grades of fish available: Grade A with protein of 50-55% and Grade B with 40-45% protein. **Fish meal is rich in both methionine and lysine, and therefore has a good-quality protein.** It supplies around 2000-2200 kcal/kg of metabolizable energy. It can be used in chick and layer feed up to 8-10% and 5-7%, respectively. Fish meal should not contain more than 3% salt, as salt produces a laxative effect in the chicken.

The oil from fish has a definite 'fishy' taste and smell. These are imparted to the poultry meat and eggs when the diet contains more than 6-10% fish meal.

## Meat Meal

Meat meal has 50-55% protein. It can be used between 3-8%, since its amino acid value is limited.

## Blood Meal

Blood meal contains ground dried blood. It has about 80% protein and is an excellent source of the amino acid **lysine**. But it is deficient in quality protein and so only small amounts can be added to the poultry feed.

## 4. Mill By-Products

### Rice Polish

Rice polish is rich in energy, containing around 2800 kcal/kg of metabolizable energy, 12% protein and 13-18% fat/oil. It can be added up to 5-12% in feed.

### De-oiled Rice Bran

When de-oiled, the energy value is reduced to around 2000 kcal/kg of feed, but protein value increases to 13-15%. Both rice polish and de-oiled rice bran are excellent sources of B-complex. De-oiled rice bran is very cheap and is used as 'filler' in poultry feed.

### Wheat Bran

Wheat bran is composed of the outer layer of wheat. It has about 15% protein and around 1800 kcal/kg of metabolizable energy. Due to its fibre content, wheat bran is not used in chick diet, and its use in layer diet is restricted to not more than 12-15% in feed.

## 5. Mineral Supplements

In addition to protein, carbohydrates, fats, and certain vitamins, **many minerals form a part of the bird's nutritional requirements.** In most cases, the necessary quantity of each is small. Many have inter-relationships with other nutrients. In some cases, amounts required are in traces and excesses are toxic. Although most of these minerals are added in the diet in their inorganic form, **sometimes organic forms are important sources.**

**Mineral supplements supply calcium and phosphorus.**

|  | Calcium (%) | Phosphorus (%) |
|---|---|---|
| 1. Mineral mixture ISI standard | 30 | 6 |
| (It also contains other trace minerals as required) | | |
| 2. **Di-calcium phosphate (DCP)** | **22** | **18** |
| 3. Bone meal | 26-30 | 13 |
| 4. Limestone powder (LSP) | 35-38 | Nil |
| 5. Oystershell grit | 35-38 | Nil |

In addition, salt and trace mineral preparations are also added, as required.

## 6. Vitamin Supplements

Various vitamin preparations, **especially manufactured for use in poultry feeds,** are available from reputed pharmaceutical companies. They are added as per manufacturer's recommendations, and include:

### Fat-Soluble Vitamins

A, D, E and K

### Water-Soluble Vitamins

C (ascorbic acid)

B group

Thiamine (B1)

Riboflavin (B2)

Pantothenic acid

Niacin

Pyridoxine (B6)

Choline

Biotin

Folic acid (Folacin)

B12 (Cobalamin)

The **fat-soluble vitamins** are often present in plants as pro-vitamins which are quickly converted to true vitamins in the body of the chicken. They are easily stored in the fat cells of the bird and excesses are excreted through the faeces. Only one vitamin, vitamin K, is synthesized in the intestinal tract.

**Chickens require all the water-soluble vitamins in their diet, except vitamin C.** When the feed contains more water soluble vitamins than the bird needs, excesses of all except B12 are excreted in the urine. **Vitamin B12 has the capacity of being stored.** Those not stored must be included in the diet, since the bird has no reservoir on which to draw.

**Vitamin preparations are administered in the feed as premix, and also through the drinking water.** A **premix** is a preparation that has to be mixed with other ingredients (such as feed) before use. ('Pre' in Latin means 'before'. Thus, 'premix' means to be mixed before use.)

# 7. Other Feed Additives

## 1. Antibiotic Growth Promoters

Antibiotic is a substance produced by a micro-organism that kills or prevents the growth of other micro-organisms. Low quantities of antibiotics are used as **'growth promoters'**. This is because they suppress disease-producing bacteria, decrease microbes that use essential nutrients and produce excess ammonia in the intestine, and increase feed and water intake. Their action is indirect. They alter the microbial environment of the intestine and lower the incidence of certain bacterial diseases. In this way they increase the availability of certain other feed constituents. **Feed levels should be those recommended by the manufacturer.** A common growth promoter used in the industry that does not appear to cause bacterial resistance is **zinc bacitracin** However, recently, Europe and United States have banned their use because of the growing concern that this practice may cause bacteria become resistant to antibiotics for the human population (see Chapter 20: **'Antibiotic growth promoters'** and Chapter 23: **'Enzymes'**).

Some of the commercially used antibiotics include bacitracin, lincomycin, virginiamycin, avilamycin, and erythromycin. At times, certain antibiotics may be used in the feed to treat an existing disease condition.

For a list of commercial antibiotic preparations currently available in the market, refer to Chapter 19 under **"Antibiotics"**.

## 2. Anticoccidials

Certain chemicals known as **'anticoccidials'** or **'coccidiostats'** are added to feeds to prevent a serious disease of poultry, known as **'coccidiosis'** (see **'coccidiosis'**). Levels of these anticoccidials should be those recommended by the manufacturer. Coccidiosis is a protozoan disease, which is common in deep litter brooding and in growers. The disease is extremely common throughout the world. Most commonly used anticoccidials are the **ionophore compounds** (maduramicin, salinomycin, monensin), clopidol, robenidine, amprolium, dinitolmide, diclazuril, etc.

For a list of commercial anticoccidial preparations available in the market, refer to Chapter 19 under **"Anticoccidials"**.

## 3. Mould Inhibitors (Antifungal Agents) and Toxin Binders

These additives are used in feed to inhibit fungal growth and resultant toxin formation (see Chapter 22: **'Mould inhibitors and toxin binders'**). These products usually contain organic acids, which are antifungal, and zeolytes (aluminosilicate) which are toxin binders. Their use is required when feed ingredients (especially cereal grains) contain high percentage of moisture (more than 10%), and also during the rainy season.

For a list of commercial mould inhibitors (antifungal agents) and toxin binders available in the market, see Chapter 19 under **"Mould inhibitors and toxin binders"**.

## 4. Enzymes

Enzymes are often added to poultry diets to increase the digestion of carbohydrates and proteins. Those enzymes are used mainly which are not found in the digestive tract of poultry. Several commercial enzymes are **'cocktails'** or combinations of enzymes that may also contain proteases to help with the digestion of proteins

Enzymes of the digestive system break down and digest dietary carbohydrate, protein and fat, so that they can be utilized by the chicken (see Chapter 23: **"Enzymes"**). **Enzyme supplementation,** that is, treatment of feeds with enzymes, **enables the birds to utilize the feed readily and more efficiently.** This is required when certain ingredients having poor digestibility are used in the feed. For example, the bird cannot utilize **non-starch polysaccharides (NSPs)** present in grain/plant ingredients. They cause sticky, wet droppings, and lead to poor feed conversion and growth. As such, addition of commercial enzymes results in better feed conversion and prevention of sticky, wet, droppings.

Use of enzymes will definitely be on an increase in the near future as more and more of poorly used ingredients are being incorporated in the feed. We can only feed the 'leftovers' following human food requirements globally. This competition between humans and animals is increasing day by day.

For a list of commercial enzyme preparations available in the market, refer to Chapter 19 under **"Enzymes"**.

## 5. Probiotics

Probiotics are a class of biological compounds which have an action opposite to that of antibiotics (see Chapter 21: **"Probiotics"**). Some useful bacterial and fungal cultures (lactobacilli, yeast, etc.) are fed to the birds which result in suppression of the harmful bacteria (e.g. *Escherichia coli*) in the intestine. Thereby the disease incidence is reduced. Probiotics are also, to some extent, immunostimulant and anti-toxic in nature.

This class of additive is gaining in popularity in all parts of the world, as it lessens the use of antibiotics whose presence in meat and egg is not desirable for human consumption.

For a list of commercial probiotic preparations available in the market, refer to Chapter 19, under **"Probiotics"**.

## 6. Antioxidants

These feed additives help to keep the feed fresh and prevent spoilage (rancidity) of fats and vitamins in the feed. Fats, particularly the unsaturated fatty acids, are prone to oxidative rancidity. To prevent oxidation antioxidants are usually added, particularly if the fats are to be stored. Fat rancidity in feed tends to destroy the fat-soluble vitamins A, D, and E. Under specific circumstances, use of antioxidants is necessary in the feed, particularly when additional fat or oil is being added. **Vitamin E is a powerful natural antioxidant along with selenium** (see 'vitamin E' and 'selenium'). Antioxidants must be added according to the manufacturer's directions.

## 7. Immuno-stimulants and other useful performance enhancers/growth promoters

Such as vitamin E with selenium, herbal liver tonics and other additives stimulate the immune system and facilitate better absorption and digestibility.

## 8. Electrolytes

Body water contains substances called **'electrolytes'**. These can be divided into two groups:

1.  **Extra-cellular:** That is, those **present outside the cells.** These include **sodium, chloride**, and **bicarbonate.**

2.  **Intra-cellular:** That is, those **present inside the cells.** These include **potassium and phosphate.**

Electrolytes regulate both enzyme activity and osmotic pressure of the body fluid, and help in controlling the body pH.

In mammals, loss of water from sweating disturbs the electrolyte balance. **But this is not so with chickens because they have no sweat glands.** However, during certain diseases such as coccidiosis and diarrhoea, there is excessive water loss from the body. Under these circumstances some improvement may be shown through the addition of electrolytes in the feed.

## Poultry Feed Formulations

1.  Feed is formulated as per the type of bird (broiler or layer), its age, and its specific requirements. Also seasonal variation has to be taken into consideration.

2.  While formulating the feed, the cost factor is also very important. **Remember that 70-80% of the total expenditure in poultry farming is on the feed.** Feed should therefore be **economical**, and at the same time well balanced with all the nutrients.

3.  **Ingredient evaluation and quality control are very important.** Ingredients should be fresh and free of mould contamination. One should be careful about adulterated feed ingredients. For example, fish is being adulterated with urea, and soyabean meal is being adulterated with rice bran, and so on.

4. To arrive at a specific formulation, it is important to know what the specifications are for a particular type of feed, and also the nutrient composition of feed ingredients being used.

5. **Usually computer aided 'least cost feed formulations' are worked out.**

6. **Seek the assistance of feed analytical labs to check the ingredient quality.**

## Analysis of Feedstuffs

In order to formulate poultry rations, it is necessary to have tables showing the analyses of the various feedstuffs. These values are necessary to build formulas that are properly balanced for the type and age of birds involved and for the environment under which they are kept.

## Feed Manufacturing

The process of manufacturing feed is relatively simple. It comprises first grinding (size reduction) of feed ingredients using a grinder (a grinding machine), and then mixing (blending) of the various ingredients as per the formula. Selected ingredients are passed through a pulverizer or a grinder to reduce the size of the particles to required mash size. Different powdered raw materials are taken by weight into mixer (blender) for uniform mixing. The vitamins and other additives are added during this stage. Mixing operation should be carried out for at least 20 minutes to ensure complete and uniform distribution.

After the above procedure, the mixed feed is stored in plastic or gunny bags, accurately weighed, and despatched to the farmer for use.

# Chapter **19**

# Continued

## NOTE

All atempts have been made to squeeze as much information as possible into the limited space available. For more details, refer to company's literature.

**Companies whose products (medicine/vaccines) have been listed include:**

1. Aamoda Pharmaceuticals
2. Advanced Biochemicals
3. Alembic
4. Alltech Inc.
5. APC Nutrients
6. Avian Remedies Ltd
7. Avians
8. Aviguard
9. AVR Industries
10. Ayurvet
11. Biomed
12. Biomin
13. Bovine Birds Pharma
14. Brihans
15. B.V. Bio-Corp
16. Caretech
17. Charak
18. Concept
19. Elanco
20. Elder
21. Elpe Labs
22. Fort Dodge
23. Golden Streak
24. Guybro
25. Harshvardhan's Lab
26. Himalaya Drug Company
27. Hitha Laboratories
28. Indian Drugs and Vitamins
29. Indian Herbs
30. Indian Immunologicals
31. Indo Bio Care (IBC)
32. Indovax
33. Intervet
34. IVPL (Intvet)
35. Jubilant Organosys
36. Kemin
37. Keypeeyes Biotech

38. Lyka Laboratories
39. Micro Labs Limited
40. Natural Herbs
41. Natural Remedies
42. Neospark
43. Nicholas Piramal
44. Novartis
45. Novo-Nordisk
46. Osco
47. Pfizer
48. Polchem
49. Premium
50. Prime
51. Qualitat Products
52. Rakshak
53. Rallis
54. Redeem
55. Sanichem Lab
56. Sarabhai Zydus
57. Stallen
58. Trichem
59. TTK
60. Uni-Sankyo (Kenko)
61. Varsha Group
62. Venky's
63. Ventri Biologicals
64. Vet Care
65. Vet Farma
66. Vet India
67. Vetline
68. Vet Med
69. Vetnex
70. Virbac
71. Wockhardt
72. Zeus Biotech

Medicines have been listed in alphabetical order. The various categories include:

# MEDICINES

1. Acidifiers
2. Amino acids
3. Ammonia binders
4. Antibiotics
5. Antibiotic growth promoters
6. Anticoccidials
7. Anti-diarrhoeals
8. Antifly agents and ectoparasiticides
9. Anti-gout drugs
10. Anti-mycoplasmal drugs
11. Antioxidants
12. Anti-stress drugs
13. Biosurfactants
14. Calcium preparations
15. Dewormers (Anthelmintics)
16. Disinfectants
17. Electrolytes
18. Enzymes

19. Hatchling supplement
20. Liver tonics
21. Male and female reproductive performance enhancers
22. Microbial environment conditioners
23. Minerals
24. Miscellaneous drugs
25. Mould inhibitors and toxin binders
26. Non-antibiotic growth promoters
27. Oligosaccharides
28. Osmoregulators and methyl donors
29. Probiotics
30. Sulpha drugs
31. Vitamins

    Vitamin A

    Vitamin $D_3$

    Vitamin E + selenium

    Vitamin K

    Vitamin $AB_2D_3EK$

    Vitamin $AD_3EC$

    Vitamin B-complex

    Vitamin $B_{12}$

    Vitamin C

    Vitamins + minerals

    Vitamins + amino acids

32. Water conditioner
33. Water sanitizers

# VACCINES

1. Avian colibacillosis vaccine
2. Avian encephalitis vaccines (AE) vaccine
3. Chicken infectious anaemia vaccine
4. Coccidiosis vaccines
5. Combined vaccines
6. Egg drop syndrome vaccines
7. Fowl cholera vaccines
8. Fowl pox vaccines
9. Fowl typhoid vaccine
10. Gumboro disease (Infectious bursal disease) vaccines
11. Infectious bronchitis vaccines
12. Infectious coryza vaccines
13. Leechi disease (Inclusion body hepatitis) vaccine
14. Marek's disease vaccines
15. Mycoplasma vaccines
16. Ranikhet disease vaccines
17. Reovaccine

# DIAGNOSTIC AGENTS

# A.
# MEDICINES

# 1. ACIDIFIERS

| S. No. | Trade Name & Company | Composition | Indications | Dosage / Administration |
|---|---|---|---|---|
| 1 | ACIDAL LACTIC (Fort Dodge) | Lactic acid 55-60%, and formic acid 11+1 %, on a Silica carrier | * Prevents the growth of pathogenic micro-organisms<br>* Improves the coagulation and enzymatic digestion of proteins<br>* Improves the growth and feed conversion rate<br>* Lowers the incidence of mortality and digestion disorders | Use at least 2 Kg / tonne. The actual inclusion rate will depend on the buffer capacity of the feed. For details refer to company's literature |
| 2 | ACID LAC DRY (Kemin) | Selected organic acids | * Regulates pH and microbial balance of the gut<br>* Promotes digestion by activating the digestive enzymes<br>* Favours mineral absorption by creating an ideal pH in the intestine<br>* Enhances nutrient utilization by birds | 3-5 Kg / tonne of feed |
| 3 | ACID LAC W Liquid (Kemin) | A synergistic combination of organic acids | * Acid Lac reduces pH in crop, intestine, gizzard<br>* Suppresses pathogenic bacteria<br>* Prevents bacterial infection through drinking water<br>* Increases body weight<br>* Improves FCR<br>* Reduces mortality | **Broilers, Layers, Breeders:**<br>0.5 ml / litre of water first two weeks continuously and then 3 days a week/alternative days. May be skipped on days of vaccination |
| 4 | ACIDOMIX (Venky's) | Blend of buffered organic acids and salts, like calcium propionate, sodium formate, propionic acid, formic acid, fumaric acid, citric acid | * Kills important pathogenic bacteria like Salmonella spp., *E. coli,* Clostridium spp., Listeria spp., Campylobacter spp. and pathogenic moulds<br>* Keeps microbial balance in the digestive system<br>* Reduces pH of the intestine. Lower gut pH results in increased size of villi. This helps in better absorption and utilization of nutrients. | **1-3 Kg / tonne of feed** depending on the microbial level in feed, kind of feed and moisture content of feed. |

| S. No. | Trade Name & Company | Composition | Indications | Dosage / Administration |
|---|---|---|---|---|
| | | | * Improves utilization of trace elements due to their chelation | |
| 5 | ACID-PAK TM 4-WAY 2X (Alltech Inc.) | A blend of organic acids, electrolytes, lactobacilli, and digestive enzymes | When changes in the bird's physical environment or physiological state alter feed intake patterns, gut pH, and gut microbial numbers such as in:<br>* Newly-placed birds<br>* Moving birds<br>* Heat-stressed birds<br>* Vaccination reactions | **Acid-pak 4 way 2 X** : 0.6 g / litre of water (It is available in two sachets of 150 g each) |
| 6 | ACIFED - FS (Neospark) | Buffered organic acids, calcium propionate, fumaric acid, sorbic acid, and citric acid | * Adds value to the feed<br>* Improves feed quality<br>* Improves performance of birds. It prevents bacteria causing intestinal disorders<br>* Useful as a feed acidifier<br>* Useful as a gut acidifier | 500 g / tonne of feed |
| 7 | ACIFIRE (Harshvardhan's Lab) | Blend of propionic acid, benzoic acid, acetic acid, sorbic acid, fumaric acid, formic acid, citric acid, phosphoric acid, and calcium propionate | * Reduces pH in feed<br>* Reduces pH in gastro-intestinal tract<br>* Controls salmonella, *E. coli*, and other bacteria<br>* Favours intestinal flora<br>* Improves litter quality<br>* Prevents lumping of feed | Mixed in finished feed of all sorts of poultry strains at the rate of 500 g / tonne of feed |
| 8 | ACIFY LIQUID (Vetcare) | A combination of organic acids, namely, lactic acid, citric acid, fumaric acid, formic acid along with most potent antifungal oxine copper, citrate, and essential oils | * To provide broad-spectrum of activity against bacteria and fungi<br>* Acidification of water to reduce pathogen load<br>* Promotes the digestive process and helps in enhanced nutrient absorption<br>* Promotes the normal gut microflora and enhances gut integrity | **Through drinking water:**<br>**Broiler / Layer / Breeder:** 0.2 ml / litre<br>**Through feed:**<br>500 ml / tonne |
| 9 | ACIPRO-WS | Concentrated | * Heat stress | **Through Water:** |

| S. No. | Trade Name & Company | Composition | Indications | Dosage / Administration |
|---|---|---|---|---|
| | (B. V. Biocorp) | live-lactic acid - producing bacteria *Pediococcus acidilactici* (MA 18/5M), organic acid, electrolyte | * New placement flock<br>* Moulting<br>* Vaccination reactions<br>* Water acidifier<br>* Birds on transport<br>* After antibiotic therapy | 0.5 g / litre of water<br>**Through Feed:**<br>2.5 – 4 Kg / tonne of feed |
| 10 | ACTIVATE - WD (Venky's) | Combination of organic acid, including HMBTA feed supplement | * Minimizes the pathologic colonization of the gastrointestinal tract<br>* Assists in elimination of salmonella, *E. coli*<br>* Reduces pathogens associated with necrotic enteritis, pH achieved is 3-4 | **Broilers:**<br>Starters: 0-21 days<br>Finishers: 10-14 days<br>Pre-slaughter calming effect, improves FCR and weight gain<br>**NE / GD Enteritis:**<br>5-7 days<br>**Normally:** 0.4 to 1 ml / litre of water<br>**Typically:**<br>0.8 ml / litre of water |
| 11 | GIT ACID – FS (Liquid Concentrate) (Neospark) | Propionic acid, acetic acid, citric acid, tartaric acid, sodium acetate, sodium citrate, buffers and stabilizers | * Acidity inhibits growth of pathogenic bacteria of the intestinal flora and stimulates the desirable lactic bacteria<br>* Improves production parameters, prevents the growth of pathogenic microorganisms i.e. *E. coli*, salmonella<br>* Stimulates enzymic activity, due to lowering of the pH in the stomach, thereby resulting in higher digestibility of feed | 1-2 ml /5-10 litres of drinking water |
| 12 | BIOTRONIC (Biomin) | Contains a balanced mixture of organic and inorganic acids ant their salts | * Decreases pH value in feed, stomach, and intestine<br>* Controls the growth of harmful bacteria<br>* Increases digestibility and improves metabolism | Dose not mentioned in the leaflet. Refer to company. |
| 13 | GUT-O-CID (Ventex) | Orthophosphoric, formic, | * It has a high acidifying power in the digestive | 500 – 1000 g /tonne of feed |

| S. No. | Trade Name & Company | Composition | Indications | Dosage / Administration |
|---|---|---|---|---|
| | | propionic acid, and their salts with natural extract of antiurease saponins | system, thereby stimulating enzymatic reactions or digestion<br>* It has a bactericidal effect which is highly boosted in the presence of a stronger acid (phosphoric acid)<br>* Reduces the pH of feed and gut content<br>* Controls the enterobacteria and clostridial infection | |
| 14 | H-PLUS (H+) (Polchem) | A blend of inorganic and organic acids | * Regulates the pH of the gut, thereby reducing the enteric problems<br>* Maintains microflora in the gut<br>* Improves digestion, as it enhances action of digestive enzymes<br>* Ensures healthy gut, leading to proper absorption of nutrients<br>* Improves mineral absorption by creating favourable pH | 1-2 Kg /tonne of feed |
| 15 | H-PLUS (Liquid) (Polchem) | Formic acid, propionic acid, specialized buffers and stabilizers | * It brings downs the pH to 4.5<br>* Improves FCR and weight gain<br>* Prevents colonization of pathogenic salmonella, *E. coli*, clostridia<br>* Maintains proper integrity of gut epithelium<br>* No resistance develops against pathogens | 1-2 ml/10 litres of water achieve the pH of 4.5. (Do not mix any water stabilizer) |
| 16 | NUTRI-TREET (Harshvardhan's Lab) | Organic acids, namely, butyric, sorbic, propionic, formic, lactic, citric and acetic acid with ammonium formate | * For action against harmful microbes<br>* For improved preconditions for digestion<br>* For feed acidification<br>* For preservation<br>* For overall performance and safety | **To check mould growth in feed:** 250 ml / tonne of feed<br>**For feed acidification:** 1-2 litre / tonne of feed<br>**To prevent salmonella:** 3-5 litres / tonne of feed |

| S. No. | Trade Name & Company | Composition | Indications | Dosage / Administration |
|---|---|---|---|---|
| 17 | POULCID (Fort Dodge) | It contains set of organic acids and mannan-oligosaccharide (MOS) | * It enhances internal integrity and prevents colonization by pathogens<br>* Improves FCR and weight gain<br>* Improves productivity<br>* Improves litter quality by reducing litter pH, ammonia and moisture | **Broilers:**<br>250 g / tonne of feed<br>**Layers:**<br>Up to 8 weeks 500 g / tonne of feed<br>After 8 weeks 250 g / tonne of feed<br>**Breeders:**<br>1 Kg / tonne of feed<br>**Premix:**<br>500 g / tonne of feed |
| 18 | POULCID LIQUID (Fort Dodge) | It contains combination of organic acids | * Reduces pH of drinking water and the entire gut of chickens<br>* Improves digestion and assimilation of nutrients<br>* Improves FCR and weight gain<br>* Reduces microbial infection<br>* Prevents formation of wet litter<br>* Improves eggshell strength | 1-2 ml / 5 litres of drinking water<br>**In feed:**<br>Add 1 litre / 20-25 litres of water and mix thoroughly in one tonne of feed |

## 2. AMINO ACIDS

| S. No. | Trade Name & Company | Composition | Indications | Dosage / Administration |
|---|---|---|---|---|
| 1 | HERBOLYSIN (Indian Herbs) | It contains lysine in conjugated dipeptide and glycopeptide form and other lysine conjugates | * For optimum growth, feed conversion, and energy utilization<br>* For optimum carcass quality<br>* For higher egg production, bigger egg size<br>* For better performance | 1 Kg Herbolysin replaces 1 Kg of synthetic lysine from poultry ration with higher and sustained lysine activity |
| 2 | HERBOMETHI-ONE PLUS (Indian Herbs) | It is a herbal feed supplement which contains methionine in a natural and bioactive form | * For maintaining optimum growth, FCR, protein and energy utilization<br>* For higher egg production<br>* As a methyl donor to help prevent fatty liver syndrome | 1 Kg Herbomethione plus replaces 1 Kg of synthetic dl-methionine in feed |
| 3 | HIM-METHIO | Naturally derived | * Quick absorption | Information not |

| S. No. | Trade Name & Company | Composition | Indications | Dosage / Administration |
|---|---|---|---|---|
| | (Himalaya) | from methionine in L-form (active form) | and transportation<br>* Does not require conversion inside the body<br>* Higher bioavailability | available. Refer to company's literature |
| 4 | LMG POWDER (Sterling Lab) | Each 100 g contains: Lysine 33 g, Methionine 16.5, Glycine 16.5 g | For better FCR, growth and production | 1 g / litre of drinking water |
| 5 | MATRIX (Avians) | Each g contains: Histidine 28 mg, Isolucine 49 mg, Lucine 64 mg, Methionine + Cystine 26 mg, Phenylalanine + tyrosine 48 mg, Threonine 48 mg, Tryptophan 11 mg, Valine 50 mg | * It is a ready source of essential amino acids<br>* It is a source of simplified protein | 10 g / 100 chicks for 3-4 days in water<br>**In gout** 1 Kg / tonne of feed<br>**In layers** 10 to 20 g / 100 birds to improve egg production |
| 6 | N-LYSINE HERBAL (Natural Herbs) | Developed from selected herbs with high lysine activity | * For better growth and feed conversion<br>* Optimum quantity obtained in breast thigh<br>* Improves egg production, egg size and weight in layers and breeders<br>* Protects the bird from stress | 1 Kg replaces 1 Kg of synthetic lysine with higher and sustained lysine activity |
| 7 | N-METHIONINE HERBAL (Natural Herbs) | It contains methionine in a sustained-release-conjugated form. It is also a rich source of **SAM** (s-adenosyl-methionine), that is, **active methionine.** | * For maintaining optimum growth, FCR, protein & energy utilization in broilers & layers<br>* For higher egg production & bigger egg size in layers & breeders<br>* For maintaining immune competence<br>* For optimum moulting & better | 1Kg N-methionine replaces 1Kg of synthetic dl – methionine from poultry ration, with higher and sustained methionine activity |

| S. No. | Trade Name & Company | Composition | Indications | Dosage / Administration |
|---|---|---|---|---|
| | | | feather quality, reduces feather pecking<br>* For better performance of breeder birds<br>* As a methyl donor to help prevent fatty liver syndrome | |
| 8 | PHYTONIN (Natural Remedies) | A herbal replacement for synthetic methionine | * For optimizing growth<br>* For better FCR<br>* To optimize egg production and egg size | **Layers:**<br>1 Kg phytonin replaces 1 Kg of synthetic methionine |

# 3. AMMONIA BINDERS

| S. No. | Trade Name & Company | Composition | Indications | Dosage / Administration |
|---|---|---|---|---|
| 1 | AMMOBLAST POWDER (Polchem) | An ammonia degrading powder | * Creates cleaner, healthier, and safer environment<br>* Reduces ammonia smell<br>* Enhances fertilizer value of manure<br>* Safe, non-toxic, odourless | **Broilers / Breeders in deep liter:**<br>**1 kg powder** over 1000 sq. ft. shed area in the litter for conventional shed.<br>**2 kg powder** over 1000 sq.ft. shed area in the environmentally controlled shed.<br>**Cage Layers/ Breeders:**<br>3 kg powder over 5000 sq. ft. shed area on manure |
| 2 | AMMOFREE PREMIX (Indian Herbs) | A herbal poultry feed supplement containing saponins and active glycol-compounds | * To minimize level of atmospheric and systemic ammonia<br>* To create healthier living conditions<br>* For better farm productivity and profitability | *100 g / tonne of feed<br>*200 g / tonne of feed when the level of ammonia is more than 25 ppm |

| S. No. | Trade Name & Company | Composition | Indications | Dosage / Administration |
|---|---|---|---|---|
| 3 | AMMONIA-BIND (Harshvardhan's Lab) | Ammonia binder | * Prevents ammonia<br>* Prevents immunosuppression<br>* Prevents diseases<br>* Lowers litter pH<br>* Reduces litter bacteria | 50 kg Ammonia-Bind to be thoroughly mixed for every 1000 sq.ft.of poultry litter. Spread slowly on litter. |
| 4 | BIO CURB DRY (Kemin) | It is an ammonia binder and contains select extracts of plant *Yucca schidigera* | For counteracting the ill effects of ammonia in poultry farms | 200-1000 g / tonne of feed |
| 5. | DE-ODORASE POWDER (Alltech Inc) | It is produced from the *Yucca schidigera* plant | * For reduction of ammonia levels in the atmosphere and in the manure to improve bird performance.<br>* For improving the efficacy of coccidiosis vaccine. | 60-120 g / tonne of feed |
| 6 | DE-ODORASE LIQUID (Alltech Inc) | It is produced from the *Yucca schidigera* plant | * For reduction in ammonia levels in the atmosphere and in the manure to improve bird performance.<br>* For improving the efficacy of coccidiosis vaccine. | **In drinking water:** 1 ml / 10 litres of water<br>**To spray on litter:** 1 ml per 1 sq. meter. (Make a solution of 100 ml in 8 litres of water and spray on 100 sq. meters) |
| 7. | ODORID-FS POWDER (Neospark) | Natural powder extract made from *Yucca schidigera* plant containing 30% yucca solids and saponins | To improve the health conditions of broilers and layers by reducing the emission of odour and ammonia | 60 g / tonne of feed |
| 8 | QUICK HEAL (Avians) | A bag containing organic matter which directly reduces ammonia levels from the | The best possible solution to keep ammonia levels at its lowest | **In Broilers:** One bag of Quickheal for 500 sq. ft for one cycle<br>**In Layers and Breeders:** One bag of |

| S. No. | Trade Name & Company | Composition | Indications | Dosage / Administration |
|--------|---------------------|-------------|-------------|------------------------|
| | | atmosphere, when hanged in the poultry sheds at the level of the brooders | | Quickheal for 60 days |

# 4. ANTIBIOTICS

| S. No. | Trade Name & Company | Composition | Indications | Dosage / Administration |
|---|---|---|---|---|
| **AMIKACIN** | | | | |
| 1 | AKAYCI INJ (Brihans) | Each ml contains : Amikacin sulphate IP 250 mg | Urogenital tract and respiratory tract infections and also infections caused by bacteria resistant to streptomycin, neomycin and gentamicin | 1 ml/100-125 chicks by subcutaneous route after dilution in 1:9 ratio with sterile water . |
| 2 | QKACIN (Inj) (Qualitat) | Amikacin sulphate 250 mg / ml | Effective against respiratory infections caused by Gram –ive and Gram +ive bacteria | **Each 30 ml vial: Up to 500 g body weight** for 2500 birds **Up to 800 g body weight** for 1500 birds **For 1 Kg body weight** for 800 birds |
| 3 | VETACIN INJ. (Indo Biocare) | Each ml contains: Amikacin sulphate 250 mg | Gram-negative septicaemic infections caused by *E.coli* , Pasteurella, Salmonella, Pseudomonas etc | 5-10 mg / Kg body weight |
| **AMOXYCILLIN** | | | | |
| 4 | AMOXISOL POWDER (Pfizer) | Amoxycillin (as amoxicillin trihydrate I.P.) 50% w/w | * Coliform infections including colisepticemia either alone or following Gumboro infections such as infectious bronchitis, infectious laryngotracheitis or CRD<br>* Infectious coryza, fowl cholera, fowl typhoid, pullorum disease, wing rot and necrotic | 40 mg / Kg body weight |

| S. No. | Trade Name & Company | Composition | Indications | Dosage / Administration | | |
|---|---|---|---|---|---|---|
| | | | enteritis | | | |
| 5 | AMOXYCILLIN POWDER (Neospark) | Amoxycillin trihydrate IP (equivalent to amoxycillin base 5% w/w) | *E. coli* infections, CRD, infectious coryza, fowl cholera, fowl typhoid, pullorum disease, wing rot and necrotic enteritis, botulism, septicaemic conditions, arthritis, stress and performance slumps | 1 g / litre of water for 5-7 days | | |
| 6 | COMOXYL POWDER (Concept) | Each 5 g contains : Amoxycillin 500 mg | * Fowl typhoid<br>* Paratyphoid<br>* Coryza<br>* Fowl cholera<br>* Necrotic enteritis<br>* Pullorum disease<br>* Gangrenous dermatitis | Weight of 1000 birds | Dose in 2 hrs drinking water (g) | Dose im 8 hrs drinking water (g) |
| | | | | 250 g | 75 g | 50 g |
| | | | | 500g | 150 g | 100 g |
| | | | | 750 g | 225 g | 150 g |
| | | | | 1 Kg | 300 g | 200 g |
| 7 | PULMOXYL – VET (Micro Labs) | Amoxycillin trihydrate IP equivalent to amoxycillin base 10% | Infections due to *E. coli,* salmonella, infectious coryza, CRD, wing rot, stress, laying slumps | 1 g / 2 litres of drinking water for 5 days | | |
| **AMOXYCILLIN + CLOXACILLIN** | | | | | | |
| 8 | AMOCLOX FORTE POWDER (Neospark) | Amoxycillin trihydrate 5% w/w, Cloxacillin sodium 5% w/w | Exerts broad bactericidal activity in fighting infections | **Prophylactic:** 1 g / 4 litres of water for 3-5 days **Therapeutic:** 1 g / 2 litres of water | | |
| 9 | PULMOCLOX VET (Micro Labs) | Amoxycillin trihydrate IP 5%, Cloxacillin sodium IP 5% | Effective in *E. coli, H. gallinarum, S. gallinarum, S. pullorum,* Staphy. Species infections, and mixed infections associated with viral | **Prevention:** 1 g / 2 litres of drinking water **Treatment:** 1 g / litre of water for 5-7 days. Only medicated water to be | | |

| S. No. | Trade Name & Company | Composition | Indications | Dosage / Administration |
|---|---|---|---|---|
| | | | and mycoplsma organisms | given throughout the treatment period |
| **AMOXYCILLIN + SULBACTAM** | | | | |
| 10 | AMOXIRUM FORTE INJ (Vetnex) | Amoxycillin + Sulbactam | Prevents early chick mortality, Coryza, *E. coli,* Necrotic enteritis, Salmonellosis | **Day-one-old chicks at hatchery:** Mix 3 g vial in 1800 ml dextrose saline and administer 0.3 ml / chick by I/M route. It is sufficient for 6000 chicks. **For broilers up to 1 Kg:** Mix 3 g vial in 125 ml dextrose saline or water for injection. 0.5 ml / bird (12 mg / Kg body weight) |
| **AMPICILLIN** | | | | |
| 11 | AMPICILLIN POWDER (Neospark) | Each g contains : Ampicillin trihydrate equivalent to ampicillin IP 50 mg | * Early chick mortality<br>* Coryza<br>* Bacillary white diarrhoea<br>* *E. coli* enteritis<br>* Colisepticaemia<br>* Clostridial enteritis | **Mix 30 g of ampicillin soluble powder to 50 litres of drinking water for Chicks :** (0-7days) – 3000 birds (1-2 weeks) – 1400 birds (2-3 weeks) – 880 birds (3-4 weeks) – 670 birds **Growers:** 250-550 birds **Pullets:** 250 birds **Layers:** 175 birds |
| 12 | ROSCILLIN ORAL POWDER | Ampicillin trihydrate 10% | * Early chick mortality<br>* Colibacillosis | 1.65 g / litre of water for 3-5 days |

| S. No. | Trade Name & Company | Composition | Indications | Dosage / Administration |
|---|---|---|---|---|
| | (Vetnex)) | | * Enteritis | |

**APRAMYCIN**

| S. No. | Trade Name & Company | Composition | Indications | Dosage / Administration |
|---|---|---|---|---|
| 13 | APRALAN SOLUBLE POWDER (Indo Biocare) | Each 100 g contains : Apramycin activity 50 g as apramycin sulphate B.P. (vet.) | Bacterial enteritis, colibacillosis, salmonellosis | **Prevention:** 500 mg / litre of water for first 3-5 days and in the 4th week for 3-5 days **Treatment:** 500 mg / litre of water for 3-5 days at the onset of the infection |

**CEFTIOFUR**

| S. No. | Trade Name & Company | Composition | Indications | Dosage / Administration |
|---|---|---|---|---|
| 14 | XCEFT Inj. (Alembic) | Ceftiofur | * Effective against salmonellosis, *E. coli* <br> * To control early chick mortality associated with *E. coli* | **Single shot treatment:** One vial = 5000 chicks @ **higher dose,** or 10,000 chicks @ **lower dose.** Use 0.20 ml / chick for **higher dose,** and 0.10 ml / chick for **lower dose** |
| 15 | XNEL Inj. (Pfizer) | Each vial contains: Ceftiofur sodium 4g sterile powder for injection | * For prevention of early chick mortality <br> * For effective control of CCRD and *E. coli* infections in adult birds | Reconstitute with sterile water before administering **Day old chicks:** 0.2 mg/chick **Adult birds:** **Normal cases:** 2 mg / Kg body weight. Repeat after 24 hours **Severe cases:** 4 mg/Kg body weight. Repeat after 24 hours |

**CEPHALEXIN**

| S. No. | Trade Name & Company | Composition | Indications | Dosage / Administration |
|---|---|---|---|---|
| 16 | CEFLAX POWDER | Cephalexin IP 7.5% w/w (equivalent to | * Prevention of early chick mortality | **Prophylactic:** 20 g / day / 3000 |

| S. No. | Trade Name & Company | Composition | Indications | Dosage / Administration |
|---|---|---|---|---|
| | (Neospark) | anhydrous Cephalexin) | * Treatment of coryza, fowl typhoid, fowl cholera, bacillary white diarrhoea, *E.coli*, gangrenous dermatitis and to combat secondary infections associated with viral diseases | **chicks** in drinking water for 5 days **Therapeutic:** 20 g / day / 1500 **chicks** for 3-5 days 20 g / day / 250 **growers** for 3-5 days 20 g / day / 100 **layers** for 3-5 days in drinking water |
| 17 | LIXEN POWDER (Virbac) | Each 20 g sachet contains: Cephalexin IP 7.5% w/w | To prevent early chick mortality, for treatment of *E.coli* and salmonella infections, fowl cholera, coryza, and gangrenous dermatitis | **To prevent early chick mortality:** 20 g sachet for 3000 chicks for 5 days in drinking water **For treatment of diseases:** 20 g sachet for 1500 chicks, 250 growers,100 layers for 3-5 days in drinking water |

**CHLORAMPHENICOL**

| S. No. | Trade Name & Company | Composition | Indications | Dosage / Administration |
|---|---|---|---|---|
| 18 | BOVICHLOR (Qualitat) | Each ml contains: Chloramphenicol – 125 mg | * Effective against *E. coli,* salmonella influenza * Necrotic enteritis | 1 ml / 2-3 litres of water for 7 days |
| 19 | CHLOROTEC-SP POWDER (Neospark) | Each g contains : Chloramphenicol IP 200 mg, Diluents q.s. | For salmonellosis, fowl cholera, colibacillosis, respiratory infections such as CRD, staphylococcal infections | 10 g / 10-20 litres of drinking water for 7 days |
| 20 | NEOCHLOR FORTE POWDER (Vetcare) | Each g contains : Chloramphenicol IP 200 mg, excipient q.s. | * Enterotoxaemia and respiratory tract infections caused by sensitive organisms * For treatment of | **Broilers and Layers: In water** – 1 g / 5 litres **In feed** – 50 g / 100 Kg |

| S. No. | Trade Name & Company | Composition | Indications | Dosage / Administration |
|---|---|---|---|---|
| | | | bacterial enteritis<br>* Bloody / loose droppings<br>* Salmonellosis and colibacillosis | **Breeders:**<br>**In water** – 2 g / 5 litres,<br>**In feed** – 100 g / 100 Kg |
| **CHLORTETRACYCLINE** | | | | |
| 21 | AUREOMYCIN SOLUBLE POWDER (Fort Dodge) | Chlortetracycline hydrochloride – soluble powder 15% | * Broad-spectrum activity against Gram +ive, Gram – ive bacteria, large viruses, and coccidia<br>* Fowl cholera, colibacillosis, infectious coryza, yolksac infection, early chick mortality<br>* Colistin sulphate can be used with aureomycin | **CRD, *E. coli*, Coryza, Early chick mortality, Yolk sac infection, Enteritis, Secondary infection:**<br>**Prevention:**<br>1 g / 2 litres of water<br>**Treatment:** 1-2 g / litre of water<br>**Synovitis:**<br>**Prevention:** 1 g / litre of water<br>**Treatment:** 2-4 g / litre of water<br>**Fowl cholera:**<br>**Prevention:**<br>1 g / 1 litre of water<br>**Treatment:**<br>5 g / litre of water |
| 22 | CTC – 150 – FS (Feed Supplement) (Neospark) | Each Kg contains: Chlortetracycline / Kg 150 g | * Growth promotion, prevention of stress, improvement in egg production<br>* To maintain health and prevent *E. coli,* Fowl cholera, and CRD<br>* To prevent early chick mortality by sensitive organisms | 335 g / tonne of feed |
| **CIPROFLOXACIN** | | | | |
| 23 | CIPROTIN FEED SUPPLEMENT (Avian Remedies) | Each g contains : Ciprofloxacin 100 mg, Tinidazole 120 mg, Vit K$_3$ 3 mg, Vit B$_1$ 5 mg, Vit C 5 mg, Excipients q.s. | For prevention and treatment of clostridial enteritis, *E. coli* infection, salmonellosis, CRD, infectious coryza, | **Prevention:**<br>0.5 g / litre drinking water or Kg feed for 5 days<br>**Treatment:**<br>1 g / litre drinking |

| S. No. | Trade Name & Company | Composition | Indications | Dosage / Administration |
|---|---|---|---|---|
| | | | fowl cholera, fowl typhoid, infectious synovitis, pullorum disease | water or Kg feed for 5 days |
| 24 | CIPROTIN POWDER (Hitha) | Each 10 g contains : Ciprofloxacin HCl 1 g, Spirulina 500 mg, Tinidazole 1 g, Base q.s. | * Effective against wide range of Gram +ve and Gram –ve bacteria<br>* Effective against CRD, fowl cholera etc<br>* Improves egg production<br>* Ensures better weight gain in broilers | 100 g / Kg weight in drinking water or 500 g / tonne of feed |
| 25 | MICROFLOX-VET (Micro Labs) | Ciprofloxacin HCl – USP 10% w/w | Mycoplasmosis, Salmonellosis, Wing rot, Arthritis, CRD, Mixed infections with *E. coli* | 1 g / 2 litres of drinking water for 5 days |
| 26 | SIPROXIN – 10% (Neospark) | Each g contains: Ciprofloxacin hydrochloride IP 100 mg, Excipients – q.s | * CRD complex<br>* Coliseptcaemia<br>* Gangrenous dermatitis (wing rot)<br>* Salmonella infection<br>* Infectious coryza | 1 g / litre of drinking water for 3-5 days |
| 27 | TRICIP-VET POWDER (Trichem) | Ciprofloxacin 10% w/w | Colisepticaemia, infectious coryza, salmonella infections, CRD and fowl cholera | 1 g / 2 litre of water |
| 28 | V-CIPROL POWDER (Varsha Labs) | Ciprofloxacin Hcl IP equivalent to Ciprofloxacin IP 10% w/w, Excipients q.s. | * Colisepticaemia, infectious coryza, salmonella infections<br>* CRD and fowl cholera | 1 g / litre of water for 3-5 days |
| **CIPROFLOXACIN + NORFLOXACIN** | | | | |
| 29 | AV-FLOXIN | Each Kg contains : | * Mycoplasma | **Broilers:** |

| S. No. | Trade Name & Company | Composition | Indications | Dosage / Administration |
|---|---|---|---|---|
| | 2000 POWDER (AVR) | Ciprofloxacin 20 g, Norfloxacin 20g | infections<br>* Coryza, wing rot<br>* Fowl cholera, fowl typhoid<br>* Colisepticaemia, Colibacillosis<br>* Paratyphoid, pullorum disease | 500 mg / tonne of feed<br>**Layers / Breeders:** 1000 g / tonne of feed a week / month |
| **COLISTIN** | | | | |
| 30 | COLISTIN SULPHATE POWDER (Vetcare) | Each g contains : Colistin sulphate U.S.P. 100 mg, Excipient q.s. | * Growth promoter<br>* Treatment of colibacillosis<br>* Useful in prophylaxis of bacterial diarrhoea, wing rot, CCRD, etc.<br>* Improves FCR | **Growth Promotion:** 50 g / tonne of feed<br>**For Colibacillosis: Treatment:** 1 g / 5 litres of water<br>**Prevention:** 60-100 g / tonne of feed for 20 days<br>**For salmonellosis: Treatment:** 1 g / 5 litres of water for 7 days |
| 31 | COLIS-V POWDER (Venky's) | Each g contains : Colistin sulphate (USP) 100 mg, Excipients q.s. | * For prevention of infection caused by *E. coli* and Gram- negative enteric problems<br>* Improves FCR and weight gain<br>* Choice for combination antibiotic | **Preventive dose:** 50 g / tonne of feed<br>**In treatment:** 200 g / tonne of feed or 2 g in 15 litres of drinking water for 75-100 birds for 3-5 days |
| **COLISTIN + DOXYCYCLINE COMBINATIONS** | | | | |
| 32 | COLIDOX POWDER (Vetcare) | Each Kg contains: Colistin sulphate 1000 mg, Doxycycline 10,000 mg, excipient q.s. | * To prevent frequent attack of *E. coli* and salmonella infection<br>* To control and prevent bacterial diarrhoea | **Broilers and Layers:** 500 g / tonne of feed<br>**Breeders:** 1 Kg / tonne of feed |

| S. No. | Trade Name & Company | Composition | Indications | Dosage / Administration |
|---|---|---|---|---|
| | | | * To improve feed efficiency<br>* As a growth promoter | |
| 33 | DOXISTIN – FS POWDER (Neospark) | Each Kg contains : Colistin sulphate 1 g, Doxycycline hydrochloride 10 g | * For improved feed conversion, increased weight gain, and improved growth<br>* For reduced incidence of mortality<br>* For increased egg production | **Broilers:**<br>500 g / tonne of feed –from day old to marketing<br>**Layers:**<br>500 g -1 Kg / tonne of feed – one week a month<br>**Breeders:**<br>2 Kg / tonne of feed |
| 34 | LAYBRO MIX POWDER (Virbac) | Each Kg contains : Colistin sulphate 1,000 mg, Doxycycline BP 10,000 mg | * Better productivity, better growth and weight gain<br>* Better FCR | **Broilers:**<br>500 g – 1Kg / tonne of feed from day one till marketing.<br>**Layers:**<br>500 g – 1 Kg / tonne of feed for seven days in a month<br>**Breeders:**<br>2 Kg / tonne of feed for 7 days in a month |
| **DOXYCYCLINE** | | | | |
| 35 | AV-DOX VET POWDER (AVR) | Doxycycline 2% w/w, base q.s. | * Bacterial infections<br>* Stress | **Broilers / Layers:**<br>250 g / tonne of feed For broilers, from day 1 till culling. For layers, a week a month programme.<br>**Breeders :**<br>500 g / tonne of feed |
| 36 | DOX-E-VET (Qualitat) | 6 Deoxy-5-hydroxytetracycline hydrochloride | * Effective against CRD, *E. coli*<br>* Effective against mycoplasma, pneumonia | **Day-old-chicks:**<br>20 g / 100 birds once a day<br>**2nd day onward:**<br>10 g / 100 birds for 5 days, once a day only |
| 37 | MEGADOX POWDER (Neospark) | Each g contains : Doxycycline hydrochloride IP | * For prevention and treatment of CRD complex, early | **Prevention:**<br>1 g / litre of drinking water for 3-5 days |

| S. No. | Trade Name & Company | Composition | Indications | Dosage / Administration |
|---|---|---|---|---|
| | | equivalent to doxycycline 2.5% | chick mortality, fowl cholera, fowl typhoid, infectious coryza, infectious sinusitis, blue comb, pullorum disease<br>* Colisepticaemia, non-specific diarrhoea, secondary bacterial infections and stress | **Treatment:**<br>2 g / litre of drinking water for 4-5 days |
| 38 | MEGADOX-FS POWDER (Neospark) | Doxycycline hydrochloride 5750 ppm, Protein hydrolysate 2500 ppm Elemental calcium 28.4% | * Improves feed efficiency<br>* Improves growth rate<br>* Increases and maintains high egg production<br>* Increases livability and weight gain in broilers<br>* Reduces susceptibility to stresses caused by diseases and environmental conditions by maintaining better health | **Broilers:**<br>500 g -1 Kg / tonne of feed<br>**In stress : 1 Kg /** tonne of feed<br><br>**Layers:**<br>1-2 Kg / tonne of feed |
| 39 | RIMODOX-FS 2% POWDER (Neospark) | Doxycycline 2% | * Improves feed efficiency, accelerates growth, reduces mortality losses<br>* Assures better health, improves feed conversion, advances onset of lay, extends peak production | **For improved growth and better feed efficiency:**<br>**Broilers / Pullets:**<br>125-250 g / tonne of feed in broilers till marketing; in pullets till onset of lay<br><br>**Hens :**<br>250 g / tonne of feed for a week every month |

| S. No. | Trade Name & Company | Composition | Indications | Dosage / Administration |
|---|---|---|---|---|
| 40 | TRIDOX PREMIX POWDER (Trichem) | Doxycycline 2% w/w | * Bacterial infections<br>* Stress | **Broilers:** 250 g / tonne of feed<br>**Layers:** 500 g / tonne of feed |
| 41 | VENDOX – VET D.S. POWDER (Venky's) | Each 100 g contains: Doxycycline hydrochloride B.P. 2.5 g, Excipient q.s. | Effective against most Gram-positive, Gram-negative bacteria, mycoplasma, some fungi which cause early chick mortality, salmonellosis, colibacillosis, fowl cholera, infectious coryza, fowl typhoid and gangrenous dermatitis | **Prevention for chicks, growers, layers:** 1st day-1 g / litre of water, 2nd day and 3rd day-1/2 g / litre of water<br>**Treatment for chicks, growers, layers:** 1st day – 2 g / litre of water, 2nd day onwards – 1 g / litre of water for 2-5 days |
| **DOXYCYLINE + NEOMYCIN** | | | | |
| 42 | BIDOX - N SOLUBLE POWDER (Wockhardt) | Each g contains : Doxycycline hydrochloride IP 100 mg, Neomycin sulphate IP 100 mg | * For prevention and treatment of early chick mortality due to a wide range of infections involving both Gram-positive and Gram-negative bacteria, mycoplasma, rickettsia, large viruses, certain protozoa and fungi<br>* For treating chronic respiratory disease with *E. coli*, coliform infections, fowl cholera and secondary bacterial infections | **In outbreak:** 1 g / 5 litres of water<br>**In stress and early chick mortality:** 1 g / 10 litres of water |

| S. No. | Trade Name & Company | Composition | Indications | Dosage / Administration |
|---|---|---|---|---|
| 43 | MEGADOX-N POWDER (Neospark) | Each g contains : Doxycycline hydrochloride IP equivalent to doxycycline 100 mg, Neomycin sulphate IP equivalent to Neomycin 100 mg | * For treatment of mixed infections specially complex CRD with *E.coli*, fowl cholera, infectious synovitis, pullorum disease<br>* Colisepticaemia, non-specific diarrhoea, secondary bacterial infections and other infections caused by Gram-positive and Gram-negative bacteria | **Prevention of early chick mortality:** 1 g / 10 litres of drinking water for 4-5 days<br>**Prophylactic:** 1 g / 10 litres of water for 4-5 days<br>**Treatment of severe outbreaks:** 1 g / 5 litres of water for 4-5 days |
| 44 | MEGADOX-N-FS POWDER (Neospark) | Each 500 g contains : Doxycycline hydrochloride 5 g, Neomycin sulphate 5 g, Elemental calcium 28.4%, Protein hydrolysate 2500 ppm | * For improved feed efficiency, fertility, hatchability<br>* Increase in egg production<br>* Prevents stress | **Broilers:** 500 g / tonne of feed<br>**In stress:** 1 Kg / tonne of feed<br><br>**Layers:** 1-2 Kg / tonne of feed |
| 45 | MICRODOX – VET (Micro Labs) | Doxycycline HCl IP 10% w/w Neomycin sulphate IP 10% w/w | Infections due to Gram +ive and Gram –ive organisms | 1 g / 5 litres of drinking water for 3-5 days |
| 46 | NYDOX POWDER (Osco) | Each Kg. Contains: Doxycycline 20 g, Neomycin 20 g, Elemental calcium 220 g, Elemental phosphorus 175 g | * Salmonellosis<br>* *E. coli* infection<br>* Necrotic enteritis<br>* Non-specific enteritis<br>* Bacterial infections<br>* Infections during stress | 250-500 g / tonne of feed |
| **ENROFLOXACIN** | | | | |
| 47 | BAYROCIN – VET (Pfizer) | Each ml contains: Bayrocin 10% oral solution. It is a clear solution containing 10 mg of enrofloxacin | * Treatment of infectious diseases caused by Gram +ive and Gram –ive bacteria and | 10 mg / Kg body weight per day for 3-5 days<br>It can be used with coccidiostats that are |

| S. No. | Trade Name & Company | Composition | Indications | Dosage / Administration |
|---|---|---|---|---|
| | | | mycoplasma<br>* It can be used in single and mixed infections of bacteria and mycoplasma<br>* Effective against CRD, colibacillosis, colisepticaemia, fowl cholera, infectious coryza, salmonellosis | used routinely in poultry |
| 48 | CONFLOX (VET) ORAL SOLUTION 10% (Concept) | Each ml contains : Enrofloxacin 100 mg | * Mycoplasmosis (CRD)<br>* CCRD<br>* Fowl cholera<br>* Colibacillosis<br>* Coryza<br>* Omphalitis<br>* Salmonellosis | **For 1000 birds:**<br><br>Weight of each bird / Conflox<br>250 g — 25 ml<br>500 g — 50 ml<br>1 Kg — 100 ml<br>2Kg — 200 ml |
| 49 | CONFLOX (VET) 5% INJ. (Concept) | Each ml contains: Enrofloxacin hydrochloride 50 mg | * Mycoplasmosis (CRD)<br>* CCRD<br>* Fowl cholera<br>* Colibacillosis<br>* Coryza<br>* Omphalitis<br>* Salmonellosis | 10 mg / Kg body weight |
| 50 | ENROCARE 10% ORAL SOLUTION (Vetcare) | Each ml contains : Enrofloxacin hydrochloride100 mg | * All forms of mycoplasmosis and complicated respiratory infections<br>* Colisepticaemia<br>* Fowl cholera<br>* Infectious coryza<br>* Salmonellosis<br>* Campylobacter infections<br>* Secondary bacterial complications due to viral diseases | **Prophylactic:**<br>1 ml / 4-8 litres of water (2.5 – 5 mg / Kg body weight)<br>**Treatment:**<br>1 ml / 2 litres of water (10 mg / Kg body weight) |

| S. No. | Trade Name & Company | Composition | Indications | Dosage / Administration |
|---|---|---|---|---|
| 51 | ENROCIN ORAL SOLUTION (Vetnex) | Each ml contains : Enrofloxacin 100 mg | For effective control of CRD, CCRD, bronchopneumonia, fowl cholera, fowl typhoid, paratyphoid, colibacillosis, colisepticaemia, infectious coryza, bacillary white diarrhoea and wing rot | **Prophylactic :** 2.5-5 mg / Kg body weight or 1 ml / 2 litres of drinking water for 7-10 days **Treatment :** 10 mg / Kg body weight or 1 ml / litre of drinking water for 3-5 days |
| 52 | ENRODAC-10 ORAL SOLUTION (Sarabhai Zydus) | Each ml contains : Enrofloxacin 100 mg | * Mycoplasmosis<br>* Colibacillosis<br>* Infectious coryza<br>* Fowl cholera<br>* Salmonellosis<br>* Staphylococcal infections<br>* Streptococcal infections<br>* Mixed bacterial infections | **Prophylactic:** 2.5-5 mg / Kg body weight or 1 ml / 4-8 litres of drinking water **Treatment:** 10 mg / Kg body weight or 1 ml / 2 litres of drinking water for 3 days |
| 53 | ENRO-S POWDER (Avian Remedies) | Enrofloxacin 12.5% w/w, Strepto-mycin sulphate equivalent to streptomycin 10% w/w | * For CRD with *E.coli* infections, coryza, fowl cholera and fowl typhoid<br>* Covers all infections caused by Gram-negative bacteria | 1 g / litre of drinking water or 1 g / Kg of feed |
| 54 | FLOCURE 10% SOLUTION (Stallen) | Each ml contains : Enrofloxacin 100 mg | * Broad-spectrum antibacterial active against Mycoplasma spp, *E. coli*, Pasteurella spp , Haemophilus spp and other bacteria<br>* Very effective against CCRD<br>* Better feed conversion rates | 10 mg / Kg body weight for 3-5 days Add 10% solution to the drinking water @ of 10 ml / 20 litres of water for 3-5 days |

| S. No. | Trade Name & Company | Composition | Indications | Dosage / Administration |
|---|---|---|---|---|
| | | | and body weights | |
| 55 | FLOXIDIN ORAL SOLUTION (Intervet) | Each ml contains : Enrofloxacin 100 mg | * Colisepticaemia, CRD, infectious coryza, fowl cholera, salmonellosis <br> * Early chick mortality <br> * Coliseptcaemia | **Prophylactic:** 1 ml / 2-4 litres of water for 3-7 days <br> **Treatment:** 1 ml / litre of water for 3-7 days |
| 56 | FLOXIDIN 10% INJ (Intervet) | Each ml contains : Enrofloxacin 100 mg | * Colisepticaemia, CRD, infectious coryza, fowl cholera, salmonellosis <br> * Early chick mortality <br> * Colisepticaemia | 10 mg / Kg body weight, or 1 ml / litre of drinking water. Dissolve 50 ml vial in 450 ml distilled water, Administer 0.04 ml / chick |
| 57 | INDOFLOX 10% ORAL SOLUTION (Indo Biocare) | Each ml contains : Enrofloxacin 100 mg | CRD complex, salmonellosis, pasteurellosis, fowl cholera, infectious coryza, secondary bacterial complications, *E coli* infections, early chick mortality | **Preventive :** 2.5-5 mg / Kg body weight or 1 ml / 4-8 litres of water <br> **Curative :** 10 mg / Kg body weight or 1 ml / 2 litres of water |
| 58 | INDOFLOX 10% INJ. (Indo Biocare) | Each ml contains : Enrofloxacin 100 mg | * Infections of GI tract <br> * Infections of upper respiratory tract <br> * Infections of urinary tract <br> * Secondary infections associated with viral infections | By I/M route. 2.5-5 mg / Kg body weight (1 ml per 20-40 Kg body weight) for 3-5 days <br> **Severe infections:** 5 mg / Kg body weight (1ml per 20 Kg body weight for 3-5 days) |
| 59 | MERIQUIN LIQUID (Wockhardt) | Each ml contains : Enrofloxacin 100 mg | For treatment and prevention of infectious diseases caused by Gram-positive and Gram-negative bacteria, Mycoplasma spp including mixed | **For treatment and prophylaxis:** 1 ml / 10 Kg body weight / day in drinking water for 3 days |

| S. No. | Trade Name & Company | Composition | Indications | Dosage / Administration |
|---|---|---|---|---|
| | | | infections, namely, CCRD, colisepticaemia, pasteurellosis and coryza | |
| 60 | QUIN INTAS INJ. / LIQUID (Intas) | Each ml contains : Enrofloxacin 100 mg | CRD complex, salmonellosis, infections coryza, secondary bacterial infections, pasteurellosis | **Prophylactic:** 1 ml / 4-8 litres of water **Curative:** 1 ml / 2-4 litres of water |
| 61 | QUINROCIN ORAL 10% SOLUTION (Neospark) | Each ml contains : Enrofloxacin 100 mg | All forms of mycoplasmosis and mixed infections of mycoplasma and bacteria, e.g., CRD, colisepticaemia, pasteurellosis (fowl cholera), infectious coryza, *Salmonella gallinarum* and other salmonellosis | **For prevention and treatment :** 10 mg / Kg body weight or 1 ml / 2 litres of water for 3 days |
| 62 | RESPINIL WS POWDER (Hitha) | Enrofloxacin 10% w/w D.O.S. 12.5% w/w | * For prevention of infectious diseases caused by Gram-positive and Gram-negative bacteria <br> * To prevent CRD with *E. coli* infections, bacterial infections, coryza, fowl typhoid, para-typhoid and pasteurellosis | 50 mg / Kg body weight or 1 g / litre of water for 4-5 days |
| 63 | VENFLOX Enrofloxacin Oral Solution 10% w/v (Venky's) | Each ml contains: Enrofloxacin – 100 mg | Infections caused by Gram –ive bacteria like E. coli, Salmonella, Haemophilus spp., Pasteurella spp., Campylobacter, Pseudomonas spp. Infections caused by Gram +ive | **Prevention:** 0.025 – 0.05 ml/ Kg body weight in drinking water (1 ml / 2-4 litres of water) **Treatment** 0.05 – 0.1ml / Kg body weight in drinking water |

571

| S. No. | Trade Name & Company | Composition | Indications | Dosage / Administration |
|---|---|---|---|---|
| | | | Strepto. Spp., Staph, Clostridium, CRD caused by *M. gallisepticum, M. synoviae and M. mealiagridis* | (1 ml / 1- 2 litres of drinking water for 3-5 days |
| 64 | V-FLOXACIN ORAL SOLUTION (Varsha Labs) | Enrofloxacin 10% w/v | * Chronic respiratory disease (CRD) in poultry associated with Mycoplasma infection<br>* Very effective against infections caused by *E. coli*, salmonella and clostridium | **Prevention:** 1 ml / 4 litres of drinking water for 3-5 days<br>**Treatment:** 1 ml / 2 litres of drinking water for 3-5 days |
| **ERYTHROMYCIN** | | | | |
| 65 | AEROCIN (Qualitat) | Erythromycin BP 2% | * Effective against Gram +ive and Gram –ive bacteria<br>* Effective against *Mycoplasma pneumoniae*<br>* For treatment of streptococcal pharyngitis | 2 Kg / tonne of feed |

ALTHROCIN SOLUBLE SP POWDER table (S. No. 66, Alembic):

| 66 | ALTHROCIN SOLUBLE SP POWDER (Alembic) | Each g contains : Erythromycin thiocyanate B.P. (vet) equivalent to 50 mg Erythromycin base, Excipients q.s. | * Prevention and treatment of CCRD<br>* Infectious coryza and infectious synovitis caused by mycoplasma spp | |

| Weeks | Broiler /1000 birds | Layer/ 1000 birds |
|---|---|---|
| 1 | 48 g | 28 g |
| 2 | 141 g | 48 g |
| 3 | 255 g | 68 g |
| 4 | 585 g | 112 g |
| 5 | 532 g | 124 - 296 g |
| 6 | 686 g | 328- 412 |
| 7 | 842g | 428 – 480 g |
| 8 | 843 g | 512 - 544 g |

| 67 | ALTHROCIN – FS | Same as above | Same as above | **High challenge area:** 1 Kg / tonne of feed |

| S. No. | Trade Name & Company | Composition | Indications | Dosage / Administration |
|---|---|---|---|---|
| | (Alembic) | | | **Week a month programme:** 500 g / tonne of feed |
| 68 | OSCOMYCIN 4% POWDER (Osco) | Each Kg contains : Erythromycin theosulphate 40 g, Elemental calcium 240 g, Elemental phosphorus 175 g | * For optimum growth promotion <br> * For improved FCR <br> * For increased egg production <br> * For increased weight gain through maximum protection and control against mycoplasma infections, respiratory disease complex, coryza, streptococcosis, necrotic dermatitis | 250 g / tonne of feed |
| **FLUMEQUINE** | | | | |
| 69 | ZYDAQUIN POWDER (Sarabhai Zydus) | Each g contains : Flumequine 100 mg | Diseases caused by Gram-negative bacteria | **In drinking water:** 100 mg / Kg body weight |
| **FURALTADONE** | | | | |
| 70 | FURASOL POWDER (Pfizer) | Furaltadone hydrochloride 20% w/w | * Coliform infections including colisepticaemia either alone or following respiratory infections, such as infectious bronchitis, infectious laryngotracheitis or CRD <br> * Salmonella infections such as bacillary white diarrhoea | **Chicks:** 0.5 g / litre of water for 10 days <br> **Adults:** 1 g / litre of water for 10 days |

| S. No. | Trade Name & Company | Composition | Indications | Dosage / Administration |
|---|---|---|---|---|
| | | | (pullorum disease) fowl typhoid and other salmonelloses affecting poultry<br>* Infectious synovitis<br>* Blackhead<br>* Caecal coccidiosis | |
| 71 | MICROSOL POWDER (Micro Lab) | Furaltadone Hcl 20% w/w | Colisepticaemia, infectious bronchitis, CRD, salmonellosis (BWD), fowl typhoid, infectious synovitis, caecal coccidiosis | **Baby chicks (up to 2 weeks):** 0.5 g / litre of drinking water for 5-7 days **Chicks / Growers / Layers:** 1 g / litre of drinking water for 5-7 days |
| **FURAZOLIDONE** | | | | |
| 72 | FURALAY-200 POWDER (Micro Lab) | Furazolidone B. P. (Vet) 20% w/w | BWD, fowl typhoid, colisepticaemia, CRD, infectious synovitis, prevention of early chick mortality | **Broilers:** 500 g / tonne of feed **Layers:** 250 g / tonne of feed regularly or 500 g / tonne of feed one week, every month |
| 73 | FURATEC-200 POWDER (Neospark) | Each Kg contains : Furazolidone 200 g, Elemental calcium 23%, Protein hydrolysate 1000 ppm | * To prevent stress from various causes<br>* To prevent loose droppings<br>* For better growth and production | **Chicks:** 2 Kg / tonne of feed for 10 days **Growers / Broilers:** 250 g / tonne of feed for 1 week in a month **Layers:** 500 g / tonne of feed for 1 week in every month **To prevent infections:** 500 g / tonne of feed for 10-14 days **Outbreak of infections:** 2 Kg / tonne of feed for 10-14 days |
| 74 | FURATIN 200 | Each Kg contains : | * Effective against | **Chicks / Broilers /** |

| S. No. | Trade Name & Company | Composition | Indications | Dosage / Administration |
|---|---|---|---|---|
| | POWDER (Avian Remedies) | Furazolidone 200 g | salmonella and *E. coli*<br>* Reduces chick mortality<br>* Reduces stress<br>* Increases FCR and weight gain in broilers and egg production in layers<br>* Improves hatchability in growers | **Growers:**<br>250 g / tonne of feed<br>**Layers:**<br>500 g / tonne of feed<br>Furatin 800 is also available |
| 75 | FURON – 200 (Qualitat) | Each Kg contains: Furazolidone – 20% w/w | * Effective against bacterial infections such as *E. coli,* fowl cholera, salmonella, and CRD<br>* Effective against diarrhoea and loose droppings | 1 – 2 Kg / tonne of feed |
| 76 | NEFTIN 200 FEED SUPPLEMENT (Pfizer) | Each Kg contains : Furazolidone 200 g | * To improve egg production<br>* To improve feed to egg ratio<br>* To increase hatchability in layers<br>* To increase weight gain in broilers and growers<br>* To improve growth rate in broilers and growers | 250 g / tonne of feed daily or 500 g / tonne of feed for 7 days every month |
| 77 | V-FUR 200 POWDER (Venky's) | Furazolidone IP 20% w/w | * In layers and breeders to increase egg production, feed efficiency and better hatchability<br>* In broilers recommended for better weight gain, | **Chicks:**<br>2 Kg / tonne of feed for 1-10 days.<br>**Broilers / Growers:**<br>250 g / tonne of feed for 1 week a month<br>**Layers:**<br>250-500g / tonne of feed |

| S. No. | Trade Name & Company | Composition | Indications | Dosage / Administration |
|---|---|---|---|---|
| | | | FCR, and fast growth | |
| **GENTAMICIN** | | | | |
| 78 | GENTAMICIN Inj (Indo Biocare) | Each ml contains : Gentamicin sulphate IP 40 mg | * Early chick mortality<br>* CRD, *E. coli* infections<br>* Infectious coryza<br>* Staphylococcal infections<br>* Salmonella infections<br>* Necrotic dermatitis | **Early chick mortality :** 2 ml of Gentamicin injection diluted in 198 ml of sterile normal saline solution. Administer 0.5 ml per chick by S/C route<br>**Egg dipping:** 100 ml of Gentamicin injection with 8 litres of clean water (Gentamicin concentration 500 ppm) for dipping 2000 hatching eggs |
| 79 | GENTAMICIN Inj (Vetcare) | Each ml contains : Gentamicin sulphate IP equivalent to 40 mg of gentamicin base | * CCRD<br>* Infectious coryza<br>* Staphylococcal infections<br>* Salmonella infections<br>* Necrotic dermatitis | **Prevention :** 2 ml Gentamicin is diluted with 198 ml of sterile physiological saline solution for 400 chicks given by S/C injection.<br>**Egg dipping:** To prepare 500 ppm concentration, 100 ml of Gentamicin Inj. Has to be diluted with 8 litres of clean water for dipping more than 2000 hatching eggs<br>**Adult birds:** 2-5 mg / bird I/M or S/C Inj. |
| 80 | GENTAMICIN Inj (Vetindia) | Each ml contains : Gentamicin sulphate IP 40 mg equivalent to gentamicin base | * CRD complex<br>* Salmonellosis<br>* Egg dipping | 0.5 ml / bird by I/M route |

| S. No. | Trade Name & Company | Composition | Indications | Dosage / Administration |
|---|---|---|---|---|
| 81 | GENTAMICIN Inj (Wockhardt) | Each ml contains: Gentamicin sulphate IP 40 mg | * For prevention of early chick mortality due to *E.coli*, salmonella spp, Pseudomonas spp, fowl typhoid, C.R.D., infectious coryza and para-typhoid infections<br>* For reduction and elimination of micro-organisms like mycoplasma and salmonella from hatching eggs by dipping them in Gentamicin medicated water before incubation | **Poultry I/M or I/V route:** 3-5 mg / kg body weight **Day-old-chick:** 0.2 – 0.4 mg / chick Add 5 ml Gentamicin to 495 ml water for injection and inject at the rate of 0.5 ml / chick |
| 82 | RANBAMYCIN Inj (Vetnex) | Each ml contains: Gentamycin sulphate IP – 40 mg | Treatment of Gram -ive bacterial infections and a few Gram +ive infections | 5-8 mg / Kg body weight once daily for 5 days |
| **GENTAMICIN COMBINATION** | | | | |
| 83 | GENDOX 10/5 FEED SUPPLEMENT (Avian Remedies) | Each g contains : Gentamycin sulphate 100 mg, Doxycycline HCl equivalent to doxycycline 50 mg, Vit $K_3$ 3 mg, Vit B1 5 mg, Vit C 5 mg, Excipients q.s. | For gastro-intestinal and respiratory infections | 1 g / 1.5 litres of drinking water or feed for 3-5 days |
| **LEVOFLOXACIN** | | | | |
| 84 | LEVOCIN (Qualitat) | Levofloxacin 10% | *Very effective against Pseudomonas *Effective against Gram +ive *Streptococcus pyogenes* and *pneumoniae*, *Staphylococcus aureus*, Gram –ive *H.* | 1 g / 2 litres of drinking water for 3-5 days |

| S. No. | Trade Name & Company | Composition | Indications | Dosage / Administration |
|---|---|---|---|---|
| | | | *influenzae or N. catarrhalis* | |
| 85 | RESTRICT – L (Venky's) | Each g contains: Levofloxacin – 100 mg | Effective against CRD, CCRD, colisepticaemia, salmonellosis, infectious coryza, necrotic enteritis, gangrenous dermatitis | **Prevention:** 20-40 mg / Kg body weight, or 2-4 g / 10 litres of water for 3-5 days **Treatment:** 40-80 mg / Kg body weight, or 4-8 g / 10 litres of water for 3-5 days |
| | **LINCOMYCIN** | | | |
| 86 | LINC (Inj) (Qualitat) | Each ml contains Lincomycin sulphate 300 mg | * Effective against Gram +ive and anaerobic bacteria * Effective to Staphylococcus, Streptococcus, and *Mycoplasma synoviae* | **30 ml vial: up to 500 g body weight** / 2500 birds **Up to 800 g body weight** / 1500 birds **Up to 1 Kg body weight** / 800 birds |
| | **NEOMYCIN** | | | |
| 87 | NUBIOTIC-100 FS POWDER (Neospark) | Each Kg contains : Neomycin sulphate 100 g, Elemental calcium 25.5%, Protein hydrolysate 1000 ppm | * For improved feed efficiency * Increases egg production, weight gain in broilers * Improves fertility and hatchability | **Broilers:** 500 g-1 Kg / tonne of feed **In stress:** 1 Kg / tonne of feed **Layers:** 1-2 Kg / tonne of feed |
| 88 | NUBIOTIC-SP POWDER (Neospark) | Each g contains : Neomycin sulphate IP 20% w/w in water soluble base | * Prevention and treatment of intestinal bacterial infections * Active against Gram –ive bacteria * Active in whole gut tract | **Broilers:** **Day-old to 5 weeks:** 1 g / 7 litres of water **6 weeks and above:** 1 g / 5 litres of water **Breeders:** 1 g / 2-3 litres of water **Feed:** 20 – 25 g / tonne of feed |

| S. No. | Trade Name & Company | Composition | Indications | Dosage / Administration |
|---|---|---|---|---|
| 89 | NEO OXY (Pfizer) | Each 100 g contains : Neomycin sulphate IP 5.506 g, Oxytetracycline hydro-chloride IP 5.507 g, Vitamins A, D3, E, B2, B12, Niacinamide, Calcium pantothenate and Sodium bisulphite | * For prevention of early chick mortality<br>* For treatment of bacterial enteritis<br>* During severe outbreaks<br>* For stress | 2 g / 10 litres of water for 3-5 days<br>**Treatment of bacterial diseases:**<br>4 g / 10 litres of water for 3-5 days<br>**During severe outbreak:**<br>8 g / 10 litres for 3-5 days |
| 90 | UNIMYCIN 50% POWDER (Vetcare) | Each 20 g contains: Neomycin sulphate IP 10 g , excipient q.s. | * To treat colibacillosis and loose droppings<br>* To treat bacterial enteritis and diarrhoea<br>* To prevent immuno-suppression | **3rd to 5th Week:**<br>1 sachet / 225 litres of water for 3-5 days<br>***E. coli* and other bacterial infections:**<br>**For chicks:** ½ sachet / 225 litres of water for 3-5 days; **For adults:** 1 sachet / 225 litres of water for 3-5 days |
| | **NEOMYCIN + DOXYCYCLINE** | | | |
| 91 | BINADOX POWDER (Stallen) | Each g contains : Neomycin sulphate IP 100 mg, Doxycycline hydrochloride IP 100 mg, Excipient q.s. | * For treatment of mixed infections especially complex CRD with *E. coli*<br>* Most infections caused by mycoplasma, Gram-positive and Gram-negative bacteria including certain fungi | **Prevention of early chick mortality:**<br>1 g / 10 litres of water for 3-4 days / 200 chicks Repeat after 4th week<br>**During stress as a prophylactic treatment:**<br>1 g / 10 litres of water for 4-5 days / **60 growers.**<br>**For adult birds:**<br>1 g / 10 litres of water for 4-5 days / **45 adult birds**<br>**In severe infection:**<br>1 g / 5 litres of water for 4-5 days |
| 92 | DOCMYCIN POWDER | Each g contains : Neomycin sulphate IP | * Colisepticaemia either alone or | **For prevention of early chick** |

| S. No. | Trade Name & Company | Composition | Indications | Dosage / Administration |
|---|---|---|---|---|
| | (Alembic) | 100 mg, Doxycycline HCl IP 100 mg, Excipients q.s. | following respiratory infections such as infectious bronchitis or complex chronic respiratory diseases (CCRD)<br>* Salmonella infections such as bacillary white diarrhoea (pullorum disease) and other salmonellosis affecting poultry<br>* Infectious synovitis<br>* Fowl cholera<br>* Non-specific diarrhoea | **mortality:**<br>1 g / 10 litres of water for 3-4 days / 200 chicks<br>**During stress as a prophylactic treatment :**<br>1 g / 10 litres of water for 4-5 days / 60 growers or 45 adult birds<br>**In acute infections:**<br>1 g / 5 litres of water for 3-4 days for 200 chicks |
| 93 | EFFIDOXYN POWDER (Hitha) | Each 50 g contains : *Lactobacillus sporogenes* 1000 million CFU, Neomycin base 5 g, Doxycycline HCl 5 g, Base fortified with BAE q.s. | * Prevents early chick mortality<br>* Lactobacillus helps to maintain intestinal flora<br>* Effective against CRD with mixed infections<br>* For better growth and better weight gain<br>* Improves the birds performance | 1 g / 10 litres of water for 4-5 days |
| 94 | NEODOX FORTE POWDER (Vetcare) | Each g contains : Neomycin sulphate IP 100 mg, Doxycycline IP 100 mg, Excipients q.s. | * Prevention of early chick mortality<br>* fowl cholera and pullorum disease<br>* Infectious synovitis<br>* Colisepticemia<br>* Non-specific diarrhoea<br>* Secondary bacterial infections<br>* For treatment of | **For prevention of early chick mortality:**<br>1 g / 5-10 litres of water for 3-5 days Repeat after 4th week<br>**For treatment :**<br>1 g / 2-4 litres of water for 4-5 days |

| S. No. | Trade Name & Company | Composition | Indications | Dosage / Administration |
|---|---|---|---|---|
| | | | mixed infections | |
| 95 | OLEDOX-N POWDER (Avian Remedies) | Each g contains : Neomycin sulphate 100 mg, Doxycycline HCl, Doxycycline 100 mg, Vit K$_3$ 3 mg, Vit B$_1$ 5 mg, Vit C 5 mg, Excipients q.s. | Gastro-intestinal and respiratory tract infections | **Prevention of early chick mortality:** 1 g / 10 litres of water / Kg feed for 200 chicks for 3-4 days. Repeat after 4$^{th}$ week **For severe cases :** 1 g / 5 litres of water / Kg feed for 4-5 days |
| 96 | RENVOX (Vetnex) | Neomycin sulphate 10% w/w, Doxycycline Hcl 10% w/w | Prevention and treatment of early chick mortality due to bacterial infections | **Prevention:** 1 g / 10 litres of water for 3-5 days **Treatment:** 1 g / 5 litres of water for 3-5 days |
| 97 | VENDOX-N POWDER (Venky's) | Each g contains : Neomycin sulphate IP 100 mg, Doxycycline base 100 mg, Excipients q.s. | * Mixed infections like CRD with *E. coli* and respiratory disease complex * Helps in most infections caused by mycoplasma, Gram-positive and Gram-negative bacteria, including certain fungi and protozoa * Prevents early chick mortality | **Prevention of early chick mortality:** 1 g / 5-10 litres of water for 3-4 days **During stress as a prophylactic treatment :** 1 g / 10 litres of water for 4-5 days **During severe infection:** 1 g / 3 litres of water for 4-5 days |
| **OFLOXACIN** | | | | |
| 98 | OFX – 10 (Qualitat) | Ofloxacin – 1% | * Effective to problems related with respiratory and intestinal system * Effective against Gram +ive and Gram –ve bacteria, aerobic and anaerobic bacteria | 10 g / tonne of feed |
| 99 | OFX – 100 | Ofloxacin – 10% | * Effective to | **Layers:** |

581

| S. No. | Trade Name & Company | Composition | Indications | Dosage / Administration |
|---|---|---|---|---|
| | (Qualitat) | | problems related with respiratory and intestinal system<br>* Effective against Gram +ive and Gram –ve bacteria, aerobic and anaerobic bacteria | 10 g / 100 birds,<br>**Chicks:**<br>5 g /100 birds,<br>**Broilers:**<br>7 g / 100 birds,<br>**Breeders:**<br>20-25 g / 100 birds |
| **OXYTETRACYCLINE** | | | | |
| 100 | OXYTETRAC YCLINE SOLUBLE POWDER (Pfizer) | Each 4 g contains : Oxytetracycline hydrochloride IP 200 mg | Chronic respiratory disease complicated with *E. coli,* heavy mortality, sudden outbreak of disease | 2-5 tsp (8-20 g) per 4.5 litres of water given for 1-2 weeks |
| 101 | OXYTETRAC YCLINE LA / OXYVET LA INJ. (Sarabhai Zydus) | Each ml contains : Oxytetracycline IP 200 mg in 2-pyrrolidone vehicle system | Mixed bacterial infections | 0.25 ml / Kg body weight by S/C route<br>**In severe infections:** A similar dose should be repeated after 3 days |
| 102 | OXY 200 MG.LA INJ. (Vetindia) | Each ml contains : Oxytetracycline IP equivalent to 200 mg of oxytetracycline on anhydrous basis in 2 pyrrolidone vehicle system | * Fowl cholera<br>* Bacterial enteritis<br>* CRD, CCRD<br>* Mycoplasmosis | 0.25 ml / Kg body weight by S/C route |
| 103 | TERRAMYCI N / LA INJ. (Pfizer) | Each ml contains : Oxytetracycline equivalent to 200 mg in 2 pyrrolidone vehicle system | For the prevention and treatment of infections susceptible to oxytetracycline, including fowl cholera, CRD, and CCRD | 0.25 ml / Kg body weight by S/C route |

| S. No. | Trade Name & Company | Composition | Indications | Dosage / Administration |
|---|---|---|---|---|
| 104 | ULTROX NUTRITIONAL FORMULA POWDER (Neospark) | Each 200 g contains : Oxytetracycline hydrochloride 12,000 mg, Vit A 6,00,000 I.U., Vit $D_3$ 72,000 I.U., Vit E 220 I.U., Vit $B_6$ 110 mg, Vit K 220 mg, Niacinamide 2,700 mg, Calcium-pantothenate 900 mg, Vit $B_2$ 600 mg, Vit $B_{12}$ 440 mcg, Folic acid 50 mg, Vit C 20 g, Sodium sulphate 23 g, Potassium chloride 23 g , Casein protein 1,000 ppm, Elemental sodium 128 mg, Elemental cobalt 180 mg, Lactose q.s. | * Optimum body weight in growers <br> * During deworming <br> * To promote growth <br> * To prevent infections | **Through drinking water : Chicks :** 5-10 g / 100 birds / day for two weeks **Growers / Broilers:** 10 g / 100 birds / day for two weeks **Layers:** 10-20 g / 100 birds / day for one week on point of lay **Breeders:** 20 g / 100 birds / day for two weeks |
| 105 | V-CYCLINE POWDER (Varsha) | Oxytetracycline hydrochloride 30% w/w | * In early chick mortality <br> * Fowl typhoid <br> * Infectious coryza <br> * *E .coli* infections <br> * Enteric infections <br> * Respiratory infections <br> * CRD and complicated mycoplasmosis | 50 mg / Kg body weight for 5-7 days |
| 106 | WOLICYCLIN DS INJ. (Wockhardt) | Each ml contains : Oxytetracycline hydrochloride IP 100 mg (10%) | For a wide range of respiratory and enteric infections, complicated chronic respiratory disease (CCRD), coryza, fowl cholera, infectious synovitis, blue comb (non-specific enteritis) | 0.25 ml / Kg body weight |
| **PEFLOXACIN** | | | | |
| 107 | PEFLACIN POWDER | Each g contains : Pefloxacin 100 mg (as | Colisepticaemia, pasteurellosis, | **Prevention:** ½ g / 2-4 litre of |

| S. No. | Trade Name & Company | Composition | Indications | Dosage / Administration |
|--------|---------------------|-------------|-------------|------------------------|
| | (Neospark) | Pefloxacin methane sulphonate) | salmonellosis, staphylococcal infections, mixed bacterial infections, secondary bacterial complications due to viral diseases, CRD complex, infectious coryza and early chick mortality | water **Treatment:** ½ g / litre of water for 3-5 days |
| **TETRACYCLINE** | | | | |
| 108 | TETRACYCLINE HYDROCHLORIDE POWDER (Intervet) | Each g contains : Tetracycline hydrochloride IP 50 mg | * To prevent infections during stress period <br> * To prevent early chick mortality <br> * To treat bacterial and rickettsial infections | **Prevention:** 2.5 g / 4.5 litres of water for 5 days **Treatment:** 5 g / 4.5 litres of water for 5 days |
| 109 | VETCLIN-112 POWDER (Sarabhai Zydus) | Each g contains : Tetracycline hydrochloride IP 112 mg | * Mixed bacterial infections <br> * To prevent early chick mortality <br> * To protect against periods of stress | **Prevention:** 5 g / 20 litres of water **Treatment:** 5 g / 10 litres of water |

# 5. ANTIBIOTIC GROWTH PROMOTERS

| S. No. | Trade Name & Company | Composition | Indications | Dosage / Administration |
|---|---|---|---|---|
| 1 | ALBAC POWDER (Vetnex) | Zinc bacitracin 15% | * Improves FCR<br>* Growth promotion<br>* Prevention and treatment of clostridial infections | 1 Kg / 3 tones of feed |
| 2 | ALBMD GRANULATED 10% PREMIX (Alembic) | Each Kg Contains : Bacitracin 100 g (42,00,000 U) | * To cure the infections caused by the penicillin resistance *Staphylococcus aureus*<br>* To promote the growth of broilers, layers and breeders<br>* To improve feed conversion ratio<br>* To prevent and cure the infective enteritis of chicken | **Broilers:** Promotes growth – 44-550 g / tonne of feed Prevents and cures infective enteritis 110-2200 g / tonne of feed **Layers :** 110-275 g / tonne of feed to increase egg production |
| 3 | ALTHROCIN FS POWDER (Alembic) | Each g contains : Erythromycin thiocyanate equivalent to 20 mg, Erythromycin base, Excipients q.s. | * As growth promoter<br>* Ensures higher weight gain<br>* Improves the feed conversion ratio<br>* As anti-stress agent | **Growth promoter:** 0.5-1 Kg / tonne of feed **Anti-stress agent:** 1-2 Kg / tonne of feed |
| 4 | AUROFAC POWDER (Fort Dodge) | Each Kg contains : Aureomycin 100 g | * Growth promotion and improved feed efficiency<br>* To prevent infections and stress<br>* For better FCR, egg production and weight gain | 500 g / tonne of feed |
| 5 | BACTOKILL – C (Indian Drugs and Vitamins) | Each g contains: Amla exrtract 10 mg, Lactic acid bacilli 18 million CFU, Ciprofloxacin 100 mg, | Animal feed supplement for effective control of: CRD, Coryza, Pullorum disease, Fowl cholera, and many other bacterial infections | For dosage, refer to company's detailed literature |
| 6 | BAMYLATE | Each g contains: | *Improves feed efficiency | **Broilers:** |

| S. No. | Trade Name & Company | Composition | Indications | Dosage / Administration |
|---|---|---|---|---|
| | (B.V. Biocorp) | Bacitracin methylene disalicylate 0.10 g | * Increases weight gain<br>* Increases egg production<br>* For better hatchability and shell quality | 125-200 g / tonne of feed **Layers:** 15-35 g / tonne of feed **Breeders:** 15-25 g / tonne of feed **Necrotic enteritis:** 500 g / tonne of feed |
| 7 | BMD POWDER (Vetnex) | Bacitracin methylene disalyicilate | Growth promotion, prevention and treatment of clostridial infections | 200-500 g / tonne of feed |
| 8 | 3-CARE SPECIAL (Vetcare) | Each Kg contains: Chlorohydroxyquinoline 55% w/w, Doxycycline hydrochloride 5% w/w | * To prevent bacterial, fungal and protozoal infections<br>* To reduce wet litter problem<br>* To improve growth and performance<br>* To extend peak production in layers | **Broilers:** **Starter/Grower/ Finisher**: 50-100 g / tonne of feed **Layers:** **Starter/Grower:** 50-100 g / tonne of feed **During lay:** 50-100 g / tonne of feed @ week a month **Breeders:** **Starter/Grower/ During lay:** 100 g / tonne of feed |
| 9 | CIPHAXIN-PLUS (Indian Drugs and Vitamins) | Each g contains: Lactobacilli 18 million CFU, Amla extract 50 mg , Neem extract 100 mg, Cephalexin 50 mg, Ciprofloxacin 50 mg, Dextrose q.s. | Controls all Gram-positive and negative aerobic bacterial infections effectively | For dosage, see company's detailed literature |
| 10 | CHLORAN | Chlortetracycline | Growth promotion, | 1 Kg / 3 tonnes |

| S. No. | Trade Name & Company | Composition | Indications | Dosage / Administration |
|---|---|---|---|---|
| | GRANULATED 15% (Vetnex) | 15% | improvement in performance, egg production and weight gain<br>* Bacterial diseases like fowl cholera, CRD, non-specific diarrhoea, secondary bacterial infections | of feed |
| 11 | CHLORTETRACYCLINE 15% POWDER (Novartis) | Each Kg contains : Chlortetracycline 152.2 g | * Growth promotion<br>* Stress prevention<br>* Improvement in egg production and general health | 1 Kg / 3 tonnes of feed or 335 g / tonne of feed |
| 12 | COLI-FEEDMIX POWDER (Vetcare) | Each 500 g contains: Colistin sulphate 5 g | * Eliminates *E. coli* and salmonella<br>* Enhances growth<br>* Improves FCR<br>* Prevents colibacillosis and salmonellosis | **Broilers and Layers:**<br>500 g / tonne of feed<br>**Breeders:**<br>1 Kg / tonne of feed |
| 13 | COLIDOX POWDER (Vetcare) | Each Kg contains: Colistin sulphate 1000 mg, Doxycycline 10,000 mg, Excipient q.s. | * As a growth promoter<br>* To improve the feed efficiency<br>* To check the pathogen count<br>* To prevent frequent attack of *E. coli* and Salmonella infections | **Broilers and Layers:**<br>500 g / tonne of feed<br>**Breeders:**<br>1 Kg / tonne of feed |
| 14 | COLINIL – PLUS (Indian Drugs and Vitamins) | Each 100 g contains: Tulsi extract 1.5 g, Amla extract 1.5 g, Copper sulphate 2 g, Lactic acid bacilli 18 million CFU, Quinoline carboxylic acid 2.5 g, Ciprofloxacin 2.5 g, Dextrose q.s. | * Yolksac infection<br>* Egg peritonitis<br>* Coligranuloma<br>* Colisepticaemia | **Below 3 weeks old:**<br>10 g / 100 birds twice daily in water for 5 days<br>**Above 3 weeks:**<br>20 g / 100 birds twice daily through water for 5 days<br>**Severe condition:**<br>Double the dose |
| 15 | COLIS-V (Venky's) | Each g contains: Colistin sulphate | * For prevention of infections caused by | **Prevention:**<br>50 g / tonne of |

| S. No. | Trade Name & Company | Composition | Indications | Dosage / Administration |
|---|---|---|---|---|
| | | (U.S.P.) equivalent to Colistin 100 mg, Excipients q.s. | *E.coli* and Gram negative enteric problems<br>* Improves FCR and weight gain<br>* Choice for combination antibiotic | feed<br>**Treatment :**<br>200 g / tonne of feed, or<br>2 g / 15 litres of water for 75-100 birds for 3-5 days |
| 16 | CTC 15% POWDER (Osco) | Each Kg contains : Chlortetracycline 150 g | * To promote growth and improve feed efficiency<br>* To prevent chronic respiratory disease, synovitis and blue comb in birds<br>* To prevent early chick mortality | 335 g / tonne of feed |
| 17 | DOXATIN PREMIX POWDER (Stallen) | Each Kg contains : Tiamulin hydrogen fumarate 33 g, Doxycycline HCl 20 g, Excipients q.s. | * It is an effective growth promoter<br>* Also used for prevention and treatement of chronic respiratory disease, complicated chronic respiratory disease, fowl cholera and infectious coryza | **Growth promotion: Layers: 2nd week:** 3 Kg / tonne of feed for 7 days. Afterwards 1.5 Kg / tonne week a month programme till culling<br>**Broilers:** 500 g / tonne of feed<br>**Breeders:** 1.5 Kg / tonne of feed |
| 18 | FURALAY – 200 (Micro Labs) | Furazolidone BP (Vet) 20% w/w | Laying slumps, late maturity, stress conditions, vaccination, debeaking, and transportation, subclinical infections | **Broilers:** 500g / tonne of feed<br>**Layers:** 250 g / tonne of feed<br>**Week a month plan:** 500 g / tonne of feed one week every month |

| S. No. | Trade Name & Company | Composition | Indications | Dosage / Administration |
|---|---|---|---|---|
| 19 | HI-FUR 200 (Hitha) | Each kg contains: Furazolidone 200 g | * Effective against Salmonella and *E. coli* <br> * Checks enteritis <br> * Reduces chick mortality <br> * Increases egg production | 250 g / tonne of feed <br> 500 g / tonne of feed |
| 20 | LAYBRO MIX POWDER (Virbac) | Each Kg contains : Colistin sulphate 1,000 mg, Doxycycline BP 10,000 mg | * For better productivity, better growth and weight gain <br> * For better FCR | **Broilers / Layers:** 500 g-1 Kg / tonne of feed <br> **Breeders:** 2 Kg / tonne of feed for 7 days |
| 21 | LINCOCIN POWDER (Avian Remedies) | Each Kg contains : Lincomycin HCl equivalent to Lincomycin base 8 g, Carrier q.s. | To increase weight gain and improve feed efficiency | 250-500 g / tonne of feed |
| 22 | LINCOMIX FEED SUPPLEMENT (Pfizer) | Each kg contains: Lincomycin hydrochloride 110 g | * Increases weight gain <br> * Improves feed efficiency <br> * Controls necrotic enteritis <br> * Ensures uniform growth in chicks and growers | 40 g / tonne of feed |
| 23 | LINCOTIN (Indian Drugs and Vitamins) | Each Kg contains: Lincomycin 2%, Tinidazole 4%, Citric acid 2% | * Improves feed efficiency <br> * Increases weight gain <br> * Controls necrotic enteritis and other infections | 250 – 500 g / tonne of feed |
| 24 | MAGNOX PREMIX FEED SUPPLEMENT (Stallen) | Each Kg contains : Lincomycin 8 g | * Promotes growth with maximum protection against necrotic enteritis <br> * Has additional activity against mycoplasma spp | **For increased weight gain:** 250-500 g / tonne of feed <br> **For control of necrotic enteritis:** 250 g / tonne of feed |
| 25 | MICRODOX PREMIX (Micro Labs) | Each Kg contains: Doxycycline hydrochloride IP – 20 g | Prevention and treatment of infection due to Gram-positive and Gram-negative bacteria | **Broilers and Layers:** 250 g / tonne of feed |

| S. No. | Trade Name & Company | Composition | Indications | Dosage / Administration |
|---|---|---|---|---|
| 26 | MYCOSAL POWDER (Golden Streak) | Zinc drug 0.25%, Enrofloxacin 2.5%, Pefloxacin mesylate 7.5%, Dihydrate | * For more eggs, better eggshell quality<br>* For better weight and uniformity<br>* For better hatchability | **For CRD prevention:** 500 g / tonne of feed<br>**For growth promotion:** 100-200 g / tonne of feed |
| 27 | NUBIOTIC-100-FS POWDER (Neospark) | Each Kg contains : Neomycin sulphate 100 g, Protein hydrolysate 1000 ppm, Calcium 25.5% | * For better FCR, egg production and weight gain<br>* To prevent infections and stress | **In stress:** 1 Kg / tonne of feed<br>**Broilers:** 500 g – 1 Kg / tonne of feed<br>**Layers:** 1-2 Kg / tonne of feed |
| 28 | OSCONITE POWDER (Osco) | Each Kg contains : 3-Nitro-4-hydroxyphenyl arsenic acid 50 g | * Stimulates growth<br>* Improves weight gain<br>* Improves feed conversion ratio | 1 Kg / tonne of feed |
| 29 | OXY-100-FS (Neospark) | Each Kg contains : Oxytetracycline hydrochloride 100 g with plant protein products as carrier and diluents | * To improve feed efficiency<br>* For higher weight gain<br>* To increase egg production<br>* To improve eggshell structure | 0.5 – 2 kg / tonne of feed |
| 30 | OXYMYCIN (Varsha Group) | Oxytetracycline hydrochloride – 3%, Neomycin sulphate 3%, Probiotics 1%, Amino acid 5%, Vit A 10 lac IU, Vit K 3750 mg, Vit E – 5000 IU, Vit C – 5 %, Electrolytes – 5%, Dextrose – q.s. | * To prevent early chick mortality<br>* To attain uniform growth<br>* For better first week body weight gain<br>* To minimize loss during debeaking, coccidiosis, etc. | 1 g / litre of water for first five days to improve livability |
| 31 | POULTRY | Each 100 g | * Stress | **Stress:** |

| S. No. | Trade Name & Company | Composition | Indications | Dosage / Administration |
|---|---|---|---|---|
| | NUTRITIONAL FORMULA (Indian Drugs and Vitamins) | contains: Neomycin sulphate 5.506 g, Oxytetracycline hydrochloride 5.6 g, Vit B12 450 mcg, Vit K3, 0.141 g, Vit D3 22000 IU, Vit E acetate 35 IU, Riboflavin 0.18 g, Niacinamide 0.885 g, Cal. Pantothenate 0.360 g, , Vit A 11,0000 IU | * Disease treatment<br>* Severe disease outbreak | 2 g / 10 litres of water<br>**Disease treatment:**<br>4 g / 10 litres of water<br>**Severe disease outbreak:**<br>8 g / 10 litres of water |
| 32 | PRIMA-DOX-20 PREMIX POWDER (Stallen) | Doxycycline 2% | Increases growth promotion and FCR | 250 g / tonne of feed |
| 33 | PRIMADOX – N POWDER (Stallen) | Neomycin 2%, Doxycycline 2% | * It has broad-spectrum activity<br>* Rapidly absorbed from intestine<br>* Very effective against mixed gastrointestinal infections | **Prevention:**<br>200 g / tonne of feed<br>**Curative:**<br>400 g / tonne of feed |
| 34 | PROFIDONE 200 POWDER (Sarabhai Zydus) | Furazolidone 20% w/w | Improves feed conversion and general health | **Chicks (1st 10 days):**<br>2 Kg / tonne of feed.<br>Thereafter, 500 g / tonne of feed for 7 days every month |
| 35 | PROGRO – VET (Vetline) | Each g contains: Colistin sulphate 1500 mg, Doxycycline 10,000 mg, base q.s. | * Better feed conversion, increased weight gain<br>* Prevents subclinical infections<br>* Prevents uneven and retarded growth | **Broilers:**<br>500 g / tonne of feed from day one till marketing<br>**Layers:**<br>500 g to 1 Kg / |

| S. No. | Trade Name & Company | Composition | Indications | Dosage / Administration |
|---|---|---|---|---|
| | | | | tonne of feed a week per month programme **Breeders:** 2 Kg / tonne of feed |
| 36 | ROXARSONE FEED SUPPLEMENT (Wockhardt) | Each Kg contains : 3-Nitro-4-hydroxy phenyl arsonic acid 50 g (5%), or 3-Nitro-4-hydroxy phenyl arsonic acid 200 g (20%) | * Helps to improve feed conversion efficiency and growth in broilers by acting as selective germicide, where it kills all harmful Gram-positive anaerobes <br> * Potentiates the action of anticoccidials when used in combination, thereby ensures better livability | Roxarsone 5%: 1 kg / tonne of feed <br> Roxarsone 20% : 250 g / tonne of feed |
| 37 | SAL CURB LIQUID / DRY (Kemin) | Organic acids, their salts and surfactants with proven anti-microbial activity | * Prevents contamination and re-contamination of feed and raw materials by salmonella, other Gram-negative organisms and moulds <br> * Controls horizontal spread of disease through arrest of shedding of organisms <br> * Helps control the contamination of feed mill and its channels <br> * Has a non-specific mode of action, hence does not develop microbial resistance <br> * It is non-corrosive, non-toxic and has no withdrawal periods <br> * Sal curb liquid is highly effective in controlling contamination and recontamination of rendering products (MBM) and animal by-products (fish meal) | **Liquid:** **Feed:** 3-5 Kg / tonne **Meat and Bone meal:** 5-10 Kg / tonne **Fish meal:** 7.5-10 Kg / tonne **Dry:** 4-5 Kg / tonne of feed |

| S. No. | Trade Name & Company | Composition | Indications | Dosage / Administration |
|---|---|---|---|---|
| 38 | SALSTOP POWDER (Fort Dodge) | A mixture of salts of Propionic, Acetic, Formic, Sorbic, Lactic and Phosphoric acid and their free acids. It contains free fatty acids on a silica carrier | For protection against salmonella in high-protein raw materials and in finished feeds | 3 Kg / tonne of feed |
| 39 | SPORIN – PLUS (Indian Drugs and Vitamins) | Each g contains: Cephalexin IP 75 mg, Lactobacilli 18 million CFU, Manganese 50 mg, Amla extract 10 mg, Tulsi extract 10 mg, Dextrose q.s. | Prevents early chick mortality and promotes growth | **To prevent early chick mortality:** 20 g daily / 3000 chicks for first 5 days in drinking water **Other diseases:** 20 g daily / 1500 chicks / 250 growers / 100 layers for 3-5 days in drinking water |
| 40 | SUPERSTART – VRS (Venky's) | Unique blend of levofloxacin, electrolytes and vitamins | * Provides supportive therapy for chicks immediately after arrival<br>* Effective against wide range of Gram-positive, Gram-negative organisms and mycoplasma spp.<br>* Vitamins, dextrose and electrolytes provide supportive therapy | **Broilers / Broiler Breeders:** 50 g daily / 1000 chicks in drinking water for first 5 days of life **Layers / Layer Breeders:** 40 g daily / 1000 chicks in drinking water for first 5 days of life |
| 41 | STAFAC 20 POWDER (Pfizer) | Each Kg contains: Virginiamycin 20 g | * Performance enhancer in layers, broilers and breeders<br>* Reduces cost in feed mills | **Broilers:** 500 g – 1 Kg / tonne of feed **Layer chicks /** |

| S. No. | Trade Name & Company | Composition | Indications | Dosage / Administration |
|---|---|---|---|---|
| | | | | **Growers:** 500 g / tonne of feed **Layers:** 250 g / tonne of feed **Breeders:** 1-2 Kg / tonne of feed |
| 42 | STAFAC – 500 (Pfizer) | Each Kg contains: Virginiamycin – 500 g | * Performance enhancer in layers, broilers, and breeders <br> * Reduces cost in feed mills | **Broilers:** 20 g / tonne of feed **Layer chicks / Growers:** 20 g up to point of lay and 10 g / tonne from point to lay till end **Breeders:** 20 – 40 g / tonne from point-of-lay to end of lay |
| 43 | STEVIMAX – 500 FS (Neospark) | Each Kg contains: Virginiamycin 500 g | * To improve growth rate and FCR <br> * To improve productivity and hatchability | **Broilers:** 40 g / tonne starter feed and 20 g finisher feed **Layers:** 40 g / tonne of feed **Breeders:** 160 g / tonne of feed |
| 44 | SURMAX 100 POWDER (Elanco) | Each Kg contains : Avilamycin 100 g | * To improve live weight gain and feed efficiency <br> * Stimulates appetite <br> * Reduces sticky droppings <br> * Improves litter dry matter content <br> * Reduces mortality from necrotic enteritis <br> * Reduces foot pad lesions | 50-100 g / tonne of feed |
| 45 | TM-100 | Each Kg | * Improves feed efficiency | **Chicks:** |

| S. No. | Trade Name & Company | Composition | Indications | Dosage / Administration |
|---|---|---|---|---|
| | FEED SUPPLEMENT (Pfizer) | contains: Oxytetracycline 100 g | * Increases growth rate<br>* Earlier marketing of broilers and reduces risks<br>* Increases egg production in layers | 1 Kg / tonne of feed<br>**Broilers:**<br>500 g / tonne of feed<br>**Pullets:**<br>(Up to the onset of egg production) 100-500 g / tonne of feed (After the onset of lay up to 1 month) 500 g – 1 Kg / tonne of feed<br>**Layers:**<br>100-500 g / tonne of feed |
| 46 | TM – 200 FEED SUPPLEMENT (Pfizer) | Each Kg contains: Oxytetracycline 200 g | Performance enhancer | **Routine:**<br>250 g / tonne of feed<br>**Treatment:**<br>500 g / tonne of feed |
| 47 | UNIMIX POWDER (Vetcare) | Each Kg contains: Lincomycin hydrochloride 8.8 g (0.88% w/w) | * For prevention and treatment of necrotic enteritis<br>* Improves weight gain and feed conversion ratio<br>* Boosts body defences | **Broilers and Layers:**<br>500 g / tonne of feed<br>**Breeders:** 1 Kg / tonne of feed |
| 48 | UNIMIX FORTE (Vetcare) | Each Kg contains: Lincomycin hydrochloride – 110 g (11%) w/w | * To prevent and control infection against staphylococcus species, strepto species, mycoplasma species<br>* To prevent and control necrotic enteritis by clostridium species<br>* To reduce bacterial endotoxin<br>* To prevent wet litter, improve CMI | **Broilers/Layers/ Breeders:**<br>20 – 40 g / tonne of feed |
| 49 | VETRADOX | Doxycycline Hcl | For preventing the | **Broilers:** |

| S. No. | Trade Name & Company | Composition | Indications | Dosage / Administration |
|---|---|---|---|---|
| | POWDER (Vetnex) | equivalent to Doxycycline 2% w/w | exponential multiplication of common disease associated bacteria like *E .coli*, *Salmonella spp.*, *Streptococcus spp.*, *Hemophilus spp.*, *Klebsiella spp.*, *Corynebacterium spp.* | 125-250 g / tonne of feed (from day one till a week before marketing) **Layers:** 250 g – 500 g / tonne of feed (for a week every month) **Pullets:** 125-250 g / tonne of feed (till onset of lay) |

# 6A. ANTICOCCIDIALS (IN WATER)

| S. No | Trade Name & Company | Composition | Indications | Dosage / Administration |
|---|---|---|---|---|
| 1 | AMPROLIUM SOLUBLE POWDER (Neospark) | Each 30 g contains; Amprolium hydrochloride B.P. Vet 6 g, Excipients q.s. | For the treatment of coccidiosis in replacement chicks, broilers, layers and breeders | **Prophylactic:** 30 g / 100 litres of water **Usual outbreaks:** 30 g / 25 litres of water **Mild outbreaks:** 30 g /50 litres of water **Severe outbreaks:** 60 g / 25 litres of water for 5-7 days |
| 2 | AMPROLIUM SOLUBLE POWDER (Wockhardt) | Each g contains : Amprolium hydrochloride B.P. Vet 200 mg | For the treatment of coccidiosis in replacement chicks, layers, broilers and breeders | **For prevention:** 30 g / 50 litres of water **For mild infection:** 30 g / 25 litres of water **For disease outbreaks:** 60 g / 25 litres of water for 5-7 days |
| 3 | AMPROLSOL / AMPROLIUM SOLUBLE POWDER (Virbac) | Each g contains: Amprolium hydrochloride IP (Vet) 200 mg | For prevention and treatment of all types of coccidiosis in chicks, growers, broilers, layers and breeders | **Mild outbreaks:** 30 g / 50 litres of water for 5-7 days **Severe outbreaks:** 30 g / 50 litres of water for 5-7 days |
| 4 | AMPROSTAT (Stallen) | Each 30 g contains: Amprolium soluble powder USP – 6 g, excipients q.s. | For prevention and treatment of cocci in replacement chicks, broilers, layers, and breeders | **Prevention:** 30 g / 50 litres of water **Mild infection:** 30 g / 25 litres of water **Outbreak:** 60 g / 25 litres of water for 5-7 days |

| S. No | Trade Name & Company | Composition | Indications | Dosage / Administration |
|---|---|---|---|---|
| 5 | BANCOXY-K POWDER (Micro Labs) | Amprolium hydrochloride 20% w/w, Vit K3 0.2% w/w | For prevention and treatment of coccidiosis | *30 g / 20 litres of drinking water for first two days<br>*30 g / 30 litres of water for the next 3 days<br>*30 g / 60 litres of water for the last 3 days |
| 6 | BANCOXY PLUS POWDER (Micro Labs) | Amprolium hydrochloride 16.67% w/w, Sulphaquinoxaline 16.67% w/w | For prevention and treatment of coccidiosis | 1 g / 2 litre of water for 5-7 days |
| 7 | BAYCOX –VET (Pfizer) | Each 100 ml contains:<br>Toltrazuril – 2.5 g<br>Excipients – q. s. | * Use for treatment of coccidiosis caused by: E. acervulina E. E. maxima, E. mitis, E. necatrix,E. tenella<br>* Baycox acts both on schizogony stages and gametogony stages of coccidia | 7 mg / Kg body weight / day for 2 days<br>This is equivalent to 28 ml of Baycox per 100 kg of live body weight / day in water |
| 8 | COCCIWIN – T Oral Solution (Sarabhai Zydus) | Each 100 ml contains:<br>Toltrazuril – 2.5 g | Caecal and intestinal coccidiosis | 7 mg (0.28 ml) / Kg body weight daily for two consecutive days |
| 9 | COMATRIL (Toltrazuril) (Vetnex) | Toltrazuril – 2.5% | Prevention and treatment of coccidiosis | 7 mg / Kg body weight for 2 days |
| 10 | COXIMAR POWDER (Virbac) | Amprolium HCL 16.67% w/w, Sulphaquinoxaline 16.67% w/w | To check mortality within a day in all stages of coccidiosis | 30 g / 50 litres of drinking water for 3-7 days |

| S. No | Trade Name & Company | Composition | Indications | Dosage / Administration |
|---|---|---|---|---|
| 11 | COXYQUIN FORTE POWDER (Vetcare) | Each g contains : Amprolium hydrochloride 20% w/w, Sulphaquinoxaline 20% w/w, Dextrose q.s. | To treat intestinal and caecal coccidiosis caused by various species of Eimeria in broilers and replacement stocks | 1 g / 2 litres of water for 5-7 days |
| 12 | Esb3 POWDER (Novartis) | Each 100 g contains: Sulphachloropyrazine 30 g | * For treatment of coccidiosis caused by all Eimeria species <br> * Fowl cholera, fowl typhoid, and other infective diseases | 1 g / litre of water for 3 days **Fowl cholera / fowl typhoid:** 1-2 g / litre of water for 5 days |
| 13 | KAMPROL (Nicholas Piramal) | Amprolium hydrochloride powder 20% w/w, Vitamin K 0.2% w/w | Caecal and intestinal coccidiosis | **Prevention:** Add 30 g / 100 litres of water, or to 60 Kg of feed continuously **Mild outbreak:** 30 g / 50 litres of water, or 30 Kg of feed for 5-7 days **Severe outbreak:** 30 g / 25 litres of water, or 15 Kg of feed for 5-7 days |
| 14 | K-FURON TABLET (Qualitat) | Each tablet contains: Furazolidone – 16 mg Nitrofurazone – 110 mg Menadione sodium-bisulphate (Vit K3) – 1 mg | * Effective against intestinal coccidiosis <br> * Effective against bacillary diarrhoea caused by *E. coli* and salmonellosis <br> * Effective against other diseases with cocci | **Curative:** 1 tablet / litre of drinking water for 7 days **Preventive:** 1 tablet /2-4 litres of drinking water for 5 days |

| S. No | Trade Name & Company | Composition | Indications | Dosage / Administration |
|---|---|---|---|---|
| 15 | RANCOX WATER SOLUBLE POWDER (Vetnex) | Each 100 g contains: Sulphaquinoxaline BP (Vet) 18.7 g, Diaveridine (as hydrochloride) 3.3 g, Excipients q.s. | * For early and effective control of intestinal and caecal coccidiosis caused by *E. tenella, E. necatrix, E. acervulina, E. praecox and E. mitis* <br> * Fowl cholera caused by *P. multocida* and fowl typhoid caused by *S. gallinarum* | *10 g / 10 litres of water for 2-3 days <br> *Afterwards give plain water for next 2 days <br> *Dissolve 10 g / 20 litres of water for 2-3 days |

## 6B. ANTICOCCIDIALS (IN FEED)

| S. No | Trade Name & Company | Composition | Indications | Dosage / Administration |
|---|---|---|---|---|
| 1 | ANACOX 1% POWDER (Stallen) | Maduramycin ammonium 1 % | Protects birds from all types of coccidiosis | 500 g / tonne of feed |
| 2 | AV-DOT-E POWDER (AVR) | Dinitolmide 25% w/w, Ethophabate 1.6% w/w, base q.s. | For prevention of coccidiosis | **Chicks (0-6 weeks):** 500 g / tonne of feed <br> **Growers (6-14 weeks):** 250-500 g / tonne of feed <br> **Broilers (0-6 weeks):** 500 g / tonne of feed |
| 3 | AVATEC (Vetnex) | Lasalocid sodium – 15% | Prevention of coccidiosis | 500 – 600 g / tonne of feed |
| 4 | AVIAX (Pfizer) | Stable premix containing 5% Semduramicin activity | To improve performance in broilers through maintaining better gut health | ½ Kg / tonne of feed to provide 25 ppm Semduramicin activity in finished broiler feeds |

| S. No | Trade Name & Company | Composition | Indications | Dosage / Administration |
|---|---|---|---|---|
| 5 | AVICOX (Pfizer) | Stable premix containing 5% Semduramicin activity | To improve performance in broilers through maintaining better gut health | ½ Kg / 1 tonne feed to provide 25 ppm Semduramicin activity in broilers |
| 6 | BAZURIL (Intervet) | Diclazuril – 0.2% w/w Zinc bacitracin – 10% w/w | * Growth promoting anticoccidial <br> * Promotes growth <br> * Prevents coccidiosis and necrotic enteritis | **Broilers:** 500 g / tonne of feed from day one to marketing age **Layers:** 500 g / tonne of feed up to 16th week of age |
| 7 | BIOCOX P/T (Natural Herbs) | A herbal preparation of anticoccidial ingredients | * Useful in coccidiosis and intestinal infections <br> * Useful in bacterial enteritis, dysentery and diarrhoea caused by *E. coli,* salmonella species, infectious coryza, caecal coccidiosis, BWD, infectious synovitis | **Prevention** **Broiler:** 0-8 week 500g / tonne of feed Over 8 week – 1Kg / tonne of feed **Layers/Breeders:** 500 g / tonne of feed **Biocox – T** **Curative dose:** **Chicks:** 25 ml / 100 birds **Broilers/Layers/Breeders:** 50 ml / 100 birds |
| 8 | C. M. P. – 1 PREMIX POWDER (Venky's) | Each Kg contains : Diclazuril 1 g, organic carrier q.s. | For prevention of coccidiosis | 1 Kg / tonne of feed |
| 9 | COBAN-100 PREMIX POWDER (Venky's) | Each Kg Contains: Active ingredient Monensin-100 g carrier q.s. | * Helps in prevention of coccidiosis <br> * For improved feed conversion ratio <br> * For better growth <br> * For improved quality of birds | **Broilers:** 1 Kg / tonne of feed from day 1 till slaughter **Layers:** **1st to 13th week –** 1 Kg / tonne of feed **13th – 16th week –** 600 g / tonne of feed |

| S. No | Trade Name & Company | Composition | Indications | Dosage / Administration |
|---|---|---|---|---|
| 10 | COCCINIL-M POWDER (Vetcare) | Each Kg contains: Maduramicin ammonium 20 g (2% w/w), excipient q.s. | For prevention of coccidiosis of all types as continuous, shuttle or rotation programme | 250 g / tonne of feed |
| 11 | COSMODOT POWDER (Neospark) | 3-5, Dinitro-o-toluamide : 25% w/w Elemental calcium: 21.5% . Protein hydrolysate: 2000 ppm. | For prevention of coccidiosis | **Broilers:** **0-8 weeks:** 500 g / tonne of feed **Replacement birds:** **0-8 weeks:** 500 g / tonne of feed **9-14 weeks:** 300 g / tonne of feed |
| 12 | COSMODOT-EP POWDER (Neospark) | 3,5 Dinitro-o-toluamide : 25% w/w Ethopabate : 1.6% w/w Elemental calcium 21.5%. Protein hydrolysate : 2000 ppm. | For prevention of coccidiosis | **Broilers:** **0-8 weeks:** 500 g / tonne of feed **Replacement birds:** **0-8 weeks:** 500 g / tonne of feed **9-14 weeks:** 300 g / tonne of feed |
| 13 | COCCIWIN POWDER (Sarabhai Zydus) | Maduramicin ammonium 1% w/w | For control of both caecal and intestinal coccidiosis | 500 g / tonne of feed |
| 14 | COXISTAC POWDER (Pfizer) | Stable premix containing Salinomycin 12% | * It is an effective aid for control of coccidiosis in broilers * Helps in improving intestinal health, weight gain and feed efficiency | 0.5 Kg / tonne of feed |

| S. No | Trade Name & Company | Composition | Indications | Dosage / Administration |
|---|---|---|---|---|
| 15 | COXISAL POWDER (Microgranulated) (Alembic) | Salinomycin sodium 12% (w/w) microgranulated | 100 For prevention of coccidiosis | **Broilers:** 500 g / tonne of feed **Layers:** **Pullets to be kept on floor: 0-6 weeks** – 500 g / tonne of feed **7-10 weeks** – 400 g / tonne of feed **11-14 weeks** – 350 g / tonne of feed **Pullets to be kept in cages:** 0-10 weeks – 500 g / tonne of feed |
| 16 | COXYCLIN POWDER (Novartis) | Each Kg contains : Diclazuril 5 g | A good anticoccidial feed additive for prevention of coccidiosis in broiler chickens | 200 g / tonne of feed |
| 17 | COZURIL (Stallen) | 0.5 % Diclazuril | * Ideal for rotation with other anticoccidials or shuttle programme * Effective against all species of Eimeria * Works as a growth promoter | **Broilers / Layers:** Replacement chickens up to 16 weeks. Thoroughly mix 200 g / tonne of feed |
| 18 | CYCOSTAT POWDER (Fort Dodge) | Robenidine 6.6% | For prevention of coccidiosis | **Broilers only:** 500 g / tonne of feed |
| 19 | CYGRO POWDER (Fort Dodge) | Maduramicin ammonium 1% | * For effective protection against intestinal and caecal coccidiosis * For best growth and feed conversion ratio | **Broilers:** 500 g / tonne of feed from day one to day of marketing |
| 20 | DINITOLMIDE POWDER (DOT) (Wockhardt) | Each Kg contains : 3,5-Dinitro-Ortho-Toluamide 250 g | Helps in prevention and control of coccidiosis | 500 g / tonne of feed |
| 21 | DURAMIX F.S. POWDER (Micro Labs) | Each Kg contains : Maduramicin ammonium 1% w/w | For treatment of coccidiosis caused by all Eimeria species | 500 g / tonne of feed |

| S. No | Trade Name & Company | Composition | Indications | Dosage / Administration |
|---|---|---|---|---|
| 22 | ELANCOBAN-200 POWDER (Elanco) | Each Kg contains : Monensin ( as Monensin sodium) 200 g | Acts early in the coccidial life cycle and is effective against all Eimeria species | **Broilers:** Mix in feed continuously from day one to culling **Layers:** Up to 10th week – 500 g / tonne of feed **Breeders:** 11th-16th week – 450 g / tonne of feed |
| 23 | ETHODOT POWDER (Rallis) | Dinitolmide 25% w/w, Ethopabate 1.6% w/w | For prevention and treatment of coccidiosis | 500 g / tonne of feed |
| 24 | GROVIRON POWDER (Virbac) | Maduramicin 1% w/w as madura-micin ammonium salt | * Effectively protects from coccidiosis * Improves growth rate * Improves FCR | **Broilers:** 500 g / tonne of feed till marketing |
| 25 | HI-DOT 25 POWDER (Hitha) | Each Kg contains : Dinitro-O-Toulamide 250 g | * Stops growth of Eimeria species causing coccidiosis * Improves intestinal environment * For better FCR * Checks mortality rate * Can be safely administered with other antibiotics and dewormers | 500 g / tonne of feed |
| 26 | INOMAX-M-FS POWDER (Neospark) | Maduramycin ammonium 1% w/w | * For effective protection against all species of Eimeria * For better growth and weight gain | **Broilers:** 500 g / tonne of feed from day one till 5 days before marketing **Growers:** 500 g / tonne of feed from day one to 16th weeks of age |

| S. No | Trade Name & Company | Composition | Indications | Dosage / Administration |
|---|---|---|---|---|
| 27 | KADIPROL POWDER (Sarabhai Zydus) | Each 100 g contains : Amprolium hydrochloride 25 g, Vit $K_3$ 250 mg | Caecal and intestinal coccidiosis | 500 g / tonne of feed |
| 28 | KAMPROL (Nicholas Piramal) | Amprolium HCL powder 20% w/w, Vitamin K 0.2% w/w | Caecal and intestinal coccidiosis | **Prevention:** 30 g / 100 litres of water or 30 g / 60 Kg of feed. Give continuously **Mild outbreak:** 30 g / 50 litres of water or 30 g of feed for 5-7 days **Severe outbreak:** 30 g / 25 litres of water or 15 Kg of feed for 5-7 days |
| 29 | KOX – CARE POWDER (Vesper) | Nitrofurazone 4.6 % w/w, Vit. K3 0.5% w/w | For prevention of coccidiosis | **Prophylactic:** 500 g / tonne of feed **Curative:** 1.5 – 2 Kg / tonne of feed |
| 30 | MACROMYCIN POWDER (Vetnex) | Salinomycin 12% | For prevention of coccidiosis | 500 g / tonne of feed |
| 31 | MADUCOX POWDER (Alembic) | Maduramicin ammonium 1.0 % w/w | * For prevention of coccidiosis * Effective against all species of Eimeria * Improves FCR * Ensures excellent growth and weight gain | **Broilers:** 200 g / tonne of feed till marketing **Layers / Breeders:** 200 g / tonne of feed, from day one to 16th week of age |
| 32 | MAXIBAN-72 POWDER (Elanco) | Narasin 80 g , Nicarbazin 80 g / Kg | * Improves overall performance * For better weight gains * Reduces oocyst output * Effective against all Eimeria species | Depending on the severity of infection of coccidiosis, dosage may vary from 337-562 g /tonne of feed |

| S. No | Trade Name & Company | Composition | Indications | Dosage / Administration |
|---|---|---|---|---|
| 33 | MERICOX (Wockhardt) | Each Kg contains 120 g (12%) of salinomycin sodium | For prevention and treatment of caecal and intestinal coccidiosis | 500 g / tonne of feed |
| 34 | MONACOX POWDER (Vetnex) | Maduramycin ammonium granulated 1% w/w | For prevention of coccidiosis caused by all Eimeria species | 500 g / tonne of feed |
| 35 | MONTEBAN-45 (Elanco) | Each Kg contains : Narasin 100 g | * Effective against all Eimeria species<br>* Better weight gain<br>* Improves feed conversion | Depending on the severity of infection of coccidiosis, dosage may vary from 540-720 g / tonne of feed |
| 36 | OCCIDAL POWDER (Vetnex) | Diclazuril 0.5% w/w | For prevention of coccidiosis caused by all Eimeria species | 200 g / tonne of feed |
| 37 | OOCOX POWDER (Stallen) | Maduramicin 1% | Effective against all pathogenic Eimeria species | 500 g / tonne of feed |
| 38 | Q – DOT (Qualitat) | Dinitro-ortho-toluamide – 25% | * Effective against *E. tenella* and mixed infections of five or more species as well<br>* Effective against intestinal and caecal coccidiosis | 250 – 500 g / tonne of feed up to 12 weeks of age |
| 39 | RACOXI PREMIX (Stallen) | Salinomycin 12% | For the prevention of coccidiosis caused by all Eimeria species | 500 g / tonne of feed |
| 40 | SULMET (Fort Dodge) | Sodium sulphadimethylpyrimidine 12.5% w/v | Effective against all strains of cocci. Acts at later stages of coccidial life cycle | 30 ml / 4 litres of water for first two days Then, 15 ml / 4 litres of water for next four days |

| S. No | Trade Name & Company | Composition | Indications | Dosage / Administration |
|---|---|---|---|---|
| 41 | SUPERCOX POWDER (Wockhardt) | Each 100 g contains : Sulphaquinoxaline 18.7 g, Diverdine 3.3 g | * For early and effective control of intestinal and caecal coccidiosis<br>* Fowl cholera caused by *Pasteurella multocida*<br>* Fowl typhoid caused by *Salmonella gallinarum* | *10 g / 10 litres of water or 100 g/ 50 Kg of feed for 2-3 days<br>*Afterwards give plain drinking water for next 2 days.<br>*Then 10 g / 20 litres of water or 100 g / 100 Kg of feed for next 2-3 days |
| 42 | VELDOT POWDER (Venky's) | Dinitolmide 25% w/w | * Helps in prevention of coccidiosis<br>* For improved feed conversion ratio | **Broilers:**<br>500 g / tonne of feed continuously<br>**Layers:**<br>500 g / tonne of feed till 14th week |
| 43 | VETSFURAN POWDER (Vets Farma) | Nitrofurazone 25% w/w, Furazolidone 3.6% w/w | For prevention of coccidiosis | **Prophylactic:**<br>125 g / 250-300 Kg feed<br>**Curative:**<br>125 g / 125 Kg feed |
| 44 | WOCOX POWDER (Wockhardt) | Each Kg contains : Diclazuril 5 g (0.5% w/w) | * Controls intestinal and caecal coccidiosis<br>* Controls subclinical and clinical coccidiosis | 200 g / tonne of feed |

# 7. ANTI-DIARRHOEALS

| S.No. | Trade Name & Company | Composition | Indications | Dosage / Administration |
|---|---|---|---|---|
| 1 | DIACONT (Polchem) | Extract of *Aegle marmelos, Holarrhena antidysentrica, Ricinus communis, Punica grantum, Scindapsus officianalis, Myristica fragrans, Magnifera indica*, natural vitamins and biominerals | * Better litter management<br>* Controls foul odour in the poultry house<br>* Controls loose droppings of non-specific cause<br>* In case of excess of water in faeces | **Feed:** 200 g / tonne of feed<br>**In Water:** 200 g /day / 10,000 broilers / 6000 layers / 4000 breeders |
| 2 | DIAREX PFS (Himalaya) | Herbal extracts | * Helps to control loose droppings due to contaminated feed, parasites<br>* Helps improve immune system<br>* Helps normalize the GI secretions<br>* Ensures better feed absorption<br>* Helps reduce morbidity and mortality | 500 g / tonne of feed<br>Higher dose may be recommended in severe conditions |
| 3 | DIAROAK (Ayurvet) | Extract of standardized herbs | To control loose droppings in poultry due to<br>* Dietary errors<br>* Mouldy and contaminated feed<br>* Infectious and parasitic diseases<br>* Non-specific causes | **For prevention:** 500 g / tonne of feed regularly<br>**For treatment:** 1 Kg / tonne of feed for 5-7 days |
| 4 | GUTMOTIL PFS (Indian Herbs) | Herbal preparation | * To maintain stable and healthy gut function, to avoid loose droppings and to keep litter in dry condition<br>* Nutritional support in infectious diarrhoeal conditions | 1-2 Kg / tonne of feed |

| | | | caused by viruses, bacteria, fungi, protozoa, parasites | |
|---|---|---|---|---|
| 5 | QUIXALUD (Novartis) | Each Kg of Quixalud contains 600 g of Chlorhydroxyquino-line 60% | * For prevention of non-specific diarrhoea<br>* Improves growth rate / egg production and feed efficiency<br>* Its anti-peristaltic action promotes nutrient absorption | **Broilers / Layers / Breeders:** 100 g / tonne of feed |
| 6 | STODI (Natural Remedies) | An effective herbal loose dropping binder | To minimize loose droppings due to peak production / growth, dietary error and high environmental temperature | 500 g – 750 g / tonne of feed |

# 8. ANTI-FLY AGENTS AND ECTOPARASITICIDES

| S. No. | Trade Name & Company | Composition | Indications | Dosage / Administration |
|---|---|---|---|---|
| 1 | CLINAR LIQUID (Virbac) | Cypermethrin High Cis 10% w/v | For control and treatment of ectoparasites like ticks, mites, lice and flies | Add 1-2 ml in 1 litre of water |
| 2 | CYROCID (Natural Remedies) | Cyromazine 2% | Cyrocid is highly effective against stable flies, house flies, and little house flies etc. | 250 g / tonne of layer feed. The laying birds are to be fed with the Cyrocid mixed feed for 4-6 weeks |
| 3 | CYROMAX 1% POWDER (Stallen) | Active ingredient : Cyromazine (feed grade) 1%, Inert ingredients :99% | For fly control around poultry | 500 g / tonne of feed |
| 4 | EKTOMIN LIQUID (Novartis) | It is a synthetic pyrethroid, containing Cypermethrin high cis | For the control of lice, ticks, mites and flies | 1 ml / litre of water (60 litres of spray mixture per 1000 birds) |
| 5 | EXO DUST (Exotic Mushrooms) | Feed supplement for control of flies and storage pests | * Fly control in dung and droppings<br>* Control of storage pests<br>* Reduces odour and moisture in dung and droppings<br>* Eliminates internal parasites without re-occurrences<br>* Reduces stress<br>* Larval control of all types of flies<br>* Acts as a broad-spectrum toxin binder | 5 Kg / tonne of feed |
| 6 | FLYBAN POWDER (Nicholas Piramal) | Cyromazine (feed grade) 1%, Inert ingredients : 99% | For control of larval stages of house fly in layer and breeder farms | 500 g / tonne of layer and breeder feed for 4-6 weeks |
| 7 | FLYCID POWDER (Virbac) | Each Kg contains : Cyromazine1% w/w | For control of larval stages of house fly in layer and breeder farms | 500 g / tonne of feed for 4-6 weeks |

| S. No. | Trade Name & Company | Composition | Indications | Dosage / Administration |
|---|---|---|---|---|
| 8 | FLYEX (Exotic Mushrooms) | Anti-fly combination | * Reduces spread of diseases<br>* Reduces the chances of avian tapeworms and caecal worms<br>* Reduces ammonia and moisture in litter | 500 g to 1 Kg per 100 sq. ft. for 10 days in a month |
| 9 | FLY – OUT (Harshvardhan's Lab) | Cyromazine 1% feed grade and 2% feed grade | * Larvacide<br>* Reduces stress on birds caused by fly infestation<br>* Checks infection due to fly borne | **Layers and Breeders** through feed when flies become active 1% 500 g / tonne of finished feed; 2% 250 g / tonne of finished feed |
| 10 | FLY – OUT (Harshvardhan's Lab) | Cyromazine 2% feed grade | * Larvacide<br>* Reduces stress on birds caused by fly infestation | 250 g / tonne of finished feed |
| 11 | LARVADEX GOLD (Feed Supplement) (Novartis) | Cyromazine (feed grade) 2%, Chlorhydroxyquinoline 24%, Excipients q.s. | Helps controlling the house fly by controlling larval stage during life cycle<br>Helps in reducing fly nuisance level in and around farm area to maintain healthy environment | 250 g / tonne of feed for 4-6 weeks until the fly population is under control |
| 12 | LARVADEX POWDER (Novartis) | Cyromazine (feed grade) 1% | For control of larval stages of house fly in layer and breeder farms | 500 g / tonne of feed |
| 13 | NO-FLY (Varsha) | Cyromazine – 1% (feed grade) | Fly menace and wet droppings | 500 g / tonne of feed Mix with normal feed and use when flies become active. Continue the application for 4-6 weeks or until fly population is under control |

# 9. ANTI-GOUT DRUGS

| S. No, | Trade Name & Company | Composition | Indications | Dosage / Administration |
|---|---|---|---|---|
| 1 | AVISOL POWDER (Venky's) | Each 100 g contains : Potassium citrate 18 g, Sodium citrate 12 g, Natural immuno-stimulant 1 g, Vit $B_1$ 0.3 g, Vit $B_2$ 0.15 g, Niacin 0.32 g, Vit $K_3$, 0.12 g, Vit C 1.1 g, Carrier q.s. | * To improve livability <br> * For prevention of stress <br> * To develop resistance against viral infection <br> * As an aid in detoxification <br> * To improve immunity <br> * To prevent gout and arthritis <br> * Relieves stress on account of IBD | 50 g / 1000 chicks to 100 g / 1000 birds in drinking water for 5 days |
| 2 | GOUT – EASE (Natural Remedies) | Biological herbal preparation | * Prevents and treats visceral and articular gout <br> * Prevents and treats urolithiasis <br> * Prevents and treats ascites <br> * Maintains normal functioning of kidney | **Prevention:** 1ml / litre of drinking water 24 hours for first two weeks <br> **Treatment:** 2 ml / litre of drinking water 24 hours for 5-7 days <br> **Powder:** **Treatment:** 350 to 500 g / tonne of feed continuously |
| 3 | GOUT- GARD (Neospark) | Natural alkaloid compounds having renal stimulants with diuretic activity | * Gout, ascites, and urinary tract infections <br> * Prevents accumulation of uric acid in the body <br> * Increases urine output and maintains kidney function | **Dosage through drinking water per day per 100 birds:** **Chicks** – 5ml **Growers** – 10 ml **Broilers/Layers** – 20 ml |
| 4 | K FLUSH LIQUID (Avians) | Maltose, Vit B complex, Lactic acid, *Saccharomyces cerevisiae* live cells | * To improve immunity and livability of chicks <br> * To prevent stress, gout and arthritis | 5 ml / 100 chicks through water for 3-4 days |

| S. No, | Trade Name & Company | Composition | Indications | Dosage / Administration |
|---|---|---|---|---|
| 5 | NEFROTEC LIQUID (Himalaya) | Herbal preparation | * Gout<br>* Ascites<br>* Urinary tract infections | **Chicks:**<br>5 ml /100 birds / day<br>**Growers:**<br>10 ml / 100 birds / day<br>**Broilers / Layers:**<br>20 ml / 100 birds / day |
| 6 | NEPHCURE (Natural Herbs) | A poly-herbal formulation of Haritiki, Bhringraj, Pasan Bhed, Gokhru, Kalmegh geloe, makoi, etc. | * Protects kidney and reduces the uric acid in blood<br>* Checks sodium bicarbonate toxicity<br>* Improves urinary flow, dissolves urate deposits in viscera, joints<br>* Diuretic action in ascites | **Broilers** (per 100 birds):<br>**0-2 weeks:**<br>Preventive 4 ml<br>Curative 8 ml<br>**3-4 weeks:**<br>Preventive 8 ml<br>Curative 16 ml<br>**5 weeks onwards:**<br>Preventive 14 ml<br>Curative 28 ml<br>**Layers** (per 100 birds):<br>**0-8 weeks:**<br>Preventive 4 ml<br>Curative 8 ml<br>**9-20 weeks:**<br>Preventive 8 ml<br>Curative 16 ml<br>**21-72 onwards:**<br>Preventive 14 ml<br>Curative 28 ml |
| 7 | NEPHTONE (Powder and Liquid) (Indian Herbs) | Herbal renal tonic and diuretic | * Visceral or articular gout<br>* Urolithiasis<br>* Ascites<br>* Acute or chronic renal insufficiency<br>* Nephrotic syndrome | **Preventive:** 1 Kg / tonne of feed<br>**Broilers:** For first 3 weeks:<br>**Layers:** Regularly during susceptible period<br>**Treatment** (per 100 birds):<br>**Broilers:**<br>**0-2 weeks:** 8 ml;  **3 – 4 weeks:** 16 ml **5 weeks onwards:** 28 ml; |

| S. No, | Trade Name & Company | Composition | Indications | Dosage / Administration |
|---|---|---|---|---|
| | | | | **Layers:** **0-8 weeks:** 8 ml **9-20 weeks:** 16 ml **21-72 weeks:** 28ml |
| 8 | UROTECH (Wockhardt) | Biologically potentiated herbal extract | * To strengthen body metabolism and kidney functions * To prevent visceral gout | 25 ml / 1000 birds / day in water 50 ml / 1000 birds during stress |

# 10. ANTI-MYCOPLASMAL DRUGS

| S. No. | Trade Name & Company | Composi-tion | Indications | Dosage / Administration |
|---|---|---|---|---|
| 1 | C.R. D. CHECK – P (Natural Herbs) | *Piper nigrum, Eucalyptus , Allium sativum, Zingiber officinale, Mentha piperita, Eucalyptus* Turmeric and Nosadar etc. | For prevention and treatment of CCRD, infectious coryza, infectious bronchitis, influenza, respiratory complex | **Preventive:**<br>1 Kg / tonne of feed<br>**Broilers:** From day one till marketing<br>**Layers:** For 15 days every month<br>**Therapeutic:**<br>2-4 Kg / tonne of feed<br>To be given for 1-2 weeks |

**Item 2:**

FORTULIN 45% GRANULES (Stallen) — Tiamulin hydrogen fumarate 45% — For effective control of chronic respiratory disease (CRD) in poultry

**Prevention for 1000 birds / day**

| Age | Broilers | Pullets | |
|---|---|---|---|
| (Weeks) | g | g | |
| 1 | 5 | 5 | 3 days |
| Day 8/9 | 5 | 5 | 2 days |
| 4 | 20 | 13 | 2 days |
| 6 | 32 | 20 | 2 days |
| 10 | - | 26 | 2 days |
| 14 | - | 32 | 2 days |
| 18 | - | 40 | 2 days |

**Treatment for 1000 broilers :**

| | | |
|---|---|---|
| 3 | 25 | 3 days |
| 4 | 40 | 3 days |
| 5 | 55 | 3 days |
| 6 | 65 | 3 days |

**Item 3:**

| 3 | FORLUTIN 80% GRANULES (Stallen) | Tiamulin hydrogen fumarate 80% | For effective control of chronic respiratory disease (CRD) in poultry | **Prophylactic:**<br>25 g / 100 Kg of feed for 2 days at interval of 3-4 weeks<br>**Curative:**<br>50 g / 100 Kg of feed for 3-5 days |
|---|---|---|---|---|

**Item 4:**

PULMOTIL-AC (Elanco) **For commercial broilers** — Tilmicosin Aqueous concentrate (as the phosphate) : 250 mg / ml

Indications:
* For easy breathing
* It can be given with other Gram negative antibiotics simultaneously
* Water sanitizer is to be avoided

Pulmotil AC dosage is calculated as tilmicosin @ 15 mg / kg body weight

| Body Wt. | Dose for 1000 birds in water |
|---|---|
| 250 g | 15 ml / day |
| 300 g | 18 ml / day |
| 350 g | 21 ml / day |
| 400 g | 24 ml / day |

| S. No. | Trade Name & Company | Composi-tion | Indications | Dosage / Administration |
|---|---|---|---|---|
| | | | while giving pulmotil | |
| 5 | PULMOTIL-AC (Elanco) **For commercial layers** | Tilmicosin (as the phosphate) : 250 mg / ml | * For easy breathing <br> * It can be given with other Gram negative antibiotics simultaneously <br> * Water sanitizer is to be avoided while giving pulmotil | Pulmotil AC dosage is calculated as tilmicosin @ 15 mg / Kg body weight on day 14 and 15. Thereafter, it is calculated 20 mg / Kg body weight <br><br> **Day / Week**    **Dose for 1000 birds in water** <br> 14 day    10 ml <br> 15 day    10 ml <br> 6$^{th}$ Week (1 day)   35 ml <br> 12$^{th}$ Week (1 day)   75 ml <br> 18$^{th}$ Week (1 day)   125 ml |
| 6 | SOLUTYL POWDER (Venky's) | Each 10 g contains: Tylosin activity 6.25 g as Tylosin tartrate IP (Vet) | * For protection against respiratory disease like CRD <br> * Effective over *Mycoplasma gallisepticum* and *Mycoplasma synoviae* <br> * For better FCR, weight gain and improved productivity | 176 mg / Kg body weight in drinking water as per recommended schedule. Refer to company's literature for details |
| 7 | TETRAMUTIN PREMIX (DENAGARD) (Novartis) | Each Kg contains : 33.3 g of Tiamulin hydrogen fumarate / 100 g of Chlortetra-cycline hydrochloride | For control of chronic respiratory disease (CRD), complicated chronic respiratory disease (CCRD), infectious coryza and fowl cholera | **Growth promotion:** <br> 0.5-1 Kg / tonne of feed <br> **Prevention:** <br> 1-1.5 Kg / tonne of feed <br> **Treatment:** <br> 3 – 4.5 Kg / tonne of feed |
| 8 | TIAMULIN 10 % PREMIX | Tiamulin hydrogen fumarate 10% | Prevention, control and treatment of | **Treatment:** <br> 100 – 300 g / tonne of feed |

| S. No. | Trade Name & Company | Composi-tion | Indications | Dosage / Administration |
|---|---|---|---|---|
| | (Vetnex) | granulated | mycoplasmal infections | |
| 9 | TIAMULIN 80% (Vetnex) | Tiamulin hydrogen fumarate 80% granulated | Prevention, control and treatment of mycoplasmal infections | **Prevention:** 12.5 mg / Kg body weight **Treatment:** 25 mg / Kg body weight |
| 10 | TIAMUTIN 10% PREMIX (DENAGAR D) (Novartis) | Each g contains : Tiamulin hydrogen fumarate 100 mg | * Highly active against mycoplasma * Improves FCR by 4.2% * Improves egg production * 4.5 % more eggs on average | 200 g / tonne of feed |
| 11 | TIAMUTIN 45% (DENAGAR D) WATER SOLUBLE GRANULES (Novartis) | Each g contains : 450 mg Tiamulin hydrogen fumarate (THF) coated | For prevention and treatment of diseases of the respiratory tract caused by mycoplasmas and complicated by secondary bacterial infections | (see table below) |

**IN WATER MEDICATION:**
**Broilers & Replacement Pullets**
**Preventive Dosage (1000 birds)**

| Age in | Qty. of Tiamutin in g / day | | |
|---|---|---|---|
| Days/ Weeks | Broilers | Replacement pullets | |
| 1st | 5 | 5 | for 3 days |
| day 8/9 | 5 | 5 | for 2 days |
| 4th | 20 | 13 | for 2 days |
| 6th | 32 | 20 | for 2 days |
| 10th | - | 26 | for 2 days |
| 14th | - | 32 | for 2 days |
| 18th | - | 40 | for 2 days |

**For Breeders:**
**Preventive Dosage (1000 birds)**

| Age in | Qty. of Tiamutin in g / day | |
|---|---|---|
| Days/ Weeks | Broiler Breeders | Layer Breeders |
| 1 | 5 | 5 |
| day 8/9 | 5 | 5 |
| 4 | 13 | 8 |

| S. No. | Trade Name & Company | Composi-tion | Indications | Dosage / Administration | | | |
|---|---|---|---|---|---|---|---|
| | | | | 8 | 26 | 16 | |
| | | | | 12 | 32 | 24 | |
| | | | | 16 | 44 | 35 | |
| | | | | 20 | 54 | 35 | |
| | | | | 24 | 73 | 37 | |
| | | | | 28 | 83 | 38 | |
| | | | | 32 | 86 | 40 | |
| | | | | 36 | 89 | 40 | |
| | | | | 40 | 92 | 40 | |
| | | | | 44 | 92 | 40 | |
| | | | | 48 | 92 | 42 | |
| | | | | 52 | 94 | 42 | |
| | | | | 56 | 94 | 43 | |
| | | | | 60 | 94 | 43 | |
| | | | | 64 | 94 | 43 | |
| | | | | 68 | 94 | 43 | |
| | | | | **Treatment : For 1000 Broilers:** | | | |
| | | | | Age in weeks | Qty. of Tiamutin in g / day | | |
| | | | | $3^{rd}$ | 25 | | |
| | | | | $4^{th}$ | 40 | | |
| | | | | $5^{th}$ | 55 | | |
| | | | | $6^{th}$ | 65 | | |
| | | | | **IN-FEED MEDICATION:** | | | |
| | | | | **Prevention :** | | | |
| | | | | 450 g / tonne of feed for 2 days | | | |
| | | | | **Treatment:** | | | |
| | | | | 900 g / tonne of feed for 3-5 days | | | |
| 12 | TIAMUTIN 80% (DENAGARD) WATER SOLUBLE GRANULES (Novartis) | Each g contains : 800 mg Tiamulin hydrogen fumarate (THF) coated | For prevention and treatment of diseases of the respiratory tract caused by mycoplasmas and complicated | **IN WATER MEDICATION :** | | | |
| | | | | **Preventive Dosage (1000 birds)** | | | |
| | | | | Age in | Qty. of Tiamutin in g / day | | |

| S. No. | Trade Name & Company | Composi-tion | Indications | Dosage / Administration | | | |
|---|---|---|---|---|---|---|---|
| | | | by secondary bacterial infections | Days/ | Broilers | Replace ment | |
| | | | | Weeks | | Pullets | |
| | | | | 1st | 3 | 3 | for 3 days |
| | | | | day 8/9 | 3 | 3 | for 2 days |
| | | | | 4th | 11 | 7 | for 2 days |
| | | | | 6th | 18 | 11 | for 2 days |
| | | | | 10th | - | 15 | for 2 days |
| | | | | 14th | - | 18 | for 2 days |
| | | | | 18th | - | 23 | for 2 days |
| | | | | **Preventive dosage (1000 birds)** | | | |
| | | | | Age in | Quantity of Tiamutin in g / day | | |
| | | | | Days/ | Broiler | Layer | |
| | | | | Weeks | Breeders | Breeders | |
| | | | | 1st | 3 | 3 | |
| | | | | day 8/9 | 3 | 3 | |
| | | | | 4 | 7 | 5 | |
| | | | | 8 | 15 | 9 | |
| | | | | 12 | 18 | 14 | |
| | | | | 16 | 25 | 20 | |
| | | | | 20 | 30 | 20 | |
| | | | | 24 | 41 | 21 | |
| | | | | 28 | 47 | 21 | |
| | | | | 32 | 48 | 23 | |
| | | | | 36 | 50 | 23 | |
| | | | | 40 | 52 | 23 | |
| | | | | 44 | 52 | 23 | |
| | | | | 48 | 52 | 24 | |
| | | | | 52 | 53 | 24 | |
| | | | | 56 | 53 | 24 | |
| | | | | 60 | 53 | 24 | |
| | | | | 64 | 53 | 24 | |
| | | | | 68 | 53 | 24 | |

| S. No. | Trade Name & Company | Composi-tion | Indications | Dosage / Administration |
|---|---|---|---|---|
| | | | | **IN FEED MEDICATION:**<br>**Prevention:**<br>250 g / tonne of feed for 2 days at interval of 3-4 weeks<br>**Treatment:**<br>500 g / tonne of feed for 3-5 days |
| 13 | TONATE 100% (Vetnex) | Tylosin tartrate 100 g powder has 98% activity | Prevention, control and treatment of mycoplasmal infections | **Treatment:**<br>1 g / litre of water |
| 14 | TOZIDEX PREMIX (Vetnex) | Tylosin phosphate 10% | Prevention, control and treatment of mycoplasmal infections | 250 to 500 g / tonne of feed |
| 15 | TROX SOLUBLE POWDER (Virbac) | Tylosin tartrate 50% w/w | For prevention and treatment of chronic respiratory disease (CRD) in poultry | *(see tables below)* |

**For Prevention: Commercial Broilers (1000 birds)**

| Age in days | Dosage |
|---|---|
| 1-3 days | 10 g daily |
| 22-26th day (1 day) | 90 g |

**Commercial Layers (1000 birds)**

| Age in days/weeks | Dosage |
|---|---|
| 1-3 days | 10 g daily |
| 26th day | 50 g |
| 70th day (10th week) | 150 g |
| 125th day (18th week) | 240 g |

**Broiler Breeders (1000 birds)**

| Age in days/weeks | Dosage |
|---|---|
| 4th, 5th, 6th, and 7th day | 14 g / day |
| 13th and 14th day | 14 g / day |
| 20th and 21st day | 70 g / day |
| 26th and 27th day | 90 g / day |
| 34th and 35th day | 110 g / day |
| 64th day (9th week) | 190 g / day |
| 85th day (12th week) | 250 g / day |
| 140th day (20th week) | 330 g / day |

| S. No. | Trade Name & Company | Composi-tion | Indications | Dosage / Administration |
|---|---|---|---|---|

| | | | | **Layer Breeders (1000 birds)** | | | | |
|---|---|---|---|---|

| Age in days/weeks | Dosage |
|---|---|
| $4^{th}$, $5^{th}$, $6^{th}$, and $7^{th}$ day | 12 g / day |
| $13^{th}$ and $14^{th}$ day | 25 g/day |
| $20^{th}$ and $21^{st\ day}$ | 50 g / day |
| $26^{th}$ and $27^{th\ day}$ | 66 g / day |
| $34^{th}$ and $35^{th\ day}$ | 82 g / day |
| $64^{th}$ day ($9^{th}$ week) | 100 g / day |
| $85^{th}$ day ($12^{th}$ week) | 200 g / day |
| $140^{th\ day}$ ($20^{th}$ week) | 290 g / day |

**For treatment 1g / litre of drinking water**

---

**16 — TROX-P (Virbac)**

Composition: Tylosin phosphate 10% w/w

Indications:
* A healthy starting feed supplement for day old chicks
* Increases weight gain
* Improves feed efficiency
* Maintains optimum egg production
* Improves hatchability

Dosage / Administration:

**For Commercial Broilers:**
Mix 200-250 g / tonne of feed from day one to marketing

**For Commercial Layers:**
*Mix 500g / tonne of feed from point of lay to $42^{nd}$ week.
*Mix 200-250 g / tonne of feed from $43^{rd}$ week to culling

**Breeders:**
500g / tonne of finished feed from point of lay to culling

---

**17 — TYLAN SOLUBLE POWDER (Indo Biocare)**

Composition: Each g contains: Tylosin as tartrate activity 100%

Indications: For rapid, powerful and cost-effective chronic respiratory disease (CRD) control

Dosage / Administration:

| Age | Broilers | Layers | Broiler breeders | Layerr breeders |
|---|---|---|---|---|
| 0-3 days | 5 | 5 | 7 | 7 |
| 13,14 days | - | - | 20.5 | 12.5 |
| 20,21/22 days | 45 | 25 | | |
| | (one day) | (one day) | 35.5 | 25 |
| 26,27 days | - | - | 45 | 33 |
| 34,35 days | - | - | 55 | 41 |
| $9^{th}$ week (0ne day) | - | 73 | 95 | 50 |

| S. No. | Trade Name & Company | Composi-tion | Indications | Dosage / Administration | | | | |
|---|---|---|---|---|---|---|---|---|
| | | | | 12th week (One day) | - | _ | 125 | 100 |
| | | | | 16 th week (One day) | - | 120 | 165 | 145 |
| 18 | TYLAN PREMIX POWDER (Indo Bio care) | Each kg contains Tylosin phosphate 100 g activity | * For superior feed efficiency <br> * For increased egg production <br> * For superior chick, egg quality <br> * For increased hatchability <br> * Prevents vertical transmission | **Broilers:** 200g / tonne of feed from day 1st to 42nd day <br> **Layers:** 500 g / tonne of feed from point of lay to 42nd week. 200g / tonne of feed from 43rd week to culling <br> **Breeders:** 500g / tonne of feed from point of lay to culling | | | | |
| 19 | TYLOMIX PREMIX (Venky's) | Each Kg contains : Tylosin as tylosin phosphate 100 g, carrier q.s. | * Better performance <br> * More quality eggs <br> * Better hatchability | 20th -40th – week 500 g / tonne of feed 41st-72nd week – 200 g / tonne of feed If hen house production is more than 285 eggs per day, use 200 g / tonne of feed from 20th- 72nd weeks <br> **Broilers:** 50 g / tonne of feed | | | | |
| 20 | TYLOMIX PLUS (Venky's) | Tylosin 25% | * Better performance <br> * More quality eggs <br> * Better hatchability | 20th -40th – week 200 g / tonne of feed 41st-72nd week – 80 g / tonne of feed If hen house production is more than 285 eggs per day, use 80 g / tonne of feed | | | | |
| 21 | TYLOTON (Neospark) | Each 100 g contains tylosin tartrate IP (Vet) equivalent to 50 g of tylosin base activity | For prevention and treatment of chronic respiratory disease (CRD) in broilers and replacement pullets | **Dosage through drinking water:** Dosage schedule for CRD prevention programme. Dosage recommended is at the rate of 110 mg tylosin per kg body weight. For details of schedule for broilers, layers and breeders, see the company's literature | | | | |
| 22 | TYLOMAX – FS (Neospark) | Each Kg contains tylosin | * Control of mycoplasma load in poultry | **Broilers:** 20 ppm (200 g / tonne of feed) from day 1 to day 45 | | | | |

| S. No. | Trade Name & Company | Composi-tion | Indications | Dosage / Administration |
|---|---|---|---|---|
| | | phosphate 100 g activity | * Increases rate of weight gain and feed efficiency<br>* In layers increases egg production and quality<br>* In breeders increases egg production, feed efficiency and hatchability | **Layers:**<br>50 ppm (500 g / tonne of finished feed ) from point of lay to 42$^{nd}$ week<br>20 ppm (200 g / per tonne of finished feed) from 43$^{rd}$ week to culling<br>**Breeders:**<br>50 ppm (500 g / tonne of finished feed) from point of lay to culling |
| 23 | TYLOVET 10% Granular Premix (Intervet) | Each 100 g contains: Tylosin phosphate equivalent to tylosin base 10 g. Excipients up to 100 g | For prevention and treatment of mycoplasmosis, and for increasing performance in chickens | *For treatment of CRD in chickens 10 Kg / tonne in feed for 3 to 7 days<br>*In stress conditions (vaccination, transporting, overcrowding, re-housing) 5 kg daily in the course of 5-10 days<br>*For increasing weight gain and improving feed efficiency 40 to 500 g / tonne of feed continuously |
| 24 | TYSIN-50 INJ (Vetindia) | Each ml contains : Tylosin – 50 mg | Particularly effective in treatment and prevention of chronic respiratory disease (CRD) and infectious sinusitis | 30 ml vial – 120 birds of below 12 weeks age for 3 days<br>30 ml vial – 90 birds of above 12 weeks age for 3 days |
| 25 | WINMYCO PREMIX (Sarabhai Zydus) | Tylosin phosphate 10% granules | * Prevention, control and treatment of mycoplasma, CRD and necrotic enteritis<br>* Improves hatchability & chick quality | **Broilers:**<br>200g / tonne of feed<br>**Layers:**<br>500 g / tonne of feed from point of lay to 42$^{nd}$ week<br>200g / tonne of feed during other periods<br>**Breeders**<br>500 g / tonne of feed |

# 11. ANTIOXIDANTS

| S.No. | Trade Name & Company | Composition | Indications | Dosage/ Administration |
|---|---|---|---|---|
| 1 | ANTIQUIN (Vetnex) | Ethoxyquin, mono and diglycerides of alimentary fatty acids, citric acid, ortho-phosphoric acid and natural silicates | * As a feedstuff protector when feed is stored for long duration(light, temperature, moisture) <br> * As a protector of animal meals (fish meal, MBM, etc.) <br> * As a fat stabilizer <br> * As a protector of vitamins (A ,D3, E), especially when they are added to mineral-vitamin premixes | 125-200 g / tonne of feed |
| 2 | BANOX – E POWDER (Alltech Inc) | BHA (butylated hydroxyanisole), BHT (butylated hydroxyl-toluene), ethoxyquin, PG (propyl gallate), and citric acid | * Broad-spectrum antioxidant to protect oxidation of fats and oils under various situations <br> * It can be applied to animal fats, vegetable oils, essential oils and flavours and also protein meals <br> * To enhance the shelf life of feed | **In Feed:** <br> **Feed stored below 15 days:** 75 g / tonne of feed. Feed through batch premix. <br> **Feed stored up to 30 days:** 100 g / tonne of feed through batch premix <br> **Feed stored beyond 30 days:** 115 g / tonne. Feed through batch premix |
| 3 | FEEDOX DRY (Fort Dodge) | It contains BHA (butylhydroxyanisole) (E-320), Ethoxyquin (E-324), Citric acid (E-330), Ortho-phosphoric acid (E-338), Emulsifiers | For protection of oxidation-sensitive feed ingredients, premixes, concentrates, and finished feeds | 100-250 g / tonne of finished feed |
| 4 | NUTRI GUARD Powder and Liquid (Harshvardhan's | Butylated hydroxyanisole, Butylated | * Protects premixes, concentrates and feeds against | **Finished Feeds (Powder):** <br> 125 g/ tonne |

| S.No. | Trade Name & Company | Composition | Indications | Dosage/ Administration |
|---|---|---|---|---|
| | Lab) | hydroxytoluene, ethoxyquin, lecithin, chelators, sequestrants, surfactants, carrier: Coated fine minerals in powder and vegetable oil in liquid | autoxidation<br>* Prevents rancidity and spoilage<br>* Prevents vitamin losses<br>* Protects unsaturated fatty acids<br>* Helps maintaining immunity<br>* Liquid protects fats and oils against autoxidation | **Premixes and Concentrates:** Incorporate required quantity to obtain 125 g / tonne of finished feeds **For Liquid: Fats and oils** 250 g /tonne. **Fish** – 500 g/tonne, **Meat and Bone** – 1 Kg/tonne |
| 5 | OXIFIN (Venky's) | Composition not given. A solution for feed oxidation | * Protects vitamins and pigments and improves shelf-life of feeds<br>* Prevents rancidity and off odours<br>* Retains palatability and feed freshness<br>* Suitable for protecting animal feeds and vitamin premixes | **Normal feed:** 125-250 g / tonne of feed **Feed premixes:** 250 – 500 g / tonne of feed **Oils and fats:** 125 to 500 g per 1000 litres |
| 6 | OXINEX – FS (Neospark) | Tertiary butyl-hydroquinone (TBHQ), butylated hydroxyanisole (BHT), butylated hydroxytoluene (BHT), ethoxyquin and citric acid | * Prevents free radical formation in the feed<br>* Absorbs any free radicals that are formed and prevents propagation<br>* Increases feed efficiency | 90-125 g / tonne of feed |
| 7 | OXISTAT (APC Nutrients) | Antioxidant containing Butylated hydroxyanisole (BHA) and Butylated hydroxytoluene (BHT) in combination with the synergistic benefits of BHT and Ethoxyquin | For prevention of rancidity in the feed | a) Long-term protection in animal feed 125 ppm b) Feather meal and meat meal 225 ppm c) In fats, oils and fish meal 800-1600 ppm |

| S.No. | Trade Name & Company | Composition | Indications | Dosage/ Administration |
|---|---|---|---|---|
| 8 | PROVIGAURD (Vetcare) | A synthetic blend of Ethoxiquin, Butylated hydroxyanisole (BHA), Citric acid and Phosphoric acid at the required levels | A synthetic blend of antioxidants and metal chelators designed to prevent oxidation of feed ingredients, premixes, and complete feed | 75 g / tonne of feed |
| 9 | VITASOL – E (Qualitat) | Each ml contains Vit E 60 mg | As a biological antioxidant to help maintain reproduction capability Useful in encephalomalacia, exudative diathesis, muscular dystrophy, lowered hatchability, abnormal embryonic development and enlarged hocks | **Chicks:** 2. 5 ml / 100 birds **Layers:** 5 ml / 100 birds |

## 12. ANTI-STRESS DRUGS

| S.No. | Trade Name & Company | Composition | Indications | Dosage / Administration |
|---|---|---|---|---|
| 1 | AUREOMYCIN NUTRITIONAL FORMULA (ANF) (Fort Dodge) | Aureomycin (chlortetracycline hydrochloride), 9 essential vitamins, sucrose, essential electrolytes | Supportive therapy in all stress conditions such as transportation, vaccination, change of temperature, debeaking, deworming, peak egg production, dehydration, overcrowding, change of house etc for chicks, broilers, laying and breeding hens | **Layers / Broilers:** 1 Kg / tonne of feed or 1 g / litre of water |
| 2 | BIOMARK LIT (Exotic Mushrooms) | Each 1 Kg contains: *Azadiraehta indica, Tinospora cordifotia,* Mannan-oligosaccharide (MOS) | *Liver tonic<br>*Immunity builder<br>*Toxin binder | 500 – 1 Kg / tonne of feed |
| 3 | BPF (Biovet Poultry Formula) (Wockhardt) | Each Kg contains: Vit A 26, 43,200 IU, Vit D3 4, 00,000 IU, Vit E 1111 IU, Vit C 5, 00,000 IU, Vit K3 1.104 g, Riboflavin 2.864, Niacin 13.52 g, Calcium pantothenate 4.408 g, Pyridoxine 552 mg, Cyanocobalamin 2.20 mg, Methyl sulphonyl methane 10 g, Non-vitamin A carotenoids 2 g, Dextran oligosaccharides 2 g, *Lactobacillus acidophilus* $50 \times 10^9$ cells, *Saccharomyces boulardii* $10 \times 10^9$ cells | *Prevents early chick mortality<br>*Stimulates immunity<br>*Useful in stress conditions<br>*Protects birds from pathogenic organisms<br>*Improves carcass grades | 1 g / litre of water |

| S.No. | Trade Name & Company | Composition | Indications | Dosage / Administration |
|---|---|---|---|---|
| | | Sodium sulphate 88.08 g, Potassium chloride 88.08 g, Carrier q.s. | | |
| 4 | GERIFORTE LIQUID (Himalaya) | A herbal preparation | * Maintains glucose homeostasis<br>* Helps increase threshold levels of stress<br>* Enhances immunity<br>* Helps fight infectious conditions<br>* Prevents accumulation of free radicals | **Per 100 birds:**<br>**Chicks:**<br>2.5 ml/day<br>**Growers:**<br>5ml/day<br>**Broilers/Layers:**<br>10 ml/day<br>**Breeders:**<br>20 ml / day |
| 5 | FIBOSEL (Venky's) | Fibosel is a cell fraction of baker's yeast strain *Saccharomyces cerevisiae* with specific beta-glucan content | * Improves immune status of the bird<br>* Better body resistance<br>* Improves feed intake<br>* Increases rate of gain<br>* Improves egg production<br>* Better hatchability | **Broilers / Layers / Breeders:**<br>50-100 g / tonne of feed |
| 6 | HERBAL STRESS FORMULA (HSF) LIQUID (Alembic) | Liquid herbal stress formula | * For all kinds of stress, especially in stress due to debeaking, vaccination, deworming, overcrowding, shifting, change in feed, peak laying and disease outbreak<br>* To reduce early chick mortality | **Chicks:**<br>5 ml / 100 birds /day<br>**Growers:**<br>7.5 ml / 100 birds / day<br>**Broilers / Layers:**<br>10 ml / 100 birds / day with drinking water to be given two days before and 5 days after the stress period |
| 7 | IMMUPLUS (Indian Herbs) | Extract of selective natural herbs in a powder form | * Maintains immune status in immuno- | **For 1000 birds:**<br>**Broilers:**<br>0-4 weeks 7.5 g |

| S.No. | Trade Name & Company | Composition | Indications | Dosage / Administration |
|---|---|---|---|---|
| | | | compromized birds<br>* Improves host defence system<br>* Increases vaccinal response<br>* Enhances microbicidal activity in neutrophils<br>* Enhances levels of immunoglobulins<br>* Potentiates macrophages and phagocytosis | 5 weeks onwards 15 g<br>**Layers:**<br>0-10 weeks. 7.5 g<br>5 weeks onward 15 g<br>More than 18 weeks, administer @ 7.5 mg / Kg body weight / day<br>Advised once daily morning in drinking water or feed for 10 days.<br>**For breeders follow the same guidelines** |
| 8 | IMMUPLUS – AFS (Indian Herbs)<br><br>Premix Powder and Water-soluble concentrate powder | A herbal feed supplement | * To optimize cellular and humoral immunity<br>* To maintain strong body defences and optimum immune functions<br>* For smooth transfer of optimum maternal immunity<br>* For optimum response to vaccination programmes<br>* For nutritional support | **For Premix:**<br>500 g / tonne of feed<br>**For Water-Soluble Powder** with drinking water for 1000 birds per day<br>**Broilers:** 1-4 weeks 5 g, 5$^{th}$ week and onward 10 g<br>**Layers:** 1-20 weeks 5 g, 21$^{st}$ week onward 10 g<br>To be given regularly, or at least for 10 days every month |
| 9 | IMMUVED (Wockhardt) | Biologically potentiated herbal extract | * Improves immune response<br>* Minimizes stress conditions<br>* Enhances vaccine performance | *25 ml/ 1000 birds for regular use<br>*50 ml/1000 birds for 3 days before and after vaccination. |

| S.No. | Trade Name & Company | Composition | Indications | Dosage / Administration |
|---|---|---|---|---|
| | | | * Improves production and productivity | |
| 10 | M. D. CARE (Vetmed) | Each 10 ml contains: Aqueous extract of: *Tinospora cordifolia* 600 mg, Gokshura 600 mg, Amalakki 600 mg, Vidanga 100 mg, *Salanum indicum* 60 mg | * Stimulates immunity<br>* Prevents stress<br>* Induces resistance to diseases<br>* Provides protection against free radicals | **Chicks:** 10 ml / 100 birds<br>**Layers:** 15-20 ml / 100 birds<br>**Breeders:** 20-30 ml /100 birds |
| 11 | MYCOSAL NUTRITIONAL FORMULA POWDER (Golden Streak) | Each 125 g contains : Mycosal (Zinc 1%, Enrofloxacin 10% and Pefloxacin 30%) 3 g, Vit C 450 mg, Vit A 4,00,000 IU, $D_3$ 40000 IU, E 150 IU, $B_6$ 75 mg, $K_3$ 140 mg, Niacin 1750 mg, Calcium pantothenate 575 mg, $B_2$ 75 mg, $B_{12}$ 275 mcg, Sodium sulphate anhydrous 12 g, Potassium chloride 12 g and Sugar q.s. | Over heating (Summer stress), dehydration, starvation, debeaking, vaccination, peak laying, drop in egg production, chilling, nutritional deficiencies, overcrowding, poor feeding, changes of house etc<br>**In Breeders:** For improving fertility and hatchability, besides egg production | **Chicks :** 1 g / litre of water for 1-2 weeks<br>**Laying hens:** 1 g / litre of water or 1260 g / tonne of feed for first 4-6 weeks of egg production |
| 12 | STI – IMMU (Natural Remedies) | Herbal preparation | * As a supportive with vaccines. Sti-immu minimizes vaccine failure<br>* To incorporate in antibiotic free feed<br>* Triggers cell-mediated immunity against conditions for which vaccines are not available | **Broilers / Layers / Breeders:** 250-500g / tonne of feed from day 1 till marketing |
| 13 | STRESS –CHECK (Indian Herbs) | Herbal anti-stress performance enhancer | * To help the bird easily adapt to | **Broilers:** 0-2 weeks – 2.5 ml |

| S.No. | Trade Name & Company | Composition | Indications | Dosage / Administration |
|---|---|---|---|---|
| | | | environmental changes, temperature extremes, and other stress conditions<br>* Maintains immune status and body's antioxidant profile at optimum levels<br>* Maintains optimum growth, FCR, under stress conditions due to heat or cold, debeaking, transportation, high stocking densities | / 100 birds<br>3-4 weeks – 5 ml / 100 birds<br>5th week and onwards – 10 ml / 100 birds<br>**Layer Chicks:** 2.5 ml / 100 birds;<br>**Growers:** 5 ml / 100 birds;<br>**Layers:** 10 ml / 100 birds<br>**Broiler breeders:** 20 ml / 100 birds<br>**Feed inclusion:** 250 g / tonne of feed |
| 14 | STRESSROAK (Ayurvet) | Herbal anti-stress adaptogen and performance enhancer | * To counteract stress due to vaccination, debeaking, disease outbreak, deworming, peak laying, shifting, change of feed, overcrowding, and similar stress conditions<br>* To counteract heat stress<br>* For reducing early chick mortality<br>* For increasing body resistance<br>* For optimum feed utilization, growth and productivity | **Liquid**<br>**Chicks:**<br>5 ml/100 birds/day<br>**Growers:**<br>7.5 ml /100 birds/ day<br>**Layers/Broilers/ Finishers:**<br>10 ml/100 birds/ day<br>**Breeders:**<br>20 ml/100 birds / day<br>**Premix:**<br>1 Kg / tonne of feed |
| 15 | STRESSBAN POWDER (Zeus Intervetcare) | Botanical extracts, Probiotics, Dextrose base | * Stimulates immune response<br>* Prevents stress<br>* Eliminates proliferation of harmful bacteria like *E. coli* and | **Broilers:**<br>0-4 weeks – 5 g / 1000 birds<br>5th week and onwards – 10 g / 1000 birds<br>**Layers:** |

| S.No. | Trade Name & Company | Composition | Indications | Dosage / Administration |
|---|---|---|---|---|
| | | | salmonella<br>* Helps to obtain optimum and sustained egg production | 0-20 weeks – 5 g / 1000 birds<br>21$^{st}$ week and onwards – 10 g / 1000 birds to be given once daily in water for 10 days or more |
| 16 | STRESSEAZE (Indian Herbs) | Herbal anti-stress adaptogen and antioxidant | * Stress management<br>* For adaptability of the body against stress<br>* To be used for its antioxidant action | **Broilers:**<br>0-4 weeks – 5 g / 1000 birds<br>5$^{th}$ week and onwards – 10 g / 1000 birds<br>**Layers:**<br>0-20 weeks – 5 g / 1000 birds<br>21$^{st}$ week and onwards – 10 g / 1000 birds to be given once daily in water for 10 days or more |
| 17 | SUPERMUNE (Sarabhai Zydus) | Potent immune-booster feed supplement of organic selenium, vitamin E and immuno-stimulant herbs | To improve immune response and vaccine performance<br>To improve overall body resistance<br>To reduce the effect and spread of viruses during outbreaks<br>To improve production and reproduction performance<br>To prevent deficiency diseases | 100 – 150 g / tonne of feed |
| 18 | VITARON | A herbal preparation: | *Prevents stress like | **Chicks:** |

| S.No. | Trade Name & Company | Composition | Indications | Dosage / Administration |
|---|---|---|---|---|
| | (Natural Herbs) | Stress reliever, Immunity booster, Growth promoter | extreme heat or cold, vaccination, debeaking, transportation, overcrowding and stress due to high production and faster growth etc<br>* Maintains feed intake and improves FCR, enhancing growth in broilers and egg production in layers. | 5-10ml / 100 birds<br>**Growers:**<br>20-25ml / 100 birds<br>**Broilers / layers:**<br>30-40 ml /100 birds |
| 19 | ZERO-STRESS (Harshvardhan's Lab) | A proprietary blend of Vit C, and iodine in natriam treated granular sucrose base | * Reduces all kinds of stresses<br>* Provides instant energy and refreshes the birds<br>* Improves liver and kidney functions<br>* Enhances immune response | **Chick arrival:**<br>25-50 g / litre of water for 12 hours<br>**Before and after handling / transportation / vaccination:**<br>10-25 g / litre of water for 24 hours |
| 20 | ZIST (Junior) (Natural Remedies) | It is a combination of extract and crude drug powder | For all kinds of stress, especially stress due to sexing, vaccination, transportation, touching, debeaking, extreme weather, diseases, etc. | 250 g / tonne of feed |
| 21 | ZIST (Senior) (Natural Remedies) | It contains crude drug powder | For all kinds of stress due to extreme weather, peak production, vaccination, diseases, shifting A. I., etc. for optimizing the | 250 g / tonne of feed |

633

| S.No. | Trade Name & Company | Composition | Indications | Dosage / Administration |
|---|---|---|---|---|
| | | | overall productivity | |
| 22 | ZIST LIQUID (Natural Remedies) | Herbal poultry feed supplement | To manage the birds from stress conditions like vaccination, debeaking, touching, extreme weather conditions, transportation, demand for higher productivity etc. To maintain the immune status and thus livability | **Mixing rate:** **Under 4 weeks:** 50 ml / 1000 birds **Above 4 weeks:** 100 ml / 1000 birds **Recommended schedule:** **Broilers and Layers:** 0-10 days – 50 ml / 1000 birds 21-30 days – 100 ml / 1000 birds **Growers and Layers:** 100 ml / 1000 birds for 10 days during peak production and to manage stressful conditions **Administration:** To be given once a day through drinking water |

# 13. BIOSURFACTANT

| S.No. | Trade Name & Company | Composition | Indications | Dosage / Administration |
|---|---|---|---|---|
| 1 | LYSOFORTE DRY (Kemin) | Hydrolysed lecithins, enriched in Lysophospholipids | * Enhances absorption of nutrients from the gut<br>* Improves feed conversion ratio and bird's performance (meat, egg)<br>* Improves livability through better nutrient availability | 500-1000 g / tonne of feed |

## 14A. CALCIUM PREPARATIONS (POWDER / GRANULES)

| S.No | Trade Name & Company | Composition | Indications | Dosage / Administration |
|---|---|---|---|---|
| 1 | AYUCAL – D (Ayurvet) | Each 5 g contains : Elemental calcium 400 mg, Elemental phosphorus 200 mg, Vit D3 6000 IU, enriched with synergistic herbs | * For better growth and egg production <br> * For better carcass and eggshell quality <br> * Ensures better bio-availability of calcium and phosphorus <br> * Prevents disorders related to deficiency of calcium and phosphorus <br> * Improves productivity | **Broilers :** 1 Kg / tonne of feed <br> **Layers and Breeders (per 100 birds):** <br> **Chicks:** 5 g <br> **Growers:** 10 g <br> **Layers:** 15 g <br> **Breeders at lay:** 30 g <br> for 7-10 days |
| 2 | CAL C CARE POWDER (Varsha) | Phytase, Calcium, Phosphorus, Vit $D_3$ in a base enriched with minerals | Phosphorus supplement for better utilization of calcium | 500 g – 1 Kg / tonne of feed |
| 3 | CALCIROYAL SOLUBLE POWDER (Concept) | Each 5 g contains : Elemental calcium 174 mg, Elemental phosphorus 50 mg, Vit $B_{12}$ 50 mcg, Vit C 30 mg, Vit $D_3$ 1000 IU, Citric acid 1g | * Ensures complete absorption of calcium and phosphorus <br> * Improves weight gain and FCR <br> * Improves egg production, hatchability and shell quality <br> * Reduces egg breakages <br> * Prevents leg weakness and *E. coli* infection <br> * Maintains peak production for longer time | **In drinking water for 5-7 days** <br> **Chicks :** 5 g / 100 birds <br> **Broilers / Growers :** 7.5 g / 100 birds <br> **Layers :** 10 g / 100 birds. <br> **Feed mix** – 250 g / tonne of feed for 5-7 days |
| 4 | CAL-V-MIX POWDER (Charak) | Each g contains : Tribasic calcium phosphate 500 mg, Vit $D_3$ 800 IU, Vit $B_{12}$ 10 mcg, Live yeast culture 500 million units | * Leg weakness, fatigue stress, prolapse, leathery eggs, for better FCR, weight gain, eggshell quality and egg production | 200 g / 100 birds daily or 200 g / tonne of feed |

| S.No | Trade Name & Company | Composition | Indications | Dosage / Administration |
|---|---|---|---|---|
| 5 | HI-CAL P GRANULES (Hitha) | Each 7.5 g contains : Calcium 1600 mg, Phosphorus 800 mg, Magnesium 1.344 mg | * For calcium and phosphorus supplementation in 2:1 ratio<br>* Prevents formation of thin-shelled eggs<br>* Strengthens bones, prevents leg weakness and lameness<br>* For better productivity, better growth and faster weight gains in broilers<br>* Magnesium helps in better absorption of calcium and phosphorus | 500-750 g / tonne of feed |
| 6 | INNOCAL (Natural Remedies) | Clear calcium and phosphorus liquid with superior bio-availability | * To overcome calcium and phosphorus deficiency<br>* To regularize calcium and phosphorus supplementation during high demand period in layers and broilers<br>* For better eggshell strength<br>* To regularize growth, weight gain, egg production and egg size | **Chicks and broilers:** 10 ml daily / 100 birds<br>**Growers:** 25 ml daily / 100 birds<br>**Layers:** 50 ml daily / 100 birds |
| 7 | KALZOL D$_3$ POWDER (Virbac) | Each 5 g contains : Calcium 1250 mg, Phosphorus 625 mg, Magnesium 1.05 mg, Vit D$_3$ 2500 IU | * For thick-shelled eggs<br>* For strong bones<br>* For better productivity<br>* For better growth<br>* For better FCR | 1 Kg / tonne of feed for 10 days every month |
| 8 | MAGACAL (Indian Herbs) | Herbal calcium tonic | * For optimum bio-availability of calcium, phosphorus and magnesium | 1 Kg / tonne of feed for at least 10 days in a month |

| S.No | Trade Name & Company | Composition | Indications | Dosage / Administration |
|------|---------------------|-------------|-------------|------------------------|
| | | | * Helps to increase the shell thickness <br> * Improves hatchability | |
| 9 | OSSOPAN GRANULES (TTK) | Each g contains : Calcium 165 mg, Phosphorus 75 mg | Osteomalacia, retarded growth, poor eggshell quality | **Chicks:** 5 g / 100 birds <br> **Growers:** 10 g / 100 birds <br> **Layers:** 15 g /100 birds |
| 10 | OSTOPHOS-FS GRANULES (Neospark) | Each 5 g contains : Calcium 165 mg, Phosphorus 75 mg, Microcrystalline appattite complex providing bone extract of young animals 1 g (5 g of dry extract of bone derived from 32.5 g of fresh bone) | * To overcome calcium and phosphorus deficiency problems like thin-shelled eggs, leathery eggs, falling of feathers etc <br> * For better growth, and to maintain optimum egg production <br> * To stimulate growth and promote weight gain in broilers | 500 – 1 Kg / tonne of feed |
| 11 | ULTRAPHOS-D$_3$ (Neospark) | Each 5 Kg contains : Calcium 1080 g, Phosphorus 780 g, Vit D$_3$ 6 Lac IU, Vit B$_{12}$ 4000 mcg, Zinc 52000 mg, Manganese 54000 mg | * Improves eggshell quality <br> * Reduces thin-shelled and broken eggs <br> * Overcomes cage fatigue <br> * Reduces prolapse of the uterus <br> * Prevents perosis <br> * Improves plumage <br> * Stops falling of feathers <br> * Helps in achieving strong bones in broilers <br> * Improves egg production and profitability <br> * Improves hatchability <br> * Prevents pecking and cannibalism | 2.5 - 5 Kg / tonne of feed |

# 14B. CALCIUM PREPARATIONS (LIQUID)

| S. No. | Trade Name & Company | Composition | Indications | Dosage / Administration |
|---|---|---|---|---|
| 1 | AQUA-CAL-PHOS-D LIQUID (Harshvardhan's Lab) | Each 20 ml contains : Calcium 400 mg, Phosphorus 200 mg, Vit $D_3$ 1600 IU, Vit $B_{12}$ 20 mcg | * To provide high concentration of calcium and phosphorus in ionic form<br>* To enhance growth, weight gain and egg production<br>* To reduce leg weakness, broken eggs, prolapse and cage layer fatigue | **Chicks / Broilers:** 10 ml / 100 birds / day<br>**Growers:** 20 ml / 100 birds / day<br>**Layers / Breeders:** 50 ml / 100 / birds / day |
| 2 | CADISOL PLUS LIQUID (Sarabhai Zydus) | Calcium gluconate, Calcium D sccharate, Cholecalciferol (Vit. $D_3$), Iron, Vit $B_{12}$ 16.7 mcg | * For higher egg production<br>* For stronger eggshell<br>* For healthy and faster growth in chicks, growers and broilers<br>* For prevention of cannibalism, prolapse and cage fatigue<br>* For prevention of calcium deficiency | **Through drinking water:**<br>**Chicks:** 10 ml / 100 birds / day<br>**Growers / Broilers:** 20 ml / 100 / birds / day<br>**Layers:** 50 ml / 100 birds / day |
| 3 | CALCICARE – C LIQUID (Brihans) | Each 20 ml contains : Calcium 325.6 mg, Phosphorus – 167.7 mg, Vit $D_3$ 1800 IU, Vit $B_{12}$ 20 mcg | * Stimulates skeletal and muscular growth<br>* Helps calcification of bones and eggs<br>* Strengthens muscles and bones<br>* Builds up calcium reserve in the body | 50 – 100 ml / 100 birds in drinking water |

| S. No. | Trade Name & Company | Composition | Indications | Dosage / Administration |
|---|---|---|---|---|
| | | | * Maintains high egg production | |
| 4 | CALCIGOLD LIQUID (Golden Streak) | Each 5 ml contains : Calcium 100 mg, Phosphorus 50 mg, Vit $D_3$ 400 IU, Vit $B_{12}$ 5 mcg | * To develop strong bones, and strong eggshell <br> * To develop resistance to diseases <br> * Helps in growth, metabolism, and erythropoiesis <br> * Prevents prolapse | **Chicks / Broilers :** 20 ml / 100 birds / 5 litres of water for 7-10 days <br> **Growers:** 50 ml / 100 birds / 7 litres of water for 7-10 days <br> **Layers:** 100 ml / 100 birds / 10 litres of water for 7-10 days |
| 5 | CALCIGUARD LIQUID / GRANULES (Vetguard) | Each 5 ml / 5 g contains : Calcium 100 mg, Phosphorus 50 mg, Vit $D_3$ 400 IU, Vit $B_{12}$ 5 mcg, Soyahydrolysate 75 mg | To improve egg quality, production, prevention of egg breakage, rickets, osteomalacia | 20-100 ml / 100 birds or 500 g / tonne of feed |
| 6 | CALDIVET $B_{12}$ LIQUID (Vetnex) | Each ml contains : Calcium lactate 250 mg, Calcium gluconate 200 mg, Vit $D_3$ 500 IU, Vit $B_{12}$ 10 mg and Choline chloride 200 mg | Stunted growth, osteomalacia, rickets, anaemia, cannibalism, thin-shelled eggs, drop in egg production, fatty liver syndrome, aflatoxicosis, and related disorders of musculoskeletal system | **Per 100 birds / day for one week:** **Chicks:** 10-12 ml **Growers:** 15 – 20 ml **Layers:** 50-100 ml |
| 7 | CASPHODIL LIQUID (Lyka Labs) | Each 5 ml provides : Calcium 100 mg, Phosphorus 50 mg, Vit $D_3$ 400 IU, Vit $B_{12}$ 5 mcg, Protein hydrolysate 75 mg | * To prevent calcium and phosphorus deficiency <br> * To prevent rickets, osteomalacia, osteoporosis and | **Through drinking water:** **Chicks / Broilers:** 20 ml / 100 birds daily **Growers:** 50 ml / 100 birds daily |

| S. No. | Trade Name & Company | Composition | Indications | Dosage / Administration |
|---|---|---|---|---|
| | | | cracking of eggs | **Layers / Breeders:** 100 ml / 100 birds daily |
| 8 | CLEARCAL LIQUID (Charak) | Each 10 ml contains : Calcium 200 mg, Phosphorus 100 mg, Vit $D_3$ 800 IU, Vit $B_{12}$ 10 mcg, Osseous tissue protein 200 mg | * Provides high concentration of phosphorus in ionic form, for improved absorption and better assimilation<br>* Enhances growth, weight gain, egg production and egg size<br>* Reduces broken eggs, leathery eggs | **Chicks / Broilers:** 20 ml / 100 birds daily<br>**Growers:** 50 ml / 100 birds / daily<br>**Layers:** 60 ml / 100 birds daily |
| 9 | DICAL LIQUID (Elpe) | Each 5 ml contains : Calcium gluconate 500 mg, Vit $D_3$ 600 IU, Vit $B_{12}$ 10 mcg, Liver extract 50 mg, Ferric ammonium citrate 50 mg | * Hypocalcaemia<br>* Reduced growth<br>* Poor feed conversion<br>* Leg-weakness<br>* Soft eggshell<br>* Osteomalacial conditions<br>* Poor hatching results<br>* Anaemic conditions | **Chicks:** 10 ml / 100 birds<br>**Growers / Broilers:** 20 ml / 100 birds<br>**Layers:** 0-50 ml / 100 birds |
| 10 | HI-CAL-D LIQUID (Hitha) | Each 5 ml contains : Calcium 100 mg, Phosphorus 50 mg, Vit $D_3$ 400 IU, Vit $B_{12}$ 5 mcg | * To provide calcium and phosphorus in the ratio of 2:1<br>* For strengthening of bones and eggshells<br>* Better egg production | **Chicks / Broilers:** 20 ml / 100 birds / day<br>**Growers:** 50 ml / 100 birds / day<br>**Layers:** 100 ml / 100 birds / day |
| 11 | NUTRICAL LIQUID FEED SUPPLEMENT (Pfizer) | Each 5 ml contains : Elemental calcium 100 mg, Elemental phosphorus 50 mg, | * For calcium and phosphorus supplementation<br>* For better skeletal growth | **Chicks / Broilers:** 20 ml / 100 birds / day<br>**Growers:** 50 ml / 100 birds / |

| S. No. | Trade Name & Company | Composition | Indications | Dosage / Administration |
|---|---|---|---|---|
| | | Vit $D_3$ 400 IU, Vit $B_{12}$ 5 mcg | * For more eggs with thicker shells <br> * For reducing incidence of cage- layer fatigue and leg-weakness syndrome | day <br> **Layers:** <br> 100 ml / 100 birds / day |
| 12 | OSTEOCALPHOS LIQUID (Harshvardhan's Lab) | Each 20 ml contains : Calcium 325.6 mg, Phosphorus 167.7 mg, Vit $D_3$ 1600 IU, Vit $B_{12}$ 20 mcg | * It helps in maintaining stronger bones <br> * It gives strength to eggshell | 10-100 ml / 100 birds daily |
| 13 | OSTOPHOS-FS LIQUID (Neospark) | Each 5 ml contains : Calcium 104 mg, Phosphorus 52 mg, Vit $D_3$ 500 IU, Vit $B_{12}$ 7.5 mcg, Predigested protein 75 mg, Elemental iron 15 mg | * Provides calcium and phosphorus in right proportion <br> * Provides higher concentrations of Vit $D_3$, and Vit $B_{12}$ <br> * Ensures complete absorption and higher bio-availability of calcium | **Through drinking water:** <br> **Chicks / Broilers:** <br> 20 ml /100 birds / 5 litres of water daily <br> **Growers:** <br> 50 ml / 100 birds / 7 litres of water daily <br> **Layers:** <br> 100 ml / 100 birds / 10 litres of water daily |
| 14 | RALCAL-DS SOLUTION (Rallis) | Each 50 ml contains : Calcium 1628 mg, Phosphorus 898.5 mg, Vit $D_3$ 8000 IU, Vit $B_{12}$ 100 mcg, Copper 8.67 mg, Cobalt 1.25 mg, Iron 27.78 mg, Zinc 59.25 mg, Chromium 0.46 mg, Selenium 22.5 mg, Manganese 33.25 mg, Magnesium 58.39 mg | A balanced nutritional supplement | 10-30 ml / 100 birds |
| 15 | RAVICAL SUSP. | **Each 20 ml contains :** | To improve growth rate, | 20-60 ml / 100 birds |

| S. No. | Trade Name & Company | Composition | Indications | Dosage / Administration |
|---|---|---|---|---|
| | (Guybro) **SOLN.** | Calcium 325.6 mg, Phosphorus 167.7 mg, Vit $D_3$ 1600 IU, Vit $B_{12}$ 20 mcg **Each 20 ml contains :** Calcium 400 mg, Phosphorus 220 mg, Vit $D_3$ 1600 IU, Vit $B_{12}$ 20 mcg | resistance against stress, egg weight / shell weight, and to prevent cannibalism and rickets | |
| 16 | SHARKOFERROL LIQUID (Alembic) | Each 15 ml contains : Calcium gluconate 360 mg, Ferric ammonium citrate 100 mg, Cholecalciferol 400 IU, Niacinamide 45 mg, Folic acid 1.5 mg, Cyanocobalamin 15 mcg, Malt extract 4.52 g | * To improve eggshell quality <br> * To combat stress of all kinds <br> * To improve egg feed ratio <br> * To boost immunity <br> * To increase the fertility of breeders | **Broilers:** 20-60 ml / 100 birds / day **Layers:** 20-40 ml / 100 birds / day **Breeders:** 40-80 ml / 100 birds / day |
| 17 | SOLUCAL LIQUID (Venky's) | Each 5 ml contains : Calcium 100 mg, Phosphorus 50 mg, Vit $D_3$ 400 IU, Vit $B_{12}$ 5 mcg | * Helps to develop strong bones and strong eggshells <br> * Helps to develop resistance to disease <br> * Helps in metabolism and erythropoiesis <br> * Prevents prolapse | **Chicks / Broilers:** 20 ml /100 birds daily **Growers:** 50 ml / 100 birds daily **Layers:** 100 ml / 100 birds |
| 18 | TRANSCAL PLUS LIQUID (Indian Herbs) | Optimum concentration of calcium, phosphorus, vitamin D3, vitamin B12 and selected herbal extracts in an acidic medium | * For improving eggshell thickness to reduce egg breakage <br> * To increase egg production and hatchability <br> * For proper development of | **Chicks and Broilers:** 20 ml / 100 birds **Growers:** 50 ml / 100 birds **Layers (commercial / breeders):** 100 ml / 100 birds |

| S. No. | Trade Name & Company | Composition | Indications | Dosage / Administration |
|---|---|---|---|---|
| | | | broilers, layers and breeders | |
| 19 | ULTRACAL-D LIQUID (Neospark) | Each 5 ml contains : Calcium gluconate 416.5 mg, Vit $D_3$ 800 IU, Stomach extract 1.65 mg, Ferric ammonium citrate 83.5 mg, Vit $B_{12}$ 8.35 mcg, Casein protein 200 ppm, Elemental iron 13.8 mg, Cobalt 5 mg | * Prevents thin-shelled eggs and drop in egg production<br>* Prevents rickets and osteomalacia<br>* Prevents macrocytic anaemia, stunted growth and hypocalcaemia<br>* Prevents leg weakness and improves weight gains in broilers<br>* Prevents prolapse and cannibalism | **Through drinking water:** **Chicks:** 10 ml / 100 birds / day **Growers / Broilers:** 20 ml / 100 birds **Layers:** 25-50 ml / 100 birds |
| 20 | XYCAL (Qualitat) | Calcium phosphate 4.8 g, Vit D3 – 8000 IU, Vit B12 – 100 mcg | * To stimulate growth<br>* To prevent lameness in growing birds<br>* To prevent cannibalism, prolapse, thin-shelled eggs and drop in egg production<br>* To prevent cage layer fatigue | **Chicks:** 20 ml / 5 litres of water **Growers:** 50 ml / 8 litres of water **Layers:** 100 ml / 10 litres of drinking water |

# 15. DEWORMERS (ANTHELMINTICS)

| S. No. | Trade Name & Company | Composition | Indications | Dosage / Administration |
|---|---|---|---|---|
| 1 | <u>ALBENDAZOLE</u> ALBOMAR POWDER (Virbac) | Albendazole 5% w/w | For control and treatment of gastrointestinal and pulmonary nematodes, cestodes and trematodes | **Layers:** **Roundworms:** 300 g / 1000 birds **Tapeworms:** 600 g / 1000 birds **Breeders:** **Roundworms:** 600 g / 1000 birds **Tapeworms:** 1200 g / 1000 birds |
| 2 | CESTONIL VET (Vetmed) | It is an Ayurvedic herbal product | * Prevents fatty liver haemorrhagic syndrome due to tapeworm infestation <br> * Improves egg production <br> * Prevents uneven size of eggs | **Layers:** One packet for 1000 birds as feed mix **Growers:** 3/4th packet for 1000 birds as feed mix **Breeders:** Two packets for 1000 birds as feed mix |
| 3 | WORMITAL SUSPENSION (Lyka Labs) | Albendazole 2.5% w/v | For control and treatment of ascaridia, capillaria and syngamus species | 10-15 ml / 100 birds as top-dressing in feed for 3 days |
| 4 | <u>CYRAMAZINE</u> LARVANIL-FS POWDER (Neospark) | Cyramazine (Feed Grade) 1%, Inert ingredients 99% | For fly control in and around : <br> * Caged or slatted flooring layer or chicken operations <br> * Breeder chicken operations | Mix 500 g / tonne of feed |
| 5 | <u>LEVAMISOLE</u> ALMIZOL POWDER (Alembic) | Each g contains : Levamisole HCl 300 mg | * Broad-spectrum anthelmintic <br> * Active against benzimidazole resistant species | 5 g / 80-100 birds / 4 litres of drinking water 100 g / 1600-2000 birds / 80 litres of drinking water |
| 6 | GOLDISOLE POWDER | Levamisole hydrochloride 30% | For deworming | 20-25 mg / Kg body weight or |

| S. No. | Trade Name & Company | Composition | Indications | Dosage / Administration |
|---|---|---|---|---|
| | (Golden Streak) | | | **Chicks:** 5 g / 5 litres of water for 500 chicks **Layers:** 5 g / 5 litres of water for 50 layers |
| 7 | LEMASOL-P POWDER (Vetnex) | Levamisole hydrochloride 30% w/w | * For deworming * Immunostimulation | **For deworming:** 30 mg / Kg body weight **For potentiation of immunity:** 7.5-15 mg / Kg body weight |
| 8 | NEMATEX-L POWDER (Neospark) | Levamisole hydrochloride 30% w/w | For deworming | **Chicks:** 50 g / 50 litres of water for 1000 chicks **Layers:** 50 g / 50 litres of water for 500 layers |
| 9 | STALMISOL (Stallen) | Levamisole hydrochloride B.P. 30% w/v | Broad-spectrum anthelmintic with immunomodulator effect | **For deworming:** 10 g / 120 birds weighing 1 Kg or 80 birds **For immunomodulation:** 10 g / 200 – 400 birds weighing 1Kg each |
| 10 | VENTRIMISOLE POWDER (Venky's) | Levamisole HCl 30% w/w | * Effective against larval and adult stages of all roundworms * Acts as an immunostimulant | **Dewormer:** 1 g / litre of water **Immunostimulant:** 15 mg / Kg body wt. in drinking water on the day of vaccination |
| 11 | WORMAL (Micro Labs) | Levamisole HCL BP (Vet) 30% w/v in water soluble base | * Roundworm infestations in poultry * Possesses immunostimulant properties * Increases resistance to infections | 100 g / 1000 birds in drinking water |

| S. No. | Trade Name & Company | Composition | Indications | Dosage / Administration |
|---|---|---|---|---|
| 12 | MEBENDAZOLE BANIF POWDER (Brihans) | Each 5 g contains : Mebendazole 500 mg | Ascarids, Capillaria, Syngamus, Moniezia etc | **Broilers / Growers:** 5-10 g / 100 birds through water **Layers:** 10-20 g / 100 birds through water |
| 13 | LEVABEND (Qualitat) | Mebendazole 10% w/w Levamisole – 2% w/w | Effective against tapeworm infections | Given for 3 days regularly and repeated after 18 days Quantity not mentioned in booklet |
| 14 | NILMINTH (Qualitat) | Mebendazole 10% w/w | Broad-spectrum anthelmintic effective against worms – roundworms, whipworms, tapewoms | 15 g / 100 birds in a day's feed |
| 15 | ZODEX POWDER (Concept) | Each 5 g contains : Mebendazole 500 mg | * Kills roundworms and tapeworms * Effective against ova, mature and immature stages of worms | 50 mg / Kg body weight |
| 16 | PIPERAZINE BRIPAZINE (Brihans) | Each ml contains : Piperazine hydrate IP 0.45 g | In roundworms, threadworms, and hookworm infestation | 30-60 ml/100 birds through drinking water |
| 17 | HARPERAZINE (Harshvardhan's Lab) | Piperazine hexahydrate – 56.35% | Highly effective against roundworms | **Birds 4-6 weeks:** 20 – 25 ml / 100 birds in 3.5 litres of water **Birds over 6 weeks:** 40 ml /100 birds 5-9 litres of water |
| 18 | KNOCK-45 LIQUID (Sarabhai Zydus) | Each 100 ml contains : Piperazine hydrate 45 g equivalent to piperazine base 19.8 g | * Effectively eradicates large roundworms in poultry * Helps growth and development * Improves feed efficiency | **Below 6 weeks:** 100 ml / 400 birds **Above 6 weeks:** 100 ml / 200 birds |
| 19 | PIPERAZINE | Each 100 ml | Control and | **Growers:** |

| S. No. | Trade Name & Company | Composition | Indications | Dosage / Administration |
|---|---|---|---|---|
| | LIQUID (Virbac) | contains : Piperazine hydrate 45 g | treatment of gastrointestinal nematodes | 40 ml / 100 birds **Layers:** 50-75 ml / 100 birds |
| 20 | PIPERAZINE HEXAHYDRATE SOLN. (Venky's) | Piperazine hydrate 56.3% w/v | Effective against Capillaria /Ascardia worms | **4-6 weeks** – 25 ml / 100 birds **6 weeks and above-** 40 ml / 100 birds in water Repeat once in a month in drinking water |
| 21 | PIPERAZINE HYDRATE LIQUID 61%, (Neospark) | Piperazine hexahydrate 61% w/v equivalent to piperazine base 26.84 w/v | A completely safe and effective oral medication for the removal of roundworms (Ascarids) in poultry | **Below 6 weeks:** 370 ml / 2000 birds **Adult birds:** 370 ml / 1000 birds |
| 22 | PIPERAZINE HYDRATE SOLUTION 56.3% w/v (Stallen) | Each 100 ml contains : Piperazine hydrate 56.3 g, equivalent to piperazine base 25% w/v, Excipients q.s. | For removal of roundworms (*Ascaridia galli*) | **Up to 4-6 weeks:** 60 ml / 10 litres of water / 300 birds **Above 6 weeks:** 60 ml / 13 litres of water / 150 birds, i. e., 40 ml / 8-9 litres of water for 100 birds |
| 23 | PIPERAZINE HYDRATE (Fort Dodge) | Piperazine hydrate 56.3% w/v, | For removal of roundworms (*Ascaridia galli*) | **Under 6 weeks:** 20 ml / 3-5 litres of water /100 birds **Above 6 weeks:** 40 ml / 5-10 litres of water /100 birds |
| **HERBAL DEWORMER AND MISCELLANEOUS** | | | | |
| 24 | AV-CESTODE (AVR) | Herbal poultry feed supplement containing Senna extract, *Embelia ribes*, base – q.s. | * Improves fatty liver syndrome due to tapeworm infestation. * Wet dropping due to worminous infestation * Regular deworming | **Layers:** 1 Kg /2000 layers as feed mix to be given in morning feed. 1 Kg / 3000 growers as feed mix to be given in morning feed. **Breeders:** 1 Kg /1000 birds. Mix in morning feed. |
| 25 | CESTONEX-N | Each g contains : | * Tapeworm | 1g for 5 adult birds |

| S. No. | Trade Name & Company | Composition | Indications | Dosage / Administration |
|---|---|---|---|---|
| | (Neospark) | Niclosamide IP 750 mg | infestation of poultry<br>* Raillientina and Davainea | (Approx. 175 mg/kg body weight) |
| 26 | CESTONIL (Vetmed) | It is an Ayurvedic herbal product | * Prevents fatty liver haemorrhagic syndrome due to **tapeworm infestation**<br>* Improves egg production<br>* Prevents uneven size of eggs | **Layers:**<br>One packet for 1,000 birds<br>**Growers:**<br>3/4th packet for 1000 birds<br>**Breeders:**<br>Two packets for 1000 birds |

## 16. DISINFECTANTS

| S.No. | Trade Name & Company | Composition | Indications | Dosage / Administration |
|---|---|---|---|---|
| 1 | ACID – A – FOAM (Venky's) | General purpose foaming acid cleaner | * Removes biofilms<br>* Quickly removes minerals, oils, soap scum, rust, scale, lime, and alkaline deposits<br>* Odourless<br>* Useful as foam, spray or soak | **General purpose cleaning:**<br>8-24 ml / litre of water<br>**Foam cleaning:**<br>16-24 ml / litre of water<br>**Farm premise wash down:**<br>1 litre / 300 litres of wash water<br>**Descaling:**<br>50-75 ml / litre of water |
| 2 | AKTICHLOR-T (Neospark) | It contains : Sodium N-Chloroparatolune sulphonamide or Chloramine-T | A fast acting ideal disinfectant | **Routine disinfection:**<br>3 g / litre<br>**Poultry houses with birds:**<br>5 g / litre<br>**Outside vehicles, footbaths, empty poultry houses:**<br>10 g / litre<br>**Gumboro & other severe viral infections:** 50 g / litre |
| 3 | AQUAMAX (+ Descaler) (Venky's) | Benzalkonium chloride Soln 6% v/v, Citric acid, 8% w/v, Inert ingredients q.s. | * Removes scale, mineral deposits, junk and slime from water lines and cooling pads<br>* Ideal for cleaning, disinfecting and descaling nipple waterers<br>* As a general purpose disinfectant<br>* Hatchery cleaning and disinfection | **Disinfection and descaling:**<br>25-50 ml / litre of water<br>**Water acidification and sanitization:**<br>1 ml / 10 litres of water |
| 4 | AQUA PLUS – 10 (Indian Drugs and Vitamins) | Benzalkonium chloride solution 10% v/v, Citric acid 8% w/v, Acetic acid 2% v/v, Inert ingredients q.s. | Biodegradable cationic, citrated disinfectant Virucidal, bactericidal, fungicidal | **For drinking water sanitization:**<br>1 ml / 20 litres of water<br>**As a general purpose cleaner:**<br>4-8 ml/ litre of water<br>**Hatchery use:**<br>8 ml / litre of water |
| 5 | AQUAQUAT | Each 100 ml | Used for | **For drinking water** |

650

| S.No. | Trade Name & Company | Composition | Indications | Dosage / Administration |
|---|---|---|---|---|
| | [+ Water sanitizer] (Polchem) | contains : Dimethyl alkyl benzalkonium chloride 5 ml | sanitization and disinfection of water | **sanitation:** 100 ml / 1000 litres of drinking water daily **To clean drinking water system in an empty shed:** 100 ml / litre in the shed overhead tank |
| 6 | ATTAK (Venky's) | Each 100 ml contains : Benzalkonium chloride soln. 5 ml, Strong glutaraldehyde soln. 7.5 ml, Formaldehyde soln. 7.5 ml, Aqueous base q.s. | * Empty shed disinfection <br> * Farm boot bath <br> * Vehicle dips <br> * Disinfecting metal and plastic equipment <br> * Incubator and setter disinfection <br> * Disinfecting stores | **Empty sheds / Incubator tank:** 4% **Plastic equipment / Incubator/ Hatchers / Vehicle dip :** 2% **Metal equipment :** 1% **Visitor shoes :** 3% or 40 ml / litre of water |
| 7 | AVIFORM POWDER (Avians) | Polyoxymethylene 91% | * For disinfection of incubators, hatchers and poultry houses <br> * For disinfection of egg storage rooms | 1 g / sq. ft. single dose 2 g / sq. ft. double dose For control of *E .coli* 1 Kg / 5000 sq ft. |
| 8 | AVIKON S (Avians) | Salts of Peroxygen compound 50% w/w, Sodium chloride 1.5% w/w, Organic acids, Surfactants, Buffer and excipients q.s. to 100% | * Terminal virus control <br> * Cleaning and disinfecting equipment <br> * Sanitizing and disinfecting equipment <br> * Continuous water sterilization | **Terminal virus control:** Dilution 1:100; 200-300 ml / $m^2$ **Cleaning and disinfecting equipment:** Dilution 1:200 – 1:100; 300-400 ml / $m^2$ **Fogging:** Dilution 1:100; Apply 1 litre of solution / 100 $m^3$ **Aerial disinfection :** Dilution 1:200; 1 litre of solution / 100 $m^3$ of air space |
| 9 | B-904 (Venky's) | Didecyl dimethyl ammonium chloride 9.2%, Alkyl(C12-61%, C14-23%, C16- | For hatchery and farm premises disinfection | 4 ml / litre of water |

651

| S.No. | Trade Name & Company | Composition | Indications | Dosage / Administration |
|---|---|---|---|---|
| | | 11%) dimethyl benzyl ammonium chloride 9.2% Alkyl (C12-40%, C14-50%, C16-10%), dimethyl benzyl ammonium chloride 4.6%, Tri butyltin oxide 1% | | |
| 10 | BIO-BUSTER (Venky's) | Potassium monopersulphate 49.8% w/w containing triple salts – Potassium monopersulphate compound, Potassium hydrogen sulphate, Sodium chloride – 1.5 % w/w, Excipients: q.s. to 100% | * Effective against bacteria, fungi, moulds, all virus families <br> * Effective on over 20 virus families, 43 bacterial genera, 27 fungal genera <br> * User and eco-friendly <br> * Non-toxic, non-irritant at user dilutions <br> * Highly effective in the presence of organic matter | **Terminal Disinfection:** 5 g / litre of water 1 lit / 25 sq. ft. carpet area <br> **Aerial / Misting Spray:** 5 g / lit of water, power spray at finest setting 1 lit / 125 sq. ft carpet area <br> **Foot / Wheel Disinfection:** 10 g / lit of water <br> **Water Sanitizer:** 1 g / 10 litres of water <br> **Disease Outbreaks:** 1 g / litre of water <br> **Vehicle Disinfection:** 5-10 g / litre of water |
| 11 | BIOCLEAN (Indian Drugs and Vitamins) | Alkyl dimethyl benzylammonium chloride, and Alkyl dimethyl ethyl benzylammonium chloride, Tri butyl tin oxide (TBTO), Aqueous base q.s. | For total water protection | **For drinking water sanitation:** 1 ml / 10 litres of drinking water daily <br> **To clean drinking water system:** 100 ml / litre of water <br> **Shed with birds:** 4 ml / 2 litres of water / spray method <br> **Empty sheds:** 4 ml / litre of water / spray method <br> **Sanitizing hatchery eggs:** 5 ml / litre of water |
| 12 | BIO-PHENE | Ortho- | * Kills all known | 4 ml / litre of water |

| S.No. | Trade Name & Company | Composition | Indications | Dosage / Administration |
|---|---|---|---|---|
| | (+ Cleaner) (Venky's) | phenylphenol 7.92% w/v, Ortho-benzyl-para-chlorophenol 9.97% w/v, Para-tertiary-amylphenol 1.95% w/v, Inert ingredients q.s. | poultry pathogens<br>* Finds excellent usage in poultry farms and hatcheries<br>* Effective in 5% organic matter and 400 ppm hard water<br>* Very high residual effect | |
| 13 | BIOSOLVE PLUS (Pfizer) | An alkaline blend of non-ionic and amphoteric surfactants in an aqueous solution incorporating a fully biodegradable sequestrant | * For washing surfaces<br>* For washing equipments | **Cleaning by Spray:** 10 ml / litre. Leave 15 – 20 min, then rinse off. **Cleaning by Foaming:** 20 ml / litre. Leave for 15-20 min, then rinse off. **Cleaning of Equipment:** 10 ml / litre of water. Make solution sufficient for cleaning all equipment |
| 14 | BROMOSEPT 50 (+ Water Sanitizer) (Sarabhai Zydus) | Each 100 ml contains : Didecyl-dimethyl-ammonium bromide (DDAB) 50 g | * General multipurpose sanitizing agent<br>* Sanitation of drinking water<br>* Washing floors, crevices, sinks, walls, furniture, food products and food processing equipment<br>* Prevention of slime formation in drinking water pipe lines | **General disinfection :** 1 ml / litre of water **General sanitation :** 1 ml / 4 litres of water **Potable water sanitation :** 1 ml / 10 litres of water **Disinfection of hatching eggs :** 5 ml / 100 litres of water |
| 15 | CHLORAMINE – T (Polchem) | It contains 20-25% w/w available chlorine | Acts as a constant reservoir releasing potent hypochlorous ion ensuring total destruction of Gumboro virus in | **Empty sheds:** 5 g / litre of water **Poultry house wth birds:** 1 g / litre of water **Outside vehicles / foot bath:** 2 g / litre of water |

653

| S.No. | Trade Name & Company | Composition | Indications | Dosage / Administration |
|---|---|---|---|---|
| | | | the environment | |
| 16 | CHLORASAN – T (Neospark) | Chloramine – T (Sodium – N – chloro-para toluene sulphonamide) | * Effective against all known viruses, bacteria, and fungi<br>* Pathogens are rapidly destroyed by irreversible oxidation of cell material. Effective against 94 bacteria, 49 viruses, 22 fungi, 6 algae, 4 yeasts and parasites<br>* Completely safe | **Spray in presence of birds:** 3 g / litre of water<br>**During disease:** 5 g / litre of water<br>**Terminal disinfection:** 5-10 g / litre of water<br>**Hatching egg sanitation:** 5 g / litre of water<br>**Equipment disinfection:** 5 – 10 g / litre of water<br>**Severe Gumboro:** 50 g / litre of water |
| 17 | CHLORASOL (Intervet) | Contains at least 98% Chloramine EP (European Pharmacopoeia) | For efficient disinfection and water sanitization | **For surface disinfection:** 3-5 g / litres of water.<br>**Contact time:** Minimum of 30 minutes<br>**For water sanitization:**<br>**Prophylactic:** 40 mg / litre of water<br>**Suspected contamination:** 100 mg / litre of water |
| 18 | DESCAL (Polchem) | Blend of descaling inorganic acids, nonionic detergents and corrosion inhibitor | * A descalant for poultry farms<br>* To remove white depositions from all surfaces<br>* To remove white scales (salt deposition) from pipelines, nipples and nozzles | **Plastic / metal equipment:** 20-30 ml / litre of water<br>**Drinking water pipelines:** 10-20 ml / litre of water<br>**Hatchery machine:** 100 ml / litre of water<br>**Nipples / Nozzles:** 40 ml / litre of water |
| 19 | DISFECT S (Pfizer) | Poly alkyl monohydric phenols 40% w/w, Dodecyl benzene sulphonic acid 24% w/w, Metacresol (40%) 5% w/w, Base | For regular disinfection of sheds and during outbreaks of viral, bacterial and fungal diseases | **For regular disinfection:** 2.5 ml / litre of water<br>**For foot and wheel dips:** 10 ml / litre of water |

| S.No. | Trade Name & Company | Composition | Indications | Dosage / Administration |
|---|---|---|---|---|
| | | q.s. | | |
| 20 | DISKOL (+ Sanitizer) (Polchem) | Benzalkonium chloride 5%, Glutaraldehyde 7.5%, Formaldehyde 7.5%, Stabilisers and Antioxidants | * Provides a combined action of disinfectant and sanitizer. It is a bactericide, fungicide and virucide<br>* Non-toxic to birds | **Empty sheds:** 800 ml / 20 litres of water<br>**Plastic equipment / Feed rooms / stores / Outside vehicles /Hatching eggs / Incubator tanks / White wash** 20 ml / litre of water<br>**Metal equipment / Foot baths:** 10 ml / litre of water<br>**Visitor shoes:** 30 ml / litre of water<br>**Incubator / Hatcher:** 40 ml / litre of water |
| 21 | DIS-N-DET (+ Sanitizer) (Polchem) | Glutaraldehyde 12.5%, Benzalkonium chloride 8%, Non-ionic detergents, Stabilizers and Antioxidants | * Provides a combined action of detergent and sanitizer. No need to use both separately<br>* Non-toxic to birds | **Incubator / Hatcher / Foot baths / Cages and Floors:** 40 ml / litre of water<br>**Metal equipment / Outside vehicles:** 10 ml / litre of water<br>**Hatching eggs / Plastic equipment:** 20 ml / litre of water |
| 22 | EZ-KLEEN (+ Cleaner) (Venky's) | Alkaline cleaner and deodorizer | * Rinses free without streaking<br>* Odourless cleaner and deodorizer<br>* Compatible with **B-904** and **safegard** | **General purpose cleaning:** 8-24 ml / litre of water<br>**Foam cleaning:** 16-24 ml / litres of water<br>**Farm premise wash down:** 1 litre / 300 litres of wash water |
| 23 | GLUFORT (Sarabhai Zydus) | Each 100 ml contains : Glutaraldehyde 7 g, 1,6 Dihydroxy 2,5 Diohexane 9.5 g, Polymethyl urea derivatives 16.3 g | * It is bactericide, virucide, fungicide and sporicide<br>* It provides protection against all bacterial, viral and fungal diseases<br>* Effective in the presence of | **For regular disinfection of sheds / Foot baths (dips):** 10 ml / litre of water<br>**Vehicle dips:** 20 ml / litre of water<br>**Visitors' shoes:** 30 ml / litre of water<br>**Sanitation of hatching eggs, hatchers and incubators:** 5 ml / litre of water |

655

| S.No. | Trade Name & Company | Composition | Indications | Dosage / Administration |
|---|---|---|---|---|
| | | | * organic matter 10 times more potent than formaldehyde alone | **For specific disinfections: Bacteria (G +ve and G –ve), Mycoplasma / Fungi:** 30 ml / litre of water **Viruses (ND and IBD and others):** 10-30 ml / litre of water **Acid-fast bacteria:** 40 ml / litre of water |
| 24 | HYPEROX ULTIMATE ('Iarshvardhan's Lab) | Peracetic acid – 5.3%, Hydrogen peroxide – 23%, Mineral acid catalyst, Surfactant stabilizer, and inert ingredients | * For water sanitization * For disinfection | **Terminal Disinfection:** 20 ml / litre. Spray using high pressure pump **Disinfection of sheds in presence of birds:** 10 ml / litre. Spray keeping nozzle towards ceiling **Plastic Equipment:** 20 ml / litre. Soak for 30 min **Metal Equipment:** 10 ml / litre. Soak for 30 min **Feed rooms / stores:** 10 ml / litre. Spray method. **Foot bath / Vehicle Dips:** 10 ml / litre. Add daily **Water sanitization: Routine:** 1 ml / 10 litre **Viral, Bacterial Infections:** 2 ml / 10 litres of water for 3 days; *E. coli* – 5 ml / 10 litres of water for 3 days **Hatching Eggs' Disinfection:** 2.5 ml / litre **Incubators and Hatchers:** 20 ml / litre by spray method |
| 25 | HYPEROX (Pfizer) | Strong hydrogen peroxide NLT – 24% | * For disinfection of water systems (overhead tanks | **Disinfection of water system:** 2 ml/ litre. Drain system and |

| S.No. | Trade Name & Company | Composition | Indications | Dosage / Administration |
|---|---|---|---|---|
| | | Peracetic acid – NLT – 4.5% | and pipelines)<br>* For terminal disinfection of sheds<br>* For foot / wheel dip disinfection | fill with the solution. Allow for 10 min contact time and flush with plain water<br>**Spray disinfection of surface and equipment:** 10 ml / litre. Spray sufficiently on clean surfaces<br>**Foot and wheel dips:** 10 ml / litre: Replenish after every 2 hours<br>**Fogging at depopulation:** 40 – 100 ml / litre. Apply at the rate of 15 ml / 10 sq. ft. with a fogging machine |
| 26 | KECIDDAL (Kemin) | Didecyl dimethyl ammonium chloride 70% sol. – 12% w/v Strong glutaraldehyde solution BP 8% w/v | * Effective in controlling major poultry viruses like avian influenza Newcastle disease virus, infectious bursal disease virus, and avian reovirus at 1:200 dilution<br>* Effective in reducing the count of bacteria and fungi at 1:200 dilution<br>* Eco-friendly and has long residual action<br>* Effective in hard water, wide range of pH and in the presence of organic matter<br>* Safe and immediate action | **Washing and cleaning surfaces:** 1 ml / litre of water. Spray 75 L solution per 1000 sq. ft. area on surfaces and wash after 30 minutes<br>**Aerial disinfection in the presence of birds:** 5 ml/ litre of water. Use fine spray/mist droplets or fogging<br>**Aerial disinfection before the placement of chicks:** 5 ml /litre of water. Use fine spray/mist droplets or fogging<br>**General disinfection (poultry houses – all surfaces, equipment, hatcheries, utensils, and flushing of water system):** 5 ml / litre of water. Wet the surfaces thoroughly with 150 to 200 ml solution per 10 sq. ft. area and leave it to dry<br>**Foot and Vehicle dips:** 20 ml/litre of water. Replace when solution starts getting dirty<br>**Disinfection of hatching** |

| S.No. | Trade Name & Company | Composition | Indications | Dosage / Administration |
|---|---|---|---|---|
| | | | | eggs:<br>5ml/litre of water. Fine spray over the hatching eggs |
| 27 | KEM<br>V 260<br>LIQUID<br>(Kemin) | It is a unique buffered soluble disinfectant based on a potentiated blend of modified phenols in a biodegradable surfactant base | * Broad-spectrum germicidal disinfectant against common bacteria, virus and other micro-organisms for adequate bio-security and disease control<br>* For terminal disinfection | **Routine disinfection:**<br>2 ml / litre of water<br>**Cross contamination :**<br>8 ml / litre of water<br>**Terminal disinfection :**<br>20 ml / litre of water |
| 28 | KLEENGUARD<br>(APC Nutrients) | It contains dioctyl dimethyl ammonium chloride | Potentiated disinfectant that can kill a wide range of bacteria, moulds, yeasts, and protozoa | **Dipping hatching eggs:**<br>15 ml / 6 litres of water<br>**Drinking water:**<br>15 ml / 30 litres of water<br>**Disinfection of skin and hands:**<br>15 ml / 10 litres of water |
| 29 | KOHRSOLIN<br>LIQUID<br>(Virbac) | Each 100 ml contains :<br>Glutaraldehyde 10 g, 1, 6 Dihydroxy 2, 5 dioxyhexane 10.4 g,<br>Polymethyl urea derivatives 7.2 g | For disinfection of sheds before chicks arrival | **For general disinfection of empty sheds:**<br>500 ml / 50 litres of water<br>**Inventory rooms and equipment, Sanitization of hatching eggs, incubators and hatchers:**<br>250 ml / 50 litres of water<br>**For specific disinfection:**<br>Bacterial, fungal and viral infections<br>1500 ml / 50 litres of water<br>**Tubercular infection:**<br>2000 ml / 50 litres of water |
| 30 | MEDDIS<br>(Varsha) | Dodecylamine sulphamate, Poly (hexamethylene) biguanide hydrochloride, Octyldecyl | * Virucidal, bactericidal, sporicidal and fungicidal<br>* Used for disinfection of empty sheds, also | **For disinfection :**<br>100 ml / 30 litres of water<br>**During disease outbreaks / Egg sanitation:**<br>200 ml / 30 litres of water<br>**For equipment / Hatchery floors:** |

| S.No. | Trade Name & Company | Composition | Indications | Dosage / Administration |
|---|---|---|---|---|
| | | dimethyl ammonium chloride, 4 Nonyl phenyl-w-hydroxy-poly (Oxyethelene) (NP9), Ethanol (DN), EDTA, Sequestrant,Corrosion Inhibitor, Demineralized water | during disease outbreak, and for equipment and egg sanitization | 100 ml / 5 litres of water |
| 31 | METAROX (Neospark) | Dihydrogen dioxide with sulphuric acid, copper (2+) salt (1:1), carbonyldi amide as activators | * As drinking water sanitizer, chlorine free<br>* As a hatchery sanitizer<br>* Removes all organic and inorganic deposits<br>* Long-lasting disinfectant action | Should be activated before application. Mix A and B part before use. Add 30 g of activator to 500 ml of metarox solution in a container. Allow 5 minutes to dissolve completely. **Drinking water treatment:** 3-4 ml / 100 litres of water **Pipeline cleaning:** 2-5 ml / litre of water **Poultry sheds / Hatchers / Setters / Hatching Eggs Spray:** 50 ml / litre of water |
| 32 | NEODINE – 2% (Neospark) | Nonyl alkyl phenoxy polyethylene oxide iodine complex providing iodine 2%, elemental potassium – 0.118%, casein protein – 1000 ppm | * Activates bactericidal, fungicidal, virucidal, and sporicidal effect<br>* Retention of biocidal activity is high<br>* Free from chlorine and phenol compounds<br>* Odourless, stainless and non-corrosive | **Drinking water sanitization:** 1 ml / 10 litres of water daily **Drinking water sanitization in disease:** 5 ml / litre of water for 5 days **Spraying of sheds:** 10 ml / litre of water. Spray at high pressure **In presence of birds:** 2 ml / 10 litres of water. Fine spray over the birds **Plastic / metal equipment:** 10 – 20 ml / litre of water |

| S.No. | Trade Name & Company | Composition | Indications | Dosage / Administration |
|---|---|---|---|---|
| | | | | Soak for 1 hour<br>**Incubators / hatchers:**<br>10-20 ml / litre of water. Spray.<br>**Hatching eggs:**<br>10-20 ml / litre of water. Dip eggs and allow to dry in air<br>**Foot baths:**<br>10 – 20 ml / litre of water.<br>**Plastic trays:**<br>20 ml / litre of water. Dip and dry.<br>**Vehicles:**<br>10 ml / litre of water. Spray |
| 33 | OMNICIDE (+ Sanitizer) (Vetcare) | Glutaraldehyde 15%, Cocobenzyl dimethyl ammonium chloride10%, added excipients q.s. | * Disinfects most of the harmful viruses /bacteria / fungi / mycoplasma, etc.<br>* Sanitizes drinking water<br>* Reduces pathogen load in the water<br>* Ensures safety even in the presence of birds | **Routine disinfection / surface disinfection / fogging :**<br>7 ml / litre<br>**Water sanitation:**<br>8 ml / 25 litres<br>**Foot dip / wheel wash :**<br>10 ml / litre |
| 34 | OXTERON (Neospark) | Balanced mixture of ethaneperoxoic acid, ethanoic acid, hydroperoxide compounds with suitable surfactants, activators and stabilizers | * Drinking water treatment<br>* Disinfectant<br>* Foot baths and vehicle spray<br>* Sanitization of hatchery eggs | **Drinking water treatment:**<br>1 ml / 10 litres of water continuously.<br>**Routine disinfection:**<br>5 ml / litre of water. Spray 300 ml /m$^2$ surface area<br>**Disinfection during diseases:**<br>10 ml/ litre of water. 300 ml / m$^2$ area<br>**Pipeline cleaning / foot baths, vehicle spray:**<br>10 ml / litre of water |
| 35 | PEROXSIL (Neospark) | Stabilized dihydrogen dioxide with noble/metal argentum | * Drinking water treatment<br>* Routine disinfection<br>* Poultry | **Drinking water treatment:**<br>3-4 ml/ 100 litres of water.<br>**Drinking water supply in pipes:**<br>2 – 5 ml / litre of water. |

| S.No. | Trade Name & Company | Composition | Indications | Dosage / Administration |
|---|---|---|---|---|
| | | | equipment cleaning<br>* Effective against virus, bacteria (Gm + and -ive), yeasts, moulds | **Poultry shed disinfection:**<br>50 ml / litre of water. Spray<br>**Hatching eggs:**<br>50 ml dilution/ litre. Spray |
| 36 | PEROX (Polchem) | Peracetic acid 12%, Hydrogen peroxide 25%, Stabilizers 0.4%. | * For terminal disinfection of empty sheds, and equipment<br>* Also may be used as a sanitizer<br>* Biodegradable and non-toxic | **Terminal disinfection of empty sheds:**<br>50 ml / 10 litres<br>**Plastic equipment / Incubator/ Hatcher:**<br>30 ml / 10 litres<br>**Metal equipment:**<br>10 ml / 10 litres<br>**Feed rooms / stores:**<br>10 ml / 10 litres<br>**Drinking water sanitation:**<br>1 ml / 40 litres of water |
| 37 | POLIDINE (Polchem) | Alkyl phenoxy polyglycol ether iodine complex, providing 1.6% available iodine | * All rounder disinfectant for poultry<br>* Compatible with water acidifiers | **Empty shed:**<br>800 ml / 20 litres of water<br>**Plastic trays / Outside vehicles:**<br>20 ml / litre of water<br>**Drinking water:**<br>1 ml / 10 litres of water<br>**Foot baths / Hatching eggs:**<br>20 ml / litre of water<br>**Incubators /Hatchers:**<br>30 ml / litres of water |
| 38 | PROTEKT (+ Cleaner) (Venky's) | Each 100 ml contains : Benzalkonium chloride solution 5 ml, Strong glutaraldehyde solution 7.5 ml, Nonionic surfactant | * Empty shed disinfection<br>* Farm boot bath<br>* Vehicle dips<br>* Disinfecting metal and plastic equipment<br>* Disinfecting stores | **Incubator / Hatcher / Incubator tank / Foot-bath:**<br>4%<br>**Hatching eggs / Plastic equipment / Feed rooms / Stores / Vehicle dip:**<br>2%<br>**Metal Equipment:**<br>1% |

| S.No. | Trade Name & Company | Composition | Indications | Dosage / Administration |
|---|---|---|---|---|
| | | 1 g, Stabilizers 1 g, Aqueous base q.s. | | **Visitors' shoes:** 3% or 40 ml / litre of water |
| 39 | QUALITROL (Vetnex) | Ortho-phenyl phenol 12%, Ortho-benzyl-para-chloro phenol 10%, Para tertiary-amylphenol 4%, and Inert ingredients 74% | * Broad-spectrum bactericidal, virucidal and fungicidal <br> * Complete protection for poultry <br> * Lowers early chick mortality | **Single dilution for all purposes :** 100 ml / 25 litres of water |
| 40 | RES-Q (Venky's) | A balanced, stabilized blend of peroxygen compounds, surfactants, organic acids, and inorganic buffering agent | * Effective against bacteria, fungi, moulds and all virus families affecting poultry <br> * Effective over 20 virus families, 43 bacterial genera, 27 fungal genera <br> * Biodegradable <br> * Non-toxic and non-irritant at user dilutions <br> * Highly effective in the presence of organic matter <br> * User and eco-friendly and ultra-fast acting <br> * Effective against biofilms | **Terminal disinfection:** 5 g / litre of water. Power spray @ 1 litre / 25 sq. ft. carpet area <br> **Aerial disinfection, Misting / Aerial spray:** 5 g / litre of water. Power spray at finest setting @ 1 litre/25 sq. ft. carpet area <br> **Cold fogging:** 10 g / litre of water. 1 litre / 125 sq. ft. carpet area <br> **Thermal fogging:** 40 g / litre of water. 1 litre / 500 sq. ft. carpet area <br> **Foot / wheel disinfection:** 10 g / litre of water. Change weekly or when visibly dirty <br> **Vehicle disinfection/ Pre-cleaned vehicles:** 5 g / litre of water. Drench wet vehicle <br> **Un-cleaned vehicles:** 10 g / litre of water. Drench wet vehicle |
| 41 | SAFEGARD (+ Water Sanitizer) (Venky's) | Iodine 1.75% w/v (as alpha-(p-nonylphenyl) – omega-hydroxypoly (oxyethylene) – | * Safe and effective poultry water sanitizer <br> * Ideal disinfectant for feeders and watering | **For spray purpose:** 8 ml / litres of water <br> **For water sanitation:** 1 ml / 10 litres of water <br> **During IBH / IBD outbreaks:** |

| S.No. | Trade Name & Company | Composition | Indications | Dosage / Administration |
|---|---|---|---|---|
| | | iodine complex) Inert ingredients q.s. | equipment<br>* Shoe bath sanitization<br>* Destroys odour as it sanitizes | 1.6 ml / litre of water |
| 42 | SUPEROX (Vetline) | Per acetic acid, hydrogen peroxide, acetic acid, sulphuric acid, stabilizer | * Control of recurrent bacterial and viral infections, such as colibcillosis, fowl cholera, coryza, IBD, RD, IB, etc.<br>* Useful at hatchery and at farms<br>* Useful in terminal disinfection and foot path | **Empty sheds:**<br>250 ml / 20 litres of water for 1000 sq. ft. surface area<br>**With birds:**<br>Use 500 ml / 20 litres of solution for 1000 sq. ft.<br>**Eggs before hatching:**<br>250 ml / 10 litres of water |
| 43 | TH 4 + (Solvay) (Fort Dodge) | Each litre contains : Didecyldimethyl ammonium chloride 18.75 g, Dioctyldimethyl ammonium chloride 18.75 g, Octydecyldimethyl ammonium chloride 37.5 g, Alkyldimethyl ammonium chloride 50 g, Glutaraldehyde 62.5 g,Pine oil 20g, Terpineol 20 g | * Broad-spectrum activity - virucidal, bactericidal and fungicidal<br>* Strong penetration power | **Spraying / Dipping (foot bath, wheel-bath):**<br>1 litre / 200 litres of water<br>**Thermo-fogging:**<br>2.5 litres / 2.5 litres of water |
| 44 | TRIGENE (Elder Pharmaceuticals) | Virucidal, bactericidal, fungicidal, sporicidal | * For disinfection of all surfaces<br>* Active against all viruses, bacterial species | **General Use:**<br>1:200<br>**For intermediate risk areas and also vehicles:**<br>1:100<br>**For high risk areas and also vehicles:** 1:50<br>**Aerial disinfection** |

| S.No. | Trade Name & Company | Composition | Indications | Dosage / Administration |
|---|---|---|---|---|
| | | | | (fogging): 1:200 |
| 45 | ULTRAXIDE (APC Nutrients) | Glutaraldehyde 15% w/v, Alkyl benzyl dimethyl ammonium chloride 10% w/v (quarternary ammonium compound) | * It is effective against all 17 virus families<br>* Kills virus, bacteria, mycoplasma, and fungi | **Dilution Rate:**<br>**Hatching room:** 1:50<br>**Egg Store:** 1:320<br>**Vehicles:** 1:400<br>**Drinking Water:** 1:3000<br>**General purpose disinfection dilution rate:** 1:150 - !:400 |
| 46 | UNIVERSAL BARN CLEANER (+ Cleaner) (Venky's) | It contains amphoteric Detergents that completely remove both organic and inorganic dirt | * For cleaning before disinfection of poultry houses, farm premises, hatcheries<br>* Exterior and interior of vehicles, trucks, cars | 1-2 ml / litre of water |
| 47 | VIRACID- S (Neospark) | A balanced, stabilized blend of peroxygen compounds, surfactants, organic acids, and an inorganic buffer system | * Effective against all virus families affecting poultry<br>* Complete control - aerial, surface and water system disinfectant<br>* Versatile and prolonged action | **Aerial spray:** 5 g / litre of water (1:200)/100 cubic meter. Spray should be twice daily<br>**Water sanitizer:** 2 g / litre of drinking water (1:500)<br>**Disease conditions:** 1:50 dilution. 20 g / litre of water during chicken infectious anaemia, Gumboro, ND, IB, AI, Marek's, ILT 1:250- 1:600 dilution. 1.5 – 4 g / litre of water |
| 48 | V-OX (Polchem) | Inorganic peroxygen compounds, salts, buffers, descalants, detergents, | * Broad-spectrum disinfectant in powder form. Can be used in presence of birds<br>* Effective against | **Environmental spray in sheds and hatchery:** 5 g / litre of water. 10 litre solution/1000 sq. ft. for terminal disinfection<br>**Spray in presence of birds:** |

| S.No. | Trade Name & Company | Composition | Indications | Dosage / Administration |
|---|---|---|---|---|
| | | stabilizers | bacteria, fungi, viruses | 3 g / litre of water. 10 litre solution /3000 sq. feet area towards ceiling of the sheds **Drinking water:** 2 g / 10 litres of drinking water |
| 49 | VIRKON S (+ Water Sanitizer) (Pfizer) | Sodium chloride 1.5% w/w, Salt containing Potassium monoper-sulphate, Potassium hydrogen sulphate, Potassium sulphate 49.6% w/w, Buffer and Excipients q.s. to 100% | * For continuous disinfection in presence of birds<br>* For terminal application (before chick replacement) | **For continuous protection / before chick replacement / disease outbreak:** 5 g / litre / Spray sufficient solution **As water sanitizer:** 2 g / litre during infection |
| 50 | WOCTANT (Wockhardt) | Poly (hexamethylene bigunide) hydrochloride 10% w/v | * Active against Gram-+ive and – negative bacteria, fungi, yeasts, enveloped and non-enveloped viruses, DNA and RNA viruses<br>* Active against waste material, such as faeces<br>* Active in presence of hard and soft water<br>Active between 1 – 11 pH | **Terminal and regular disinfection for farm surfaces and equipment:** 2 ml / 6 litres of water for 5 minutes **Aerial disinfection/ fogging:** 4 ml / litre of water for 25 minutes **Egg wash:** 2 ml / litre of water for 3 minutes **Hatchery disinfection/ hatching egg sanitizer:** 2 ml / litre of water for 3 minutes **Incubator disinfection:** 2 ml / litre of water for 5 minutes **Foot dip:** 6 ml / litre of water for 30 seconds **Descaling:** 8 ml / 14 litres of water for 24 hours |
| 51 | X-185 (Venky's) | Cresylic acid saponified 30% | Bactericidal, fungicidal, | 4 ml / litre of water |

| S.No. | Trade Name & Company | Composition | Indications | Dosage / Administration |
|---|---|---|---|---|
| | | v/v,Ortho-benzyl-para-chlorophenol 3% w/v, Ortho-phenylphenol 4% w/v, Bis-n-tributyltin oxide 0.5% v/v, Inert ingredients q.s. | virucidal, tuberculocidal, mycoplasmicidal, oocidal | |
| 52 | ZOACID – CP (Neospark) | Coccidial disinfectant with virucidal and bactericidal action | * Coccidial disinfectant with virucidal and bactericidal action<br>* Coccidiocidal, effective against all species of oocysts of Eimeria<br>* Effective against viruses, bacteria, fungi | **Two packs of Zoacid-CP:**<br>1. Coccidiocide source, and<br>2. Coccidiocide activator<br>Remove old litter and debris and thoroughly clean the area.<br>*Dissolve **Pack 1** dissolve in 30 litres<br>of water (1:20 dilution). Spray floor area, posts, walls up to a height of 0.5 metre using a coarse spray, thoroughly wetting all surfaces.<br>*Immediately dissolve **pack no. 2** in 30 litres of water (1:20 dilution). Spray entire area previously treated with pack 1, while it is wet.<br>Treated area will turn pink. |

# 17. ELECTROLYTES

| S. No. | Trade Name & Company | Composition | Indications | Dosage / Administration |
|---|---|---|---|---|
| 1 | AQUALYTE-C (Harshvardhan's Lab) | Each 100 g contains : Dextrose anhydrous 50 g, Potassium chloride 15 g, Sodium chloride 25 g, Sodium bicarbonate 0.5 g, Vit-C (Coated) 1.2 g | * In heat stress<br>* In the presence of diseases such as diarrhoea, which result in dehydration<br>* Prior to and after transportation<br>* Other areas of stress | 1/2 g / litre of water |
| 2 | ELECTROCARE PLUS (+ PROBIOTICS) (Vetcare) | Each 100 g contains : Sodium chloride 0.8 g, Potassium chloride 5 g, Sodium bicarbonate 3 g, Sodium acid phosphate 0.8 g, Sodium citrate 6.5 g, Calcium lactate 1.7 g, Magnesium sulphate 1 g, Lactose 25 g, Ascorbic acid (coated) 1.2 g, Lactobacillus viable spores 3000 million CFU,· Dextrose anhydrous q.s. | * For treating stress due to heat, transportation, liver damage, post-antibiotic / coccidial therapy<br>* To prevent dehydration due to heat stress<br>* To prevent stress from transportation, vaccination, debeaking,<br>* To reduce mortality | 1 g / 2 litres of water for 3-5 days or, 1 Kg / tonne of feed |
| 3 | ELECTROL PLUS POWDER (Avian Remedies) | Each Kg contains : Sodium chloride 10 g, Potassium chloride 60 g, Sodium bicarbonate 40 g, Sodium citrate 66 g, Calcium gluconate 17 g, Magnesium sulphate 15 g, Lactose 25 g, Dextrose anhydrous 700 g, Vit C 12 g, Lactobacillus spores 30,000 million spores, Organic nutritive | * Dehydration due to diarrhoea, stress, heat and humidity<br>* Prior and subsequent to transportation, shifting<br>* High temperatures | **Broilers:** 10 g / litre of water for 100 birds **Layers:** 15 g / litre of water for 100 birds |

| S. No. | Trade Name & Company | Composition | Indications | Dosage / Administration |
|---|---|---|---|---|
| | | carrier q.s. | | |
| 4 | ELECTROL PLUS POWDER (AVR) | Each 100 g contains : Sodium chloride 1 g, Potassium chloride 4.5 g, Sodium bicarbonate 3 g, Sodium acid phosphate 0.75 g, Sodium citrate 7 g, Calcium lactate 1.8 g, Magnesium sulphate 1 g, Vit C 2 g, Lactose 30 g, Lactobacillus viable spores 3500 million, Dextrose anhydrous q.s. | * Poultry feed supplement electrolytes and probiotics with vitamin C<br>* Prevents all kinds of stress | 1 Kg / tonne of feed or 1 g / 2 litres of water |
| 5 | GTROSE (Golden Streak) | Each 200 g contains : Calcium lactate 2 g, Potassium chloride 8 g, Magnesium sulphate 1 g, Sodium chloride 1.6 g, Sodium bicarbonate 2 g, Sodium hydrogen phosphate 1.4 g, Sodium citrate 6 g, Dextrose 80 g, *Lactobacillus sporogenes* 3000 million viable spores, Vit C 4 g, Water soluble carbohydrate q .s. | * Prior to and after transportation<br>* In summer to avoid dehydration and heat<br>* For energy and as supportive therapy in diarrhoea and dysentery<br>* To maintain correct osmotic pressure, acid-base equilibrium | **Chicks:** 10 g / litre of water **Growers / Layers:** 15 g / litre of water for 5 days |
| 6 | C –LYTE (Sarabhai Zydus) | Each 250 g contains : Sodium chloride 2 g, Potassium chloride 12.5 g, Sodium bicarbonate 7.5 g, sodium acid phosphate 2 g, Sodium citrate 16.25 g, Calcium lactate 4.25 g, Magnesium sulphate 2.5 g, Vit C (coated) 2.91 g, Dextrose 195 g Lactobacillus | * Maintains osmotic balance in body and alleviates stress conditions caused by heat, transportation, diseases, medication, vaccination, debeaking and moulting<br>* Increases FCR and growth<br>* Enhances body resistance | 1 g / 2 litres of water for 5-7 days |
| 7 | HI-LYTES FEED | Each g contains : Dextrose 760 mg, Sodium | Stress in birds during summer, | 1-2 g / litre of water or 500 g / |

| S. No. | Trade Name & Company | Composition | Indications | Dosage / Administration |
|---|---|---|---|---|
|  | SUPPLEMENT (Hitha) | chloride 75 mg, Sodium citrate 103 mg, Potassium chloride 50 mg, Vit C 12 mg | overcrowding, pecking, debeaking, transportation, vaccination, bacterial, viral and parasitic infections | tonne of feed |
| 8 | INDOLYTE (Indian Drugs and Vitamins) | Each 100 g contains: Sodium chloride 0.8 g, Potassium chloride 5 g, Sodium bicarbonate 3 g, Sodium acid phosphate 0.8 g, Sodium citrate 6.5 g, Calcium lactate 1.7 g, Magnesium sulphate 1 g, Vit C 1.3 g, Lactic acid bacilli, Dextrose q.s. | * Prior and after transportation<br>* In extreme temperatures (high or low)<br>* Other areas of stress | 1 Kg / tonne of feed, or 1 g / 2 litres of water for 3-5 days |
| 9 | PRIMELYTE C FEED SUPPLEMENT (Prime) | Each 100 g contains: Sodium chloride 0.80 g, Potassium chloride 4.5 g, Magnesium sulphate 1 g, Sodium bicarbonate 3 g, Sodium acid phosphate 0.75 g, Sodium citrate 5 g, Calcium lactate 1.7 g, Lactose 25 g, Lactobacillus (Spores) 3000 billion, Ascorbic acid (coated) 3 g, Dextrose q.s. | * Poultry feed supplement containing electrolytes and probiotics with desired level of Vitamin C<br>* Prevents all kinds of stress | 1 g / 2 litres of water or 1 Kg / tonne of feed |
| 10 | REHYDRAL (Vetline) | Each 100 g contains: sodium chloride 8.250 g magnesium sulphate 1 g, calcium gluconate 2 g, potassium sulphate 1 g, vitamin C 1 g, Lactobacillus viable spores 3200 million, and dextrose anhydrous q.s. | * Recommended for all kinds of stresses, including heat stress<br>* Prior to and after transportation | 1 Kg / tonne of feed or 1 g in 2 litres of water for 3-5 days |
| 11 | REHYDRAL + (Vetline) | Each 100 g contains: sodium chloride 8.250 g , magnesium sulphate 1 g, calcium gluconate 2 g, potassium sulphate 1 g, vit C 1g, Lactobacillus viable spores 3200million, glycine | For treating any kind of stress due to extreme climatic conditions, transportation including liver damage, diarrhoea | 1kg/tonne of feed<br>**In water**: 1g in 2 litres for 2-3 days |

| S. No. | Trade Name & Company | Composition | Indications | Dosage./ Administration |
|---|---|---|---|---|
| | | 12.5g , biotin 0.005 g, Dextrose anhydrous q.s. | and post antibiotic / coccidial therapy | |
| 12 | SOLMIN COOL (Qualitat) | Each 100 g contains: CuSo4 – 125 mg, ZnSo4 –- 1.25 g, MgSo4 -1.25 g, Mn – 1.25 g, Kcl – 18.8 g, NaHCo3 –.21 g, Nacl – 25g, FeSo4 – 500 mg, Citric acid – 6.5 g. Vit. C – 1.5 g, Vit B12 – 2 mg, Dextrose – q.s. | * Effective against summer stroke stress<br>* Gout<br>* Helps in recovering dehydration due the heat of the brooder<br>* Better weight gain | **Chicks:** 10 – 20 g / 100 chicks / day<br>**Broilers / Layers:** 40 g / 100 birds |
| 13 | STRESS CARE (Varsha) | Each 10 g contains: Sodium chloride – 300 mg, Potassium chloride – 100 mg, Glycine – 75 mg, Manganese sulphate – 30 mg, Sodium bicarbonate – 2000 mg, Sod. citrate – 350 mg, Vit C -100 mg Calcium hypophosphite – 100 mg, Lactic acid bacteria – 120 x $10^6$ | * Replenishes electrolyte balance<br>* Better Ca mobilization and utilization<br>* Better shell quality, increased fertility and hatchability<br>* Better immunity<br>* Establishes gut microflora which get depleted during stress | 1 g / 2 litres of water, or 0.75 – 1 Kg / tonne of feed |
| 14 | ULTRALYTE-C (Neospark) | Each 100 g contains : Sodium chloride 1 g, Potassium chloride 5 g, Sodium bicarbonate 3 g, Sodium acid phosphate 0.8 g, Sodium citrate 6.5 g, Calcium lactate 1.7 g, Magnesium sulphate 1 g, Vit-C (coated) 1.2 g, DFM (probiotic) CFU 3300 million, Casein protein 200 ppm, Elemental sodium 3.05 g, Elemental potassium 2.62 g, Lactose 40 g, Dextrose anhydrous q.s. | * Poultry supplement containing electrolytes and probiotics with Vitamin C<br>* Prevents all kinds of stress | **Chicks :** 1000 g / 1000 chicks / day for 3-5 days<br>**Broilers:** 100 g / 1000 birds / day for 5-7 days<br>**Growers:** 100 g / 750 birds / day for 3-5 days<br>**Layers:** 100 g / 500 birds / day for 3-5 days<br>**Breeders:** 100 g / 500 birds / |

| S. No. | Trade Name & Company | Composition | Indications | Dosage / Administration |
|---|---|---|---|---|
| | | | | day for 5-7 days, all through water |
| 15 | VENLYTE (Venky's) | Each 100 g contains : Sodium chloride 1 g, Calcium lactate 1.1 g, Calcium gluconate 1.1 g, Magnesium sulphate 0.9 g, Potassium chloride 3 g, Sodium bicarbonate 1 g, Sodium citrate 2.5 g, Vit C 1 g, Dextrose mono-hydrate 58.4 g, Carriers q.s. | * Provides energy and supportive therapy for chicks immediately after arrival at farm<br>* For energy and supportive therapy during diseases<br>* In summer to avoid dehydration and heat stroke<br>* In diarrhoea and dysentery<br>* To maintain correct osmotic pressure and precise acid base equilibrium | 1-2 g / litre of water for 5 days or 200 g / tonne of feed |
| 16 | VITOSEL (Brihans) | Each 100 g contains : Sodium chloride 24 g, Potassium chloride 2.5 g, Calcium gluconate 4.71 g, Magnesium chloride 1.72 g, Sodium bicarbonate 9.4 g, Magnesium sulphate 11 g, Vit $B_1$ 281.8 mg, Vit $B_2$ 340.4 mg, Vit $B_6$ 15.7 mg, Niacin 1.04 g, Vit B12 1.43 mg, Vit E 340.4 mg, Choline chloride 510.3 mg, Folic acid 81.6 mg, Inositol 877.5 mg, Rutoside (Vit P) 1.766 mg, Dextrose anhydrous q.s. | For dehydration in stress of all kinds | **Chicks:** 3-4 g / litre of water<br>**Growers / Broilers:** 2-3 g / litre of water<br>**Layers:** 1-2 g / litre of water, or 10-30 g daily / 100 birds<br>All for 3-5 days |

671

## 18. ENZYMES

| S. No. | Trade Name & Company | Composition | Indications | Dosage / Administration |
|---|---|---|---|---|
| 1 | AFLAANIL (Avians) | Hydrolyzing enzymes. Organic metabolites, Citric acid | * Improves general metabolism<br>* Improves production in layers<br>* Improves body weight in broilers<br>* Improves liver and kidney function | 0.5 ml / litre of water, or 200 ml / 1000 birds daily |
| 2 | ALVIZYME PLUS (Alembic) | It is a combination of nine cozy enzymes for enzymatic action Prebiotic + Probiotic for microbial digestion | * Improves energy utilization of feedstuffs<br>* Decreases gut viscosity<br>* Improves absorption<br>* Improves quality of litter<br>* Reduces faecal loss of phosphorus | 500 g / tonne of feed |
| 3 | ALLZYME PS (Alltech Inc) | Amylase, protease, lipase, xylanase, beta-glucanase, cellulase | * Improves FCR, weight gain and uniformity in broilers<br>* Improves energy, protein and amino acid release<br>* Improves bird performance<br>* Improves litter quality | 500 g / tonne of feed |
| 4 | ALLZYME SSF (Alltech Inc) | Amylase, protease, pectinase, phytase, xylanase, beta-glucanase, cellulase | * Reduces feed cost<br>* Improves FCR, weight gain and uniformity in broilers<br>* Improves energy, calcium and phosphorus release<br>* Improves litter quality | **In Feed:**<br>**Broilers:** 200 g / tonne of feed<br>**Layers and Broilers:** 150 g / tonne of feed |
| 5 | ANAZYME (Varsha Group) (Aamoda Pharmaceutical) | Alpha-amylase, beta-mananase, cellulase, beta-glucanase, hemicellulase, xylanase, pectinase, lipase, protease, phytase | * Releases available phosphorus from phytate hydrolysis<br>* Eliminates anti-nutritional properties of certain dietary components<br>* Improves utilization of non-starch | 500 g / tonne of feed |

| S. No. | Trade Name & Company | Composition | Indications | Dosage / Administration |
|---|---|---|---|---|
| | | | polysaccharides, fat, protein, and phytates | |
| 6 | AV-ZYME – Spl. POWDER (AVR) | Beta-glucanase, Cellulase, Hemicellulase, Protease, Amylase, Xylanase, Pectinase, Phytase, Lipase, Beta-mannase, Galactosidase Live yeast Culture (*Saccharomyces cerevisiae*), Lactobacillus, *Spirulina algae,* Performance promoters | * Improves growth rate, feed efficiency, and egg production<br>* Reduces wet droppings and odour<br>* Improves nutrient utilization<br>* Decreases nutrient and water excretion | **Broilers / Layers :** 500 g / tonne of feed **Breeders:** 500 g / tonne of feed |
| 7 | BEETAZYME POWDER (Kaypeeyes Biotech) | Each g contains : Beta-Glucosidases 2000 IU, Cellulases a) F Pase (Exo-cello-biohydrolase) 20 IU b) Endo-Beta-D-gluconases 60 IU, Amylases 500 IU, Proteases 15000 IU, Phytases 1200 IU Pectinases 200 IU, Amyloglucosidases 6000 IU, Xylanase 200 IU | **In Broilers:**<br>* For faster growth and more body weight<br>* Improves productive value of feed<br>* For better feed conversion ratio<br>* For complete phosphorus and mineral assimilation<br>* Controls tibial dyschondroplasia<br>**In Layers:**<br>* Improves bioavailability of energy<br>* For better egg / feed ratio in controlled feeding<br>* Increases egg production<br>* Maintains good shell thickness<br>* Reduces wet droppings | 250 – 500 g / tonne of feed |
| 8 | BEETAZYME-L LIQUID (Kaypeeyes | Each ml contains : Beta-glucosidases 600 IU, | **In Broilers:**<br>* For faster growth and more body weight | **Through drinking water: Chicks :** |

| S. No. | Trade Name & Company | Composition | Indications | Dosage / Administration |
|---|---|---|---|---|
| | Biotech) | Cellulases : a) F Pase (Exo-cello biohydrolase) 20 IU b) Endo-Beta-D-gluconases 60 IU Amylases 500 IU, Proteases 600 IU, Phytases 600 IU, Amyloglucosidases 6000 IU | * Improves productive value of feed <br> * For better feed conversion ratio <br> * For complete phosphorus and mineral assimilation <br> * Controls tibial dyschondroplasia <br> **In Layers:** <br> * Improves bioavailability of energy <br> * For better egg / feed ratio of controlled feeding <br> * Increases egg production <br> * Maintains good shell thickness | 5 ml / 100 birds **Broilers:** 0-3 weeks – 5ml / 100 birds 4-8 weeks – 10 ml / 100 birds **Growers / Layers :** 10 ml / 100 birds |
| 9 | BIO-FEED PHYTASE (Novo Nordisk) a. Coated Granulate (CT) b. Aqueous liquid (L) | Bio-feed phytase is a phytase from *Peniophora lycii* | * To improve phosphorus utilization in feed <br> * Bio-feed phytase breaks phytates and thereby increases the availability of phosphorus and other nutritional components | **Bio-feed Phytase (CT):** 200-400 g / tonne of feed, mixed into the feed before any pelleting of the feed **Bio-feed Phytase (L) :** 100-200 g / tonne of feed, sprayed on the feed pellets after cooling and de-dusting |
| 10 | BIO FITASE 1600 (Indian Herbs) | Contains natural phytase with significant enzyme activity (NLT 1600 FYT/g) | * Increases bioavailability and utilization of phytic acid bound dietary phosphorus as well as calcium, iron, and zinc contained in feed <br> * It contains natural | 250 – 500 g / tonne of feed depending upon reduction of DCP |

| S. No. | Trade Name & Company | Composition | Indications | Dosage / Administration |
|---|---|---|---|---|
| | | | vitamin D3 metabolites | |
| 11 | BIOMIN PHYTASE 5000 (Biomin) | Biomin phytase 5000 is a new generation of phytase derived from *E. coli.* It is highly efficient in releasing digestible phosphorus and other nutrients | * Improves phytate phosphorus utilization by breaking down phytic acid in digestive tract<br>* Improves bioavailability of calcium, zinc, copper, magnesium, and other minerals | **Laying hens:** 60 g / tonne of finished feed (300 FTU / Kg)<br>**Broilers:** 100 g / tonne of finished feed (500 FTU / Kg) |
| 12 | BIOPHOS-P-FS (Neospark) | It contains 1800 phytase units (FTU) per gram | * Reduces accumulation of phosphorus in the environment<br>* Reduces excretion of nitrogen<br>* Improves nutrient digestibility | **Layers:** 26.5 – 31.5 g can spare 1 Kg of DCP<br>**Broilers:** 44 – 56 g can spare 1 Kg of DCP |
| 13 | CAPLIX FEED SUPPLEMENT (Wockhardt) | Cellulase, Amylase, Arabinase, Pectinase, Phytase, Protease, Lipase,Xylanase, Beta-Glucanase, Galactosidase | Multi-enzyme feed supplement for proper utilization of feed ingredients | 500 g / tonne of feed |
| 14 | CAPLIX LIQUID (Wockhardt) | Each litre contains: Cellulase 10,00,00,000 U, Amylase 1, 25, 000 U, Arabinase 7000 U, Pectinase 30,000 U, Protease 1, 50, 000 U, Lipase 10,000 U, Xylanase 15, 00,000 U, Beta-Glucanase 10,000 U, Alpha-Galactosidase 10,000 U | For better feed utilization, upgrading lower quality feedstuffs, better performance , better biosecurity, assurance of compensatory growth | 1 ml / 4 litres of water |
| 15 | ENZIVER (Vetnex) | Each g contains: Pectinase 900 IU, Cellulase 10,000 IU, xylanase 5000 IU, protease 5500 IU, phytase 1000 FYT, | For releasing phytate-bound phosphorus, energy, and protein from poultry feed, and reducing wet droppings | **Broilers and Breeders:** 250 g / tonne of feed<br>**Layers:** 200 g / tonne of |

| S. No. | Trade Name & Company | Composition | Indications | Dosage / Administration |
|---|---|---|---|---|
| | | beta-glucanase 800 IU, amylase 7500 IU, | | feed |
| 16 | ENZYMEX (Exotic Mushrooms) | Blend of 8 enzymes, alpha-amylase, protease, xylanase, beta-gluconase, Cellulase, phytase, pectinase, lipase | * Enzyme complex designed to digest maize, jowar/ soya based feed<br>* Effectively gets lowest FCR | 500 g / tonne of fee |
| 17 | HIFEED BGX (Jubilant Organosys) | A feed grade thermo-stable fungal multi-enzyme preparation for broilers | * Improvement in FCR<br>* Extra live weight gain per bird<br>* Saving on feed | 400-450 g / tonne of broiler mash feed, or 500 g / tonne of pellet feed |
| 18 | HIFEED – PC (Jubilant Organosys) | Each g contains: Xylanase 3000 U, Beta-Glucanase 1200, Carboxy methyl Cellulase (CMCase) 3400 U, Amylase 500 U, Protease 400 U, Lipase 500 U, Phytase 1000 FYT | Reduces the inclusion of inorganic phosphorus and calcium by 0.1% (available phosphorus) Reduces the energy level of the diet by 2.5 % of the metabolizable energy per kg of the diet in corn and soya based diets | **Broilers:** 200 g / tonne of feed<br>**Layers:** 150 g / tonne of feed |
| 19 | HIFEED-PHYTASE 5000 (Jubilant Organosys) | Hi-performance thermotolerant micro-granulated phytase | * Ensures optimum performance<br>* Quality assurance<br>* Effective in broad range of pH | **Broilers:**<br>**Mash feed:** 100 – 120 g / tonne to replace 50% DCP<br>**Pellet feed:** 110 – 130 g / tonne to replace 50% DCP<br>**Layers:**<br>Mash feed: 75 – 100 g / tonne to replace 50% DCP<br>**Pellet feed:** 80-110 g / tonne to replace 50% DCP |
| 20 | KEMZYME P | Cellulase, | * Liberates phytate bound | 250 g – 1000 g / |

| S. No. | Trade Name & Company | Composition | Indications | Dosage / Administration |
|---|---|---|---|---|
| | DRY POWDER (Kemin) | Hemicellulase, Betaglucanase, Phytase, Amylase, Lipase and Protease | phosphorus from plant raw materials <br> * Helps effective utilization of less conventional feed raw materials <br> * Improves health and hygiene of litter through better utilization of nutrients <br> * Improves performance of birds (FCR, egg production) | tonne of feed |
| 21 | KEMZYME CS DRY POWDER (Kemin) | Alpha-galactosidase, Protease, Cellulase, Xylanase | * Helps optimal utilization of corn soya rations <br> * Helps digestion of fibre and protein fraction of corn soya rations <br> * Spares no sugars for fermentation by pathogenic microflora of hind gut, thus controls their proliferation <br> * Improves performance of birds (FCR, egg production) | 500 g – 1000 g / tonne of feed |
| 22 | MAXIGRAIN (Polchem) | Amylase, xylanase, beta-glucanase, cellulase, pectinase, protease, phytase, lipase | * Improves FCR <br> * Improves weight gain in broilers <br> * Improves litter quality and dropping consistency <br> * Improves egg production and shell quality <br> * Reduces level of DCP incorporation in the feed | Dosage not available. **Maxgrain 'B'** for broilers; **'L'** for layers , and **'LP'** for layers with phytase |
| 23 | MAXIGEST (Advanced Biochemicals) | Alpha-amylase, pectinase (polygalacturonase), acid protease, lipase, | * Improves FCR <br> * Improves uniformity of flock and weight gain <br> * Reduces wet droppings | 500 g to 1 Kg / tonne of feed |

| S. No. | Trade Name & Company | Composition | Indications | Dosage / Administration |
|---|---|---|---|---|
| | | xylanase, hemicellulase, phytase, alpha-galactosidase, invertase | * Gives energy boost in feed by 7 to 12%<br>* Reduces fat level in feed up to 5%<br>* Improves absorption of antibiotics, methionine | |
| 24 | MAXIGRO (Vetcare) | Cellulase, pectinase, protease, xylanase, beta-glucanase, alpha-amylase, *Lactobacillus acidophilus*, *Lactobacillus sporogenes*, *Saccharomyces cervisiae* | * Improves FCR and production<br>* Reduces wet litter<br>* Reduces ammonia excretion<br>* Reduces disease incidence | **Chicks:** 250 g / tonne of feed<br>**Broilers, Layers:** 500 g / tonne of feed<br>**Breeders:** 1 Kg / tonne of feed |
| 25 | MAXIPHOS (Polchem) | Phytase containing minimum – 2500 FTU / g | * Increases phosphorus availability from feed grains<br>* Substantially reduces incorporating level of DCP bringing down the cost of feed<br>* Improves eggshell quality | 125-250 g / tonne of feed |
| 26 | MULTIZYME – PLUS (Bovine Birds Pharma) | Alpha-amylase, Cellulase, Alpha-galactosidase, Glucanase, Lipase, Phytase, Pectinase, Protease, Xylanase, Lactobacillus, yeast | * Increases absorption<br>* Improves FCR<br>* Reduces intestinal disorders<br>* Improves eggshell quality | **Broilers and Layers:** 500 to 1000 g / tonne of feed<br>**Breeders:** 1000 to 1500 g / tonne of feed |
| 27 | NATUZYME POWDER (Novartis) | Contains: Cellulase, Xylanase, Beta-glucanase, Alpha amylase, Pectinase<br>Also contains : Acid phytase, Protease, Hemicellulase, Aminoglycosidase,, and acid phosphatase | * Improves the digestibility of all key feed components<br>* Gives better growth performance and improves FCR<br>* Fat level in the diet can be reduced by 4%<br>* Decreases fat storage in broilers<br>* Reduces wet droppings and odour | 350 g / tonne of feed |

| S. No. | Trade Name & Company | Composition | Indications | Dosage / Administration |
|---|---|---|---|---|
| | | | * For better pellet quality<br>* For better nutrient retention<br>* Inactivates mycotoxins in feed<br>* Improves antibiotic absorption (25-50%)<br>* Increases energy availability<br>* Increases amino acid availability in feed | |
| 28 | NICOPHYT – PLUS (Nicholas Piramal) | Phytase – 2500 FTU Probiotic and yeast culture | * Helps to improve digestion<br>* Increases weight gain<br>* Improves laying performance<br>* Improves immunity power | **Broilers:** 200 g / tonne of feed to replace 7 Kg of DCP<br>**Layers:** 175-200 g / tonne of feed to replace 7-10 Kg of DCP |
| 29 | NICOZYME POWDER (Nicholas Piramal) | Cellulase, Amylase, Protease, Beta-glucanase, Xylanase, Phytase Lactobacillus, Yeast culture | * Improves the nutritive value of feed ingredients<br>* For better FCR, better egg laying performance<br>* For drier and hence more hygienic litter<br>* For reduced number of dirty eggs | 250-300 g / tonne of feed |
| 30 | NR – PHYTASE 5000 ((Natural Remedies) | Contains 5000 phytase units (FTU) / g. Analysis as per AOAC (2005) Test Protocol | * To reduce the level of DCP in the feed<br>* To improve the overall productivity of birds<br>* To improve the bioavailability of phosphorus available in grains and oil seeds<br>* To reduce the environmental hazard by reducing the phytate excretion | **Broilers:** Broilers (commercial) 100 g / tonne of feed<br>**Layers:** **Chicks and Growers:** (commercial and breeders) 100 g / tonne of feed<br>**Laying birds** (commercial and breeders): 70 g / tonne of feed |

| S. No. | Trade Name & Company | Composition | Indications | Dosage / Administration |
|---|---|---|---|---|
| 31 | NUTRIZYME P FORTE POWDER (Vetcare) | Each g contains: Phytase 2500 FYT | * Hydrolyzes phytase phosphorus making it available for absorption<br>* Releases phytate bound minerals, protein, amino acids and starch<br>* Improves FCR<br>* Improves shell strength<br>* Improves laying performance<br>* Improves body weight<br>* Effectively replaces DCP | **Layers:** 175-200 g / tonne<br>**Broilers:** 200 g / tonne |
| 32 | NUTRIZYME SPL LAY POWDER (Vetcare) | Cellulase, xylanase, amylase, pectinase, protease, glucanase and *Saccharomyces cerevisiae* | * Degrades fibre<br>* Reduces viscosity<br>* Reduces wet litter condition<br>* Maintains gut integrity<br>* Improves nutrient utilization | 500 g / tonne of feed |
| 33 | OPTIPHOS PREMIX (Venky's) | Each g contains: Phytase enzyme with activity equivalent to 2500 PPU | * Improves FCR<br>* Improves body weight gain<br>* Improves laying performance<br>* Improves shell strength<br>* Reduces environmental pollution<br>* Reduces cost of production | To replace 8.5 Kg of DCP, use 175 g of Optiphos per tonne of feed |
| 34 | PEPTIZYME POWDER (Kaypeeyes Biotech) | Protein hydrolysate from vegetable origin 20%, Single cell protein 17.5%, Vit $D_3$ 350 IU / g | * A rich protein supplement for chicks<br>* Improves digestion and mineral assimilation<br>* Prevents early chick mortality<br>* Prevents leg weakness<br>* Weight gain in broilers<br>* Improves egg production<br>* Increases eggshell thickness<br>* Improves fertility in | 500 g / tonne of feed |

| S. No. | Trade Name & Company | Composition | Indications | Dosage / Administration |
|---|---|---|---|---|
| | | | breeders<br>* Uniform flock size<br>* Improves productive value of feed | |
| 35 | PEPTIZYME – L LIQUID (Kaypeeyes Biotech) | Protein hydrolysate from vegetable origin 20.0%, sing. Cell protein 17.5%, Vitamin D3 350 IU/g Digestive enzymes: amylase, cellulases, and proteases | * A rich protein supplement as chick nutrition<br>* Improves digestion and mineral assimilation<br>* Intestinal tract developing nourishment in starters and growers<br>* Pronounced bone growth, prevents leg weakness<br>* Weight gain in broilers<br>* Improves egg production<br>* Increases eggshell thickness<br>* Improves fertility in breeders<br>* Uniform flock size<br>* Improves productive value of feed | In drinking water for 100 birds:<br>**Chicks:** 5 ml<br>**Growers and Layers:** 10 ml<br>**Broilers:** 0-3 weeks 5 ml<br>4-8 weeks 10 ml |
| 36 | PHYTOPHOS POWDER (Kaypeeyes Biotech) | Phytase obtained from *Aspergillus niger* | * For utilization of phytate phosphorus from the feed<br>* Increases phosphorus availability of the feed up to 70%<br>* For feed cost saving in the form of reduced DCP requirement<br>* Releases minerals for assimilation<br>* For higher growth rate in broilers<br>* Improves the shell thickness<br>* Prevents the production drop in layers<br>* For prevention of leg | **Layers:** 150 g / tonne of feed<br>**Broilers:** As recommended by the nutritionist |

| S. No. | Trade Name & Company | Composition | Indications | Dosage / Administration |
|---|---|---|---|---|
| | | | weakness<br>* In the treatment of phosphorus deficiency related diseases | |
| 37 | PHYTASE -2500 (Varsha Group) | Contains 2500 units of phytase activity per g. Each 300 units of phytase activity is equal to 1 g of phosphorus as provided by DCP | * Better development of bones<br>* Releases bound phosphorus, calcium, zinc, iron, magnesium, protein<br>* Reduction in ration cost | 150 – 225 g / tonne of feed depending on the reduction of DCP |
| 38 | PROVIZYME POWDER – BRO (Vetcare) | Amylase, xylanase, pectinase, cellulase, glucanase, protease, enzyme activity enhancers | * Improves body weight gain<br>* Improves FCR<br>* Improves litter quality<br>* Reduces ammonia excretion | **Broilers:** 500 g / tonne of feed |
| 39 | SEBPHYTASE (Advanced Biochemicals) | It is a heat-stable and highly active phytase enzyme produced from thermostable organism and can withstand pelleting temperatures | Net variable cost (or savings) with phytase supplementation<br>Net cost change equals summation of added cost and added returns | **Sebphytase MG:** 150-200 g / tonne of feed<br>**Sebphytase 2 MG:** 75-125 g / tonne of feed<br>*Phytase can be used to replace DCP in poultry feed, possibly to the level of 50 to 60% |
| 40 | SYNERZYME-FS POWDER (Neospark) | Each Kg of Premix contains :<br>Amylase 24,00,000 units, Hemi-Cellulase 54,00,000 units, Cellulase 1,20,00,000 units, Protese – 24,00,000 units, Beta-glucanase 1,06,000 units, Phosphorus | * For better feed utilization<br>* For improved performance in poultry | 500 g / tonne of feed |

| S. No. | Trade Name & Company | Composition | Indications | Dosage / Administration |
|---|---|---|---|---|
| | | 1,38,000 ppm, Calcium 1,84,000 ppm, Elemental sodium 500 ppm | | |
| 41 | SYNERZYME-P-FS (Neospark) | Amylase, Hemicellulase, Xylanase, Galactosidase, Cellulase, Protease, Betaglucanase, Phytase | * For better feed utilization <br> * For improved performance in poultry | 500 g / tonne of feed |
| 42 | UNIZYME – 5 Spl (Vet Med) | It contains: Amylase, protease, xylanase, Cellulase, hemi-cellulase, phytase, beta-glucanase, beta-mannase, lipase, pectinase, arabinase, galactosidase, *Saccharomyces cerevisiae, Lactobacillus acidophilus* | * Improves fertility and hatchability in breeders <br> * Prevents wet droppings <br> * Improves digestibility of fibre <br> * Reduces mortality <br> * Improvement in egg production and quality of eggs in layers | **Breeders/ Broilers/ Layers:** 500 g / tonne of feed |
| 43 | VENZYME – CB (Venky's) | Alpha-amylase, cellulase, alpha-galactosidase, beta-glucanase, beta-mannanase, xylanase, pectinase, protease, lipase, phytase, bile extract | * Improves weight gain <br> * Improves FCR <br> * Reduces cost of feed per Kg of meat produced <br> * Reduces environmental pollution | 500 g / tonne of feed |
| 44 | VENZYME – CL (B. V. Biocarp/ Venky's) | Alpha-amylase, Alpha-galactosidase, Beta-glucanase, Beta-mannanase, Pectinase, Cellulase, Xylanase, Protease, Phytase | * Improves egg production <br> * Improves eggshell quality <br> * Reduces feed cost per egg produced <br> * Reduces environmental pollution | 500 g / tonne of feed |
| 45 | VENZYME YE (B. V. Biocorp/ Venky's) | Alpha-amylase, Beta-glucanase, Cellulase, Protease, | Improves FCR <br> Improves body weight gain | 500 g / tonne of feed |

| S. No. | Trade Name & Company | Composition | Indications | Dosage / Administration |
|---|---|---|---|---|
| | | Alpha-galactosidase, Beta-mannanase, Pectinase, Xylanase | Enhances the immunity Decreases the incidence of coccidiosis, *E. coli,* Salmonella | |
| 46 | WOKASE (Wockhardt) | Each g contains: 2,500 I. U. of phytase | Provides phosphorus Breaks phytate | **Add 200 g /** tonne of broiler feed (mash) **Add 250 g /** tonne of broiler feed (pellets) **Add 150 g /** tonne layer feed (mash) **Add 150 g /** tonne of layer feed (pellets) |
| 47 | XYLANASE-PC POWDER (Kaypeeyes Biotech) | Contains: Xylanases, Polygalacturonase, Phytase, Proteases, Pectinase, Cellulase and other digestive enzymes | * For prevention of wet droppings<br>* For higher energy gain and mineral assimilation<br>* Reduces stress on birds | **Broilers:** 500 g / tonne of feed **Layers / Breeders:** 750 g / tonne of feed during first week and 500 / tonne of feed during subsequent weeks |

## 19. HATCHLING SUPPLEMENT

| S. No. | Trade Name & Company | Composition | Indications | Dosage/ Administration |
|---|---|---|---|---|
| 1 | OASIS (Venky's) | Nutrients: Crude protein – 20%, Crude fat – 0.5%, Crude fibre – 3%, Moisture minimum – 25%, pH between 4 and 5 | * A better start for better bird<br>* Stimulates gut growth<br>* It delivers complete nutrition and greater flexibility<br>* Benefits to immune system<br>* Increases initial body weight and improves growth<br>* Improves pullet uniformity<br>* Improves livability<br>* Improves egg production | 1. Chicks are fed Oasis either **at hatchery** in the transport box, or 2. At the farm as a top-dressing application over starter feed **In Transport Box:** 200 – 250 g / 100 chicks. Distribute evenly as the box is sub-divided into quadrants. **Farm (Top-dress application):** Between 200-250 g / 100 chicks / day for first 2-3 days. Distribute evenly on the top of the starter feed. Do not mix. |

# 20A. LIVER TONICS

| S.No. | Trade Name & Company | Composition | Indications | Dosage / Administration |
|---|---|---|---|---|
| 1 | AN LIV CARE (Vetmed or VM) | Each Kg contains: Tricholine citrate, Lecithin, Protein hydrolysate, Methyl donors, Selenium, Vit B12, Vit E, Biotin, Inositol, Base enriched with liver stimulants, mould inhibitors and toxin binders | * Better fat metabolism<br>* Better FCR and body weight in broilers<br>* Increased performance and production in layers<br>* Reduced incidence of fatty changes, gout, ascites, leechi disease and MD | **Chicks / Growers**<br>**Layers:**<br>500 g / tonne of feed<br>**Broilers:**<br>500 g to 750 g / tonne of feed<br>**Breeders:**<br>500 g to 1 kg / tonne of feed |
| 2 | BIO-LIV LIQUID/ POWDER/ (Polchem) | Each 10 ml contains: Liver extract 500 mg (derived from 12.5 g of fresh liver), Choline chloride 1000 mg, Lysine 100 mg, DL-Methionine 100 mg, Biotin 50 mcg, Inositol 35 mg, Nicotinamide 45 mg, Ferric chloride 80 mg, Vit $B_1$ 4 mg, Vit $B_{12}$ 4 mcg, Panthenol 4 mg | * Prevents fatty degeneration of liver<br>* Prevents fatty liver and kidney syndrome<br>* Corrects niacin deficiency and improves hock and leg strength<br>* Controls protein synthesis and improves liver health | **LIQUID:**<br>**Chicks:**<br>5 ml / 100 chicks daily<br>**Broilers:**<br>10 ml / 100 birds daily<br>**Growers / Layers:**<br>20 ml / 100 birds daily<br>**Breeders:**<br>25 ml / 100 birds daily<br>**POWDER:**<br>500 g to 1 Kg / tonne of feed |
| 3 | BROTONE LIQUID (Virbac)) | Each 10 ml contains : 1.25 g of liver fraction 1 (Soluble liver fraction from 31.25 g of fresh liver) with Vit $B_{12}$ activity equivalent to 7.5, Yeast extract 0.4 g, Nicotinic acid 24 mg, Alcohol 1 ml, Aqueous base 10 ml, Alcohol | * Helps liver to function at optimum levels<br>* Ensures healthy growth and productivity<br>* Improves FCR and achieves an additional weight gain<br>* Improves digestion<br>* Acts as supportive treatment in aflatoxicosis and | **Broilers :**<br>5-10 ml / 100 birds daily from 3rd to 4th week<br>**Layers :**<br>20 ml / 100 birds daily for 7 days 16th – 18th week of age<br>200 ml / 100 birds daily for 7 days during 32nd – 34th week of age. |

| S.No. | Trade Name & Company | Composition | Indications | Dosage / Administration |
|---|---|---|---|---|
| | | content 9.4% v/v | prevents fatty liver syndrome | |
| 4 | GOLDLIV PLUS POWDER (Golden Streak) | Each Kg contains : Liver extract 15 g, Tricholine citrate 20 g, Inositol 5 g, DL-Methionine 30 g, Vit C 5 g, Vit $B_{12}$ 300 mcg, Niacin 5 g, Selenium 100 mg, base q.s. | * Stimulates liver functions<br>* Corrects liver dysfunctions<br>* Optimizes liver activity under conditions of aflatoxicosis<br>* Improves efficiency of digestion and feed conversion | Broilers / Layers : 1.5-2 Kg. / tonne of feed |
| 5 | HEPATO – CARE (Varsha Group) | Liver stimulants, tricholine citrate, inositol, Vit B12, biotin, protein hydrolysate, methyl donors, Vitamin E and selenium, mould inhibitors and toxin binders (organic acid, HSCAS, MOS) | * Improves body weight, FCR<br>* Improves egg production<br>* Improves shell quality<br>* Improves hatchability and fertility,<br>* Uniform growth and speedy recovery from diseases<br>* Enhanced immunity | **Broilers:** 1 Kg / tonne of feed 10 ml / 100 birds 2days / week **Layers:** 500 g / tonne of feed 10 ml / 100 birds as week a month programme **Breeders:** 1 Kg / tonne of feed 25 ml / 100 birds as week a month programme |
| 6 | KIKK OFF LIQUID (Novartis) | Each 10 ml contains : Choline chloride 2000 mg, Liver extract 125 mg, Yeast extract 40 mg, Vit $B_1$ 2.5 mg, Vit $B_{12}$ 0.75 mcg, Niacin 24 mg, DL-Panthenol 2.5 mg, Inositol 35 mg | * Improves liver function<br>* Enhances performance like better weight gain in broiler and production in layers<br>* Protects birds from toxins in contaminated feeds | **Broilers:** 5-10 ml / 100 birds daily **Layers:** 20 ml / 100 birds daliy |
| 7 | LIPO-CARE (Varsha Group) | It is a combination of lecithin (PC), emulsifiers and lipase promoting factor (LPF) to provide safe and better replacement of | * Better digestion and utilization of fat<br>* Better and effective replacement of choline chloride<br>* Better absorption of fat soluble vitamins | **Broilers:** 1000 to 1500 g / tonne of feed **Growers / Layers:** 250 – 500 g / tonne of feed **Breeders:** |

| S.No. | Trade Name & Company | Composition | Indications | Dosage / Administration |
|---|---|---|---|---|
| | | choline chloride | | 1500 g / tonne of feed |
| 8 | LIVERACT PLUS SOLUTION (AVR) | Each 10 ml contains : Choline chloride 2.2 g, Liver extract 150 mg, Thiamine 20 mg, Cyano-cobalamin 0.95 mg, Nicotinic acid 25 mg, DL-Methionine 1 g, Inositol 15 mg, Protein hydrolysate 100 mg, Ascorbic acid 75 mg | * Stimulates liver functions<br>* Prevents fatty liver and kidney syndrome<br>* Improves efficiency of digestion and feed conversion<br>  5-□ Controls ascites | **Broilers:**<br>5-10 ml / 100 birds daily<br>**Layers:**<br>20 ml / 100 birds daily<br>For 3-5 days |
| 9 | LIVER PLUS LIQUID (Elpe Labs) | Each 10 ml contains : Choline chloride 1500 mg, L-Lysine 125 mg, DL-Methionine 125 mg, D-Biotin 50 mcg, Inositol 50 mg, Vit $B_{12}$ 100 mcg | * Acute fatty liver and kidney conditions<br>* Retarded growth, specially in broilers<br>* Low feed conversion<br>* Reduced fed intake<br>* Aflatoxicosis<br>* Perosis | **Prophylactic:**<br>10 ml / 100 birds<br>**For growth:**<br>20 ml / 100 birds<br>**In acute cases:**<br>2-3 ml / litre of water per day for 5-7 days |
| 10 | LIVOGUARD (Indian Drugs & Vitamins) | Each 10 ml contains: Vitamins, chelated minerals, electrolytes, various amino acids, liver extract, and yeast extract | It stimulates appetite, corrects anorexia rapidly, improves feed intake, FCR, and weight gain | **Broilers:**<br>10 ml / 100 birds / day from 7th day till marketing<br>**Layers:**<br>15 ml /100 birds for liver stimulation<br>**Breeders:**<br>20 ml / 100 birds for liver stimulation |
| 11 | LIVOTAL (Qualitat) | Each 10 ml contains: Tricholine citrate – 100 mg, choline chloride – 1000 mg, methionine – 10 mg, liver extract 50 mg, protein hydrolysate – 50 mg, inositol – 2 mg | * Detoxifies the aflatoxins<br>* Enhances immune system<br>* Regulates rapid body weight<br>* Improves FCR | **Chicks:**<br>5 ml / 100 birds<br>**Broilers / Growers:**<br>15 ml / 100 birds<br>**Layers:**<br>20 – 25 ml / 100 birds |
| 12 | LIVOTAL FORTE Inj (Qualitat) | Each ml contains: Vitamin B1 25 mg, Vit. B2, 1.37 mg, Vit. | * It is very useful for non-specific anorexia and liver | **Use one 30 ml vial:**<br>Up to 500 g body weight |

| S.No. | Trade Name & Company | Composition | Indications | Dosage / Administration |
|---|---|---|---|---|
| | | B12 30 mcg, Choline chloride 15 mg, D – Pantothenol 5 mg, Nicotinamide 100 mg, Lignocaine HCL 100 1% w/v, Liver injection crude 0.66 ml | disorders<br>* Prevents liver damage due to mycotoxins, pesticide residues and bacterial toxins<br>* Stimulates liver functions<br>* To combat stress<br>* Provides additional nutrients in the form of choline chloride and vitamins | for 2500 birds<br><br>Up to 800 g body weight for 1500 birds<br><br>Up to 1000 g body weight for 800 birds |
| 13 | LIVTON – S (Vetline) | Each 10 ml contains: Choline chloride 2000 mg, liver extract 125 mg, yeast extract 40 mg, Vitamin B1 2.5 mg, Vitamin B12 0.75 mcg, niacin 24 mg, dl – panthenol 2.5 mg, and inositol 35 mg | As a general liver tonic to boost liver functions | **Broilers:**<br>5-10 ml / 100 birds $2^{nd}$ to $6^{th}$ week<br>**Growers / Layers:**<br>20 ml for 10 days |
| 14 | NUTRILIV FORTE LIQUID (Vetcare) | Each 10 ml contains : Choline chloride 2000 mg, Liver extract 125 mg, Yeast extract 40 mg, Vit $B_1$ 2.5 mg, Vit $B_{12}$ 0.75 mcg, Niacin 24 mg, DL-Panthenol 2.5 mg, Inositol 35 mg, Solubilizing agents added | * Prevents liver damage due to mycotoxins, pesticide residues, and bacterial toxins<br>* Stimulates liver functions<br>* To combat stress<br>* Provides additional nutrients in the form of choline chloride and vitamins | **Broilers:**<br>5-10 ml / 100 birds from $2^{nd}$ – $6^{th}$ week<br>**Layers :**<br>20 ml / 100 birds daily for 7 days<br>**In case of liver damage:**<br>10-20 ml / 100 birds for 5-7 days |
| 15 | UPLIV-FORTE LIQUID (Venky's) | Each 10 ml contains: Choline chloride 2000 mg, Liver extract 175 mg, Yeast | * Keeps liver healthy from ill- effects of toxins<br>* For supplementation | 15-20 ml / 1,000 birds 5 days in a month |

| S.No. | Trade Name & Company | Composition | Indications | Dosage / Administration |
|-------|---------------------|-------------|-------------|------------------------|
| | | extract 50 mg, Vitamin B$_1$ 2.5 mg, Vit B$_{12}$ 0.75 mcg, Niacin 24 mg, D-Panthenol 2.5 mg, Inositol 35 mg, DL-Methionine 25 mg, L-Lysine 150 mg, Manganese 7.68 mg, Zinc 4.3 mg | in toxic condition, fatty liver condition and other hepatic irregularities <br> * For supplementation in deficiencies <br> * As general liver toner to use regularly to enhance liver functioning <br> * Improves FCR and weight gain | |

# 20B. HERBAL LIVER TONICS

| S. No. | Trade Name & Company | Composition | Indications | Dosage / Administration |
|--------|---------------------|-------------|-------------|------------------------|
| 1 | DETOX-FS LIQUID CONCENTRATE (Neospark) | Each 100 g contains : *Aphanamixis polystachia* 2 g, *Phyllanthus niruri* 5 g, *Eclipta alba* 5 g, *Andrographis paniculata* 5 g, *Picrorhiza kurroa* 01 g, *Tinospora cordifolia* 15 g, *Naregamia alata* 2g, *Emblica offcinalis* 5 g, Excipient q.s. | * Aflatoxicosis, leg weakness and diffuse diseases of liver <br> * For improved livability, increased body resistance feed efficiency, higher egg production in layers and more weight gains in broilers <br> * Against all types of stress | **Broilers:** **Starters:** 10 ml / 100 birds **Finishers:** 20 ml / 100 birds **Layers:** **Chicks:** 5 ml / 100 birds **Growers:** 15 ml / 100 birds **Layers:** 20 ml / 100 birds |
| 2 | DETOX-FS POWDER (Neospark) | Extract of 11 herbs : 99% Calcium : 450 ppm Phosphorus : 340 ppm Polysaccharides with Predigested protein : 10,000 ppm | * Aflatoxicosis, leg weakness and diffuse diseases of liver <br> * For improved livability, increased body resistance, feed efficiency, higher egg production in layers and more weight gains in broilers <br> * Against all types of stress | **Chicks / Growers / Layers:** 2.5-5 Kg / tonne of feed **Broilers/Starters/ Finishers:** 2.5-5 Kg / tonne of feed for 5-7 days |
| 3 | ENLIV HP POWDER | Each 100 g contains : *Aphanamixis polystachia* | * Prevents aflatoxicosis <br> * Improves liver | 250 g / tonne of feed |

| S. No. | Trade Name & Company | Composition | Indications | Dosage / Administration |
|---|---|---|---|---|
| | (Sarabhai Zydus) | 2 g, *Phyllanthus niruri* 5 g, *Eclipta alba* 5 g, *Andrographis paniculata* 5 g, *Picrorhiza kurroa* 0.1 g, *Tinospora cordifolia* 15 g, *Naregamia alata* 2 g, *Emblica officinalis* 5 g, *Excipient q.s.* | function<br>* Prevents fatty liver syndrome<br>* Maximizes utilization of feed<br>* Improves production performance in layers and broilers | |
| 4 | GEOLIV (Guybro) | Herbal ingredients with hydro-biotite base | * To protect liver from hepatotoxins<br>* For better feed assimilation and immune response<br>* For restoration of health and production | 500 g – 1 Kg / tonne of feed |
| 5 | GOLDLIV HERBAL LIQUID / POWDER (Golden Streak) | Each 5 ml contains : *Tephrosia purpurea* 800 mg, *Eclipta alba* 400 mg, *Phyllanthus niruri* 400 mg, *Andrographis paniculata* 200 mg, *Terminalia chebula* 200 mg, *Oscimum sanctum* 200 mg | * Protects the liver from aflatoxins<br>* Helps to treat and prevent enlarged liver and kidney<br>* Increases egg production in layers and weight gain in broilers<br>* Improves feed efficiency | LIQUID:<br>**Broilers:**<br>0-4 weeks 10 ml / 100 birds<br>5-8 weeks 20 ml / 100 birds<br>**Layers:**<br>**Chicks:**<br>5 ml / 100 chicks<br>**Growers:**<br>15 ml / 100 birds<br>**Layers:**<br>20 ml / 100 birds<br>**POWDER:**<br>500 g / tonne of feed |
| 6 | HARSH-O-LIV-LIQUID (Harshvardhan 's Lab) | *Boerhaavia diffusa* – 10% *Picrorhiza kurroa* – 7.5% *Terminalia chebula* 10%, *Amoora rohituka* 7.5%, *Eclipta alba* -10% *Embelia ribes* – 5% Aloe – 5% Licorice – 5% *Ocimum sanctum* – 5% Indian celery seed oil – 0.25 % Sua oil – 0.25% | * To control toxins in aflatoxicosis<br>* To improve body resistance<br>* To attain uniform growth<br>* To boost up liver<br>* To check leg weakness<br>* Improve FCR<br>* For better livability | **Chicks:**<br>5 ml / 100 birds / day<br>**Growers:**<br>7.5 ml / 100 birds / day<br>**Layers:**<br>10 ml / 100 birds / day<br>**Broiler starters:**<br>5 ml / 100 birds / day<br>**Broiler finishers:** |

| S. No. | Trade Name & Company | Composition | Indications | Dosage / Administration |
|---|---|---|---|---|
| | | | | 10 ml / 100 birds / day |
| 7 | HARSH – O – LIV PREMIX (Harshvardhan 's Lab) | Polyherbal formulation containing: *Andrographis paniculata, Azadirachta indica, Boerhaavia diffusa, Picrorrhiza kurroa, Swertia chirata, Phyllanthus niruri* | * Hepato-protective<br>* Enhances growth, weight gain, FCR, livability<br>* Enhances liver metabolism and reduces ill effects of aflatoxins, pesticides, antibiotics | 250 g / tonne of feed |
| 8 | HEPACEF LIQUID (Concept) | Contains 16 unique herbal aqueous extracts: Kutaki 12.5 mg, Bhringaraj 375mg, Sariva 437.5 mg, Ashwagandha 187.5 mg, Yashthimadhu 750 mg, Sarapunkha 750 mg, Shatavari 187.5 mg, Pippali 125, Maricha 125 mg, Shunthi 125mg, Vacha 125 mg, Rohitak 375 mg, Chitraka 125 mg, Punarnava 375 mg, Bhumyamalaki 375 mg, Trifala 750 mg | * Protects liver from aflatoxicosis<br>* Provides higher immune status<br>* Assures increased weight gain in broilers and improves egg production in layers<br>* Ensures better FCR | **Broilers:**<br>**1ˢᵗ week** – 2 ml / 100 birds in drinking water (add 2 ml for each week)<br>**Layers:**<br>**1ˢᵗ week** – 1 ml / 100 birds in drinking water (add 1 ml for each week) |
| 9 | HEPACEF VET POWDER FEED-SUPPLEMENT (Concept) | Contains 16 unique herbal aqueous extracts. Each 100 g contains: Kutaki 1.5 mg, Bhringaraj 0.5 g, Sariva 1.3 g, Ashwagandha 1 g, Yashthimadhu 3.75 g, Sarapunkha 3.75 g, Shatavari 1 g, Pippali 0.62 g,Maricha 0.62 g, Shunthi 0.62 g, Vacha 0.62g, Rohitak 1.9 g, Chitraka 0.62 g, Punarnava 1.9 g, Bhumyamalaki 1.9 g, Trifala 3.75 g | * Higher weight gain<br>* Increased egg production<br>* More chick per breeder bird<br>* Improved flock performance | **Broiler Feed:**<br>250 – 500 g / tonne of feed<br>**Layer Feed:**<br>**Chicks:**<br>250 g / tonne of feed<br>**Growers / Layers:**<br>250 g – 500 g / tonne of feed<br>**Breeder Feed:**<br>500-1000 g/ tonne of feed |
| 10 | HEPAGEST LIQUID / | LIQUID:<br>Each 100 ml contains : | * Aflatoxicosis<br>* Anorexia | LIQUID:<br>Chicks: |

| S. No. | Trade Name & Company | Composition | Indications | Dosage / Administration |
|---|---|---|---|---|
| | POWDER (Alembic) | Kalmegh (S) *Andrographis paniculata* (L) 10 g, Bhringraj (S) *Eclipta elba* (L) 10 g, *Bakul chal (S) Mimusops elen (L)* 20 g, *Punarnava mool (S) Boerhavia diffusa (L)* 10 g, water q.s. **POWDER :** Each 100 g contains : Kalmegh (s) *Andrographis paniculata (L)* 20 g, Bhringraj (S) *Eclipta elba (L)* 20 g, *Bakul chal (S) Mimusops elen* (L) 40 g, *Punarnava mool* (S) *Boerhavia diffusa (L)* 20 g, excipients q.s. | * Fatty liver<br>* As a growth promoter | 3 ml / 1000 chicks / day **Growers:** 7 ml / 1000 birds / day **Broilers / Layers:** 10 ml / 1000 birds / day **POWDER:** 500 g – 1 Kg / tonne of feed |
| 11 | HI-LIV LIQUID (Hitha) | Rare combination of selected herbs | * General liver disorders<br>* Fights against aflatoxins<br>* Antiviral<br>* Increases resistance against diseases<br>* Better FCR<br>* Rejuvenator | **Through drinking water:** **Chicks:** 2 ml / 100 birds / day **Broilers:** 0-4 weeks – 3 ml / 100 birds / day 5th – 8th week – 6 ml / 100 birds/day **Growers:** 4 ml / 100 birds / day **Layers:** 6 ml / 100 birds / day |
| 12 | LIMEX POWDER (Indo Biocare) | A herbal liver tonic | * Neutralizes the damaging effects of aflatoxins<br>* Fatty liver infiltration | 500-750 g / tonne of feed |

| S. No. | Trade Name & Company | Composition | Indications | Dosage / Administration |
|---|---|---|---|---|
| | | | * Anorexia<br>* Malnutrition<br>* Acts as growth promoter in young birds<br>* Helps in better weight gain in broilers | |
| 13 | LIV-52 PROTEC LIQUID (Himalaya) | A herbal liver tonic | * Protects liver from various toxins, chemicals, etc.<br>* Useful in aflatoxicosis, hepatitis, ascites, fatty liver disease and toxaemia<br>* Growth promoter, production enhancer, and hepatic stimulant | **Chicks:**<br>5 ml / 100 birds / day<br>**Growers:**<br>10 ml / 100 birds / day<br>**Layers / Broilers:**<br>20 ml / 100 birds / day |
| 14 | LIV-52 PROTEC FEED SUPPLEMENT (Himalaya) | Each g contains :<br>**Pdrs:**<br>Nimba 270 mg,<br>Bhringaraja 135 mg<br>Bhumyaamlaki 135 mg,<br>Haritaki<br>135 mg, Yasada bhasma<br>100 mg<br>**Exts:**<br>Kasani 113 mg, Arjuna 56 mg,<br>Kakamachi 56 mg | * Useful in aflatoxicosis, hepatitis, ascites, fatty liver disease and toxaemia<br>* Growth promoter, production enhancer, and hepatic stimulant | **Chicks:**<br>250 g / tonne of feed<br>**Broilers / Layers:**<br>250 g / tonne of feed<br>**Breeders:**<br>500 g / tonne of feed |
| 15 | LIVER ACT VET (AVR) | *Tephrosia purpurea, Emblica officinalis, Ocimum sanctum, Sida rbombifolia,* | * A powerful hepato-stimulator and removes congestion of liver<br>* Protects liver from harmful toxins<br>* Prevents fatty liver kidney syndrome,<br>* A powerful performance booster, increases body weight and egg production<br>* Fights aflatoxins, improves liver's | 1 Kg / tonne of feed |

| S. No. | Trade Name & Company | Composition | Indications | Dosage / Administration |
|---|---|---|---|---|
| | | | detoxification capacity and increases body resistance | |
| 16 | LIVEROLIN LIQUID (Vetnex) | *Solanum nigrum* 3%, *Tephrosia purpurea* 4%, *Fumaria parviflora* 2%, *Cichorium intybus* 2.5%, *Andrographis paniculata* 3%, *Terminalia chebula* 2%, *Eclipta alba* 2%, *Swertia chirata* 1%, *Glycyrrhiza glabra* 1%, *Tachyspermum ammi* 2%, *and Boerhavaaia diffusa* 2% | For liver disorders and as a liver rejuvenating performance enhancer | 5-10 ml / 100 birds daily in drinking water |
| 17 | LIVEROLIN FORTE ( Vetnex) | A concentrate for use as feed additive with 21 herbs including Silymargin | For liver disorders and as a liver rejuvenating performance enhancer | 250 g / tonne of feed |
| 18 | LIVER-UP LIQUID (Sarabhai Zydus) | Each 5 ml contains (extract of): *Andrographis paniculata* (Kalmegh) 400 mg, *Eclipta alba* (Bhringaraja) 300 mg, *Phyllanthus niruri* (Bhumyaamalaki) 250 mg, *Boerhaavia diffusa* (Punarnava) 200 mg, *Picrorhiza kurroa* (Kutki) 100 mg, *Chicorium intybus* (Kasni) 166.75 mg | * FCR, growth and production failure, Immuno-suppression<br>* Hepatic dysfunction<br>* Hepatic damage due to fungal and other hepatotoxins<br>* Fatty liver disease<br>* Prophylaxis against drug- induced hepatotoxicity | **Broilers:** 5-10 ml / 100 birds daily<br>**Layers:**<br>**Chicks** – 5 ml /100 birds daily<br>**Growers** – 7.5 ml / 100 birds daily<br>**Layers** – 10 ml / 100 birds daily |
| 19 | LIVFIT VET LIQUID / PREMIX (Ayurvet) | Major herbs : *Andrographis paniculata, Eclipta alba, Picrorhiza kurroa,* | * Fights aflatoxins<br>* Improves FCR<br>* Enhances growth rate<br>* Improves egg | **Premix:** 2 Kg / tonne of feed<br>**Liquid:**<br>**Chicks:** |

| S. No. | Trade Name & Company | Composition | Indications | Dosage / Administration |
|---|---|---|---|---|
| | | *Phyllanthus niruri* | production in layers<br>* Helps in increasing body weight in broilers<br>* Increases disease resistance | 5 ml / 100 birds / day<br>**Growers:**<br>10 ml / 100 birds / day<br>**Broilers / Layers:**<br>20 ml / 100 birds / day for 7 days |
| 20 | LIVGROW (Natural herbs) | Each 10 ml contains: Ecliptaalba, *Picrorrhiza, kurroa, Andrographis paniculata, Tephrosia purpurea, Emblica officinale, Phyllanthus niruri, Terminalia arjuna, Zingiber officinale, Ocimum sanctum* | * Stimulates hepatic microsomal enzyme system<br>* Improves weight gain, and growth<br>* Protects liver against mycotoxins, antibiotics, anthelmintic | **Chicks:**<br>5 ml / 100 birds / day<br>**Growers:**<br>10 ml / 100 birds / day<br>**Layers/Broilers:**<br>20 ml / 100 birds day |
| 21 | LIVITO (Natural herbs) | A herbal combination | * Enhances growth, weight gain, FCR,<br>* Maintains digestion, absorption, and health<br>* Protects hepatic functions<br>* Inhibits growth of toxins in feed<br>* Counteracts on ill effects of chemical toxins | 250 g / tonne of feed |
| 22 | LIVOMARK (Exotic Mushrooms) | Each 1 Kg contains: *Azardirachta indica Tinospora cordifolia Tephrosia purpurea* Choline chloride | * Regains the tone of sluggish liver and repairs hepatic cells<br>* Choline chloride mobilizes the fat from the liver to make it metabolically active | 500 g – 1 Kg / tonne of feed |
| 23 | LIVOL PFS CONCENTRATE LIQUID (Natural Remedies) | *Andrographis paniculata, Boerhaavia diffusa, Eclipta alba, Phyllanthus amarus* | * To counteract ill effects of aflatoxins and other hepato-toxins<br>* To improve FCR, growth, performance and productivity | **Broilers:**<br>0-2nd week – 2 ml / 100 birds<br>3rd – 4th week – 4 ml / 100 birds<br>5th week onwards – 7 ml / 100 birds |

| S. No. | Trade Name & Company | Composition | Indications | Dosage / Administration |
|---|---|---|---|---|
| | | | * To improve livability | **Layers:** **Chicks : 0-2ⁿᵈ week** 2 ml / 100 birds **Growers: 3ʳᵈ-4ᵗʰ week** 4 ml / 100 birds **Layers: 21ˢᵗ – 72ⁿᵈ week** 7 ml / 100 birds |
| 24 | LIVOLIV 250 POWDER (Indian Herbs) | A herbal preparation | * Liver tonic and growth promoter <br> * Digestive and metabolic stimulant <br> * Mould inhibitor and mycotoxin binder | **Broilers:** 250 g / tonne of feed from day one till marketing **Layers:** 250 g / tonne of feed 0-20 weeks and 21-72 weeks |
| 25 | LIVOLIV LIQUID (Indian Herbs) | A herbal preparation | * Liver tonic and growth promoter <br> * Digestive and metabolic stimulant <br> * Mould inhibitor and mycotoxin binder | **Broilers:** 0-2 week – 5 ml / 100 birds 3-4 week – 10 ml / 100 birds 5ᵗʰ week & onwards – 20 ml / 100 birds **Layers:** **Chicks:** 5 ml / 100 birds **Growers:** 10 ml / 100 birds **Layers:** 20 ml / 100 birds |
| 26 | LIVOPLEX (Qualitat) | Each litre contains: Kasaundi -7000 mg, Makoh – 7000 mg, Choline chloride – 2500 mg, Methionine – 1000 mg, Zinc – 1250 mg, Vit B12 – 666 mcg, Vit B1 – 180 mg, Folic acid – 135 mg | * Overcomes aflatoxin toxicity <br> * Improves FCR <br> * Overcomes all stress | **Chicks:** 5 ml / 100 birds **Broilers / Growers:** 10 ml / 100 birds **Layers:** 20 ml / 100 birds |
| 27 | LIVOTOX (Indian Herbs) | Herbal preparation | * Counteracts mycotoxins and | 500 g / tonne of feed |

| S. No. | Trade Name & Company | Composition | Indications | Dosage / Administration |
|---|---|---|---|---|
| - | | | improves liver functions <br> * Improves FCR <br> * Prevents damages caused by mycotoxins | |
| 28 | NATURALIV (Natural Remedies) | Productivity booster | * To optimize the egg production, body weight gain, FCR, and livability <br> * To maintain proper digestion and absorption of nutrients <br> * To optimize liver functions and helps in better utilization of fat and fat-soluble vitamins | **Powder:** 250 g / tonne of feed **Liquid:** 0 - 2 week 10 ml / 100 birds; 3rd - 4th week in 15 ml / 100 birds, 5th week onwards 25 ml / 100 birds **Layers:** **Chicks:** 10 ml / 100 birds **Growers:** 15 ml / 100 birds **Layers:** 25 ml / 100 birds |
| 29 | NUTRILIV HERBAL LIQUID (Vetcare) | Each 10 ml contains: Choline chloride1000 mg, Liver extract 75 mg, Yeast extract 40 mg, Vit B1 2500 mcg, Vit B120.45 mcg, Niacin 25, mg, DL-Panthenol 2.5 mg Inositol 20 mg, **Herbal extract of** *Phyllanthus niruri, Andrographis paniculata, Tinospora cordifolia* q.s. | * To minimize and prevent liver damage <br> * To prevent fatty changes of liver <br> * To neutralize hepatic intoxication <br> * To correct hepatic insufficiency | **Layers and Breeders:** 20 ml / 100 birds as a week a month **Broilers:** 10 ml / 100 birds from $2^{nd}$ to $3^{rd}$ week 20 ml / 100 birds from $4^{th}$ <br><br> week onwards |
| 30 | NUTRILIV HERBAL POWDER (Vetcare) | Each Kg contains: Choline chloride 30 g, Niacin 1 g, Liver extract 10 g, Yeast extract 15 g, Herbal extract q. s. containing: *Phyllanthus niruri, Andrographis paniculata, Tinospora cardifolia, Piper longum* | * To optimize liver functions <br> * To protect from hepatic damage due to various reasons Improves liver secretions for better digestion | 250 – 500 g / tonne of feed |

| S. No. | Trade Name & Company | Composition | Indications | Dosage / Administration |
|---|---|---|---|---|
| 31 | REJU LIV FORTE (Vetmed) | Each 10 ml contains: Liver extract 125 mg, Yeast extract 40 mg, Choline chloride 2 g, Vitamin B1 2.5 mg, Vitamin B12 0.75 mg, Niacin 24 mg, Inositol 35 mg, DL-panthanol 2.5 mg, Biotin 25 mcg | * Strongly stimulates liver function<br>* Enhances immune response<br>* Protects liver from effects of toxins<br>* Treats the fatty liver condition | **Growers / Layers:** 20 ml / 100 birds daily for 10 days<br>**Broilers:** 5-10 ml daily from $2^{nd}$ to $6^{th}$ week / 100 birds |
| 32 | SUPERLIV LIQUID / PREMIX (Ayurvet) | A polyherbal formulation containing extract of herbal ingredients | * Improves growth rate, body weight and egg production<br>* Improves Feed Conversion Ratio (FCR)<br>* Reduces incidence of liver disorders | **Liquid:**<br>**Chicks:** 5 ml / 100 birds / day<br>**Growers:** 10 ml / 100 birds / day<br>**Layers / Finishers:** 20 ml / 100 birds / day<br>**Premix:** 500 g / tonne of feed |
| 33 | SUPERLIV DS PREMIX (Ayurvet) | Fortified and improved formula. Active ingredients are in higher strength | * Improves growth rate, body weight and egg production<br>* Improves Feed Conversion Ratio (FCR)<br>* Reduces incidence of liver disorders | 250 g / tonne of feed |
| 34 | TEPHROMIX POWDER (Polchem) | *Tephrosia purpurea* (Sharpunka), *Ocimum sanctum* (Tulsi), *Andrographic paniculata* (Kalmegh), *Azadirachta indica* (Neem), *Tinospora cordofolia* (Gulvel Amruta), *Boerhaavaia diffusa* (Punarnava), and *Picrorhiza kurrow* ('Kutki') | * Protects and corrects liver and promotes growth<br>* To increase FCR in broilers<br>* To increase egg production in layers<br>* Severe stress conditions<br>* Mortality due to fatty liver condition<br>* Neutralizes toxic effects | 150 g / tonne of feed |

| S. No. | Trade Name & Company | Composition | Indications | Dosage / Administration |
|---|---|---|---|---|
| 35 | VENTRILIV LIQUID (Venky's) | Extracts of herbs, Sodium Taurocholate, Sodium glycocholate, and Activated atapulgite | * Improves digestion and feed conversion<br>* Improves detoxification, keeps liver healthy<br>* Acts as a toxin binder | 15-20 ml / 100 birds 5 days in a month |
| 36 | VENTRILIV FORTE POWDER (Venky's) | Extracts of herbs, Sodium Taurocholate, Sodium glycocholate, and Activated atapulgite | * Improves digestion and feed conversion<br>* Improves detoxification, keeps liver healthy<br>* Acts as a toxin binder | 500 g – 1 Kg / tonne of feed daily |
| 37 | VENTRILIV PLUS CONCENTRATE (Venky's) | Herbal feed concentrate exhibiting hepatogenic, hepatoprotective, digestive, and metabolic stimulant properties | * For effective liver function and metabolism<br>* Supports optimal growth and in-time maturity<br>* To counteract the damaging effect of mycotoxins / chemicals / drugs<br>* For improving livability, production, resistance and better FCR | 500 g / tonne of feed continuously for broilers, layers, and breeders |
| 38 | X-LIVPRO PREMIX (Ayurvet) | *Andrographis paniculata*<br>*Azadirachta indica*<br>*Tinospora cordifolia*<br>*Solanum nigrum*<br>*Boerhaavia diffusa*<br>*Eclipta alba*<br>*Phyllanthus niruri*<br>*Phyllanthus emblica* | * For maintaining and improving liver functions<br>* For protecting and correcting the damaging effects of aflatoxins<br>* Improves growth rate<br>* Improves FCR, meat yield, and livability | 250 g / tonne of feed |

# 21. MALE AND FEMALE REPRODUCTIVE PERFORMANCE ENHANCERS

| S. No. | Trade Name & Company | Composition | Indications | Dosage / Administration |
|---|---|---|---|---|
| 1 | EGUP (Natural Remedies) | A herbal preparation | To optimize egg production after 45th week | **Broiler Breeders:** 60 g / 1000 birds per day for 10 days through feed **Layer Breeders:** 45 g / 1000 birds per day for 10 days through feed |
| 2 | LIBIDO-ON (Natural Herbs) | Ashvagandha, Shilajeet, Safed Musli, Satavar, Kesar, Almond oil | * Improves libido, sexual function and semen quality <br> * Useful in development and maturity of sex organs <br> * Enhances spermatogenesis and fertility index of spermatozoa | 50 g / 100 birds for 7 – 10 days every month |
| 3 | PROLIBID (Indian Herbs) | A herbal preparation | * To improve semen volume with proper viscosity <br> * For full development and functional maturation of sexual organs <br> * For improving libido and sexual behaviour | 50 g / 100 birds for 7-10 days every month |
| 4 | SPEMAN FORTE VET (Himalaya) | It is a herbal preparation, and includes four important herbs namely Gokshura, Jivanti, Kumkuma and Ashvagandha | * Improves semen quality and quantity <br> * Improves fertility and hatchability <br> * Improves libido | 0.5 g / bird / day for 10 days, to be repeated every month |
| 5 | SPEMAN VET (Himalaya) | Each g contains : **Pdrs:** Salabmisri *(Orchis* | To increase sperm count, sperm motility, seminal | 0.5 g / bird for at least 1 week every month |

701

| S. No. | Trade Name & Company | Composition | Indications | Dosage / Administration |
|---|---|---|---|---|
| | | *mascula)* 0.253 g, Vanya kahu *(Lactuca scariola)* 0.062 g, *Hygrophila spinosa* 0.125 g, *Kapikachchhu (Mucuna-pruriens)* 0.062 g, Suvarnavang *(Mosaic gold)* 0.062 g **Exts:** Shaileyam *(Parmelia perlata)* 0.062 g, Vriddadaru*(Argyreia speciosa)* 0.125 g, Gokshura *(Tribulus terrestris)* 0.125 g, Jeevanti *(Leptadenia-□eticulate)* 0.062 g | volume and viscosity and viability of spermatozoa | |
| 6 | TENTEX FORTE VET (Himalaya) | A herbal preparation containing 14 herbs | To increase sperm count, sperm motility, volume and viability of the spermatozoa | 0.5 g / bird for at least 1 week every month |

## 22. MICROBIAL ENVIRONMENT CONDITIONER

| S.No. | Trade Name & Company | Composition | Indications | Dosage / Administration |
|---|---|---|---|---|
| 1 | SANIPRO (Intvet IVPL) | Indigenous, beneficial, naturally occurring environmental bacteria, with beneficial Lactobcillus | * Reduces pathogenic bacterial load in environment<br>* Reduces pathogenic bacterial load in litter<br>* Reduces bad odour<br>* Stabilizes and balances external ecosystem | After disinfection, mix 1 litre Sanipro in 25 litres of water. Liberally spray in brooders / roofs / cages / litter in approximately 9000 sq. ft. area Absolutely safe for birds. Can be sprayed when birds are housed. |

# 23. MINERALS

| S. No. | Trade Name & Company | Composition | Indications | Dosage / Administration |
|---|---|---|---|---|
| 1 | AQUAMIN-VET LIQUID (Elpe) | Each 5 ml contains : Copper sulphate 50 mg, Cobalt chloride 1 mg, Ferrous sulphate 300 mg, Manganese sulphate 800 mg, Potassium iodide 30 mg, Magnesium sulphate 100 mg, Zinc sulphate 800 mg, Sodium selenite 100 mcg | * Muscular weakness<br>* Anaemic conditions<br>* Retarded growth<br>* Poor feather or hair growth<br>* Leg weakness<br>* Soft shell | 12-15 ml / 100 birds for 7-10 days |
| 2 | AV – MIN LIQUID (AVR) (Mineral + amino acid) | Each 500 ml contains: Methionine -- 118 g, Lysine – 62 g, Choline chloride  - 62 g, Sodium – 450 mg, Phosphorus – 150 mg, Magnesium 575 mg, Zinc – 210 mg, Calcium 900 mg, Iron – 220 mg, Copper – 155 mg, Cobalt – 200 mg, Manganese – 380 mg | * To improve growth and for better weight gains<br>* To overcome leg weakness<br>* To minimize the loss of body weight during summer stress<br>* To make up amino acid and mineral deficiencies | **Broilers:** 5-10 ml / 100 birds |
| 3 | ALKOSEL (B.V. Bio-Corp) | An inactivated whole cell yeast (*Saccharomyces cerevisiae*) containing elevated levels of selenium in its natural food form L (+) selenomethionine | * Improves hatchability<br>* Improves egg shelf life<br>* Enhances passive immunity<br>* Better resistance against stress<br>* Improves meat and egg quality | **Broilers / Layers / Breeders:** 150 g / tonne of feed |
| 4 | AVR TRCEMIN POWDER (AVR) | Each Kg contains – **According to one leaflet:** Manganese 150 g, Zinc 120g, Iron 90 g, Copper 15 g, Iodine 1.5 g, Selenium 150 mg **According to another leaflet:** Zinc 6.0%, Manganese 4.8%, Ferrous 2.0%, Copper 0.5% , Sodium 110 mg, Iodine 1.5 % | Trace mineral deficiency conditions | 1 Kg / tonne of feed |

| S. No. | Trade Name & Company | Composition | Indications | Dosage / Administration |
|---|---|---|---|---|
| 5 | BIOPLEX POULTRY PAK (Alltech Inc) | A complete package of organic minerals from Alltech (Biolpex Zn, Mn, Fe, Cu, EDDI – Iodine, Sel – plex, Se and organic chromium) | * As a replacement for inorganic trace minerals in all species of poultry<br>* To enhance poultry performance when used on top of inorganic trace minerals | **In Feed:** Complete replacement of inorganic minerals **Breeders:** 1 Kg / tonne of feed **Layers:** 350 – 500 g / tonne of feed **Broilers** 500 g / tonne of feed **On top of inorganic minerals:** 250 – 500 g / tonne of feed |
| 6 | BREEDER-TM POWDER (Harshvardhan's Lab) | Each Kg contains: Manganese 100 g, Zinc 75 g, Iron 100 g, Copper 10 g, Iodine 1.1 g, Cobalt 0.39 g, Selenium 0.28 g, Molybdenum 1 g | Minerals recommended for all kinds of breeder strains including chicks, growers and adults | 1 Kg / tonne of feed |
| 7 | BROILER-TM POWDER (Harshvardhan's Lab) | Each Kg contains: Manganese 70 g, Zinc 65 g, Iron 15 g, Copper 5 g, Iodine 0.5 g, Cobalt 0.3 g, Selenium 0.15 g, Molybdenum 1 g | Minerals recommended for all kinds of commercial broiler strains | 1 Kg / tonne of feed |
| 8 | BROILER TM FORTE (Harshvardhan's Lab) | Each Kg contains: Manganese 90 g, Zinc 80 g, Iron 90 g, Copper 15 g, Iodine 2 g, Selenium 0.3 g | Minerals recommended for all kinds of commercial broiler strains | 1 Kg / tonne of feed |
| 9 | EGGSHELL 49 (Alltech Inc) | Highly bioavailable trace mineral proteinates and enzyme activators | * To improve eggshell quality and strength, particularly in hens | **In Feed:** 500 g / tonne on top of inorganic |

| S. No. | Trade Name & Company | Composition | Indications | Dosage / Administration |
|---|---|---|---|---|
| | | | more than 45 weeks of age<br>* To improve hatchability in breeders<br>* Reduction in bucket eggs, down grades and cracks in layers | minerals after 45 weeks of age in layers and breeders |
| 10 | HITHA-TM POWDER (Hitha) | Each Kg contains:<br>Manganese 52 g, Zinc 35 g, Iron 20 g, Copper 5 g, Iodine 300 mg, Calcium 120 g | Helps to overcome trace mineral deficiency disorders like:<br>* Retarded growth<br>* Perosis<br>* Ruffled feathers<br>* Premature moulting<br>* Bare back | 1 Kg / tonne of feed |
| 11 | HITHA TM DS POWDER (Hitha) | Each Kg contains:<br>Manganese 104 g, Zinc 70, Iron 40 g, Copper 10 g, Iodine 600 mg, Calcium 120 g | Helps to overcome trace mineral deficiency disorders like:<br>* Retarded growth<br>* Perosis<br>* Ruffled feathers<br>* Premature moulting<br>* Bare back | 500 g / tonne of feed |
| 12 | HITHA TM + POWDER (Hitha) | Each 500 g contains :<br>Manganese 34 g, Zinc 32.5 g, Iron 12.5 g, Copper 1.25 g, Iodine 1.25 g, Calcium 60 g, Selenium 50 mg | Helps to overcome trace mineral deficiency disorders like:<br>* Retarded growth<br>* Perosis<br>* Ruffled feathers<br>* Premature moulting<br>* Bare back | 100 g / 100 kg of feed |
| 13 | IMMUNOVET LIQUID (Caretech) | Each 10 ml contains:<br>Glycine 60 mg, Vit E 27 mg, Selenium 1.2 ppm, Sodium chloride 13 mg, Potassium chloride 10 mg, Manganese sulphate 12 mg, Yeast extract 20 mg | * To tone up and maintain immune system<br>* To prevent stress | **Chicks / Growers / Broilers:**<br>5-7 ml / 100 birds<br>**Layers:**<br>10 ml / 100 birds |
| 14 | KUKKUT MIN. MIX | Calcium 30%, Phosphorus 6%, Manganese 0.32%, Zinc | High quality mineral mixture for poultry | 2.5-3% of the compounded |

| S. No. | Trade Name & Company | Composition | Indications | Dosage / Administration |
|---|---|---|---|---|
| | (Harshvardhan's Lab) | 0.32%, Copper 0.06 %, Iron 0.24%, Iodine 0.004 %, Selenium 0.0012%, Cobalt 0.0012%, Molybdenum 0.0033%, Fluorine 0.03% | | poultry feed under normal feeding conditions |
| 15 | LAYER TM FORTE (Harshvardhan's Lab) | Each Kg contains: Manganese 80 g, Zinc 80 g, Iron 60 g, Copper 15 g, Iodine 1 g, Selenium 0.3 g | Trace mineral deficiency conditions | 1 Kg / tonne of feed |
| 16 | LAYER-TM POWDER (Harshvardhan's Lab) | Each Kg contains : Manganese 40 g, Zinc 30 g, Iron 30 g, Copper 4 g, Iodine 0.5 g, Cobalt 0.3 g, Selenium 0.1 g, 100 Molybdenum 1 g | Recommended for all kinds of commercial layer strains including chicks, growers and layers | 1 Kg / tonne of feed |
| 17 | MAXMIN – B (**For broilers**) (Vetmed) | Each 1 Kg contains: Manganese 90 g, Zinc 80 g, Copper 15 g, Iron 90 g, Iodine 2 g, Cobalt 0.60 g, Selenium 0.30 g | Highly concentrated trace mineral mixture for **broilers** | 1 Kg / tonne of feed |
| 18 | MAXMIN-BR (**For breeders**) (Vetmed) | Each 1 kg contains: Manganese 100 g, Zinc 80 g, Copper 20 g, Iron 110 g, Iodine 2.50 g, Cobalt 0.60 g, Selenium 1 g | Highly concentrated trace mineral mixture for **breeders** | 1 Kg / tonne of feed |
| 19 | MAXMIN – L (**For layers**) (Vetmed) | Each 1 Kg contains: Manganese 80 g, Zinc 80 g, Copper 10 g, Iron 50 g, Iodine 0.60 g, Selenium 0.06 g | Highly concentrated trace mineral mixture for **layers** | 1 Kg / tonne of feed |
| 20 | MINADEX-P POWDER (Virbac) | Copper 0.075%, Iodine 0.01%, Iron 0.75%, Manganese 0.5625% Selenium 0.00075%, Zinc 0.625% Calcium 29%, Phosphorus 9% | * Complete mineral mixture for layer feeding<br>* To improve FCR, general health and weight gain<br>* To improve utilization of fat, carbohydrate and protein | 20 Kg / tonne of feed |

| S. No. | Trade Name & Company | Composition | Indications | Dosage / Administration |
|---|---|---|---|---|
| 21 | MULTIMIX -TM POWDER (Trichem) | Each Kg contains : Manganese 108 g, Zinc 104 g, Iron 40 g, Iodine 4 g, Copper 4 g, Cobalt 2 g, Selenium 100 mg | * Stress <br> * Deficiency conditions | **Routine use:** 500 g / tonne of feed <br> **Broilers / Breeders:** 1 Kg / tonne of feed <br> **During stress:** 1 Kg / tonne of feed |
| 22 | NUTRIMAR K (Exotic Mushrooms) | Proteins – 25.17%, Crude fibre – 19.48%, Calcium - 4.29%, Phosphorus – 0.68%, Magnesium – 0.36%, Potassium – 1.20%, Nitrogen – 4.02%, Sodium – 0.93%, Sulphur – 0.01%, Iodine – 0.05%, Iron – 0.11%, Zinc – 0.02%, Copper – 120 ppm, Cobalt – 55 ppm, Boron – 80 ppm, Manganese – 40 ppm, Selenium – 40 ppm, Vit A 70 IU / g, Vit C – 120 ppm, Vit E – 200 mg / Kg, Choline – 275 mg / Kg, Cytokinins – trace | * In the deficiency of macro and micro minerals <br> * Builds up defence mechanism of the body <br> * Improves fertility in males and females <br> * Increases hatchability and checks mortality <br> * Layers produce eggs with stronger shells, maintain longer peak production period and withstand stress <br> * Improves FCR and weight gain in broilers | **Chicks / Broilers / Layers / Breeders:** 1.5 Kg / tonne of feed |
| 23 | POUL TM DS (Harshvardh an's Lab) | Each Kg contains: Manganese 140 g, Zinc 100 g, Iron 80 g, Copper 10 g, Iodine 1.6 g, Selenium 0.3 g | * Ensures adequate supply of high quality minerals <br> * Ensures rapid growth <br> * Increases fertility, hatchability and livability <br> * Builds up resistance to infections and worm infestations | 500 g / tonne of feed |
| 24 | SEL-PLEX (Alltech Inc) | Organic selenium (Selenomethionine and Selenopeptides) | * To improve hatchability, chick viability and male fertility | **Inclusion: Broilers – Starter / Growers / Finishers:** |

| S. No. | Trade Name & Company | Composition | Indications | Dosage / Administration |
|---|---|---|---|---|
| | | | * Has effective antioxidant properties<br>* To improve storage life of hatching eggs | 0.2-0.3 ppm<br>**Layers:**<br>Laying period – 0.15 to 0.3 ppm<br>**Broiler Breeders:**<br>Egg production – 0.3 ppm |
| 25 | SOLMIN CAP (Qualitat) | Each 100 g contains:<br>Ca – 6 g, Phosphorus – 3.3 g, Iron – 2.14 g, Copper – 750 g, Cobalt – 1.29 g, Zn – 136 g, Manganese – 123.5 g, Sodium – 1.25 g, Potassium – 5.90 g, Sulphur – 9.26 g | * Very effective in prolapse<br>* Better shell quality<br>* Avoids lameness in chicks. Reduces mortality<br>* Better FCR, weight gain<br>* Reduces early chick mortality | 100 g / 1000 layers or,<br>100 g / 3000 chicks, broilers/ day for 2-3 days |
| 26 | SUPPLIMIN POWDER (Sarabhai Zydus) | Calcium 32%, Phosphorus 6%, Manganese 0.27%, Iodine 0.01% Zinc 0.26%, Fluorine 0.03%, Copper 100 ppm, Iron 1000 ppm Moisture 3% | * Improves feed efficiency<br>* Enhances growth and weight gain<br>* Produces better hatchability and strong eggshells<br>* Prevents mineral deficiencies | 2.5 Kg / 100 Kg of feed |
| 27 | SUPPLIMIN -P POWDER (Sarabhai Zydus) | Calcium 30%, Phosphorus 9%,<br>Iron 2000 ppm, Iodine 0.01%, Copper 500 ppm, Manganese 0.4%, Fluorine 0.05%, Zinc 0.4%<br>Acid insoluble ash 3%, Moisture 3% | * Optimizes feed efficiency<br>* Enhances growth and weight gain<br>* Improves egg production<br>* Produces better hatchability and strong eggshells<br>* Prevents mineral deficiencies | 2.5 Kg / 100 Kg of feed |
| 28 | SUPPLIMIN – TM (Sarabhai – Zydus) | Each Kg contains:<br>Manganese – 54 g, Zinc sulphate – 52 g, Ferrous sulphate 30 g, Copper sulphate 4 g, Potassium iodide 1 g, Cobalt sulphate – 0.1 g, | * Protects mineral deficiencies<br>* Improves immunity, growth, FCR, egg production, fertility, hatchability, energy utilization, | **Broilers / Layers:**<br>1 Kg / tonne of feed<br>**Breeders:**<br>1.5 – 2 Kg / tonne of feed |

| S. No. | Trade Name & Company | Composition | Indications | Dosage / Administration |
|---|---|---|---|---|
| | | Chromium chloride – 0.2 g, Selenomethionine – 100 ppm | feathering, meat and egg quality | |
| 29 | TRACEMIN BB (**For breeders**) (Venky's) | Each Kg contains: Manganese 50 g, Zinc 40 g, Iron 55 g, Copper 10 g, Iodine 1.25 g, Selenium 250 mg | * Prolapse<br>* Stress condition<br>* Disease (CRD, coryza, etc.)<br>* Lameness<br>* Moulting of feathers | **Normal course:** 2 Kg / tonne of feed **Deficiency:** 3 Kg / tonne of feed |
| 30 | TRACEMIN CB (**For commercial broilers**) (Venky's) | Each Kg contains: Manganese 90 g, Zinc 80 g, Iron 90 g, Copper 15 g, Iodine 2 g, Selenium 300 mg | * Stress condition<br>* Disease (CRD, coryza, etc.)<br>* Poor productivity<br>* Poor feed intake | **Normal course:** 1 Kg / tonne of feed **Deficiency:** 2 Kg / tonne of feed |
| 31 | TRACEMIN CL (**For commercial layers**) (Venky's) | Each Kg contains: Manganese 80 g, Zinc 80 g, Iron 60 g, Copper 15 g, Iodine 1 g, Selenium 300 mg | * Prolapse<br>* Stress condition<br>* Disease (CRD, coryza, etc.)<br>* Lameness<br>* Moulting of feathers | **Normal course:** 1 Kg / tonne of feed **Deficiency:** 2 Kg / tonne of feed |
| 32 | TRACEMIN FORTE POWDER (Avian Remedies) | Each Kg contains : Copper 10 g, Manganese 120 g, Iodine 1.6 g, Selenium 0.3 g, Iron 80 g, Zinc 100 g, Cobalt 0.1 g | * Prevents perosis, poor hatchability, anaemia, goitre, poor feathering, slow growth, short bones<br>* Prevents mortality<br>* Increases feed efficiency | **In normal course:** 50 g / 100 Kg feed **During deficiency:** 100-200 g / 100 Kg feed |
| 33 | TRACEMIN POWDER (Venky's) | Copper 1%, Iodine 0.16%, Iron 8%, Manganese 12%, Selenium 0.02%, Zinc 9.2% | For the requirements of copper, iodine, iron, manganese, selenium and zinc | 500 g / tonne of feed |
| 34 | TRACE MINERALS (Vetline) | Contains manganese, zinc, iron, copper, cobalt, selenium, molybdenum and iodine | For the requirements of trace minerals for layers and broilers | 1 Kg / tonne of feed |
| 35 | ULTRAMIN -LAYER POWDER (Neospark) | Calcium 32%, Phosphorus 6%, Manganese 0.27%, Zinc 0.26%, Copper 100 ppm, Iron 1000 ppm, Iodine 0.01%, Fluorine 0.03% | The complete mineral feed supplement for optimum production in poultry | **Chicks / Growers / Layers:** 20 Kg / tonne of feed |

| S. No. | Trade Name & Company | Composition | Indications | Dosage / Administration |
|--------|----------------------|-------------|-------------|--------------------------|
| 36 | ULTRA – TM PLUS Liquid Concentrate (Mineral + amino acid) (Neospark) | Each 500 ml contains: Magnesium – 616.21 mg, Zinc – 221.34 mg, Ferrous (iron) – 230.16 mg, Copper – 163.25 mg, Cobalt – 212.95 mg, Manganese – 395.12 mg, Sodium – 482.00 mg, Phosphorus – 158.40 mg, MHA (methionine activity) – 130.30 g, Choline chloride – 63 – 125 g, Lysine hydrochloride – 63 – 125 g | * MHA (Methionine hydroxyl analogue) protects and carries trace minerals for effective absorption and utilization<br>* An ideal source for methionine in poultry | **Layers:** 10 to 20 ml / 100 birds through water<br>**Broilers:** 5 to 10 ml / 100 birds through water |
| 37 | ULTRA-TM POWDER (Neospark) | Each 100 g contains: Manganese 10.8 g, Zinc 10.4 g, Iron 4 g, Iodine 0.4 g, Copper 0.4 g, Cobalt 0.2 g | Concentrated trace mineral feed supplement for poultry | **Regular use:** 500 g / tonne of feed<br>**Stress / Breeders:** 1 Kg / tonne of feed |

# 24. MISCELLANEOUS DRUGS

| S.No. | Trade Name & Company | Composition | Indications | Dosage / Administration |
|---|---|---|---|---|
| 1 | ANIMUNIN POWDER / LIQUID (Indian Herbs) | A herbal preparation | * To maintain a clear respiratory system<br>* To maintain respiratory health and production performance in the presence of microbes<br>* To facilitate easy breathing<br>* As a supportive to antibiotics for fast and complete recovery from severe respiratory infections | **Prevention: Powder:** 750 g / tonne of feed **Broilers:** To be given regularly **Layers:** Regularly or 15 days every month **Treatment: Liquid: Broilers:** 3-4 weeks 160 ml / 1000 5$^{th}$ week onwards – 320 ml / 1000 birds **Layers:** 3-8 weeks – 80 ml / 1000 birds; 3-20 weeks 160 ml / 1000 birds; 5$^{th}$ week onwards – 320 ml / 1000 birds |
| 2 | AVILON (Indian Herbs) | A herbal preparation | * To control loose droppings<br>* To accommodate healthy gut function<br>* To improve FCR and production | 2 Kg / tonne of feed In severe conditions 4 Kg / tonne of feed for first 7 days The same dose is recommended for breeders |
| 3 | BUTOX LIQUID ((Intervet) | Each ml contains : Deltamethrin 12.5 mg, Solvent and emulsifiers q.s. | For prevention and control of ectoparasitic infestations like ticks, mites, lice and flies | **Spray / Dip charging: Ticks / Flies:** 2 ml / litre of water **Mites:** 4 ml / litre of water **Lice:** 1 ml / litre of water **Topping up: Ticks / Flies:** 3 ml / litre of water **Mites:** 6 ml / litre of water **Lice:** 1.5 ml / litre of water |
| 4 | CAFLON (Natural Remedies) | *Adathoda vasica, Hedychium spicatum, Ocimum sanctum,* | Supportive treatment in respiratory diseases like | 5 Kg / tonne of feed for 7-10 days |

| S.No. | Trade Name & Company | Composition | Indications | Dosage / Administration |
|---|---|---|---|---|
| | | *Solanum xanthocarpum* | coryza, CRD, IB, ND, etc | |
| 5 | DEFENSE UP (Indian Herbs) | A herbal feed supplement | A herbal preventive against VVND | 1 Kg / tonne of feed |
| 6 | DERMAGON (Polchem) | Extracts of *Azardirachta indica, Glycyrrhiza glabra, Lawsonia alba, Thuja occidentalis, Ocimum sanctum,* natural vitamins and biominerals | Useful against dermatitis in poultry | *200 g / tonne of feed<br>*200 g / day in water for 10,000 broilers, 6000 layers, and 4000 breeders |
| 7 | IMMUPLUS POWDER (Indian Herbs) | It contains the extracts of selected natural herbs in a powder form. An immune potentiator | * To strengthen body defences<br>* To improve and maintain humoral and cell-mediated immunity<br>* To increase the vaccinal response<br>* To minimize the incidence of diseases and mortality | **Broilers:**<br>0-4 weeks 7.5 g / 1000 birds<br>5 weeks onwards 15 g / 1000 birds<br>**Layers:**<br>0-10 weeks 7.5 g / 1000 birds<br>10-18 weeks 15 g / 1000 birds<br>More than 18 weeks 7.5 mg / Kg body weight / day |
| 8 | IMMUTON POWDER (Zeus Intervetcare) | Pepto-nucleotides, carotenoids, phytomolecules | To improve immunity | **Through drinking water:**<br>**Broilers:**<br>5 g / 1000 birds daily<br>**Layers:**<br>5 g / 1000 birds daily (till 6th week). 10-20 g / 1000 birds (during vaccination and stress conditions)<br>**Breeders:**<br>10 g / 1000 birds daily. 15-30 g / 1000 birds (during vaccination and stress conditions<br>**In Feed:**<br>**Broilers / Layers:**<br>100 g / tonne of feed<br>**Breeders:**<br>150 g / tonne of feed |

| S.No. | Trade Name & Company | Composition | Indications | Dosage / Administration |
|---|---|---|---|---|
| 9 | NICOLI POWDER (Zeus Intervetcare) | Phytomolecules, Quinoline carboxylic acid, Probiotics | To prevent *E. coli*, Salmonella, and other bacterial infections in poultry | **Through drinking water:** **Below 3 weeks old:** 10 g / 100 birds twice daily **Above 3 weeks old:** 20 g / 100 birds twice daily **Severe conditions:** Double the dose **For prevention:** 5 g / 100 birds twice daily for 3 days **Feed Mix:** 500 g / tonne of feed |
| 10 | RESPIRON (Polchem) | Each 10 ml contains: Extracts of *Allium cepa, Azadirachta indica, Glycyrrhiza glabra,* natural vitamins and biominerals | * Routinely as a precaution to exposure of respiratory infections * During infection for rapid recovery * Post-infection for normalization of respiratory function | *200 g / tonne of feed *200 g per day in water for 10,000 broilers, 6000 layers, 4000 breeders |
| 11 | TOPICURE (Natural Remedies) | Each 10 ml contains : Extracts and distillates (in g) *Pinus longifolia* 1.5, *Eucalyptus* spp 1.25, *Cedrus deodara* 1, Excipients q.s. | To treat the wounds due to physical injury, pecking, cannibalism, gangrenous dermatitis or any other etiology | Spray in sufficient quantity once or twice daily until complete cure is achieved |
| 12 | V-COFEX SOLUTION (Varsha Labs) | Each 5 ml contains : Diphenhydramine HCl IP 8 mg Bromohexine HCl IP 4 mg, Ammonium chloride IP 100 mg, Sodium citrate IP 50 mg, Menthol IP 1 mg | Supportive along with antibiotics in respiratory infections such as bronchitis CRD, Coryza to reduce mortality rate | 1 ml / litre of water for 3-5 days |

# 25. MOULD INHIBITORS AND TOXIN BINDERS

| S.No. | Trade Name & Company | Composition | Indications | Dosage / Administration |
|---|---|---|---|---|
| 1 | AFLASIL FORTE (Jubilant Organosys)` | A highly adsorbent aflatoxin binder and anti-caking agent | * Prolongs the duration to act inside the body and bind the toxins like aflatoxin B1, B2, G1 and G2, and ochratoxins and T-2 toxins<br>* Ensures uniform mixing with the feed<br>* It ensures non-sticking of the finished feed in the mixer/blender | **Up to 12% moisture level:**<br>0.1% of the finished feed<br>**At moisture level of 12%:**<br>0.25% of the finished feed |
| 2 | ALTIMATE ZM PLUS POWDER (Alembic) | Hydrated sodium, Calcium aluminosilicate, activated charcoal, organic acid, dried neem leaf powder | * Effective against many mycotoxins<br>* Low inclusion level<br>* Wide spectrum affinity<br>* Positive impact of FCR<br>* Does not bind nutrients, vitamins or minerals | **Moisture content up to 15 %:**<br>1 Kg / tonne of feed<br>**Moisture content above 15%:**<br>1.5 – 2 Kg / tonne of feed |
| 3 | AGRIMOS (B.V. Bio-Corp) | A specific combination of manno-oligosaccharides (MOS) and glucans extracted from the cell wall of yeast *Saccharomyces cerevisiae* | * A potent and effective pathogen binder<br>* Prevents colonization of pathogens<br>* Ensures optimum flowability, homogeneous repartition into premixes and finished feeds | **Broilers / Chicks / Growers:**<br>1 Kg / tonne of feed<br>**Finishers / Breeders / Layers:**<br>500 g / tonne of feed |
| 4 | ALUSIL PREMIX MOS POWDER (Stallen) | MOS (mannan oligosaccharides), HSCAS, activated charcoal, copper oxinates, organic acids, lipotropic agent, and herbal ingredients | To maintain rate of weight gain, FCR and egg production in the presence of aflatoxins, ochratoxin, toxin $T_2$, fumonisin and zearalenòne | **Moisture up to 14%:**<br>1 Kg / tonne of feed<br>**Moisture above 14%:**<br>2 Kg / tonne of feed |
| 5 | ALUSIL PREMIX – PC POWDER (Stallen) | Hydrated sodium calcium aluminosilicates, Activated charcoal, Organic acids, Natural | * For the control and elimination of mycotoxins in feed<br>* For blocking the toxic effects at the digestive tract of birds that | 1 Kg / tonne of feed |

715

| S.No. | Trade Name & Company | Composition | Indications | Dosage / Administration |
|---|---|---|---|---|
| | | herbal ingredients | ingested contaminated feed | |
| 6 | ATB (Vetline) | A unique blend of organic acids and hydrated sodium, calcium, alumino silicates | * Binds and neutralizes mycotoxins<br>* Inhibits mould growth<br>* For better FCR and increased productivity | **Moisture content up to 15%:**<br>1.5 to 2 Kg / tonne of feed<br>**Moisture content above 15%:**<br>2.5 to 3 Kg / tonne of feed |
| 7 | AVSORB + POWDER (Avitech) | Organic acids, Hydrated sodium calcium aluminosilicate, Activated charcoal | * For the prevention of moulds in feed<br>* For the adsorption of toxins thereby restricting the bio – availability of toxins to poultry<br>* As an anticaking agent<br>* To reduce microbial contamination in feed | 2 Kg / tonne of feed<br>High risk conditions:<br>4-8 Kg / tonne of feed |
| 8 | BAN-TOX POWDER (Venky's) | Propionic acid, Acetic acid, Citric acid, 3-p cymenol, Potassium sorbate, Pyropylene glycol, Silicon dioxide, Essential oil extracts, Zeolites | * To provide broad-spectrum mould inhibition<br>* To bind mycotoxins<br>* For better growth and production<br>* For better FCR<br>* For better immunity<br>* For better response to vaccination | 1 Kg / tonne of feed (1.5 Kg if moisture is more) |
| 9 | BIO-BANTOX (Venky's) | Formulated dipolar phyllo-silicates | Broad-spectrum mycotoxin adsorbent for all types of feed | **For normal level of mycotoxin:** 1 Kg / tone of feed<br>**For high level of mycotoxin:** 1.5 Kg / tonne of feed |
| 10 | CHECK-O-TOX POWDER (Vetnex) | Organic acid salts like Propionates, Benzoates , Sorbates and Acetates together with specially treated hydrated sodium calcium, aluminosilicates | * Broad-spectrum mould inhibitor<br>* Mycotoxin binder<br>* Feed acidifier and strong gut-acting antibacterial agent | **Moisture content in feed up to 15%:**<br>1 Kg / tonne of feed<br>**Moisture content more than 15%:**<br>2 Kg / tonne of feed |

| S.No. | Trade Name & Company | Composition | Indications | Dosage / Administration |
|---|---|---|---|---|
| | | (HSCAS) | | |
| 11 | CHECK-O-TOX BIOPLUS (Vetnex) | Mannan-oligosaccharides (MOS), oxine copper, propionic acid, benzoic acid, sorbic acid, acetic acid, hydrated sodium calcium aluminium silicates (HSCAS) | * Broad-spectrum mould inhibitor<br>* Mycotoxin binder<br>* Feed acidifier and strong gut-acting antibacterial agent | **Moisture content in feed up to 15%:**<br>500 g / tonne of feed<br>**Moisture content in feed more than 15%:**<br>1 Kg / tonne of feed |
| 12 | DETOX POWDER (Aamoda Pharmaceuticals) (Varsha Group) | Hydrated sodium calcium aluminosilicates (HSCAS), Mould inhibitors and Yeast cell wall (MOS) and Activated charcoal | To eliminate mycotoxins | 1-2 Kg / tonne of feed |
| 13 | DETOX – FS LIQUID CONCENTRATE (Neospark) | Extract of 11 proven herbs in right levels | * Useful in conditions like aflatoxicosis, hepatitis, jaundice, leg weakness and diffuse diseases of liver<br>* Improves body resistance, feed efficiency, egg production in layers, and weight gain in broilers | **Layers:**<br>**Chicks:** 5 ml / 100 birds<br>**Growers:** 15 ml / 100 birds<br>**Layer:** 20 ml / 100 birds<br>**Broilers:**<br>**Starters:** 10 ml / 100 birds<br>**Finishers:** 20 ml / 100 birds |
| 14 | DETOX PLUS (AVR) | HSCAS (Hydrated sodium calcium aluminosilicate), free organic acids, kaolins, activated charcoal | * Absorbs moisture in feed, arrests mould growth and mycotoxin production<br>* Detoxicates all mycotoxins<br>* Helps to reduce caking of feed and improves | **Up to 1% moisture:**<br>1 Kg / tonne of feed<br>**12-15% moisture:**<br>2 Kg / tonne feed<br>**16-18% moisture:**<br>3 Kg / tonne feed |

| S.No. | Trade Name & Company | Composition | Indications | Dosage / Administration |
|---|---|---|---|---|
| | | | flowability of feed<br>* Improves growth and feed conversion<br>* Checks the growth of pathogenic bacteria in the feed and gut | |
| 15 | EXOSORB (Exotic Mushrooms) | Combination of mineral and non-mineral toxin binders | * Binds the mycotoxins<br>* Improves FCR, weight gain<br>* High stability over wide pH range in the gut | 500 g – 2Kg / tonne of feed |
| 16 | GENVET (Antifungal feed supplement) (Qualitat) | Activated gentian violet – 2% | * Prevents the growth of fungus or aflatoxins in feed<br>* Safe chemical; can be given to chicks from day one | 1 Kg / tonne of feed |
| 17 | HBC – bio POWDER (Nicholas Piramal) | HSCAS – plus, Na – bentonite, organic acids, activated charcoal, MOS, *Bacillus subtilis* | * Feed contaminated by moulds<br>* Depressed immune response due to mycotoxicosis | **Routine mixing:** 500 g / tonne of feed<br>**High risk conditions:** 1 Kg / tonne of feed |
| 18 | HSCAS POWDER (Harshvardhan's Lab) | Hydrated sodium calcium aluminosilicate | * Detoxifies feeds and raw materials<br>* Neutralises mycotoxins and free radicals<br>* Improves bird's immune response to medication | **In humid season:** 2.5 Kg / tonne of finished feed<br>**In dry season:** 1-1.5 Kg / tonne of feed |
| 19 | MOLDSTOP MYCO-PLUS (Fort Dodge) | Its 50% contains : Propionic acid and its salt ammoniumpropionate, Natural extracts, Emulsifiers Its remaining 50% contains : Hydrated sodium calcium aluminium silicates (HSCAS) | * Prevents the formation of moulds<br>* Prevents and treats mycotoxins in feed<br>* Prevents feed spoilage and preserves full nutritive value<br>* Increases feed and production efficiency | **Prevention:** 1 Kg / tonne of feed.<br>**In contaminated feed with moisture content of max 13%,** use 2-3 Kg / tonne of feed |

| S.No. | Trade Name & Company | Composition | Indications | Dosage / Administration |
|---|---|---|---|---|
| 20 | MOLD-ZAP POWDER (Alltech Inc) | Diammonium propionic acid | * Kills a wide range of moulds in feed<br>* Has a prolonged action<br>* Enhances the shelf life of feed | **In feed:**<br>500 g / tonne of feed |
| 21 | MYCO CURB DRY (Kemin) | Calcium propionate, Organic acids and their salts with potent inhibitory activity against a wide range of moulds | For effective control of a wide range of moulds infesting feed | 500 g -1Kg / tonne of feed |
| 22 | MYCOFIX PLUS 3.0 (Biomin) | BBSH 797, Phytogenic substances | * Complete solution to mycotoxin related problem<br>* Stimulates immune system to compensate the suppression, caused by toxins<br>* Reduces mycotoxin related fertility problems | **Breeders:**<br>1.5 Kg / tonne of finished feed |
| 23 | MYCOSORB POWDER (Alltech Inc) | Glucomannan polymer derived from inner cell wall of yeast | Provides protection against various mycotoxins like aflatoxin, ochratoxin, $T_2$ toxin, DON, zearalenone, fumonisins, etc. | **In feed:**<br>0.5 to 2 Kg / tonne of feed |
| 24 | OLIGOTOX POWDER (Polchem Lab) | Each Kg contains : Zeolite (HSCAS) 90%, activated charcoal 10%, Yeast cell wall oligosaccharides 1000 ppm, Acetic acid 5000 ppm, Propionic acid 10,000 ppm, Fumaric acid 5000 ppm, Formic acid 5000 ppm | * Provides protection against various mycotoxins like aflatoxin, ochratoxin, $T_2$ toxin, etc.<br>* Effectively prevents mould growth in the feed | 1 Kg / tonne of feed |

| S.No. | Trade Name & Company | Composition | Indications | Dosage / Administration |
|---|---|---|---|---|
| 25 | PRETOX – PLUS POWDER (Premium) | Hydrated sodium calcium aluminosilicate, Acetic acid, Organic acid, Propionic acid, Activated charcoal | * To arrest mould growth and mycotoxin production<br>* For effective binding of mycotoxins, like aflatoxin | 1 Kg / tonne of feed |
| 26 | PURE MOS (Animal feed supplement) (Exotic Mushrooms) | Derived from cell wall of *Saccharomyces cerevisiae* Sc 47 MOS | * Most efficient toxin binder<br>* Prevents adherence and colonization of pathogens in the gut | 250 – 500 g / tonne of feed |
| 27 | T-LOC-PLUS POWDER (Polchem) | Each Kg contains : **Zeolites** (Hydrated sodium calcium aluminosilicate) $SiO_2$-64.2%, $Fe_2O_3$-3.4%, $MgO$-2.6%, $K_2O$-0.4%, $P$-0.015%, $Al_2O3$-19.45%, $CaO$-5.6%, $Na_2O$-4.1%, $Mn$-0.03%. **Organic acids:** Acetic acid, Citric acid, Propionic acid. **Probiotics**: *Lactobacillus sporogenes* $5x10^{10}$ *Saccharomyces cerevisiac* $2x10^{12}$ *Bacillus coagulans* $5x10^{10}$ *Streptococcus faecium* $5x10^{10}$ | * Acts as a selective toxin binder<br>* Inhibits mould growth<br>* Improves flow property of feed<br>* Probiotics result in lactate production thereby establish healthy gut flora<br>* Competitive exclusion of entero-invasive and enterotoxic bacterial pathogens from the gut<br>* Enhances biosynthesis of digestive enzymes | **Up to 15% moisture:** 1 Kg / tonne of feed **Above 15% moisture:** 1.5 Kg / tonne of feed |
| 28 | TOXIBIND DRY POWDER (Kemin) | Silicates, organic acids, their salts and surfactants | * Binds mycotoxins and prevents their absorption<br>* Arrests mould growth<br>* Prevents immunosuppression caused by mycotoxins | 2.5 Kg / tonne of feed |
| 29 | TOXI-BOND PLUS | Hydrated sodium calcium aluminium | * A mycotoxin binder, mould inhibitor, potent | 1 Kg / tonne of feed |

| S.No. | Trade Name & Company | Composition | Indications | Dosage / Administration |
|---|---|---|---|---|
| | (Indian Drugs and Vitamins) | silicates (HSCAS) blended with propionic acid, citric acid, acetic acid, benzoic acid, and sorbic acid | antifungal, and anti-bacterial<br>* A feed acidifier, and preservative for vitamins and other macro-nutrients in feed | |
| 30 | TOXICHECK (Indian Herbs) | A unique herbal poultry feed supplement | * Inhibits mould growth and prevents the production of mycotoxins<br>* Improves FCR, weight gain, and egg production | **Contamination less than 200 ppb @ 0.5 Kg / tonne of feed Contamination level more than 200 ppb @ 1 Kg / tonne of feed** |
| 31 | TOXICURB POWDER (Polchem) | Each Kg. Contains : **Zeolites (HSCAS) such as:** $SiO_2$-64.2%, $Fe_2O_3$-3.4%, MgO-2.6%, $K_2O$-0.4%, P-0.015%, $Al_2O_3$ – 19.45%, CaO-5.6%, $Na_2O$-4.1%, Mn-0.03% **Organic acids:** Propionic acid 10000 ppm, Fumaric acid 5000 ppm, Formic acid 5000 ppm, Acetic acid 5000 ppm | * To arrest mould growth and mycotoxin production<br>* For effective binding of mycotoxins, like aflatoxin<br>* To prevent immunosuppression and damage to the liver and the kidney | 1 – 2 Kg / tonne of feed depending on moisture content of ingredients |
| 32 | TOXYBIND FORTE POWDER (Avian Remedies) | A synergistic blend of select broad-spectrum, potent antifungal organic acid salts like propionates, benzoates, sorbates, acetates stabilized on HSCAS | * To arrest mould growth and mycotoxin production<br>* For effective binding of mycotoxins, like aflatoxin | 1 Kg / tonne of feed |
| 33 | TOXICARE PLUS (Vetmed) | Tricholine citrate, Vit B1, Vit B12, Vit E, biotin, inositol, selenium, liver stimulants, methyl donors, protein hydrolysate | * Protects liver from feed contaminated with aflatoxins, trichothecenes, ochratoxins A, zearalenone, fumonisins<br>* Checks growth of pathogenic bacteria | **Weekly once programme: Broilers:** 10 / 100 birds in water **Layers:** 10 / 100 birds **Layer breeders:** 25 ml / 100 birds |

| S.No. | Trade Name & Company | Composition | Indications | Dosage / Administration |
|---|---|---|---|---|
| | | | * Increases FCR and weight gain | **Broiler breeders:** 25 ml / 100 birds **Disorders:** 20-30 / 100 birds for 5-7 days |
| 34 | TOXIDEX (Wockhardt) | Each Kg contains: Phyllosilicates 800 g, Mycotoxin destroyer complex and surfactant 200 g | * Broad-spectrum toxin binder<br>* Protects from mycotoxins without affecting beneficial nutrients<br>* Toxidex acts as an absorbent of mycotoxins, destroys and eliminates mycotoxins through faeces of birds | **Broilers/Layers:** 1 Kg / tonne of feed **Breeders:** 3 Kg / tonne of feed |
| 35 | TOXIMAR POWDER (Virbac) | Natural hydrated sodium calcium aluminium silicate (HSCAS) | * For binding and neutralizing mycotoxins<br>* For inhibition of mould growth<br>* For better FCR<br>* For increased productivity (weight gain, eggs) | **Moisture content up to 15%:** 1 Kg / tonne of feed **Moisture content above 15%:** 1.5 Kg – 2 Kg / tonne of feed |
| 36 | TOXINEX POWDER (Feed Supplement (Novartis) | Propionic acid, Benzoic acid, Sorbic acid, Acetic acid, Hydrated sodium calcium aluminium silicate (HSCAS), Mannan-oligosaccharide (MOS), B-glucan | * Feed contaminated with aflatoxin, trichothecenes, ochratoxins A, zearalenone and fumonisins<br>* Depressed immune response due to mycotoxicosis<br>* Depressed feed consumption and weight gai | **Moisture content up to 14%:** 2.5 Kg / tonne of feed **Moisture content 15%:** 5 Kg / tonne of feed. **Moisture content 16%:** 10 Kg / tonne of feed |
| 37 | TOXINIL HERBAL (Natural Herbs) | Herbal preparation of antitoxin ingredients | * To inhibit mould growth and prevent mycotoxins<br>* To absorb mycotoxins from feed and prevent | **For mycotoxin levels less than 200 ppb:** 500 g / tonne of feed **For mycotoxin levels** |

| S.No. | Trade Name & Company | Composition | Indications | Dosage / Administration |
|---|---|---|---|---|
| | | | absorption from intestine<br>* To prevent the damage caused by mycotoxins<br>* To maintain growth, FCR, egg production, hatchability, immunocompetence | **more than 200 ppb:**1 Kg / tonne of feed |
| 38 | TOXIROAK POWDER (Ayurvet) | A herbo-mineral toxin binder | * Checks the growth of fungus in feed<br>* Inhibits the biosynthesis of aflatoxin from fungus<br>* Inactivates toxin by chemosorption in gut<br>* Bio-neutralizes the aflatoxin reaching liver | **For low risk periods:** 500 g / tonne of feed **For high risk periods :** 1.25 Kg / tonne of feed |
| 39 | TOXISORB PREMIUM (Pfizer) | Originally modified mont morillonite | Mycotoxicosis | 500 g to 1 Kg / tone of feed (under local conditions) |
| 40 | TOXIWIN POWDER (Sarabhai Zydus) | Blend of hydrated sodium calcium aluminosilicates (zeolites) with oxides of sodium, calcium, magnesium and iron | * Effectively binds mycotoxins<br>* Increases feed conversion ratio<br>* Increases growth and productivity<br>* Increases immune response<br>* Increases eggshell quality<br>* Increases fertility and hatchability | 500 g / tonne of feed |
| 41 | TOXORID POWDER (Wockhardt) | Hydrated Sodium calcium alumino-silicates (HSCAS ), activated charcoal, organic acids, herbal ingredients | * Checks the growth of fungus in feed<br>* Inhibits the biosynthesis of aflatoxin from fungus<br>* Inactivates toxin by chemosorption in gut<br>* Bio-neutralizes aflatoxin reaching liver | **Routine:** (less than 15% moisture) 1 Kg / tonne of feed **High risk conditions:** (more than 15% moisture) 2 Kg / tonne of feed |
| 42 | TURBOSIL POWDER (Guybro) | Hydrated sodium calcium alumino-silicate, sodium oxide, calcium oxide, | * For binding and neutralizing mycotoxins<br>* For inhibition of mould growth | 250 g / tonne of feed regularly 500 g / tonne of feed with moisture 12- |

| S.No. | Trade Name & Company | Composition | Indications | Dosage / Administration |
|---|---|---|---|---|
| | | magnesium oxide, iron oxide, and other mineral oxides | * For increased productivity (weight gain, eggs) | 15% 1 Kg / tonne of feed with moisture 15-18% |
| 43 | ULTRASIL-TCF POWDER (Neospark) | Sodium aluminosilicate 95.25%, with gentian violet and organic acids, predigested protein 1000 ppm, cobalt 100 ppm | Prevents mycotoxin poisoning and promotes growth | 0.5-2.5 Kg / tonne of feed |
| 44 | US CURATOX – FS POWDER (Neospark) | Hydrated sodium calcium aluminosilicate (HSCAS), Mould inhibitors, Organic acids, Cross linked insoluble vinyl pyrrolidone homopolymer, Mannan-oligosaccharide (MOS), activated charcoal along with Lipotropic factors | * Provides protection against various mycotoxins like aflatoxin, ochratoxin, $T_2$ toxin, etc <br> * Effectively prevents mould growth in the feed <br> * By virtue of having MOS, it helps in pathogen shedding through competitive exclusion <br> * Potentiates the immune response of the birds | **When moisture content is below 15% :** 0.5 Kg / tonne of feed **When moisture content is between 15-17%:** 1 Kg / tonne of feed **When moisture content above 17% :** 1.5 Kg / tonne of feed |
| 45 | UTPP- 5 POWDER (Vetcare) | Buffered organic acids and specially treated hydrated sodium calcium aluminosilicates | * To arrest mould growth and mycotoxin production <br> * For effective binding of myco- toxins, like aflatoxin <br> * Lowers PH of feed and gut <br> * To improve protein digestion <br> * To check the growth of pathogenic bacteria and fungi in the feed gut <br> * To control and reduce feed contamination | **Moisture content up to 15% :** 2.5 Kg / tonne of feed **Moisture content above 15%:** 5 Kg / tonne of feed |
| 46 | UTPP BIOTECH POWDER | Mannan-oligosaccharide (MOS), HSCAS | * To prevent aflatoxicosis <br> * To reduce pH of gut and feed | 1 Kg / tonne of feed |

| S.No. | Trade Name & Company | Composition | Indications | Dosage / Administration |
|---|---|---|---|---|
| | (Vetcare) | oxine copper, activated charcoal, buffered organic acids, lipotropic agents | * To prevent pathogen population<br>* To prevent ochratoxicosis<br>* To prevent immune stress | |
| 47 | UTPP SPECIAL (Vetcare) | HSCAS, buffered organic acids, MOS | * Effectively binds aflatoxins<br>* Prevents / controls multiple mycotoxicoses<br>* Ensures effective and irreversible toxin binding<br>* Protects immunity<br>* Reduces stress on liver<br>* Eliminates harmful pathogens | ! Kg / tonne of feed |
| 48 | VARISHTA (Varsha) | Buffered organic acids, HSCAS, MOS, charcoal, , antioxidants, *Picrorhiza kurroa* | Multi-spectrum toxin binder to prevent and protect the birds from the damaging effects of multiple mycotoxicoses | 1 Kg / tonne of feed |

## 26. NON-ANTIBIOTIC GROWTH PROMOTERS / PERFORMANCE ENHANCERS

| S.No. | Trade Name & Company | Composition | Indications | Dosage / Administration |
|---|---|---|---|---|
| 1 | AMNOVIT POWDER (Intervet) | Each 100 g contains : Vit A 5 lacs IU, Vit $D_3$ 29000 IU, Vit E 200 mg, Vit $B_2$ 300 mg, Vit $B_6$ 60 mg, Vit $B_{12}$ 400 mcg, Vit K 40 mg, Niacinamide 1.32 g, Calcium pantothenate 440 mg, Folic acid 10 mg, Choline chloride 150 mg, L-Lysine 1 g, L-Methionine 2 g, L-Tryptophan 20 mg, Excipients qs | * Stress conditions, before and after deworming and vaccinations<br>* To improve productivity in broilers, layers and breeders<br>* Deficiency diseases due to vitamins and amino acids | **In Water:** 1 g / litre of water for 3-4 days a week<br>**In Feed:** 500 g / tonne of feed |
| 2 | BIOMIN PLUS (Vetmed) | Each 5 ml contains: DL-methionine 3.82 g, Choline chloride 1.89 g, L-Lysine 1.89 g, Protein hydrolysate 300 mg, Yeast autolysate 600 mg, **Chelated minerals:** Calcium 40 mg, Magnesium 20 mg, Iron 1.5 mg, Manganese 11.25 mg, Zinc 3 mg, Copper 4.5 mg, Cobalt 6 mg, Sodium chloride 30 mg, Potassium chloride 10 mg | * Enhances body weight<br>* Improves health of birds and feed efficiency<br>* Higher egg production | **Chicks:** 5 ml / 100 birds<br>**Broilers / Growers / Layers:** 5-10 / 100 birds<br>**Breeders:** 10-12 ml / 100 birds |
| 3 | BIOSPARK V LIQUID (Venky's) | Each 15 ml contains : Protein hydrolysate liquid 5.4 g, Sodium 30 mg, Magnesium 25 mg, Potassium 10 mg, Chloride 41.6 mg, Manganese 0.25 | * To promote growth and performance<br>* The best energizer and supportive in malnutrition<br>* Prevents stress during summer<br>* Provides functional | 15-30 ml / 100 birds for 5 days Repeat after 10 days or as required |

| S.No. | Trade Name & Company | Composition | Indications | Dosage / Administration |
|---|---|---|---|---|
| | | mg, Iron 0.3 mg, Copper 0.06 mg, Zinc 0.1 mg, Cobalt 0.06 mg, Iodine 32.45 mg, Carbohydrates 2.5 g, L-lysine 60 mg, Yeast 30 mg, Papain 15 mg, High energy 14 Kcal, High protein | nutrients for better FCR | |
| 4 | BIOSPARK V POWDER (Venky's) | Each 100 g contains : Protein hydrolysate 32 g, Manganese 5.56 mg, Sodium 667 mg, Magnesium 556 mg, Potassium 223 mg, Chloride 1020 mg, copper 1.33 mg, Iron 6.66 mg, Cobalt 1.34 mg, Zinc 2.23 mg, Carbohydrates 56 g, Iodine 728 mg, Yeast 667 mg, L-lysine 1400 mg, Calcium 56mg, Papain 333mg High energy 313 Kcal, High protein | * To promote growth and performance<br>* The best energizer and supportive in malnutrition<br>* Prevents stress during summer | 500 g / tonne of feed or Mix 500 g x 3 packs in 4.2 litres of distilled water and administer 15-30 ml / 100 birds for 5 days. Repeat after 10 days or as required |
| 5 | BIOSTIM POWDER (Zeus Intervetcare) | Herbal extracts, Probiotics, Nucleotides, Dextrose base | * Prevents early chick mortality<br>* Stimulates antibody production<br>* Prevents stress and rejuvenates the chicks<br>* Improves feed conversion<br>* Stimulates growth | 1 g / 100 chicks daily through drinking water for 5 days |
| 6 | BIO-MOS (Pathogen Binder) | Mannan-oligosaccharides derived from outer cell | * For effective pathogen binding<br>* To modulate immune | **Broilers:** **Starter** – 2 Kg / tonne of feed |

| S.No. | Trade Name & Company | Composition | Indications | Dosage / Administration |
|-------|----------------------|-------------|-------------|-------------------------|
| | (Alltech Inc) | wall of yeast | response<br>* To improve gut health | **Grower** – 1 Kg / tonne of feed<br>**Finisher** – 0.5 Kg / tonne of feed<br>**Layers and Breeders:**<br>1 Kg / tonne of feed |
| 7 | CHQ-60 POWDER (Sarabhai Zydus) | Halquinol 12% w/w | Optimizes feed conversion and improves production | **Broilers:**<br>250 g / tonne of feed<br>**Layers:**<br>500 g / tonne of feed |
| 8 | COLINIL – FEED MIX (Indian Drugs and Vitamins) | Each g contains:<br>Tulsi extract 25 mg, Amla extract 1.20 mg, Quinoline carboxylic acid 25 mg, Mineral mixture; base | * To prevent *E. coli,* salmonella, mycoplasma, Haemophilus and other bacterial infections<br>* To improve FCR and growth promotion | **Broilers:**<br>250 g / tonne of feed from day one till slaughter<br>**Layers:**<br>250 g / tonne of feed for 10 days in a month<br>**Breeders:**<br>500 g / tonne of feed for 10 days in a month |
| 9 | DIMBPRO (Ayurvet) | A herbal premix for layer birds | * To increase egg production at various stages<br>* To restore egg production during convalescence period | 50 g / 100 Kg for 10 days |
| 10 | G-PRO MIN LIQUID (Vetcare) | Each 500 ml contains :<br>Methionine activity (MHA) 127.6 g, Lysine hydrochloride 63.125 g, | * Prevents production failure related to nutritional deficiencies<br>* Improves size, production and quality | **Broilers:**<br>5-10 ml / 100 birds through water<br>**Layers:**<br>20 ml / 100 birds |

| S.No. | Trade Name & Company | Composition | Indications | Dosage / Administration |
|---|---|---|---|---|
| | | Choline chloride 63.125 g, Sodium 459 mg, Phosphorus 154.16 mg, Magnesium 595.4 mg, Zinc 215.7 mg, Iron 223.4 mg, Copper 158.8 mg, Cobalt 206.25 mg, Manganese 384.55 mg | of eggs<br>* Improves fertility and hatchability in breeders<br>* Reduces mortality<br>* Compensates for loss of nutrients especially during 'summer'. | through water |
| 11 | HERBIOTIC FS (Indian Herbs) | It is a herbal antimicrobial feed supplement | * To improve FCR, growth and body weight<br>* To reduce the incidence of infections and mortality<br>* To protect from enteric bacterial diseases | **For growth promotion:** 200-250 g / tonne of feed<br>**For control of necrotic enteritis, salmonellosis:** 500 g / tonne of feed |
| 12 | HIVIT-MIN POWDER (Hitha) | **VITAMINS**<br>Each Kg contains :<br>Vit A 100,00,000 IU, Vit $D_3$ – 20,00,000 IU, Vit $B_2$ 5.5 g, Vit $B_1$ 1.1 g, Vit $B_6$ 2 g, Vit $B_{12}$ 15 mg, Calcium pantothenate 9 g, Niacinamide 33 g, Vit C 7.5 g, Vit E 18 g, Vit K 3 g, Folic acid 0.6 g, Selenium 100 mg<br>**MINERALS**<br>Each 2 Kg contains :<br>Choline chloride 500 g, Manganese 95 g, Zinc 60 g, Iron 40 g, Copper 5 g, Iodine 1.2 g, Cobalt 0.5 g | Poultry feed supplement for improved performance and production | 1 Kg of vitamin and 2 Kg of mineral to be added per tonne of feed for broilers |

| S.No. | Trade Name & Company | Composition | Indications | Dosage / Administration |
|---|---|---|---|---|
| 13 | PROMIN LIQUID (Polchem) | Each 15 ml contains: **AMINO ACIDS:** Lysine 86.4 mg, Methionine 35.76 mg, Arginine 82.84 mg, Aspartic acid 71.40 mg, Threonine 45.96 mg, Serine 69.36 mg, Glutamic acid 213 mg, Proline 139.56 mg, Glycine 21.48 mg, Alanine 22.72 mg, Valine 78.6 mg, Histidine 32.64 mg, Isoleucine 76.56 mg, Leucine 102 mg, Tyrosine 65.28 mg, Phenylalanine 64.32 mg, Trypto-phan 18.80 mg, cystine 18 mg **CHELATED MINERALS** Calcium 45 mg, Magnesium 24 mg, Iron 1.5 mg, Manganese 11.25 mg, Zinc 3 mg, copper 4.5mg, Cobalt 6 mg **ELECTROLYTES** Sodium as chloride 30 mg, Potassium as chloride 10 mg, Yeast autolysate 600 mg | * To improve the amino acid profile to ensure better utilization and conversion of dietary protein into body proteins<br>* Also supplies chelated minerals, electrolytes and yeast autolysate<br>* Higher egg production<br>* Enhanced body weight in broilers and growers<br>* Improved feed efficiency<br>* Healthier birds | **Chicks:** 15 ml / 100 birds / day for 5 days to be repeated after every 10 days **Broilers:** $2^{nd}$ and $3^{rd}$ week : 15 ml / 100 bird / day $5^{th}$, $6^{th}$, $7^{th}$, week : 30 ml / 100 birds / day **Growers:** 15 ml / 100 birds / day for 5 days to be repeated after every 10 days **Layers:** 30 ml / 100 birds / day for 7 days in a month **Breeders:** 20 ml / 100 Kg body weight / day for 5 days to be repeated after every 10 days |
| 14 | PROMIN PLUS POWDER (Sanichem Labs) | Each Kg contains : Partially hydrolyzed proteins (Casein and vegetable proteins) 300 g **ENZYMES :** | A feed supplement containing hydrolyzed proteins, enzymes, chelated minerals and electrolytes to give maximum feed efficiency | 500 g / tonne of feed |

| S.No. | Trade Name & Company | Composition | Indications | Dosage / Administration |
|---|---|---|---|---|
| | | Alpha amylase 65,000 IU, Phytase 6,500 IU, Alpha galactosidase 9,900 IU, Acid proteases 2,60,000 IU **CHELATED MINERALS :** Calcium 20 g , Iron 5 g, Magnesium 10 g, Mineral mixture 100 g **ELECTROLYTES** Sodium as chloride 20 g, Potassium as chloride 10 g | | |
| 15 | QUINCARE – FS (Feed supplement) (Neospark) | Each Kg contains: 600 g of chlorohydroxy quinoline | * Gut-acting growth promoter <br> * Reduces pathogen load in intestine and feed <br> * It is non-absorbent in gut, hence non-toxic | **For growth promotion: Broilers / Layers / Breeders 50-100 g** / tonne of feed **To overcome wet droppings:** 200-250 g / tonne of feed |
| 16 | SENAB-GP (Neospark) | Combination of natural non-antibiotic and competitive exclusion compounds | * Reduces salmonella and *E. coli* load in the intestine <br> * Improves gut health and prevents diarrhoea <br> * Improves daily growth and FCR | **Prevention:** 1 Kg / tonne of feed as week a month programme |
| 17 | SPIRUMAX PREMIX (Ayurvet) | Micronutrients, Unidentified growth promoting factors, Biological antioxidants and Free radical scavengers and Select herbs | * Promotes digestibility by improving the utilization of nutrients <br> * Optimizes the health status during various stages of life by providing superior nutritional support <br> * Minimizes the incidence of infections | 500 g / tonne of feed |

| S.No. | Trade Name & Company | Composition | Indications | Dosage / Administration |
|---|---|---|---|---|
| | | | by stimulating the immune system<br>* Ensures better growth, livability, improved nutrient utilization and FCR | |
| 18 | STAQUINOL 12% and 60% (Stallen) | Each Kg contains : Halquinol 60 g | * Improves growth rate and feed conversion efficiency<br>* Active against fungi, Gram- positive and Gram-negative bacteria and against protozoa<br>* Prevents and cures many types of diarrhoea | **Staquinol 12%:** 500 g – 1 Kg / tonne of feed<br>**Staquinol 60%:** 50 – 100 g / tonne of feed |
| 19 | TURBO (Liquid Feed Supplement) (Polchem) | Each 500 ml contains: Methionine activity (MHA) 127.6 g, choline chloride 63.125 g, Lysine hydrochloride 63.125 g, **Chelated minerals:** calcium 1.5 g, magnesium 0.8 g, iron 0.217 g, manganese 0.375 g, zinc 0.2 g, copper 0.15 g, cobalt 0.2 g **Electrolytes:** sodium chloride 1 g, potassium chloride 0.333 g, Yeast autolysate 20 g, | * Improved FCR<br>* Rapid and uniform growth<br>* Improved and stabilized egg production in layers and breeders<br>* Less pullet eggs<br>* Rapid onset of production and extended peak production<br>* Successful sustenance to heat and other stress | **Chicks:** 5 ml / 100 chicks<br>**Growers:** 10 ml / 100 birds<br>**Layers:** 20 ml / 100 birds<br>**Broilers:** 2nd and 3rd week 10 ml / 100 birds 4th and 5th week 15 ml / 100 birds<br>**Broiler breeders:** 15 ml / 100 Kg body weight |

# 27. OLIGOSACCHARIDES

| S.No. | Trade Name & Company | Composition | Indications | Dosage / Administration |
|---|---|---|---|---|
| 1 | BIO-MOS (Alltech Inc) (Pathogen binder) | Mannan-oligosaccharides derived from outer cell wall of yeast | * For effective pathogen control in broilers, layers and breeders <br> * To improve weight gain and FCR <br> * To modulate the immune response <br> * To protect the intestinal membrane | **Broilers:** <br> Starter – 2 Kg / tonne <br> Grower – 1 Kg / tonne <br> Finisher – 0.5 Kg / tonne <br> **Layers and Breeders:** <br> 1 Kg / tonne of feed |
| 2 | FERMENTO-MOS (Sanichem Labs) | Each Kg contains : Mannan and glucan oligo-saccharides 5000 ppm, *Saccharomyces cerevisiae* 1000 billion, *Candida rugosa* 1000 billion, *Bacillus subtilis* 1000 billion | * For stabilization and establishment of healthy gut microflora <br> * To enhance immunity <br> * To reduce GI tract related problems e.g. enteritis <br> * To improve FCR | 1 Kg / tonne of feed |

## 28. OSMOREGULATORS AND METHYL DONORS

| S. No. | Trade Name & Company | Composition | Indications | Dosage / Administration |
|---|---|---|---|---|
| 1 | BEETAFIN (Finnfeeds) | Betaine | * To maintain cell water balance under periods of stress<br>* For reducing feed cost by sparing methionine / choline<br>* For consistent bird performance and increased profitability | 700 g / tonne of feed<br>**In severe osmotic stress** 1-1.5 Kg / tonne of feed |
| 2 | BIOMETH (Varsha) | Methyl donor | Alternative source of methionine | Replacement of synthetic methionine in feed on equal weight basis |
| 3 | NICOMIX BETAINE (Nicholas Piramal) | Each g contains: Vit A 20,000 IU, Vit $D_3$ 3,000 IU, Vit $B_1$ 1.6 mg, Vit $B_2$ 10 mg, Vit $B_6$ 3.2 mg, Vit $B_{12}$ 41 mcg, Niacin 24 mg, Calcium pantothenate 16 mg, Vit K 2 mg, Vit E 16 mg, Folic acid 1.6 mg, Betaine hydrochloride 600 mg | * It is a better methyl donor than choline and methionine<br>* To maintain cell water and ion balance due to its osmolytic action<br>* To improve action of coccidiostats<br>* To reduce wet droppings due to its osmoprotective action<br>* To replace choline chloride and part of methionine in feed, thereby reducing feed cost | 500 g / tonne of feed |
| 4 | RECYMETH (Wockhardt) | Methyl donors and methyl group recycling agents are easily bioavailable with organic sulphur base, fortified with short chain fatty acids, chelated minerals and amino nitrogen | * A better alternate source of methionine<br>* Conserves methionine<br>* Reduces sulphate production<br>* Supports metabolic enzymes | Replaces synthetic methionine in feed on equal weight basis |

# 29. PROBIOTICS

| S. No. | Trade Name & Company | Composition | Indications | Dosage / Administration |
|---|---|---|---|---|
| 1 | AVR PROBIOTIC (AVR) | Each g contains: $2.5 \times 10^9$ Lactobacillus species with Vitamin C | * Helps to maintain healthy gastrointestinal tract after antibiotic therapy<br>* Reduces the incidence of chick mortality<br>* Inhibits the growth of pathogenic organisms by means of competitive inhibition, by lowering the pH of the surroundings, which is not conducive for the growth of pathogens. | **Through feed**<br>**Broilers/Layers:** 100g/tonne of feed<br>**Breeders:** 200g/tonne of feed<br>**Through water:**<br>**Chicks:** 1g/ 2 litres of drinking water for first 5-7 days.<br>**Adult Birds:** 1 g in 4 litres of water for 5 days |
| 2 | BACTOSACC (Bio-Corp) | *Pediococcus acidilactici* (MA 18/5 M) and *Saccharomyces cerevisiae* (CNCM1 – 1079) | * Improves growth performance and FCR<br>* Improves disease resistance and overall viability<br>* Improves the resistance towards pathogens<br>* Lowers mortality rate and cost of medication | 500 g / tonne of feed |
| 3 | BIOBOOST POWDER (Lyka Labs) | Each Kg contains: Live yeast culture 25 g, live *Lactobacillus sporogenes* culture 200 million CFU, amino acid 25 g, liver extract 500 mg | To improve FCR, growth, weight gain, egg production and hatchability | 1- 1.5 Kg / tonne of feed |
| 4 | BIOBOOST FORTE POWDER (Lyka Labs) | Each 200 g contains: Live yeast culture of *Saccharomyces cerevisiae* 50 g, live culture of *Bacillus* | * To prevent early chick mortality, stress, diarrhoea<br>* For better weight gain and egg | **Chicks:** 1-3 g / 100 chicks / day or 100 – 150 g / tonne of feed<br>**Layers:** |

| S. No. | Trade Name & Company | Composition | Indications | Dosage / Administration |
|---|---|---|---|---|
| | | *coagulans* 6000 x 18 million CFU | production, | 10- 12 g / 1000 birds / day **Breeders:** 16-18 g / 1000 birds/ day |
| 5 | BIOMARK-SA (Exotic Mushrooms) | Each Kg contains: *Bacillus subtilis*-500 billion c.f.u. , *Lactobacillus acidophilus* 500 billion /c.f.u. | * Probiotic growth promoter <br> * Improves FCR, keeps intestine free from pathogens and helps better digestion and absorption of feed. | 500 g – 1 kg / tonne of feed |
| 6 | BIOMARK – SB (Exotic Mushrooms) | Each 500 g contains: *Saccharomyces boulardii* 200 billion CFU. | * To check loose droppings from 1<sup>st</sup> day <br> * Builds up immunity <br> * Provides growth of friendly bacteria and removes harmful pathogens like *E. coli, s*almonella spp. <br> * Neutralizes toxins <br> * It can be given with antibiotics | 500 g / tonne of feed |
| 7 | BIOPRIME FEED Supplement (Prime) | Each 1 kg of Bioprime provides live yeast culture SC-47 9 (French strain) *Saccharomyces cerevisiae* 5 billion CFU/ gram | * Better FCR, growth in chicks and growers <br> * Improves disease resistance <br> * Improves egg production <br> * Better weight gain in broilers <br> * Better hatchability <br> * Enhances growth of beneficial gut bacteria, and maintains an efficient digestive system for peak performance | 100g / tonne of feed |
| 8 | BIOVET – YC FEED | Each kg contains: *Lactobacillus* | * To balance and harmonize | **Chicks, Growers and Broilers : 500 g** |

736

| S. No. | Trade Name & Company | Composition | Indications | Dosage / Administration |
|---|---|---|---|---|
| | SUPPLEMENT (Wockhardt) | *sporogenes* 7500 million CFU, *L.acidophilus* 30000 million CFU, live yeast culture of *Saccharomyces cerevisiae* SC-47 125,000 million CFU, alpha amylase 5 g, sea weed extract 100g excipient q.s. | operations of digestive system. <br> * To improve intestinal ecology <br> * To proliferate useful intestinal microflora <br> * To prevent digestive upsets and prevent diarrhoea. | / tonne of feed **Layers and Breeders:** 1 kg / tonne of feed. |
| 9 | BROLAC (IVPL) | Each 150 g contains: $36 \times 10^{11}$ CFU *Lactobacillus acidophilus, L. casei, Bifidobacterium bifidus, Enterococcus faecium, L. salivarius, L. reuteri, L. lactis, L. cellobiosus, L. animalis,* oligosaccharides, fortified with N.M.B. complex and acidifiers. | * Better livability <br> * Reduces fat deposition <br> * Eliminates bacterial diseases <br> * Improves immunity <br> * Improves weight gain and FCR | **Broilers /Breeders:** 150 g / 5000 birds **Broilers** from 1st day -- alternate weeks. Use continuously for minimum 7 days in first drinking water. |
| 10 | E – MICROBES (Twin pack liquid) (Neospark) | **Pack -1 liquid contains:** *Lactobacillus acidophilus, L. bulgaricus, L lactis, L. fermentum, L. rhamnose,L. Streptococcus thermophilus S.. faecium.* **Pack-2 liquid contains:** *L. sporogenes, Bacillus subtilis, B.licheniformis, Saccharomyces boulardii* | * Highly concentrated live microbial cultures for use as **Direct Feed Microbial** (Probiotic) feed supplement for poultry | 1. Take 1 litre water. Make it into 2 parts of 500 ml each. 2. Add 5ml of pack 1 liquid with one part of 500 ml of water and mix with 500 g of **DORB** (de-oiled rice bran). 3. Add 5 ml of pack 2 liquid with second part of 500 ml of water and mix with 500 g of DORB. 4. Mix together these two parts of DORB. 5. Incubate for 3 days at room temperature in an airtight polythene |

737

| S. No. | Trade Name & Company | Composition | Indications | Dosage / Administration |
|---|---|---|---|---|
| | | | | bag. **6.** Finished product of DORB probiotic culture should be used on the same day. **7.** Each g of finished DORB contains 2 billion CFU **Regular Use** 500 g /finished DORB per tonne of feed. **Stress conditions:** 1 Kg /finished DORB per tonne feed. **Each 500 ml twin pack is sufficient for 100 tonne of feed** |
| 11 | FIBOSEL (B.V. Biocorp) | It is a cell fraction of baker's yeast strain *Saccharomyces cerevisiae* with specific beta-glucan content | * Improves immune status of the bird<br>* Better body resistance<br>* Improves feed intake and production<br>* Better hatchability | **Broilers, Layers and Breeders:** 50-100g/tonne of feed |
| 12 | GALLIPRO ( Jubilant Organosys) | A preparation of beneficial bacteria to gut | * Improves FCR<br>* Improves body weight gain | Dose not mentioned in the literature |
| 13 | G-PROBIOTIC – SPL (Vetcare) | Each kg contains: *Saccharomyces cerevisiae* 1,25,000 million CFU, *Lactobacillus acidophilus* 15,000 million CFU, *Bacillus coagulans* 15,000 million CFU, *B. subtilis* 15,000 million CFU, *B. licheniformis* 15000 million CFU, protease, phytase, fibre degrading enzyme, liver extract q.s. | * To improve weight gain<br>* For better feed conversion ratio<br>* To reduce mortality<br>* For improved performance<br>* To improve growth rate<br>* Reduces loose droppings | 500g/ tonne of feed |

| S. No. | Trade Name & Company | Composition | Indications | Dosage / Administration |
|---|---|---|---|---|
| 14 | IMPROLAY (IVPL) | Each 150 g contains: $18 \times 10^{11}$ CFU of: *L. acidophilus, L. casei, Bifidobacterium bifidus, Enterococcus faecium, Lsalivarius, Lreuteri, L. lactis, L. fermentum, Saccharomyces cremoris, L. bulgaricus,* oligosaccharides, fortified with N.M.B. complex with acidifiers | * Prevents bacterial diseases <br> * Relieves stress conditions <br> * Improves antibody titres <br> * Improves immunity <br> * Better absorption of nutrients <br> * Better FCR, increases egg production | **Use for Layers and Layer Breeders:** Make stock solution: 150 g for 5000 birds – week a month. Use minimum for 7 days in first drinking water . |
| 15 | IMPROVAL POWDER (Sarabhai Zydus) | Each Kg contains: *Saccharomyces cerevisiae* $1.5 \times 10^{11}$ CFU, *Lactobacillus sporogenes* 30,000 million CFU, fortified with phytase, and enriched with calcium, phosphorus, proteins, carbohydrates ,vitamins and UGF | * To prevent early chick mortality <br> * To prevent diarrhoea and wet droppings <br> * To improve FCR <br> * To improve weight gain in broilers <br> * To prevent disease and improve body resistance <br> * To increase bioavailability of calcium and phosphorus <br> * To improve fertility and hatchability <br> * Also useful as a growth promoter | 500 g – 1 Kg / tonne of feed |
| 16 | INTELZYME POWDER (Guybro) | Alpha- amylase, beta-glucanase, phytase, galactosidase, alkaline protease, acid protease, Cellulase, xylanase, *Lactobacillus acidophilus, Lactobacillus sporogenes, Streptococcus* spp, *Saccharomyces cerevisiae* | * For proper feed utilization, digestion, metabolism <br> * For increased weight gain and production | 250-500 g / tonne of feed |

| S. No. | Trade Name & Company | Composition | Indications | Dosage / Administration |
|---|---|---|---|---|
| 17 | LACTO-SACC POWDER (Alltech Inc.) | *Saccharomyces cerevisiae, Lactobacillus acidophilus* 50,000 million (50 x $10^9$), *Streptococcus faecium* 50,000 million (50 x $10^9$) | * As an alternative to antibiotic growth promoters<br>*During periods of stress<br>* To improve gut health *When birds go off feed. | **Broilers and Layers:** 250-500 g / tonne of feed<br>**Breeders:** 500 -1 Kg / tonne of feed |
| 18 | LEVUCELL – SB (B.V. Biocorp.) | Each g contains : $2 \times 10^9$ CFU of live yeast *Saccharomyces boulardii* (sub-species of *Saccharomyces cerevisiae*) | * Enhances nutrition and health of birds<br>* Optimizes and maintains the ecological balance of gut microflora<br>* It is a potential and satisfactory alternative growth promoter<br>* For better productivity performance | 250g / tonne of feed |
| 19 | MAXIGRO FEED SUPPLEMENT (Vetcare ) | *Lactobacillus acidophilus, Lactobacillus sporogenes, Saccharomyces cerevisiae,* phytase, alpha- amylase, cellulase, beta-glucanase, pectinase, protease, xylanase, | * Improves FCR, egg quality and flock uniformity<br>* Prevents loose droppings and sub-clinical infections like *E. coli* and salmonella<br>* Reduces effects of anti- nutritional factors | **Chicks:** 250 g / tonne of feed<br>**Broilers and Layers** : 500 g / tonne of feed<br>**Breeders** : 500 g – 1 Kg / tonne of feed |
| 20 | MICROGUARD (Zeus Intervetcare) | Lactic ferments, Specially cultured live yeast cells | Selective and effective microflora for the gut to achieve maximum biosecurity in the gastro-intestinal tract | **Through drinking water: Chicks:** 10 g / 1000 chicks from day one for 7 days<br>**Broilers:** 5 g / 1000 birds daily till marketing<br>**Growers / Layers:** 10 g / 1000 birds for 3 days<br>**Feed mixing:** 100 g / tonne |

| S. No. | Trade Name & Company | Composition | Indications | Dosage / Administration |
|---|---|---|---|---|
| 21 | NICOPROTIC (Nicholas Piramal) | It contains: *Lactobacillus acidophilus, L. sporogenes*, Yea-sacc, Biomos and Betaine Total viable count of Nicoprotic is 400 x $10^9$ CFU per Kg | * Improves FCR, growth, and stimulates immunity <br> * Reduces mortality, protects from *E. coli*, salmonella, and *Clostridium perfringens* <br> * Helps during summer stress <br> * Makes the gut balance its pH <br> * Reduces feed contamination, and environmental stress <br> * Also reduces vaccination and deworming stress, and stress caused during shifting and transportation | 500 g / tonne of feed |
| 22 | PROBENZ PREMIX POWDER (Stallen) | *Bifidobacterium bifidum, Lactobacillus acidophilus, Lactobacillus bulgaricus, Lactobacillus casei, Lactobacillus plantarum, Streptococcus faecium, Saccharomyces cerevisiae.* **Yeasts:** *Torulopsis spp. Aspergillus oryzae* fortified with phytase and *Spirulina* | * Minimizes different kinds of stress such as debeaking, vaccination and summer stress <br> * Helps to maintain healthy gastrointestinal tract after antibiotic therapy <br> * Reduces the incidence of chick mortality, <br> * Quicker detoxification of mycotoxins <br> * Produces more metabolizable energy through its positive effect on starch and fat digestibility | **Broilers and Layers** : 250 g / tonne of feed <br> **Breeders:** 250-500 g / tonne of feed |

741

| S. No. | Trade Name & Company | Composition | Indications | Dosage / Administration |
|---|---|---|---|---|
| 23 | PROBIOLAC (IVPL) | Each 100 g contains: Minimum 32 billion CFU of *Lactobacillus acidophilus, L. reutri, L. fermentum L.. lactis. L. casei, Bifidobacterium bifidus, Streptococcus faecium, Apergillus oryzae and* Torulopsis | * Relieves stress conditions<br>* Improves resistance to bacterial diseases<br>* Improves feed efficiency<br>* Reduces egg breakage<br>* Improves protective effect of vaccination | 100g/tonne of compound feed |
| 24 | PROBIOS SOLUBLE – POWDER (Stallen) | Each g of Probios contains : $2 \times 10^9$ CFU of *Bifidobacterium bifidum, Lactobacillus acidophilus, Lactobacillus bulgaricus, Lactobacillus casei, Lactobacillus plantarum, Streptococcus faecium, Streptococcus thermophilus,* and Yeasts : *Torulopsis* spp *Aspergillus oryzae* | * Improves enzyme activity in the gut<br>* Improves litter condition<br>* Improves feed efficiency, organic phosphorus utilization and fibre digestion due to yeasts<br>* Improves protein and fat synthesis<br>* Improves egg production, egg quality and shell quality in layers and breeders<br>* Improves weight gain and FCR in broilers | **In Water:** **Chicks :** 1 g / litre of water for first 5-7 days of life **Adult birds :** 1 g / 4 litres of water for 5 – 7 days **In Feed:** **Broilers:** **Pre-starter:** 150 g / tonne **Starter:** 100 g / tonne **Finisher:** 50 g / tonne **Layers and Breeders:** 50-100g / tonne |
| 25 | PROBIOS-PREMIX (Stallen) | Each g of Probios contains: $2 \times 10^9$ CFU of *Bifidobacterium bifidum, Lactobacillus acidophilus, Lactobacillus bulgaricus, Lactobacillus casei, Lactobacillus plantarum, Streptococcus faecium, Streptococcus thermophilus,* and | * Improves enzyme activity in the gut<br>* Improves litter condition<br>* Improves feed efficiency, organic phosphorus utilization and fibre digestion due to yeasts<br>* Improves protein and fat synthesis<br>* Improves egg production, egg | **Broilers, Starters:** 100 g / tonne of feed **Growers, Finishers** : 50 g / tonne of feed **Layers , Breeders:** 50-100 g / tonne of feed |

| S. No. | Trade Name & Company | Composition | Indications | Dosage / Administration |
|---|---|---|---|---|
| | | **Yeasts:**<br>*Torulopsis* spp<br>*Aspergillus oryzae* | quality and shell quality in layers and breeders<br>* Improves weight gain and FCR in broilers | |
| 26 | PROCID (Avians) | Each g contains: $6 \times 10^9$ CFU:<br>*Saccharomyces boulardii,*<br>*Propionibacterium freudenriichii,*<br>*Lactobacillus acidophilus,*<br>*Lactobacillus sporogenes,*<br>*Lactobacillus bulgaricus,*<br>*Lactobacillus plantarum,*<br>*Streptococcus faecium,*<br>and *Pediococcus acidilactici* | * Maintains G.I. tract microflora<br>* Decreases concentration of several pathogenic microbes and their toxins<br>* Improves growth rate and FCR | 500 g – 1 Kg / tonne of feed |
| 27 | PROMIX-Y FORTE (Alembic) | Each 500 g contains:<br>Live yeast culture<br>*Saccharomyces cerevisiae* (SC-47) 62,500 million CFU,<br>*Lactobacillus sporogenes* 15,000 million CFU,<br>*Lactobacillus acidophilus* 7,500 million CFU,<br>*Streptococcus* spp 7,500 million CFU,<br>Beta-gluconase 5 g,<br>Alpha- amylase 2.5 g,<br>Liver extract 250 g,<br>*Hawaiian spirulina* (Blue green algae) 25 g. | * Improves growth and feed conversion<br>* Inhibits growth of disease – producing organisms<br>* Protects against *E. coli* and salmonella infections<br>* Improves metabolism of carbohydrates and starch<br>* It also acts as an immunomodulant | **Broilers: 0-4 weeks-** 500 g / tonne of feed **4-6 weeks-** 250 g / tonne of feed<br>**Layers: 0-20 weeks** – 250-500 g / tonne of feed 20-72 weeks – 250 g / tonne of feed<br>**Breeders:** 0-72 weeks – 500 g / tonne of feed |
| 28 | PROSAC (Kaypeeyes | *Lactobacillus acidophilus,* | * Improves FCR<br>* Improves immune | **Broilers:**<br>0-4 weeks – 100 g / |

| S. No. | Trade Name & Company | Composition | Indications | Dosage / Administration |
|---|---|---|---|---|
| | Biotech) | *Lactobacillus casei, Lactobacillus bulgaricus, Streptococcus lactis, Bacillus subtilis Saccharomyces cerevisiae* varieties 3000 million CFU/g | status<br>* Creates healthy gut environment | tonne of feed<br>4-6 weeks – 75 g / tonne of feed<br>**Layers:**<br>0-20 weeks – 100 g / tonne of feed<br>20 – 72 weeks – 75 g / tonne of feed<br>**Breeders:** 0-72 weeks – 150g / tonne of feed |
| 29 | PROSOL WATER SOLUBLE POWDER (Intvet) | Each 100 g contains: $5 \times 10^7$ CFU *Lactobacillus acidophilus, L. casei, Bifidobacterium bifidum, Streptococcus faecium Vit* C, and UGF | * To reduce early chick mortality<br>* To prevent intestinal bacterial diseases<br>* To improve absorption of nutrients<br>* For more weight gain<br>* To improve FCR<br>* For better utilization of nutrients<br>* For increased egg production | 100 g / 5000 chicks / birds. Use in first drinking water for minimum 7 days |
| 30 | PROTEXIN SOLUBLE POWDER (Novartis) | Each g contains: *Lactobacillus plantarum* $1.26 \times 10^8$ CFU, *Lactobacillus bulgaricus* $2.06 \times 10^8$ CFU, *Lactobacillus acidophilus,* $2.06 \times 10^8$ CFU, *Lactobacillus casei* $2.06 \times 10^8$ CFU, *Streptococcus thermophilus* $4.10 \times 10^8$ CFU, *Streptococcus faecium* $5.40 \times 10^8$ CFU, *Bifidobacterium bifidum* $2.00 \times 10^8$ CFU. **Yeasts:** *Torulopsis* spp $5.32 \times 10^8$ CFU | * An ideal stress reliever after vaccination and antibiotic therapy<br>* Reduces mortality when used in cases of mycotoxicosis along with toxin binders in feed<br>* Establishes sufficient microbial flora in gut and ensures optimal competitive exclusion in the early stages of life<br>* Improves immune status in disease conditions | **Chicks:** 1 g / litre of water for 5-7 days<br>**Adults:** 1 g / 4 litre of water for 5 days |

| S. No. | Trade Name & Company | Composition | Indications | Dosage / Administration |
|---|---|---|---|---|
| | | *Aspergillus oryzae* $5.32 \times 10^8$ CFU Total viable count $2 \times 10^9$ CFU | | |
| 31 | PROTEXIN IN-FEED (Novartis) | Each g contains : *Lactobacillus plantarum* $1.26 \times 10^8$ CFU, *Lactobacillus bulgaricus* $2.06 \times 10^8$ CFU, *Lactobacillus acidophilus*, $2.06 \times 10^8$ CFU, *Lactobacillus casei* $2.06 \times 10^8$ CFU, *Streptococcus thermophilus* $4.10 \times 10^8$ CFU, *Streptococcus faecium* $5.40 \times 10^8$ CFU, *Bifidobacterium bifidum* $2.00 \times 10^8$ CFU. **Yeasts:** *Torulopsis* spp $5.32 \times 10^7$ CFU *Aspergillus oryzae* $5.32 \times 10^7$ CFU Total viable count $2 \times 10^9$ CFU | * An ideal probiotic for feed mill operations <br> * Produces 120 g extra weight in broilers in 42 days <br> * Conditions bird before it comes in lay <br> * Ensures steady and higher egg production throughout the laying cycle <br> * No cracked or thin-shelled eggs | **Broilers:** 0-4 weeks-100 g / tonne of feed 4-6 weeks-75 g / tonne of feed **Layers:** 0-20 weeks-50-100 g / tonne of feed 20-72 weeks-50 g / tonne of feed **Breeders:** 0-72 weeks-100 g / tonne of feed |
| 32 | PROVILACC (Vetcare) | Each Kg contains: *Saccharomyces cerevisiae* 5855 billion CFU, *Lactobacillus sporogenes* 14040 billion CFU, *Lactobacillus acidophilus*-14040 million CFU, *Bacillus subtilis* 15000 million CFU | * To prevent and reduce colonization of harmful pathogens <br> * To reduce ammonia excretion <br> * To maintain intestinal integrity <br> * To reduce wet litter problem <br> * To prevent stress | **Broilers / Layers:** 500 g / tonne **Breeders:** 1 Kg / tonne |
| 33 | PROVISACC (Vetcare) | Each g contains: Live yeast culture of (*Saccharomyces cerevisiae*) 5000 million CFU | * To increase egg production <br> * For better FCR and weight gain <br> * To reduce post antibiotic stress | **Broilers:** 500 g / tonne of feed **Layers:** 250 g / tonne of feed **Breeders:** 1 Kg / tonne of feed |

| S. No. | Trade Name & Company | Composition | Indications | Dosage / Administration |
|---|---|---|---|---|
| | | | * To decrease disease outbreaks by improving body resistance <br> * To improve the semen quality in male birds <br> * To improve fertility and hatchability in breeders | |
| 34 | REDEEM VIT – DS POWDER (Redeem) | Each g contains: Vit A 82,500 IU, Vit $B_2$ 50 mg, Vit $D_3$ 12.5 lac IU, Vit K 10 mg, *Lactobacillus* 15 billion CFU | * To prevent rickets and leg weakness <br> * To improve hatchability and fertility | 100-200 g / tonne of feed |
| 35 | REDEEPLEX (Probiotics + B-complex) (Redeem) | Each 5 ml contains: Vit $B_1$ 4 mg, Vit $B_2$ 2.25 mg, Vit $B_{12}$ 6.25 mcg, Vit $B_6$ 0.65 mg, Niacinamide 30 mg, D-pantothenol 1.2 mg, DL-methionine 7 mg, Biotin 15 mg, Probiotics 9 types- 15 billion CFU | * To improve growth and production in stress conditions <br> * To reduce post-antibiotic stress | **Chicks:** 10 ml / 100 birds <br> **Growers:** 15 ml / 100 birds <br> **Broilers:** 15-20 ml / 100 birds <br> **Layers:** 20 ml / 100 birds <br> Breeders : 30-35 ml / 100 birds |
| 36 | SPECTRA-DFM (Neospark) | Each 100 g contains: Lyophilized viable organisms – *Lactobacillus acidophilus, Lactobacillus bulgaricus, Lactobacillus cellobiosus, Lactobacillus casei, Lactobacillus plantarum, Bifidobacterium bifidum, Streptococcus faecium, Torulopsis, Aspergillus oryzae* total viable count of $30 \times 10^9$ CFU | * Prevention and treatment of digestive disorders induced by stress due to changes of accommodation, feed and transportation <br> * Improves weight gain and feed conversion <br> * Prevents *E. coli* invasion and decreases problems of diarrhoea <br> * Better egg production | **Regular usage:** 100 g / tonne of feed In stress conditions : 200 g / tonne of feed |

| S. No. | Trade Name & Company | Composition | Indications | Dosage / Administration |
|---|---|---|---|---|
| 37 | SPECTRASOL-DFM (Neospark) | Each 100 g contains: Lyophilized viable organisms – *Lactobacillus acidophilus*, *Lactobacillus bulgaricus*, *Lactobacillus cellobiosus*, *Lactobacillus casei*, *Lactobacillus plantarum*, *Bifidobacterium bifidum*, *Streptococcus faecium*, *Torulopsis*, *Aspergillus oryzae* total viable count of 150x10$^6$ CFU | * Prevention and treatment of digestive disorders induced by stress due to changes of accommodation, feed and transportation<br>* Improves weight gain and feed conversion<br>* Prevents *E. coli* invasion and decreases problems of diarrhoea<br>* Better egg production | **Chicks, Broilers and Layers (Starter):** 2 g / 250 chicks for 1$^{st}$ 7 days<br>**Broiler (finisher):** 1 g / 250 birds<br>**Layers:** 2 g / 250 birds (during stress) |
| 38 | SPORICH – PLUS (Uni-Sankyo) (Kenko) | *Saccharomyces boulardii, Bacillus subtilis*, Lactic acid bacillus Total potency > 4.5 x 10$^9$ / g | * Improves growth rate, body weight gain, and FCR<br>* Improves resistance to disease<br>* Helps to control loose droppings | **Broilers / Layers:** 100 g / tonne of feed<br>**Breeders:** 100 – 150 g / tonne of feed |
| 39 | SPORICH PLUS WATER-SOLUBLE (Uni-Sankyo) (Kenko) | *Saccharomyces boulardii, Bacillus subtilis*, Lactic acid bacillus Total potency: > 4.5 x 10$^9$ / g | * Improves growth rate, body weight gain and feed efficiency<br>* Improves resistance against diseases | 100 g / 5000 chicks / birds 7 – 10 days from day-old chick, or during any stress condition |
| 40 | SPORICH-Y 1500 and 3000 (Uni-Sankyo) (Kenko) | Lactic acid bacillus 1500/3000 million spores per gram in Yeast base Potency: 1.5 x 10$^9$ : 3 X 10$^9$ | * Improvement in growth rate<br>* Improvement in body weight gain and feed efficiency<br>* Improved digestion and feed utilization<br>* Improved resistance to diseases<br>* Improved production | **Sporich – Y 1500:**<br>**Broilers:** 50 – 100 g / tonne of feed<br>**Layers:** 100 g / tonne of feed<br>**Breeders:** 100 – 150 g / tonne of feed<br>**Sporich – Y 3000:**<br>**Broilers / Layers:** 50 – 75 g / tonne of feed<br>**Breeders:** 75 – 100 g / tonne of feed |

| S. No. | Trade Name & Company | Composition | Indications | Dosage / Administration |
|---|---|---|---|---|
| 41 | TCL-MIX POWDER (Trichem) | Each g contains : Vit $B_1$ 8 mg, Vit $B_6$ 16 mg, Vit $B_{12}$ 80 mcg, Vit E 80 mg, Calcium pantothenate 40 mg, Niacin 120 mg, Folic acid 8 mg, DL-Methionine 10 mg, L-Lysine 10 mg, Calcium 260 mg, *Lactobacillus* 35 million | * For better growth and egg production | 100 g / tonne of feed |
| 42 | YEAMARK (Exotic Mushrooms) | Contains *Saccharomyces cerevisiae* SC 47 5 billion CFU / g | * Stimulates brush border disaccharides<br>* Stimulates immunity<br>* Antioxidant activity (removes free radicals from the body)<br>* Balances gut microflora. Keeps gut healthy for maximum absorption of nutrients<br>* Checks mortality, morbidity, and enhances production and profitability | 250 – 500 g / tonne of feed |
| 43 | YEA-SACC[1026] (Alltech Inc) | Each g contains: Yeast culture of *Saccharomyces cerevisiae* strain 1026 $5 \times 10^9$ cells | * To improve FCR, weight gain and egg numbers<br>* To reduce post-antibiotic stress<br>* To improve fertility and hatchability in breeder stock<br>* To increase sperm cell counts in males | **Broilers/Layers:** 250-500 g / tonne of feed |

# 30. SULPHA DRUGS

| S. No. | Trade Name & Company | Composition | Indications | Dosage / Administration |
|---|---|---|---|---|
| 1 | BIOTRIM ORAL LIQUID (Vetnex) | Each ml contains : Sulphadiazine 200 mg, Trimethoprim 40 mg | * For treating conditions like enteritis due to *E. coli*, Clostridia and Salmonella<br>* Fowl cholera, fowl typhoid and infectious coryza | 25-30 mg of combined activity per Kg body weight for 3-5 days |
| 2 | COSUMIX PLUS POWDER (Novartis) | Each 100 g contains: Sulphachloropyridazine sodium 10 g, Trimethoprim 2 g | For treatment of colibacillosis and salpingitis, fowl cholera, paratyphoid infection, infectious coryza, staphylococcal infection | **Chicks up to one week:** 50 g / 100 litres of water **Broilers: 1 to 4 weeks** -100 g / 100 litres of water **5-8 weeks** – 150 g / 100 litres of water **Layers: Above 20 weeks** – 100-150 g / 100 litres of water **Breeders: 1 to 8 weeks** -100 g / 100 litres of water **9-20 weeks** – 150 g / 100 litres  of water |
| 3 | DUAPRIM (Brihans) | Each 5 g contains : Sulphamethoxazole 2000 mg, Trimethoprim 400 mg | For the prevention and treatment of CRD, coryza, diarrhoea, enteritis, salmonellosis, coccidiosis, fowl typhoid, fowl cholera, dermatitis, foot rot and other microbial infections | **Through drinking water or with feed for 3-5 days:** **Chicks:** 2.5 g / 100 birds **Broilers / Growers:** 5 g / 100 birds **Layers:** 10g / 100 birds |
| 4 | DUXPRIM (Neospark) | Sulphamethoxazole 10% w/w, Trimethoprim 2% w/w | Infectious coryza, enteritis, bacillary white diarrhoea, colisepticaemia, coccidiosis with mixed bacterial infections, early chick mortality, | **Chicks:** 0.5 g / Litre of water for 5-7 days |

| S. No. | Trade Name & Company | Composition | Indications | Dosage / Administration |
|---|---|---|---|---|
| | | | secondary bacterial infections associated with viral infections | |
| 5 | ENTRADIN SOLUTION (Neospark) | Sodium sulphadimethylpyrimi dine 12.5% w/v, (equivalent to 11.579% of Sulphadimethylpyrim idine) | Infectious coryza, coccidiosis, acute fowl cholera, pullorum disease | 30 ml / 4 litres of water. Treat for 2-6 days |
| 6 | GOLDIPRIM (Golden Streak) | Sulphamethoxazole 10%, Trimethoprim 2% | Coliform infections either alone or in complicated forms of CRD, infectious coryza, fowl cholera, salmonella, coccidiosis with mixed bacterial infections, early chick mortality | 1-2 g / litre of water or 0.5 – 1 Kg / tonne of feed for 5 days |
| 7 | MORTIN-VET POWDER (Micro Labs) | Trimethoprim IP 2.0% w/w Sulphsamethoxazole IP 10% w/w | * Broad-spectrum potentiated bactericidal, chemotherapeutic agent <br> * For chronic respiratory disease, infectious coryza, fowl cholera, coli-septicaemia, coccidiosis with mixed bacterial infections | **Chicks:** 1g/ litre of drinking water continuously for a maximum of 5 days at a time . **Broilers and Layers :** 1g/ litre of drinking water continuously for 5 -7 days |
| 8 | ORIPRIM POWDER (Sarabhai Zydus) | Each g contains : Sulphamethoxazole 500 mg, Trimethoprim 100 mg, Excipients q.s. | * Primary infections like colibacillosis, infectious coryza, bacillary white diarrhoea, coccidiosis <br> * Secondary bacterial infections in CRD | **In drinking water:** 1 g / 4 litres of water **In feed:** 100 g / 100 Kg of feed |

| S. No. | Trade Name & Company | Composition | Indications | Dosage / Administration |
|---|---|---|---|---|
| | | | * Respiratory, urogenital and GI tract infections | |
| 9 | REDEEPRIM POWDER (Redeem) | Sulphamethoxazole 10% w/w, Trimethoprim 2% w/w | * Primary infections like colibacillosis, infectious coryza, bacillary white diarrhoea, coccidiosis<br>* Secondary bacterial infections in CRD | 1500 g / tonne of feed |
| 10 | SULMET (Fort Dodge) | Sodium sulphadimethylpyrimidine 12.5% w/w | * For immediate control of coccidiosis<br>* To minimize losses from secondary bacterial infections | *30 ml / 4 litres of water for 2 days and 15 ml / 4 litres of water for next 4 days<br>*Also add Aureomycin soluble powder 1 g / litre of water throughout treatment |
| 11 | STERBAC POWDER (Sterling Lab) | Sulphamethoxazole 10% w/w, Trimethoprim 2% w/w | * Primary infection like colibacillosis, infectious coryza, bacillary white diarrhoea, coccidiosis<br>* Secondary bacterial infections in CRD | 1 g / litre of water |
| 12 | SULCOPRIM POWDER (Concept) | Each 5 g contains : Sulphamethoxazole 2 g, Trimethoprim 400 mg | * *E.coli*<br>* Fowl typhoid<br>* Fowl cholera<br>* Coryza<br>* Bacillary white diarrhoea | **Chicks:** 2.5 g / 100 birds daily<br>**Broilers / Growers:** 5 g / 100 birds<br>**Layers:** 10 g / 100 birds daily for 3-5 days |
| 13 | V-COZINE POWDER (Varsha Labs) | Sulphadiazine 10% w/w, Trimethoprim 2% w/w | To prevent early chick mortality, BWD, CRD, coryza, colisepticaemia, and respiratory infections | 1-2 g / litre of water |

# 31. VITAMINS

| S. No. | Trade Name & Company | Composition | Indications | Dosage / Administration |
|---|---|---|---|---|
| 1 | ANICHOL – 60 (Jubilant Organosys) | 60% Choline chloride-dry (on a cereal carrier, a feed grade) | * Treatment of fatty liver syndrome<br>* For an overall increase in the hen day egg production by 2-3% in the winter season | **Broiler:** 1000 g / tonne of feed **Layer:** 500 g / tonne of feed **Breeder:** 1200 g / tonne of feed |
| 2 | ANICHOL – 75 (Jubilant organosys) | 75% Choline chloride – aqueous | * Treatment of fatty liver syndrome<br>* For an overall increase in the hen day egg production by 2-3% in the winter season | Dosage not given in the literature |
| 3 | BIOCARE POWDER (Vetcare) | Each 50 g contains : Biotin (Vitamin H) 20 mg, Water soluble carrier q.s. | * Prevents dermatitis of:<br>1. Foot pad<br>2. Skin around the beak<br>3. Eyes<br>* Improves hatchability<br>* Improves weight gain<br>* To enhance feathering in birds | **In Water:** 1 g / 2 litres of water **In Feed:** **Chicks:** 500 / tonne of feed **Layers:** 400 g / tonne of feed **Breeders:** 500 g / tonne of feed |
| 4 | BIO CHOLINE (Indian Herbs) | A unique combination of natural and highly bioavailable biotin and choline. Also contains herbal constituents | * As a feed supplement to provide optimum quantity of natural biotin and choline<br>* To maintain optimum mobilization of liver fat<br>* To maintain secretion of bile at optimum level<br>* To maintain growth, FCR, egg production, livability and hatchability | 500 g / tonne of feed |

| S. No. | Trade Name & Company | Composition | Indications | Dosage / Administration |
|---|---|---|---|---|
| 5 | BIO-H POWDER (Elpe) | Each 10 g contains : Biotin 6 mg, Dextrose monohydrate q.s. | * Acute fatty liver and kidney conditions<br>* Leg weakness<br>* Flip over conditions (sudden death syndrome)<br>* Reduced feed conversion<br>* Reduced hatching results | **Chicks / Growers:** 40-60 g / 100 Kg of feed or 1 g / litre of water<br>**Broilers:** 50-75 g / 100 Kg of feed or 1-2 g / litre of water<br>**Layers:** 30-50 g / 100 Kg of feed or 0.5 g – 1 g / litre of water |
| 6 | BIOTIN F-2 POWDER (Novartis) | Each g contains : D-biotin 20 mg | For better FCR, growth and production | **Broilers / Layers (0-6 weeks):** 150 mcg / Kg feed<br>**Broilers/Layers (6-20 weeks):** 100 mcg / Kg feed<br>**Breeders:** 150-300 mcg / Kg feed |
| 7 | BREEVIT (For Breeders) (Venky's) | Each Kg contains: Vit A 20 MIU, Vit $D_3$ 4 MIU, Vit E 60 g, Vit $K_3$ 8 g, Vit $B_1$ 4 g, Vit $B_2$ 20 g, Vit $B_6$ 6 g, Vit $B_{12}$ 30 mg, Niacin 60 g, Cal-D-pantothenate 30 g, Folic acid 4 g, Biotin 200 mg, Vit C 100 g, Antioxidant q.s., Carrier q.s. | * For better chick quality<br>* For better nutrient digestion and availability<br>* For vitamin supplementation | 1000 g / tonne of feed |
| 8 | BROLAY – CLP (Jubilant Organosys) | Each 500 g contains: Vit A – 10,000000 IU,Vit D3 – 250000 IU, Vit E – 8 g, Vit K3 – 1 g, Vit B1 – 0.8 g, Vit B2 – 5 g, Vit 6 – 1.5 g, Vit B12 – 8 mg, Niacin – 12 g, Pantothenic acid – 8 g, Folic acid – 0.8 g, Lactose and Calcium carbonate as carrier | * To ensure high bioavailability of vitamins<br>* To maintain potency of vitamins under practical storage conditions<br>* To maintain potency and stability of vitamins | 500 g / tonne of feed |

| S. No. | Trade Name & Company | Composition | Indications | Dosage / Administration |
|---|---|---|---|---|
| 9 | BROVIT PREMIX (For Commercial Broilers) (B. V. Bio-Corp) | Each Kg contains: Vit A 25 MIU, Vit $D_3$ 5 MIU, Vit E 24 g, Vit $K_3$ 3g, Vit $B_1$ 3 g, Vit $B_2$ 10 g, Vit $B_6$ 4 g, Vit $B_{12}$ 30 mg, Niacin 30 g, Cal-D- pantothenate 20 g, folic acid 1 g , Organic nutritive, Carrier q.s. | * For vitamin supplementation of broiler's diet <br> * Enhances profitability | 500 g / tonne of feed |
| 10 | BROVIT PLUS PREMIX (For Commercial Broilers) (B.V. Bio-Corp) (Vitamin enriched premix) | Each Kg contains : Vit A 25 MIU, Vit $D_3$ 5.6 MIU, Vit E 60 g, Vit $K_3$ 4 g, Vit $B_1$ 4 g, Vit $B_2$ 10 g, Vit $B_6$ 6 g, Vit $B_{12}$ 30 mg, Niacin 80 g, Cal-D-pantothenate 30 g, Folic acid 2 g, Biotin 160 mg, Organic nutritive, carrier q.s. | * For vitamin supplementation of broiler's diet <br> * For better livability and optimum FCR | 500 g / tonne of feed |
| 11 | BV – 250 (Varsha Group) | Each 250 g contains: Vit A – 12500000 IU, Vit B2-5000 mg, Vit D3 – 2500000 IU, Vit K3, 1000 mg, Vit B1 – 800 mg, Vit B6 – 1600 mg, Vit B12 – 25000 mcg, Niacin – 12000 mg, Biotin – 10000 mcg, Calcium pantothenate – 8000 mg, Vit E – 8000 IU, Folic acid – 800 mg, Yeast 250000 CFU, Sorbitol 10000 mg | Unique combination of premix | 250 g / tonne of feed |
| 12 | COMPLIVITE – BFS (Neospark) | Each 500 g contains: Vit A – 12.5 MIU, Vit D3 – 3.0 MIU, Vit E – 12 g, Vit K3 – 1.5 g, Vit B12 – 15 mg, Vit B1 – 1.5 g, Vit B2 – 7.5 g, Vit B6 – 2.0 g, Niacin – 15 g, Calcium | Vitamin premix for use in broilers | 500 g / tonne of feed |

754

| S. No. | Trade Name & Company | Composition | Indications | Dosage / Administration |
|--------|----------------------|-------------|-------------|-------------------------|
| | | pantothenate 10 g, Folic acid – 0.5 g, Biotin – 50 mg | | |
| 13 | COMPLIVITE – LFS (Neospark) | Each 500 g contains: Vit A – 10 MIU, Vit D3 – 2.5 MIU, Vit E – 8 g, Vit K3 – 1 g, Vit B12 – 10 mg, Vit B1 – 1 g, Vit B2 – 5 g, Vit B6 – 1.5 g, Niacin – 12 g, Calcium pantothenate 8 g, Folic acid 0.5 g | * For layers<br>* Vitamin premix | 500 g / tonne of feed |
| 14 | HERBAL E – 50 (Indian Herbs) | Natural and stable vitamin E | * To improve health, growth, and production<br>* To improve broiler and layer performance<br>* To overcome stress | 100 g / tonne of feed |
| 15 | KAY-BEEMIX (Hitha) | Each g contains : Vit A 82,500 IU, Vit $B_2$ 50 mg, Vit $D_3$ 12,000 IU, Vit K 10 mg, Vit $B_1$ 8 mg, Vit $B_6$ 16 mg, Vit $B_{12}$ 120 mcg, Vit E 80 mg, Calcium pantothenate 80 mg, Niacin 120 mg | * Improves metabolism in the body<br>* Promotes growth<br>* For better weight gain<br>* Guaranteed potency | 100 g / tonne of feed |
| 16 | LAYVIT (For Layers) (Venky's) | Each Kg contains : Vit A 20 MIU, Vit $D_3$ 5 MIU, Vit E 16 g, Vit $K_3$ 2 g, Vit $B_1$ 2 g, Vit $B_2$ 10 g, Vit $B_6$ 3 g, Vit $B_{12}$ 16 mg, Niacin 24 g, Cal-D-pantothenate 16 g, Antioxidant q.s., Carrier q.s. | * For vitamin supplementation of layers<br>* To enhance profitability | 500 g / tonne of feed |
| 17 | LINE – H (Vetline) | Each 50 g contains: Biotin (Vit 'H') 20 mg, Water soluble carrier q.s. | Poor feathering in birds, loss of appetite, delayed growth, and reduced hatchability of eggs | **Chicks:** 50 g / 100 Kg of feed<br>**Growers and Layers:** 40 g / 100 Kg of feed<br>**Breeders:** 250 / 100 |

| S. No. | Trade Name & Company | Composition | Indications | Dosage / Administration |
|---|---|---|---|---|
| | | | | Kg of feed **In water:** 1 g / 2 litres of water Double the dose in severe deficiency |
| 18 | HIGHIMMUNE LIQUID (Aviguard) | Each ml contains : Vit A 3500 IU, Vit E 30 IU, Vit H 12.5 mg, Vit B$_6$ 1 mg, Vit C 100 mg | * For reducing stress * For better production, growth and fertility | **Chicks: Below 1 week:** 10 ml / 100 chicks for 5 days **2-6 weeks:** 3 ml / 100 chicks for 5 days **Pullets (7-18 weeks)** : 5 ml / 100 birds for 5 days **Broilers / Breeders:** 10 ml / 100 birds for 5 days **Layers:** 5-7 ml / 100 birds for 5 days |
| 19 | NATCHOL (Natural Remedies) | A natural alternative to synthetic choline chloride and equivalent | * To maintain growth, FCR, egg production, hatchability and livability * To prevent fatty liver condition | 300 g of Natchol replaces 1 Kg of synthetic choline chloride |
| 20 | N-CHOLINE (Natural Herbs) | It provides the required quantity of biotin and also contains herbal constituents | * Prevents the incidence of fatty liver syndrome * Helps to significantly reduce abdominal and carcass fat in broilers * To maintain growth, FCR, egg production and hatchability | 500 g / tonne of feed |
| 21 | NICOMIX AD3 500/100 (Nicholas Piramal) | Each g contains : Vit A 500,000 IU, Vit D$_3$ 100,000 IU | To improve growth, production and fertility | 15-20 g / tonne of feed |
| 22 | NICO-STRONG – B POWDER (Nicholas Piramal) | Each 100 g contains: Vit B2 – 1.25 g, Vit B6 – 0.62 g, Vit B12 – 12.6 mg, Niacin – 37.5 g, L-lysine – 10 g, | * For better growth and production * Improves metabolism and FCR | *Add 100 g of powder to 5 litres of fresh water and mix it to make a uniform solution. |

| S. No. | Trade Name & Company | Composition | Indications | Dosage / Administration |
|---|---|---|---|---|
| | | Choline bitartarate – 15.82 g, Calcium D-pantothenate – 3 g, DL-methionine 5 g, Excipients – q.s. | * Initiates faster recovery of weaker birds <br> * To prevent polyneuritis and paralysis <br> * Builds resistance | *Administer 15 – 20 ml solution per 100 birds daily through drinking water for 5-7 days |

# VITAMIN A

| S. No. | Trade Name & Company | Composition | Indications | Dosage / Administration |
|---|---|---|---|---|
| 1 | NICOSOL A ORAL LIQUID [Type 100] (Nicholas Piramal) | Each ml contains : Vit A 1,00,000 IU | To improve hatchability, fertility and egg production | **Chicks / Broilers:** 5 ml / 100 birds **Growers:** 8 ml / 100 birds **Layers:** 12 ml / 100 birds |
| 2 | SPARKSOL-A-LIQUID (Neospark) | Each ml contains : Vit A 1,00,000 IU, Casein protein 500 ppm, Elemental sodium 1mg, Elemental chloride 1.54 mg | * Increases egg production and hatchability<br>* Improves growth and weight gains<br>* Helps to build resistance<br>* Prevents blood spots in eggs | **Per 100 birds in drinking water:** **Chicks:** 5 ml / day for 7-10 days **Broilers:** 5 -7.5 ml / day for 7-10 days **Growers / Layers:** 5-10 ml / day for 7-10 days |
| 3 | VENTRI FORTE-A LIQUID (Venky's) | Each ml contains : Vit A 1,00,000 IU | * Helps in conditions like enteritis, coccidiosis, helminthiasis<br>* For tissue repair | 2 ml / 100 birds / 10 days a month |
| 4 | VITABLEND WM FORTE LIQUID (Virbac) | Each ml contains : Vit A 1,00,000 IU | * Increases egg production and hatchability<br>* For better growth<br>* For healthy chicks | **Chicks:** 2 ml / 100 birds **Growers:** 5 ml / 100 birds **Layers:** 5-10 ml /100 birds regularly for 10 days in drinking water |
| 5 | VITASOL – A (Qualitat) | 1 lac IU / ml | * Increases egg production and hatchability<br>* Better immune response and prevents blood spots in eggs<br>* Helps build resistance during coryza, CRD, enteritis, coccdiosis, helminthiasis<br>* To overcome stress | Administer once a day in drinking water for 7 days in a month per 100 birds as follows: **Chicks** 7 days: 1-2 ml **Growers** 7 days: 5ml **Broilers** 5 days: 5-7.5 ml **Layers** 5 days:10 ml |

# VITAMIN D$_3$

| S. No. | Trade Name & Company | Composition | Indications | Dosage / Administration |
|---|---|---|---|---|
| 1 | AV-FEROL-D$_3$ GRANULES (AVR) | Each g contains : Vit D$_3$ 6,00,000 IU | * Thin-shelled eggs<br>* Decreased egg production<br>* Low hatchability | 5 g / tonne of feed |
| 2 | DEESOL (Qualitat) | Each g contains : Vit D$_3$ 6,00,000 IU | * To improve eggshell quality, wing lameness, leg lameness<br>* To improve egg production and hatchability,<br>* It helps in better absorption of calcium. | **For regular use:** 5 g / tonne of feed **Curative:** 5 g / 2500 birds in drinking water **Preventive:** 5g / 5000 birds in drinking water |
| 3 | D-MIX 60 POWDER (Nicholas Piramal) | Each g contains : Vit D$_3$ 60,000 IU (Cholecalciferol) | * Thin-shelled eggs<br>* Decreased egg production<br>* Low hatchability | **Layers and Breeders:** 20 – 30 g / tonne of feed **Broilers:** 15 – 20 g / tonne of feed |
| 4 | DILVIT D$_3$ POWDER (Wockhardt) | Each g contains : Vit D$_3$ activity of 2,00,000 IU | * Protects from vitamin D$_3$ deficiency and rickets development<br>* Optimizes calcium-phosphorus metabolism<br>* Results in strong bones and hard eggshell<br>* Higher body weight gain and better FCR<br>* Reduces cost of feeding<br>* Increases productivity and profitability per bird | 10-15 g / tonne of feed |
| 5 | DVITOL-PLUS (Neospark) | Each 250 g contains: Vitamin D3 activity 4 MIU, fortified with manganese, zinc, natural alkaloids | * Formation of strong bones, hard eggshells<br>* Improves plumage<br>* Maintains egg production<br>* Improves productivity<br>* Better feed conversion ratio | **Preventive:** 125 g / tonne of feed **Curative dose:** 250 g / tonne of feed |

759

# VITAMIN – E + SELENIUM

| S. No. | Trade Name & Company | Composition | Indications | Dosage / Administration |
|---|---|---|---|---|
| 1 | BIO-SEL-E POWDER (Polchem) | Each g contains : Biotin (Vit H) 20 mcg, Selenium 200 mcg, Vit E 100 mg, Carrier q.s. | * Activates immune system and gives good immune response after vaccination<br>* Marked impact on general health and growth<br>* Elevates natural resistance power of bird<br>* Helps in preventing dermatitis, encephalomalacia, exudative diathesis, muscular myopathies and acute death syndrome<br>* Increases fertility and reduces embryonic mortality | **Chicks / Growers / Layers:**<br>5 g / 200 birds through water or 150-250 g / tonne of feed<br>**Broilers:**<br>5 g / 50 birds through water<br>**Breeders:**<br>10 g / 50 birds through water |
| 2 | BIOSTAR – VET (Micro Labs) | Vit E 10% w/w Selenium – 0.01% | * Reduces stress, leg weakness<br>* Improves fertility and hatchability<br>* Improves FCR | **Layers:**<br>150 – 250 g / tonne of feed<br>25 g / 1000 birds in drinking water<br>**Broilers:**<br>25 g / 250 birds in drinking water<br>**Breeders:**<br>20 g / 100 birds in drinking water |
| 3 | CHARAK-E-SEL POWDER (Charak) | Each g provides: Vit E 100 mg, Selenium 200 mcg, Biotin 20 mcg | * Improves strength and stamina to withstand stress<br>* Promotes immune response<br>* Protects from muscular dystrophy, crazy chick disease and | **Chicks / Growers / Layers:**<br>5 g / 200 birds or 150-250 g / tonne of feed<br>**Broilers:** 5 g / 50 birds |

| S. No. | Trade Name & Company | Composition | Indications | Dosage / Administration |
|---|---|---|---|---|
| | | | exudative diathesis<br>* Enhances fertility and hatchability<br>* Improves feather conditions | |
| 4 | E-CARE Se POWDER (Vetcare) | Each 200 g contains : Vit E 20 g, Selenium 200 ppm, Inert carrier q.s. | * Crazy chick disease<br>* Exudative diathesis<br>* Muscular dystrophy<br>* To improve fertility and hatchability<br>* Leg weakness<br>* Ascites | **Chicks / Growers / Layers:** 5 g / 200 birds through water<br>**Broilers:** 5 g / 50 birds through water |
| 5 | E-CARE Se FORTE POWDER (Vetcare) | Each Kg contains: Vit E 200 g, Selenium 400 mg, Inert carrier q.s. | * Nutritional encephalomalacia, twisted neck, prostration, curled toes and crazy chick disease<br>* Exudative diathesis<br>* Male sterility<br>* Impaired egg production and hatchability<br>* Increased embryonic mortality | **Chicks / Growers / Layers:** 75-125 g / tonne of feed<br>**Broilers / Breeders:** 250 g / tonne of feed |
| 6 | E-CARE Se HERBAL LIQUID (Vetcare) | Each ml contains: Vit E 100 mg, Selenium 0.5 mg, *Ocimum sanctum* extract q.s. | * During first week to boost immunity<br>* Pre and post-vaccination<br>* During outbreaks of immuno-suppressive problems like IBD, IBH, mycotoxicoses<br>* To overcome vaccination failure<br>* To minimize stress of transportation, debeaking, etc. | **Through drinking water for 5-7 days twice daily:**<br>**Chicks / Growers:** 2 ml / 100 birds<br>**Breeders:** 4 ml / 25-50 birds<br>**Layers / Broilers:** 2 ml / 75 birds |
| 7 | E-CARE Se HERBAL POWDER | Each g contains: Vit E 100 mg, Selenium 0.5 mg, | * Improves weight of bursa, spleen and thymus | Through drinking water for 5-7 days twice daily: |

| S. No. | Trade Name & Company | Composition | Indications | Dosage / Administration |
|---|---|---|---|---|
| | (Vetcare) | *Ocimum sanctum* extract q.s. | * Maintains immunity<br>* Improves vaccination titres against ND and IBD<br>* Increases leukocyte counts | **Chicks:** 1 Kg / tonne of feed<br>**Layers:** 250 g / tonne of feed<br>**Broilers / Breeders:** 500 g / tonne of feed |
| 8 | E-Se POWDER (Golden Streak) | Each 250 g contains : Vit E 25 mg, Selenium 50 mg (200 ppm) | * For better fertility and production<br>* For treatment of leg weakness, exudative diathesis and encephalomalacia | **Chicks / Growers / Layers:** 150-250 g / tonne of feed<br>**Broilers:** 1-1.5 Kg / tonne of feed |
| 9 | ESEL LIQUID (Elpe) | Each ml contains : Vitamin E 100 mg, Sodium selenite 500 mcg | * Leg weakness (muscular dystrophy)<br>* Exudative diathesis<br>* Encephalomalacial conditions<br>* Reduced fertility<br>* Reduced immunity<br>* Lower hatching results | 1-2 ml / litre in drinking water |
| 10 | E SOL B (Vetmed) | Each 10 ml contains: Vit E 1000 mg, Biotin 50 mcg, Selenium 200 ppm | * Boosts egg production, fertility, and hatchability<br>* Prevents muscular dystrophy and leg weakness<br>* Treats exudative diathesis and encephalomalacia | **Chicks:** 0.5 – 1 ml / litre of water<br>**Broilers:** 2 ml / litre of water<br>**Layers:** 1-2 ml / litre of water |
| 11 | E VET Se (AVR) | Each 200g contains: Vitamin E 20,000 IU, Selenium 200 ppm Base q.s. | * Immune potentiation<br>* Improves fertility/ hatchability in breeders.<br>* Improves muscle tone,<br>* Antioxidant | **Layers:** 150-250 g /tonne of feed. 5g / 200 birds in drinking water<br>**Broilers:** 5 g / 50 birds in drinking water |

| S. No. | Trade Name & Company | Composition | Indications | Dosage / Administration |
|---|---|---|---|---|
| | | | | **Breeders:** 10 g / 50 birds in water. |
| 12 | INDO-E-SEL-H (Indian Drugs and Vitamins) | Ecah g contains: Vit E 100 mg, Selenium 200 mcg, Biotin 20 mcg, Carrier q.s. | * Improves strength to withstand stress<br>* Promotes immune response<br>* Protects from muscular dystrophy, crazy chick disease, and exudative diathesis<br>* Improves general health and growth | **Chicks / Growers / Layers:** 5 g / 200 birds daily through water, or 150-250 g / tonne of feed<br>**Broilers:** 5 g / 50 birds daily through water<br>**Breeders:** 10 g / 50 birds daily through water |
| 13 | NEOSEL-E (Vetline) | Each g contains: Vit E 100 mg, Selenium 200 ppm, Biotin 20 mcg | * For immune potentiation against various viral diseases, coccidiosis, and also post-vaccination<br>* To overcome stress of deworming, vaccination and debeaking | **Chicks / Growers / Layers:** 150-250 / tonne of feed, or 5 g / 200 birds through water<br>**Broilers:** 5 g / 50 birds through water |
| 14 | NUTRI-SHIELD-P POWDER NUTRI-SHIELD-L LIQUID (Harshvardhan's Lab) | Vit E, Selenium and Biotin | A caretaker in the problem of immunosuppression | **Powder:** 200-250 g / metric tonne of feed<br>**Liquid:** 1-2 ml / litre of water |
| 15 | OLESEL-E DS FEED SUPPLEMENT (Avian Remedies) | Each g contains : Vit E 200 mg, Selenium 400 ppm, inorganic nutritive carrier q.s. | * For prevention and treatment of encephalomalacia (crazy chick disease), muscular dystrophy and exudative diathesis<br>* To improve fertility in the breeders and avoid the stress of deworming, vaccination and | **Chicks / Growers / Layers:** 100-125 g / tonne of feed<br>**Broilers:** 1 Kg / tonne of feed |

| S. No. | Trade Name & Company | Composition | Indications | Dosage / Administration |
|---|---|---|---|---|
| | | | debeaking<br>\* For immune potentiation against various viral diseases, coccidiosis and also post- vaccination | |
| 16 | PERIVAC PLUS (Neospark) | Each 200 g contains: Vit E 20 g, Biotin 160 g, Selenium 50 g | It is a potent combination of vit E, selenium, and biotin. It increases antibody production to enhance both humoral and cell-mediated immunity | **Chicks / Growers / Layers / Commercial Broilers:** 200 g / tonne of feed for 5 days **Breeders:** 500 g – 1 Kg / tonne of feed for 5 days |
| 17 | PERIVAC PLUS LIQUID CONCENTRATE (Neospark) | Each 10 ml contains : Vit E 250 mg, Biotin 2 mg, Selenium 1 mg | Stress, deficiency diseases, debility, encephalomalacia, exudative diathesis, to improve fertility and hatchability | **Chicks:** 5 ml / 100 birds / day **Broilers / Layers:** 10 ml / 100 birds / day **Breeders:** 20-40 ml / 100 birds / day |
| 18 | PERIVAC PLUS FORTE-FS POWDER (Neospark) | Each 200 g contains : Vit E 40 g, Biotin 320 mg, Selenium 100 mg, Carrier q.s. | \* It is a potent combination of Vit E, selenium and biotin. It increases antibody production to enhance both humoral and cell-mediated immunity | **Chicks / Growers / Layers:** 100 g / tonne of feed for 5 days **Broilers:** 500 g / tonne of feed for 5 days |
| 19 | SELE-H POWDER (Elpe) | Each 250 g contains : Vit E 20,000 mg, Selenium 150 mg, Biotin 80 mg | \* Leg weakness (muscular dystrophy)<br>\* Dermatitis<br>\* Exudative diathesis<br>\* Encephalomalacial conditions<br>\* Reduces immune response<br>\* Reduces feed conversion<br>\* Poor quality of | **Chicks:** 200-250 g / tonne of feed **Growers:** 150-200 g / tonne of feed **Broilers:** 250-500 g / tonne of feed **Layers:** 200-250 g / tonne of feed |

| S. No. | Trade Name & Company | Composition | Indications | Dosage / Administration |
|---|---|---|---|---|
| | | | chicks<br>* Lower hatching results<br>* Acute fatty liver / kidney conditions | |
| 20 | SELVIT-E POWDER (Venky's) | Each g contains :<br>Vit E 100 mg,<br>Selenium 200 mcg | * Enhances immune response<br>* Prevents encephalomalacia | **Chicks / Growers / Layers:**<br>200 g / tonne of feed or 5 g / 200 birds in drinking water<br>**Broilers:**<br>5 g / 50 birds in drinking water |
| 21 | SELVIT E D. S. POWDER (Venky's) | Each g contains :<br>Vit E 200 mg,<br>Selenium 400 mcg | * Enhances immune response<br>* Prevents encephalomalacia | 100 g / tonne of feed |
| 22 | SELVIT-E GREEN POWDER (Venky's) | Each g contains :<br>Vit E 100 mg,<br>Selenium 200 mcg,<br>Herbal immuno-stimulant compound 25 mg, Organic carrier q.s. | * Early embryonic deaths, gizzard damage, hatchability, exudative diathesis, muscular dystrophy and encephalo-malacia<br>* To potentiate immune response against various viral diseases and during post-vaccinal periods<br>* Improves fertility and hatchability | 5 g / 100 chicks, or in feed @ 200 g / tonne<br>Recommended for 10 days course |
| 23 | STARBLEND POWDER (Virbac) | Each 100 g contains :<br>Vit E 20,000 IU,<br>Selenium 20,000 mcg | * For fertility and hatchability in breeders<br>* For immunity<br>* Acts as an immunostimulant during post-vaccination period, reduces stress during deworming, debeaking, weather | **Through water:**<br>**Chicks / Growers / Layers:**<br>2.5 g / 200 birds<br>**Broilers:**<br>5 g / 100 birds<br>**Through feed:**<br>75-125 g / tonne of feed |

| S. No. | Trade Name & Company | Composition | Indications | Dosage / Administration |
|---|---|---|---|---|
| | | | changes and vaccination | |
| 24 | SUPERMUNE (Sarabhai Zydus) | Vitamin E, Selenium, Herbs | * Immunomodulator, removes immunosuppression<br>* Antistress<br>* Removes ascites | 100g/ tonne of feed |
| 25 | TRA-E-SEL POWDER (Rallis) | Each 25 g contains : Vit E 1000 IU, Selenium 20 mg, Cobalt 100 mg, Copper 900 mg, Iron 3 g | * To improve production, fertility, hatchability<br>* To potentiate immune response and overcome stress | **Broilers / Breeders:** 25 g / 25 Kg feed **Layers:** 25 g / 100 Kg feed |

# VITAMIN K

| S. No. | Trade Name & Company | Composition | Indications | Dosage / Administration |
|---|---|---|---|---|
| 1 | AV-SOL K₃ POWDER (AVR) | Each 50 g contains : Vit K₃ 500 mg, Vit C 250 mg | * To be given after the stress of debeaking <br> * To reduce blood loss in coccidiosis | **Preventive:** 50 g / 3200 birds / day **Therapeutic:** 1 g / 5 litres of water |
| 2 | KAYSOL FORTE SOLUBLE POWDER (Vetcare) | Each 50 g contains : Vit K₃ 500 mg w/w, Inert carrier q.s. | * To reduce blood loss in coccidiosis <br> * After debeaking <br> * To improve laying in peak production | **Chicks / Growers** : 50 g / 3000 birds / day for 5-7 days in water **During coccidiosis:** 1 g / 5 litres of water |
| 3 | SOLVI-K (Vetline) | Each 50 g contains: Vit K3 500mg , Base (water soluble) q.s. | * To reduce blood loss during coccidiosis <br> * To reduce stress due to blood loss <br> * To improve laying in peak production after debeaking | **Chick/growers** : 50 g/day for 3200 birds for 5 days **During coccidiosis** : 1 gm/5litre of water |

# VITAMIN AB$_2$D$_3$EK

| S. No. | Trade Name & Company | Composition | Indications | Dosage / Administration |
|---|---|---|---|---|
| 1 | AFFOMIN (Qualitat) | Each Kg contains: Vit A 20,00,000 IU, Vit D3 4,00,000 IU, Vit B2 1 g, Vit E 300 mg, Vit K 0.4 g, Calcium pantothenate 1 g, Niacin 6 g, Vit B12 4 mcg, Choline chloride 120 g, Calcium 320 g, Gentian violet 4 g | * Combating aflatoxin <br> * Better resistance to infections, <br> * Gentian violet acts as antifungal <br> * Increases body weight | 2.5 Kg / tonne of feed |
| 2 | ALVIMIX-FORTE (Alembic) | Vit A – 10,00,0000 IU, Vit D3 – 25,00000 IU, Vit E – 8 g, Vit K3 – 1 g, Vit B1 – 0.8 g, Vit B2 – mg, Vit B12 – 20.5 mg, Calcium-D-pantothenate – 8 g, Niacinamide – 12 g, Vitamin B6 – 1.6 g, Folic acid – 0.8 g, | Prevents soft-shelled eggs, cage layer paralysis and rickets | 250 g / tonne of feed |
| 3 | AV-MIX AB$_2$D$_3$K POWDER (AVR) | Each g contains : Vit A 82,500 IU, Vit B$_2$ 50 mg, Vit D$_3$ 16,500 IU, Vit K 10 mg | * Stress <br> * Retarded growth <br> * Deficiency syndrome <br> * Off feed | 100 – 150 g / tonne of feed |
| 4 | AV-PREMIX- L (AVR) | Each Kg contains: Vit A – 5,00,000 IU, Vit D3 – 1,00,000 IU, Vit E – 32 g, Vit K3 – 4 g, Vit B1 – 4 g, Vit B2 – 20 g, Vit B6 – 6 g, Vit B12 – 38 mg, Nicotinates – 48 g, Pantothenic acid – 32 g, Folic acid – 2.4 g, | * Improves the egg laying capacity <br> * Improves shell strength and egg size | **Layers:** 250 g / tonne of feed |
| 5 | AV-PREMIX- B (AVR) | Each Kg contains: Vit A – 2.5 lac IU, Vit D3 – 5 lac IU, Vit E – 24 g, Vit K3 – 3 g, Vit B1 3 g, Vit B2 – 10 g, Vit B6 – 4 g, Vit B12 – 30 g, Nicotinamide – | * Complete source of vitamin supplement as per requirement of the bird <br> * Improves shell strength and egg size | **Broilers:** 500 g / tonne of feed |

| S. No. | Trade Name & Company | Composition | Indications | Dosage / Administration |
|---|---|---|---|---|
| | | 30 g, Pantothenic acid – 20 g, Folic acid – 1 g, Antioxidants q.s., Carrier q.s. | | |
| 6 | BROLAY CLP (Jubilant Organosys) | Each 500 g contains: Vit A 1,00,00000 IU, Vit D3 25,00000IU, Vit E 8 g, Vit K3 1 g, Vit B1 0.8 g, Vit B2 5 g, Vit B6 1.5 g , Vit B12 8 mg, Niacin 12 g, Pantothenic acid 8 g, Lactose and Calcium carbonate as carrier | * Ensures high bioavailability of vitamins<br>* Maintains potency of vitamins under practical storage conditions<br>* Maintains potency and stability of vitamins | 500 g / tonne of layer feed |
| 7 | COMPLIVITE – BFS (Neospark) | Each 500 g contains: Vit A 12.5 MIU, Vit D3 3 MIU, Vit E 12 g, Vit K3 1.5 g, Vit B12 15 mg, Vit B1 1.5 g, Vit B2 7.5 g, Vit B6 2 g, Niacin 15 g, Calcium pantothenate 10 g, Folic acid 0.5 g, Biotin 50 mg | Vitamin premix for use in broilers | 500 g / tonne of feed |
| 8 | COMPLIVITE – LFS (Neospark) | Each 500 g contains: Vit A 10 MIU, Vit D3 2.5 MIU, Vit E 8 g, Vit K3 1 g, Vit B12 10 mg, Vit B1 1 g, Vit B2 5 g, Vit B6 1.5 g, Niacin 12 g, Calcium pantothenate 8 g, Folic acid 0.5 g | Vitamin premix for use in poultry | 500 g / tonne of feed |
| 9 | DAILYMIX (Brihans) | Each g contains : Vit A 82,500 IU, Vit $B_2$ 50 mg, Vit $D_3$ 12,000 IU, Vit K 10 mg, Vit $B_{12}$ 15 mcg | * Provides all essential vitamins<br>* Builds resistance against infections and parasites<br>* Stimulates growth and production<br>* Improves hatchability | 100 g / tonne of feed |
| 10 | HI-PERFORMANCE | Each 250 g contains: Vit A- 10 MIU, Vit D3 | For deficiency of vitamins | 250 g / tonne of feed |

| S. No. | Trade Name & Company | Composition | Indications | Dosage / Administration |
|---|---|---|---|---|
| | PREMIX (Nicholas Piramal) | – 2 MIU, B1 – 0.8 g, Vit B2 – 5 g, Vit B6 – 1.60 g, Vit B12 – 20.50 mg, Niacin – 12 g, Calcium pantothenate – 8 g, Vit K3 – 1 g, Vit E – 8 g, Folic acid – 0.8 g | | |
| 11 | HI-VEEMIX POWDER (Hitha) | Each g contains : Vit A 82,500 IU, Vit B$_2$ 50 mg, Vit D$_3$ 12,000 IU, Vit K 10 mg | * Improves growth rate through proper feed utilization <br> * Improves egg production | 1 Kg / 10 tonnes of feed |
| 12 | HIVIT INJECTION (Vetnex) | Each ml contains: Vit A 2000 IU, Vit D3 2000 IU, Vit E acetate 4 mg, Nicotinamide 10 mg, Thiamine Hcl, 10 mg, Pyridoxine Hcl 5 mg, Riboflavin 1 mg, D-Panthenol 1 mg, Vit B12 10 mcg, d-Biotin 10 mcg, Calcium glycerophosphate 10 mg | Multivitamin supplement for better livability of chicks and vitamin deficiency disorders | 1 ml / Kg body weight. For day-old chicks, mix 100 ml of normal saline and give this to 2500 chicks at the dose rate of 0.2 ml per chick |
| 13 | HYBLEND POWDER (Virbac) | Each g contains : Vit A 82,500 IU, Vit B$_2$ 50 mg, Vit D$_3$ 12,000 IU, Vit K 10 mg | * Improves growth rate through proper feed utilization <br> * Improves egg production | 1 Kg / 10 tonnes of feed |
| 14 | MERIVITE AB$_2$D$_3$K POWDER (Wockhardt) | Each g contains : Vit A 82,500 IU, Vit B$_2$ 52 mg, Vit D$_3$ 12,000 IU, Vit K 10 mg, Calcium 166 mg, Phosphorus 129 mg | * Helps to maintain growth and production by improving the feed conversion efficiency <br> * Helps to improve resistance to fight infections <br> * Helps to prevent curled toe paralysis and rickets | 100 g / tonne of feed |
| 15 | NICOMIX AB2D3 POWDER | Each gm contains: Vit A 40,000 IU, Vit | * Prevents early chick mortality | 200 – 250 g / tonne of feed |

| S. No. | Trade Name & Company | Composition | Indications | Dosage / Administration |
|---|---|---|---|---|
| | (Nicholas Piramal) | B2 20 mg, Vit D3 5000 IU | * For better fertility, hatchability<br>* Increases resistance to infections<br>* Increases weight gain | |
| 16 | NICOMIX AB2D3K (Nicholas Piramal) | Each g contains: Vit A – 82,500 IU, Vit B2 – 50 mg, Vit D3 – 12,000 IU, Vit K – 10 mg, | * Improves weight gain, hatchability and fertility<br>* Improves resistance to infections | 100 g / tonne of feed |
| 17 | NICOMIX SUPER (Nicholas Piramal) | Each 500 g contains: Vit A – 12.50 MIU, Vit D3 – 2.5 MIU, Vit B1 – 2g, Vit B2 – 8 g, Vit B6 – 3 g, Vit B12 15 mg, Niacin – 30 g, Calcium pantothenate – 10 g, Vit K3 – 2 g, Vit E – 40 g, Folic acid 1 g, Biotin 20 mg | For additional nutritional requirement of layers | 500 g / tonne of feed |
| 18 | NICOMIX SUPER LAY (Nicholas Piramal) | Each 500 g contains: Vit A – 12.50 MIU, Vit D3 – 3.0 MIU, Vit B1 – 0.8 g, Vit B2 – 5 g, Vit B6 – 1.6 g, Vit B12 20 mg, Niacin – 12 g, Calcium pantothenate – 8 g, Vit K3 – 1 g, Vit E – 8 g, Folic acid 0.8 g, Biotin 100 mg | * Fatty acid synthesis<br>* Synthesis of glucose<br>* Fast and uniform growth<br>* Improves hatchability | 500 g / tonne of feed |
| 19 | NUTRIVITE-AB$_2$D$_3$K POWDER (Harshvardhan's Lab) | Each g contains : Vit A 82,500 IU, Vit B$_2$ 50 mg, Vit D$_3$ 16,500 IU, Vit K 10 mg | * Increases calcium and phosphorus assimilation<br>* For better mobility of calcium in the bones<br>* For lesser leg weakness<br>* For better bone growth | **Chicks:** 150 g / tonne of feed<br>**Growers / Broilers / Layers:** 100 g / tonne of feed |

| S. No. | Trade Name & Company | Composition | Indications | Dosage / Administration |
|---|---|---|---|---|
| 20 | OLEMIX POWDER (Avian Remedies) | Each g contains : Vit A 82,500 IU, Vit B$_2$ 50 mg, Vit D$_3$ 16,000 IU, Vit K 10 mg, Calcium 260 mg, Organic nutrient carrier q.s. | * Improves shell strength and egg size<br>* Helps in stress situations<br>* Prevents appearance of blood spots in eggs<br>* For better egg production<br>* Reinforces resistance to disease | 100 g / tonne of feed |
| 21 | OLEMIX FORTE POWDER (Avian Remedies) | Each g contains : Vit A 2,47,500 IU, Vit B$_2$ 150 mg, Vit D$_3$ 48,000 IU, Vit K 30 mg, Calcium 260 mg, Organic nutrient carrier q.s. | * Improves shell strength and egg size<br>* Helps in stress situations<br>* Prevents appearance of blood spots in eggs<br>* For better egg production<br>* Reinforces resistance to disease | 35 g / tonne of feed |
| 22 | OSCO AB$_2$D$_3$K (Osco) | Each g contains : Vit A 82,500 IU, Vit B$_2$ 50 mg, Vit D$_3$ 16,000 IU, Vit K 10 mg | * Helps to build resistance to fight infections<br>* Helps to stimulate growth and production by improving the feed conversion efficiency<br>* Helps to prevent curled-toe paralysis and rickets<br>* Helps to increase egg production<br>* Helps to prevent haemorrhagic syndrome and blood loss specially | 100 g / tonne of feed |

| S. No. | Trade Name & Company | Composition | Indications | Dosage / Administration |
|---|---|---|---|---|
| | | | during coccidiosis | |
| 23 | PENTAFORTE BROILER DS (Vetnex) | Each Kg contains: Vit A 50 MIU, Vit D3 12 MIU, Vit E 120 g, Vit K3 8 g, Vit B1 8 g, Vit B2 20 g, Vit B6 12 g, Vit B12 0.06 g, Niacin 120 g, Pantothenic acid 60 g, Folic acid 4 g, Biotin 0.32 g | Multivitamin feed supplement | 250 g / tonne of feed |
| 24 | PENTAFORTE LAYER 1 (Vetnex) | Each Kg contains: Vit A 40 MIU, Vit D3 10 MIU, Vit E 40 g, Vit K3 4 g, Vit B1 4 g, Vit B2 20 g, Vit B6 6 g, Vit B12 0.032 g, Niacin co-pantothenate 32 g, folic acid | Multivitamin feed supplement | 250 g / tonne of feed |
| 25 | PENTAFORTE LAYER 2 | Each Kg contains: Vit A 50 MIU, Vit D3 14 MIU, Vit E 20 g, Vit K3 8 g, Vit B1 3.2 g, Vit B2 32 g, Vit B6 3.6 g, Vit B12 0.024 g, Niacin 28 g, Pantothenate 16 g, Folic acid 5.6 g | Multivitamin feed supplement | 250 g / tonne of feed |
| 26 | SIMVITE – B (Vetline) | Each 500 g contains: Vit A 10 mlu, Vit D3 3.3 mlu, Vit E 15 g, Vit K 1.6 g, Vit B1 0.5 g,Vit B2 6 g, Vit B6 1 g, Vit B12 12 mg, calcium pantothenate 10 g, niacin 30 g, folic acid 1 g, biotin 25 mg, base q.s. | * For healthy and faster growth in chicks, growers and broilers <br> * Improves feed utilization and feed conversion efficiency <br> * Prevents nutritional imbalances in deficiency diseases | **For Broilers:** 500 g / tonne of feed |
| 27 | SIMVITE-L (Vetline) | Each 500 g contains: Vitamin A 8.25 mlu,Vit D3 3.3 mlu,Vit E 5 g, Vit K 1 g, Vit B1 0.2 g, Vit B2 5 g, | * Prevents nutritional imbalances and deficiency diseases <br> * Improves shell quality and | **For Layers:** 500 g / tonne of feed |

| S. No. | Trade Name & Company | Composition | Indications | Dosage / Administration |
|---|---|---|---|---|
| | | Vit B6 0.5 g, Vit B12 5 mg, calcium pantothenate 3 g, niacin 6 g, folic acid 0.2 g, base q.s. | thickness<br>* Reduces the chances of leg weakness | |
| 28 | SPECTRO BE (Vetnex) | Each g contains:<br>Vit B1 8 mg, Vit B6 16 mg, Vit B12 80 mcg, Niacin 120 mg, Ca-pantothenate 80 mg, Vit E 160 mg, Lysine 10 mg, DL-methionine 10 mg | Multivitamin feed supplement | 100 g / tonne of feed |
| 29 | SPECTRO MIX POWDER (Vetnex) | Each g contains :<br>Vitamin A 82,500 IU, Vit $B_2$ 50 mg, Vit $D_3$ 12,000 IU, Vit K 10 mg | * Improves feed conversion ratio<br>* Increases egg production<br>* Provides additional weight gain<br>* Promotes growth<br>* Facilitates immune response<br>* Helps proper skeletal develop-ment<br>* Prevents rickets and curled toe  paralysis | 100 g / tonne of feed |
| 30 | SUPER BLEND POWDER (Hitha) | Each g contains :<br>Vit A 82,500 IU, Vit $B_2$ 50 mg, Vit $D_3$ 12,000 IU, Vit K 10 mg, Vit $B_1$ 2 mg, Vit $B_6$ 4 mg, Vit $B_{12}$ 30 mcg, Niacin 30 mg, Calcium pantothenate 20 mg | * Maintains growth, better FCR<br>* Improves metabolism in the body<br>* Prevents curled toe paralysis,  rickets and dermatitis<br>* Ensures proper coagulation of blood<br>* Builds resistance to fight against diseases<br>* Prevents embryonic mortality  and anaemia<br>* Improves feathering | 100 g / tonne of feed |

| S. No. | Trade Name & Company | Composition | Indications | Dosage / Administration |
|---|---|---|---|---|
| 31 | SUPER BLEND FORTE + FEED SUPPLEMENT (Hitha) | Each g contains : Vit A 82,500 IU, Vit $B_2$ 50 mg, Vit $D_3$ 12,000 IU, Vit K 10 mg, Vit $B_1$ 2 mg, Vit $B_6$ 4 mg, Vit $B_{12}$ 30 mcg, Niacin 30 mg, Calcium pantothenate 20 mg, Vit E 40 mg, Vit C 20 mg | * For better growth, FCR<br>* Improves immunity<br>* Prevents embryonic mortality<br>* Helps in proper coagulation of blood<br>* Helps to overcome stress conditions | 100 g / tonne of feed |
| 32 | TCL-$AB_2D_3K$ POWDER (Trichem) | Each g contains : Vit A 82,500 IU, Vit $B_2$ 50 mg, Vit $D_3$ 12,000 IU, Vit K 10 mg | For better growth, production and fertility | 100 g / tonne of feed |
| 33 | ULTRABLEND A + $B_2$ + $D_3$ POWDER (Vitamin + Mineral) (Neospark) | Each g contains : Vit A 40,000 IU, Vit $B_2$ 25 mg, Vit $D_3$ 6,000 IU Calcium 184 mg, Phosphorus 138 mg, Elemental sodium 500 ppm | * For better growth, production and fertility<br>* For mineral deficiency diseases and poor eggshell | 200 g / tonne of feed |
| 34 | ULTRABLEND A + $B_2$ + $D_3$ + K POWDER [Vitamin + Mineral] (Neospark) | Each g contains : Vitamin A 82,500 IU, Vit $B_2$ 50 mg, Vit $D_3$ 12,000 IU, Vit K 10 mg, Calcium 184 mg, Phosphorus 138 mg, Elemental sodium 500 ppm | * For better growth, production and fertility<br>* For mineral deficiency diseases and poor eggshell | 100 g / tonne of feed |
| 35 | VENTRIMIX D.S. POWDER (Venky's) | Each g contains : Vit A 82,500 IU, Vit $B_2$ 50 mg, Vit $D_3$ 12,000 IU, Vit K 10 mg | * For better growth and production<br>* To build resistance<br>* To prevent curled toe paralysis | 100 g / tonne of feed<br>**In summer :** 200 g / tonne of feed |
| 36 | VITAMIN PREMIX (Indian Drugs and Vitamins) | Each Kg contains: Vit A 48 MIU, Vit D3 11 MIU, Vit E 200 g, Vit K3 6.4 g, Vit B1 10 g, Vit B2 30 g, Vit B6 | * Ensures full potency of all vitamins<br>* Vitamin supplementation as | 250 g / tonne of feed |

| S. No. | Trade Name & Company | Composition | Indications | Dosage / Administration |
|---|---|---|---|---|
| | | 14 g, Vit B12 0.08 g Cal-D-pentothenate 44 g, Niacin 160 g, Folic acid 4.8 g, Biotin 0.4 g, Anti-caking 10 g, Preservatives 2.5 g | per requirement of birds<br>* Cost-effective feed formulation<br>* Homogeneous mixing in feed | |
| 37 | VITASOL ABDEC (Qualitat) | Each 5 ml contains: Vit A – 2, 50, 000 IU, Vit D3 – 25000 IU, Vit E – 150 mg, Vit C – 500 mg, Vit B12 – 100 mcg | * Helps in fast recovery from infections<br>* Stimulates growth and production<br>* Provides strength during vaccination, debeaking, deworming, stress and fatigue<br>* Maintains fertility in males and females | **Chicks (5-7 days):** 3-5 ml / 100 birds<br>**Growers (5-7 days):** 5 – 7 ml / 100 birds<br>**Broilers (0-4 weeks):** 3-5 ml / 100 birds<br>**Layers (5-7 days):** 7- 10 ml / 100 birds |
| 38 | VM MIX-ABDK POWDER (Vetmed) | Each g contains : Vit A 82,500 IU, Vit $B_2$ 50 mg, Vit $D_3$ 16,500 IU, Vit K 10 mg | * For better FCR, growth and production<br>* To prevent deficiency conditions | 10 g / tonne of feed |

# VITAMIN AD₃EC

| S. No. | Trade Name & Company | Composition | Indications | Dosage / Administration |
|---|---|---|---|---|
| 1 | ALVITON LIQUID (Alembic) | Each 5 ml contains : Vit A 2,50,000 IU Vit D₃ 25,000 IU, Vit E 150 IU, Vit C 500 mg | * Alleviates stress<br>* Increases body resistance<br>* Improves fertility<br>* Improves FCR | 5-10 ml / 100 birds |
| 2. | BIOSOL ORAL (Vetmed) | Each 10 ml contains: Vit A 5,00,000 IU, Vit D3 50,000 IU, Vit E 300 mg, Vit C 1000 mg | * Prevents stress<br>* Accelerates growth<br>* Enhances higher egg production<br>* Increases weight gain | **Broilers:** 3-5 ml / 100 birds<br>**Layers:** 10-15 ml / 100 birds<br>**Breeders:** 20 ml / 100 birds |
| 3 | BONNYSOL AD₃ECB₁₂ LIQUID (Neospark) | Each 5 ml contains : Vit A 2,50,000 IU Vit D₃ 25,000 IU, Vit E 150 IU, Vit C 500 mg, Vit B₁₂ 100 mcg, Protein hydrolysate 20 mg, Elemental sodium 19.67 mg, Elemental cobalt 4.5 mg | * For uniform and rapid growth in chicks, increased body resistance, improved egg production, more weight gain and improved feed efficiency in broilers<br>* During all kinds of stress | **Chicks:** 5 ml / 100 chicks / day<br>**Broilers / Growers / Layers:** 5-10 ml / 100 birds / day |
| 4 | CAPOVIT LIQUID (Indian Immunologicals) | Each ml contains : Vit A 12,000 IU, Vit D₃ 6,000 IU, Vit E 48 mg, Vit B₁₂ 20 mcg | * To promote growth, resistance to infections and fertility<br>* To overcome stress | **Chicks:** 5 ml / 100 chicks<br>**Growers:** 7 ml / 100 birds<br>**Layers:** 10 ml / 100 birds |
| 5 | CAPOVIT FORTE LIQUID (Indian Immunologicals) | Each 5 ml contains : Vit A 2,50,000 IU, Vit D₃ 25,000 IU, Vit E 150 mg, Vit C 500 mg | * To improve growth, resistance to infections, eggshell quality, fertility and hatchability<br>* To overcome stress | **For 1000 birds:**<br>**Period  Broilers  Layers**<br>1-3 wks  10 ml  15 ml<br>4-6 wks  20 ml  35 ml<br>7-9 wks  30 ml  45 ml<br>10-12 wk  -  35 ml<br>13-18 wks    50 ml |

| S. No. | Trade Name & Company | Composition | Indications | Dosage / Administration |
|---|---|---|---|---|
| | | | | Above 18 wks  90 ml |
| 6 | CONCITONE (Concept) | Each 5 ml contains : Vit A 60,000 IU, Vit $D_3$ 30,000 IU, Vit E 240 mg, Vit C 5 mg, Vit $B_2$ 5 mg, Vit $B_6$ 5 mg, Vit $B_{12}$ 125 mcg, Nicotinamide 35 mg, D. panthenol 10 mg, Elemental sodium 1.48 mg, Elemental phosphorus 1 mg, Elemental potassium 1.10 mg, Elemental chloride 1 mg. | * Improves immunity<br>* Improves feed consumption<br>* Improves FCR<br>* Improves weight gain / egg production<br>* Reduces mortality | **Chicks:** 5 ml / 100 birds **Broilers / Growers:** 7.5 ml/100 birds **Layers:** 10 ml / 100 birds for 5-7 days |
| 7 | CURATONE LIQUID (Indo Biocare) | Each 5 ml contains : Vit A 60,000 IU, Vit $D_3$ 30,000 IU, Vit E 240 mg, Vit C 100 mg, Vit $B_{12}$ 100 mcg | * Alleviates stress<br>* Improves disease resistance<br>* Ensures intensive growth<br>* Improves immunity<br>* For proper bone calcification | **Chickens:** 5 ml / 100 birds **Growers / Broilers :** 7 ml / 100 birds **Layers:** 10 ml / 100 birds |
| 8 | FAMITONE LIQUID (Vetnex) | Each 5 ml contains : Vit A 2,50,000 IU, Vit $D_3$ 25,000 IU, Vit E 150 IU, Vit C 500 mg | For all types of stress like heat stress, production stress, transport stress, handling stress, vaccination stress, deworming stress, antibiotic therapy stress, vitamin deficiency stress and in mycotoxicosis | 5-10 ml / 100 birds, once daily for a week, in drinking water |
| 9 | GOLDISTRESS LIQUID | Each 5 ml contains : Vit A 62,500 IU, Vit | * Reduces stress due to vaccination, | **Chicks:** 3-5 ml / 100 chicks |

| S. No. | Trade Name & Company | Composition | Indications | Dosage / Administration |
|---|---|---|---|---|
| | (Golden Streak) | $D_3$ 25,000 IU, Vit E 150 IU, Vit C 500 mg | deworming, transportation, debeaking etc. <br> * Improves growth, production, fertility and hatchability <br> * Enhances laying performance reduced from intense heat, illness, cold, and fatigue in cages <br> * Corrects calcium and phosphorus metabolism <br> * Improves bone and eggshell quality | **Broilers / Growers:** 5-7 ml / 100 birds <br> **Layers:** 7-10 ml / 100 birds |
| 10 | HI-TONE LIQUID (Hitha) | Each 5 ml contains : Vit A 2,50,000 IU, Vit $D_3$ 25,000 IU, Vit E 150 mg, Vit C 500 mg | * Maintains growth, better FCR <br> * Improves resistance against infections <br> * Enhances fertility and hatchability of breeder flocks <br> * Increases egg production <br> * Prevents xerophthalmia <br> * Provides strength and stamina during stress | **Chicks:** 0.5-1 ml / 100 birds <br> **Broilers / Growers:** 1-2 ml / 100 birds <br> **Layers:** 2-5 ml / 100 birds |
| 11 | HI-TONE (Natural Herbs) | Herbal combination of vitamin A, C, D3, E, Selenium oxalate and Bromide | * Boosts immune response <br> * Improves fertility and hatchability in breeders <br> * Overcomes stress during vaccination, deworming, and transportation <br> * Improves | **Chicks:** 2-3 ml / 100 birds <br> **Broilers:** 4-6 ml / 100 birds <br> **Growers / Layers:** 6-10 ml / 100 birds |

| S. No. | Trade Name & Company | Composition | Indications | Dosage / Administration |
|---|---|---|---|---|
| | | | productivity in broilers, layers, and breeders | |
| 12 | HI-VITONE LIQUID (Hitha) | Each 5 ml contains : Vit A 12,000 IU, Vit D$_3$ 6,000 IU, Vit E 48 mg, Vit B$_{12}$ 20 mcg | * Maintains growth, better FCR <br> * Increases egg production <br> * Enhances fertility and hatchability of breeder flocks <br> * Improves resistance against infections <br> * Prevents xerophthalmia | 5-10 ml / 100 birds daily |
| 13 | NICOSOL AD$_3$EC ORAL LIQUID FEED SUPPLEMENT (Nicholas Piramal) | Each ml contains : Vit A 50,000 IU, Vit D$_3$ 5,000 IU, Vit E 30 IU, Vit C 100 mg | * Removes stress associated with weather changes, particularly heat stress <br> * Improves fertility and hatchability <br> * Prevents encephalomalacia and exudative diathesis | **Chicks:** 3-5 ml / 100 birds <br> **Broilers / Growers:** 5 ml / 100 birds <br> **Layers:** 10-15 ml / 100 birds |
| 14 | RECOVIT LIQUID (Brihans) | Each ml contains : Vit A 50,000 IU, Vit D$_3$ 5,000 IU, Vit E 50 mg, Vit C 100 mg, Vit B$_{12}$ 25 mcg | * Provides strength and stamina during vaccination, debeaking, and deworming <br> * Stimulates growth and production <br> * Builds body resistance to infections | **Chicks:** 1-2 ml / 100 chicks <br> **Broilers / Growers:** 2-3 ml / 100 birds <br> **Layers:** 4-5 ml / 100 birds for 7-10 days every month |
| 15 | STADEC LIQUID (Stallen) | Each ml contains: Vit A 50,000 IU, Vit D3 5,000 IU, Vit E 30 IU, Vit C 100 mg, Excipients q. s. | * To increase the resistance against diseases <br> * For quicker growth, increase egg production and fertility rate | **For 100 birds:** <br> **Broilers:** 3-5 ml <br> **Layers:** 10 – 15 ml <br> **Breeders:** 20 ml |

| S. No. | Trade Name & Company | Composition | Indications | Dosage / Administration |
|---|---|---|---|---|
| | | | * Avitaminosis A D E and C | |
| 16 | STRESVEL LIQUID (Venky's) | Each ml contains : Vit A 50,000 IU, Vit $D_3$ 5,000 IU, Vit E 30 IU, Vit C 100 mg | * Reduces stress<br>* Enhances immune response | **Chicks:**<br>4-5 ml / 100 chicks for 5-7 days<br>**Broilers / Layers:**<br>5 ml / 100 birds for 5-7 days |
| 17 | VIMERAL LIQUID (Virbac) | Each ml contains: Vit A 12,000 IU, Vit $D_3$ 6,000 IU, Vit E 48 mg, Vit $B_{12}$ 20 mcg | * Removes stress<br>* For better growth<br>* For better egg production<br>* For strong shelled eggs<br>* For strong bones | **Chicks:**<br>5 ml/100 birds<br>**Growers:**<br>7 ml/100 birds<br>**Layers:**<br>10 ml/100 birds |
| 18 | VITALIZER (Harshvardhan's Lab) | Each ml contains: Vitamin A 50000 IU, Vit D3 5000 IU, Vit E 30 IU, Vit C 100 mg | * Maintenance of health, performance and fertility<br>* Elimination of deficiencies<br>* In all situations of stress | **Chicks:**<br>2-3 ml / 100 chicks for 5-7 days<br>**Broilers / Layers:**<br>4-5 ml / 100 broilers / layers for 5-7 days |
| 19 | VITAMAX – ORAL LIQUID (Elpe) | Each ml contains : Vit A 12,000 IU, Vit $D_3$ 6,000 IU, Vit E 50 mg, Vit $B_{12}$ 20 mcg, Selenium 50 mcg | * For retarded growth<br>* For low egg production and hatchability<br>* For poor fertility and formation of eggshell<br>* Rickets<br>* Nutritional encephalomalacia | **Broilers:**<br>10 ml / 100 birds<br>**Layers:**<br>5-7 ml / 100 birds |

# VITAMIN B – COMPLEX

| S. No. | Trade Name & Company | Composition | Indications | Dosage / Administration |
|---|---|---|---|---|
| 1 | AMBIPLEX LIQUID (Brihans) | Each 5 ml contains : Vit $B_1$ 7 mg, Vit $B_2$ 2.5 mg, Vit $B_6$ 1 mg, Vit $B_{12}$ 12.5 mcg, Biotin 25 mcg, Calcium panto-thenate 2.5 mg, Niacin 75 mg, Choline chloride 10 mg, Methionine 10 mg, Lysine 20 mg | * Stimulates natural immunity to protect from non-specific chick mortality <br> * Stimulates growth <br> * Improves feed utilization and weight gain <br> * Improves digestion and corrects chronic diarrhoea <br> * Stimulates egg production <br> * Improves hatchability <br> * Prevents untimely moulting <br> * Prevents FLK disease | **Chicks:** 5 – 6 ml / 100 birds <br> **Growers / Broilers:** 8-10 ml / 100 birds <br> **Layers:** 10-15 ml / 100 birds |
| 2 | AMINOMIX-VM POWDER (VM) | Each 100 g contains : Vit A 5 lacs IU, Vit D 1 lac IU, Vit E 200 mg, Vit $B_2$ 300 mg, Vit $B_6$ 60 mg, Vit $B_{12}$ 400 mcg, Vit K 50 mg, Niacinamide 1.5 g, Calcium pantothenate 500 mg, Folic acid 10 mg, Choline chloride 200 mg, L-Lysine 2g, DL-Methionine 3 g, Tryptophan 20 mg | Stress, retarded growth, deficiency syndrome, off feed | 10 g / 25 litres of water or 1 Kg / tonne of feed |
| 3 | AQUAPLEX-L LIQUID (Harshvardhan's Lab) | Each 5 ml contains : Vit $B_1$ 4 mg, Vit $B_2$ 1.25 mg, Vit $B_6$ 0.62 mg, Vit $B_{12}$ 6.25 mcg, D-panthenol 1.25 mg, Niacinamide 37.5 mg, Vit C 5 mg, L-Lysine 4.5 mg, DL-Methio-nine 4.5 mg | * Improves growth rate during chick and grower stages through proper feed utilization <br> * Improves egg production in layers and weight gain in broilers | 15-20 ml / 100 birds / day |

782

| S. No. | Trade Name & Company | Composition | Indications | Dosage / Administration |
|---|---|---|---|---|
| | | | * Increases resistance to diseases<br>* For better health | |
| 4 | AQUAPLEX – P (Harshvardhan's Lab) | Each 65 g contains: Vit. B1 4000 mg, B2 – 1250 mg, B6 – 620 mg, B12 – 6250 mg, D-panthenol – 1250 mg, niacinamide – 37500 mg, vit. C – 5000 mg, L-lysine – 4500 mg, DL-methionine – 4500 mg | * Improves growth rate in chick and grower<br>* Improves weight gain and FCR in broilers<br>* Improves egg production in layers<br>* Increases resistance<br>* Prevents stress | 15 – 20 ml / 100 birds / day |
| 5 | AV-MIX BEE PLUS POWDER (AVR) | **Single Strength:** Each g contains: Vit $B_1$ 4 mg, Vit $B_6$ 8 mg, Vit $B_{12}$ 40 mcg, Calcium pantothenate 40 mg, Niacin 60 mg, Vit E 40 mg, Folic acid 4 mg<br>**Double Strength:** Each g contains: Vit $B_1$ 8 mg, Vit $B_6$ 16 mg, Vit $B_{12}$ 80 mcg, Calcium pantothenate 80 mg, Niacin 120 mg, Vit E 80 mg, Folic acid 8 mg | * Improves egg production, fertility and hatchability<br>* Stimulates growth<br>* Works against loss of vitamins due to improper feed storage conditions | **Single Strength:** 200-250 g / tonne of feed<br>**Double Strength:** 100 – 120 g / 10 tonne of feed |
| 6 | BECOMIX POWDER (VM) | Each g contains : Vit $B_1$ 4 mg, Vit $B_6$ 8 mg, Vit $B_{12}$ 60 mcg, Vit E 40 mg, Folic acid 4 mg, Niacin 60 mg, Calcium pantothenate 40 mg, Vit C 2 mg. | To improve appetite, growth, fertility and production | 200 g / tonne of feed |
| 7 | B COMPLEX ORAL – 5 X (Vetnex) | Each ml contains: Vit B2 2 mg, Vit B6 0.62 mg, Vit B12 6.25 mcg, D-panthenol 1.25 mg, niacinamide 37.5 mg, DL-methionine 5 mg, L- | Vitamin B deficiency diseases | **Through drinking water:**<br>**Broilers:** 2.5 ml / 100 birds<br>**Layers:** 3-6 ml / 100 birds |

| S. No. | Trade Name & Company | Composition | Indications | Dosage / Administration |
|---|---|---|---|---|
| | | lysine 5 mg, choline chloride 5 mg | | |
| 8 | BEVISOL – FS (Powder) (Neospark) | Each 100 g contains: Vit B2 – 1.25 g, Vit B6 – 0.62 g, Ca. pantothenate – 1.25 g, Niacinamide – 37.50 g, Vit B12 – 6.25 mg, Lysine monohydrochloride – 5.00 g, , DL-Methionine – 5.00 g, Choline bitartrate – 5.00 g | * Stress conditions like vaccination, deworming, debeaking<br>* Poor growth due to improper nutrition<br>* B-complex deficiencies<br>* Improves fertility and hatchability<br>* Stimulates energy | Mix 100 g / 5 litres of water. Give 15 to 20 ml / 100 birds for 7 – 10 days |
| 9 | BIOMEX LIQUID (Indo Biocare) | Each 5 ml contains : Choline chloride 5 mg, Vit B$_2$ 1.25 mg, Vit B$_6$ 0.62 mg, Niacinamide 37.5 mg, DL-Panthenol 1.25 mg, Vit B$_{12}$ 6.25 mcg, Methionine 5 mg, Lysine 5 mg. | * Increases feed conversion<br>* Improves egg production<br>* Enhances weight gain<br>* Imparts higher disease resistance | 10-20 ml / 100 birds daily in drinking water |
| 10 | BRIPLEX POWDER (Brihans) | Each g contains : Vit B$_1$ 8 mg, Vit B$_2$ 4 mg, Vit B$_6$ 16 mg, Vit B$_{12}$ 80 mcg, Niacinamide 120 mg, Calcium pantothenate 80 mg, folic acid 3.6 mg, Vit E 80 mg. | * Unique combination of all essential B vitamins and Vit E<br>* Keeps birds healthy<br>* Improves feed conversion<br>* Stimulates growth and production<br>* Improves hatchability | 100 g / tonne of feed |
| 11 | CADIPLEX FORTE Water soluble granules (Sarabhai Zydus) | Each g contains: Vit B2 12.5 mg, Vit B6 5 mg, B12 62.5 mcg, Nicotinamide 250 mg, D-panthenol 6.5 mg, Biotin 100 mcg, Choline bitartrate 60 mg, L-lysine monohydrochloride 40 mg, DL-methionine | * To improve metabolism<br>* To improve feed efficiency<br>* To improve growth and weight gain<br>* To improve egg production and hatchability<br>* To improve feathering | To be given daily as fresh supplementation through drinking water at the rate of 1 to 2 g per 500 birds |

| S. No. | Trade Name & Company | Composition | Indications | Dosage / Administration |
|---|---|---|---|---|
| | | 20 mg, | * To prevent and correct the deficiency disorders<br>* To improve farming profits | |
| 12 | CADIPLEX-L LIQUID (Sarabhai Zydus) | Each 5 ml contains : Riboflavin 1.25 mg, Vitamin $B_6$ 0.62 mg, Vit $B_{12}$ 6.25 mcg, Nicotinamide 25 mg, D-Panthenol 0.62 mg, Choline chloride 10 mg, Lysine monohydrochloride 5 mg | * Results in proper digestion and metabolism<br>* Helps in effective feed utilization<br>* Enhances growth<br>* Increases body resistance<br>* Stimulates growth of gut microflora after oral antibiotic or sulphonamide therapy<br>* Helps in increasing production of egg and meat | 10-20 ml / 100 birds daily through drinking water |
| 13 | CHARAKPLEX POWDER (Charak) | Each g contains : Vit $B_1$ 8 mg, Vit $B_6$ 16 mg, Vit $B_{12}$ 80 mcg, Cal-D-Pantothenate 25 mg, Niacin 120 mg, Vit E 40 mg, Active live yeast 600 million units, Lactobacillus 12 million units, Proteolytic enzymes 5 mg, Folacin 1 mg, Calcium 130 mg, Phosphorus 60 mg | * Deficiency disease syndromes, stress, weakness<br>* For better FCR, weight gain, eggshell quality, production and hatchability | 100 g / tonne of feed |
| 14 | ELPLEX LIQUID (Elpe) | Each 5 ml contains : Thiamine mononitrate 3.75 mg, Pyridoxine hydrochloride 0.62 mg, Riboflavin 1.25 mg, D-Panthenol 1.25 mg, Niacinamide 37.5 mg, Cynocobalamin 6.25 mcg, Biotin 5 | * B-complex deficiencies<br>* Poor growth due to improper nutrition and feed utilization<br>* Lower egg yield<br>* Fatty liver syndrome<br>* Poor feather growth<br>* Cannibalism | 15-20 ml / 100 birds |

| S. No. | Trade Name & Company | Composition | Indications | Dosage / Administration |
|---|---|---|---|---|
|  |  | mcg, DL-Methionine 12 mg, Choline chloride 20 mg, L-Lysine hydrochloride 5 mg | * Loss of weight and strength |  |
| 15 | GROVIPLEX LIQUID (Virbac) | Each 5ml contains: Vit B$_2$ 1.25 mg, D-Panthenol 0.65 mg, Vit B$_6$ 0.62 mg, Vit B$_{12}$ 6.25 mcg, Nicotinamide 18.75 mg, Choline chloride 10 mg, Lysine mono hydrochloride 10 mg | * Improves growth rate by proper feed utilization<br>* Improves egg production | **Liquid:** 15-20 ml / 100 birds daily through drinking water for 7-10 days |
| 16 | GROVIPLEX POWDER (Virbac) | Each 100 g contains: Nicotinamide 18.75 g, Vit B2 1.25 g, Vit B6 0.62 g, Vit B12 6.25 mcg, Calcium pantothenate 1.51 g, Lysine monohydrochloride 10g, Choline bitartrate 15.82 g | * For better growth and productivity<br>* For better FCR<br>* For better egg production<br>* Improves hatchability | 100g / 5 litres of water |
| 17 | HI-BEEPLEX LIQUID (Hitha) | Each 10 ml contains : Vit B$_2$ 2.5 mg, Vit B$_6$ 1.24 mg, Vit B$_{12}$ 12.5 mcg, D-Panthenol 2.5 mg, Niacinamide 75 mg, Choline chloride 10 mg, L-Lysine HCl 10 mg, DL-Methionine 10 mg | * Improves hatchability in breeder<br>* Prevents embryonic mortality<br>* Better development<br>* Better metabolism<br>* Better rate of growth and production | **Chicks up to 2 weeks:** 15 ml / 100 birds / day<br>**Above 2 weeks:** 20 ml / 100 birds / day |
| 18 | HI B-PLEX CONCENTRATE (Hitha) | Each 10 ml contains : Vit B$_2$ 12.5 mg, Vit B$_6$ 6.2 mg, Vit B$_{12}$ 62.5 mcg, D-Panthenol 12.5 mg, Niacinamide 375 mg, Choline chloride 50 mg, L-Lysine HCl 50 mg, DL-Methionine 50 mg | * Improves hatchability<br>* Prevents embryonic mortality<br>* For better development<br>* For better metabolism<br>* For better growth and production | **Chicks up to 2 weeks:** 30 ml / 1000 birds / day<br>**Above 2 weeks:** 40 ml / 1000 birds / day |

| S. No. | Trade Name & Company | Composition | Indications | Dosage / Administration |
|--------|----------------------|-------------|-------------|-------------------------|
| 19 | HIVITABEE POWDER (B COMPLEX + VITAMIN E) (Hitha) | Each g contains : Vit $B_1$ 4 mg, Vit $B_6$ 8 mg, Vit $B_{12}$ 60 mcg, Vit E 40 mg, Niacin 60 mg, Calcium pantothenate 40 mg | * Improves metabolism in the body<br>* Promotes growth and stimulates appetite<br>* Improves weight gain<br>* Builds resistance<br>* Enhances hatchability and fertility | 200 g / tonne of feed |
| 20 | HIVITABEE DS POWDER (B COMPLEX + VITAMIN E DOUBLE STRENGTH) (Hitha) | Each g contains : Vit $B_1$ 8 mg, Vit $B_6$ 16 mg, Vit $B_{12}$ 120 mcg, Vit E 80 mg, Niacin 120 mg, Calcium pantothenate 80 mg | * Improves metabolism in the body<br>* Promotes growth and stimulates appetite<br>* Improves weight gain<br>* Builds resistance<br>* Enhances hatchability and fertility | 100 g / tonne of feed |
| 21 | HIVITABEE PLUS POWDER (Hitha) | Each g contains : Vit $B_1$ 4 mg, Vit $B_6$ 8 mg, Vit $B_{12}$ 60 mcg, Vit E 40 mg, Niacin 60 mg, Calcium pantothenate 40 mg, Folic acid 2 mg | * Improves metabolism in the body<br>* Promotes growth and stimulates appetite<br>* Improves weight gain<br>* Builds resistance<br>* Enhances hatchability and fertility<br>* Prevents embryonic mortality and anaemia<br>* Improves feathering | 200 g / tonne of feed |
| 22 | MERIPLEX POWDER (Wockhardt) | Each g contains : Vit $B_1$ 4 mg, Vit $B_6$ 8 mg, Vit $B_{12}$ 40 mcg, Vit E 40 mg, Niacin | * For growth & production<br>* Builds resistance against infections | 200 g / tonne of feed |

787

| S. No. | Trade Name & Company | Composition | Indications | Dosage / Administration |
|---|---|---|---|---|
| | | 60 mg, Calcium pantothenate 40 mg, Calcium 188 mg, Phosphorus 145 mg | * Improves egg production and hatchability<br>* Prevents encephalomalacia in hens | |
| 23 | MERIPLEX DS POWDER (Wockhardt) | Each g contains : Vit $B_1$ 8 mg, Vit $B_6$ 16 mg, Vit $B_{12}$ 80 mcg, Vit E 80 mg, Niacin 120 mg, Calcium pantothenate 80 mg, Calcium 125 mg, Phosphorus 98 mg | * For growth and production<br>* Builds resistance against infections<br>* Improves egg production and hatchability<br>* Prevents encephalomalacia in hens | 100 g / tonne of feed |
| 24 | MERIPLEX-F DS POWDER (Wockhardt) | Each g contains : Vit $B_1$ 8 mg, Vit $B_6$ 16 mg, Vit $B_{12}$ 80 mcg, Vit E 80 mg, Niacin 120 mg, Calcium pantothenate 80 mg, Calcium 125 mg, Phosphorus 98 mg, Folic acid 8 mg | * For growth and production<br>* Builds resistance against infections<br>* Improves egg production and hatchability<br>* Prevents encephalomalacia in hens<br>* Folic acid prevents feather loss and perosis and helps in fat metabolism | 100 g / tonne of feed |
| 25 | MERIPLEX FORTE POWDER (Wockhardt) | Each g contains : Vit $B_1$ 16 mg, Vit $B_6$ 32 mg, Vit $B_{12}$ 160 mcg, Vit E 160 mg, Niacin 240 mg, Calcium panto-thenate 160 mg, Calcium 35 mg, Phosphorus 26 mg, Folic acid 16 mg | * For growth and production<br>* Builds resistance against infections<br>* Improves egg production and hatchability<br>* Prevents encephalomalacia in hens<br>* Folic acid prevents feather loss and perosis and helps in fat metabolism | 50 g / tonne of feed |

| S. No. | Trade Name & Company | Composition | Indications | Dosage / Administration |
|---|---|---|---|---|
| 26 | MERIPLEX-K (Wockhardt) | Each g contains : Vit A 40,000 IU, Vit D$_3$ 6000 IU, Vit B$_1$ 3.2 mg, Vit B$_2$ 20 mg, Vit B$_{12}$ 82 mcg, Niacin 48 mg, Calcium pantothenate 32 mg, Vit K$_3$ 4mg, Vit E 32 mg, Folic acid 3.2 mg, carriers q.s. | * For growth and production<br>* Builds resistance against infections<br>* Improves egg production and hatchability<br>* Prevents encephalomalacia in hens<br>* Folic acid prevents feather loss and perosis and helps in fat metabolism | 250 g / tonne of feed |
| 27 | MULTI VIT PREMIX (Stallen) | Each g contains: Vit A, 40,000 IU, Vit D3 10,000 IU, Vit B1 3.2 mg, Vit B2 20 mg Vit B12 82 mcg, Niacin 48 mg, Calcium pantothenate 32 mg, Vit K3 4 mg, Vit E 32 mg, Folic acid 3.2 mg, carriers q.s. | * For improving feed conversion efficiency<br>* For quicker growth, to improve egg production and hatchability<br>* As immunity system enhancer | 250 g / tonne of feed |
| 28 | OLEBEE-PLUS FEED SUPPLEMENT (Avian Remedies) | Each g contains : Vit B$_1$ 4 mg, Vit B$_6$ 8 mg, Vit B$_{12}$ 40 mcg, Vit E 40 mg, Calcium D-Pantothenate 40 mg, Niacin 60 mg, Folic acid 4 mg, Calcium 26 mg, Organic nutritive carrier q.s. | * Improves egg production, fertility and hatchability<br>* Stimulates growth and reduces mortality<br>* Works against poor bioavailability of chemically bound nutritients, e.g., niacin | 20-25 g / 100 Kg of feed |
| 29 | OLEBEE-PLUS DS FEED SUPPLEMENT (Avian Remedies) | Each g contains : Vit B$_1$ 8 mg, Vit B$_6$ 16 mg, Vit B$_{12}$ 80 mcg, Niacin 120 mg, Calcium D-pantothenate 80 mg, Vit E 80 mg, Folic acid 8 mg, Calcium 52 | * Improves egg production, fertility and hatchability<br>* Stimulates growth and reduces mortality<br>* Works against poor bioavailability of | 10-15 g / 100 Kg of feed |

| S. No. | Trade Name & Company | Composition | Indications | Dosage / Administration |
|---|---|---|---|---|
| | | mg, Organic nutritive carrier q.s. | chemically bound nutrients, e. g., niacin | |
| 30 | OLEBEE-FORTE FEED SUPPLEMENT (Avian Remedies) | Each g contains : Vit B$_1$ 16 mg, Vit B$_6$ 32 mg, Vit B$_{12}$ 160 mcg, Niacin 240 mg, Calcium D-Pantothenate 160 mg, Vit E 160 mg, Folic acid 16 mg, Calcium 104 mg, Organic nutritive carrier q.s. | * Improves egg production, fertility and hatchability<br>* Stimulates growth and reduces mortality<br>* Works against poor bioavailability of chemically bound nutrients, e. g., niacin | 5-10 g / 100 Kg of feed |
| 31 | OSCO BF-DS FEED SUPPLEMENT (Osco) | Each g contains : Vit B$_1$ 8 mg, Vit B$_6$ 16 mg, Vit B$_{12}$ 80 mcg, Niacin 120 mg, Calcium pantothenate 50 mg, Folic acid 4 mg, Vit E 50 mg, Calcium 180 mg, Phosphorus 140 mg | * Increases egg production<br>* Enhances hatchability and fertility of breeder flocks<br>* Improves metabolism<br>* Promotes growth<br>* Prevents crazy chick disease and leg weakness | 100 g / tonne of feed |
| 32 | OSCO BF-SS FEED SUPPLEMENT (Osco) | Each g contains : Vit B$_1$ 4 mg, Vit B$_6$ 8 mg, Vit B$_{12}$ 40 mcg, Niacin 60 mg, Calcium pantothenate 25 mg, Folic acid 4 mg, Vit E 25 mg, Calcium 180 mg, Phosphorus 140 mg | * Increases egg production<br>* Promotes growth<br>* Prevents crazy chick disease and leg weakness<br>* Enhances hatchability and fertility of breeder flocks | 200 g / tonne of feed |
| 33 | PLEXA BC - FORTE (D.S.) POWDER (Concept) | Each g contains : Vit B$_1$ 8 mg, Vit B$_6$ 16 mg, Vit B$_{12}$ 80 mcg, Vit E 80 mg, Niacinamide 120 mg, Calcium pantothenate 80 mg, Folic acid 15 mg | * Improves productivity<br>* Promotes growth<br>* Helps in building resistance<br>* Enhances hatchability and fertility in breeders | 100 g / tonne of feed |

| S. No. | Trade Name & Company | Composition | Indications | Dosage / Administration |
|---|---|---|---|---|
| 34 | PREMIPLEX LIQUID (Premium) | Each 5 ml contains : Vit B$_2$ 1.25 mg, Vit B$_6$ 0.62 mg, Vit B$_{12}$ 6.25 mcg, Calcium pantothenate 1.25 mg, Niacinamide 37.5 mg, Choline chloride 5 mg, L-Lysine 5 mg, DL-Methionine 5 mg | * For increased egg production<br>* For better growth and weight gain<br>* For effective feed utilization and absorption<br>* Prevents crazy chick disease and leg weakness | **Broilers / Layers:** 15-20 ml / 100 birds / day |
| 35 | PRIME BIOBEE FEED SUPPLEMENT (Vit B-complex + Minerals) (Prime) | Each g contains : Vit B$_1$ 8 mg, Vit B$_6$ 16 mg, Vit B$_{12}$ 80 mcg, Niacin 120 mg, Calcium pantothenate 40 mg, Folic acid 4 mg, Vit E 40 mg, Lactobacillus 7 types 13 billion, Yeast 2 types 20 billion, Calcium 180 mg, Phosphorus 140 mg | * For increased egg production<br>* For better growth and weight gain<br>* For effective feed utilization and absorption<br>* Prevents crazy chick disease and leg weakness | 100 g / tonne of feed |
| 36 | SIMPLEX – DS (Vetline) | Each Kg contains: Vit B1 8 g, Vit B6 16 g, Vit B12 80 g, Vit E 80 g, Cal. D-pantothenate 80 g, Folic acid 4 g | * Provides nutrients required by poultry for growth and development<br>* Improves egg production and hatchability | 100 g / tonne of feed |
| 37 | SOLEX-M POWDER (Venky's) | Each g contains : Vit B$_2$ 12.5 mg, Vit B$_6$ 6.2 mg, Vit B$_{12}$ 63 mcg, Calcium D-pantothenate 29 mg, Niacin 375 mg, DL-methionine 50 mg | * For better metabolism, production and hatchability<br>* For normal development and feathering<br>* To prevent embryonic mortality | **Up to 2 weeks of age:** 15 ml / 100 chicks<br>**Above 2 weeks of age** 20 ml / 100 birds |
| 38 | SPECTROBE POWDER (Vetnex) | Each g contains : Vit B$_1$ 8 mg, Vit B$_6$ 16 mg, Vit B$_{12}$ 80 mcg, Niacinamide 120 mg, Calcium pantothenate 1.25 mg, L-Lysine 10 | * Improves growth<br>* Builds resistance to fight against diseases<br>* Improves feed conversion | 100 g / tonne of feed |

| S. No. | Trade Name & Company | Composition | Indications | Dosage / Administration |
|---|---|---|---|---|
| | | mg, DL-Methionine 10 mg, Calcium 260 mg | * Prevents perosis and paralysis caused by vitamin deficiency<br>* Increases hatchability and fertility | |
| 39 | SUPRAPLEX-AA POWDER (Neospark) | Each 5 g contains : Vit B$_1$ 25 mg, Vit B$_6$ 40 mg, Vit B$_{12}$ 300 mcg, Vit E 300 mg, Calcium pantothenate 225 mg, Niacinamide 300 mg, Folic acid 20 mg, Choline chloride 1000 mg, DL-Methionine 1000 mg, L-Lysine 1000 mg, Vit C 1000 mg, Vit A 16000 IU, Vit B$_2$ 12.5 mg, Vit D$_3$ 2400 IU, Calcium 5 mg, Protein hydrolysate 50 ppm, Cobalt 500 mcg | * During stress<br>* At the time of deworming<br>* In caged layers<br>* During vaccination and debeaking<br>* In laying slumps | 200-250 g / tonne of feed |
| 40 | SUPRAPLEX-FS-LIQUID (Neospark) | Each 5 ml contains : Vit B$_1$ 3.75 mg, Vit B$_2$ 1.25 mg, Vit B$_6$ 0.62 mg, Vit B$_{12}$ 6.25 mcg, D-Panthenol 1.25 mg, Niacinamide 37.5 mg, DL- Methionine 5 mg, L-Lysine 5 mg, Choline chloride 5 mg, Casein protein 200 ppm, Cobalt 5 mg, Elemental sodium 5 mg | * Stress conditions like vaccination, deworming and debeaking<br>* Poor growth due to improper nutrition<br>* B-complex deficiencies<br>* Lower egg yield<br>* Feather growth<br>* Cannibalism | **Up to 2 weeks:** 15 ml / 100 chicks daily<br>**Above 2 weeks:** 20 ml / 100 birds daily<br>**Stress condition:** 100 ml / 100 birds daily |
| 41 | SUPRAPLEX-SS-FS (Neospark) | Each g contains: Vit B1 4 mg, Vit B6 8 mg, Vit B12 40 mcg, Nicotinic acid 60 mg, Pantothenic acid 40 mg, Vit E 40 IU | * During stress<br>* At the time of dewoming<br>* In caged layers<br>* During vaccination and debeaking<br>* In laying slumps | 200 g / tonne of feed |

| S. No. | Trade Name & Company | Composition | Indications | Dosage / Administration |
|---|---|---|---|---|
| 42 | TOXOL POWDER (Vitamin B-complex + Amino Acids) (Vesper) | Each 10 g contains : Tricholine citrate 100 mg, Methionine 10 mg, Inositol 2 mg, Vit B$_{12}$ 0.33 mcg fortified with pre-digested protein and amino nitrogen | * Fatty liver and debility <br> * To improve FCR <br> * For better immunity and growth | **Prophylactic:** 1 Kg / tonne of feed or 1/2 g / litre of water **Curative:** 2.5 Kg / tonne of feed or 1 g / litre of water. |
| 43 | TRIPLEX LIQUID (Trichem) | Each 5 ml contains : Thiamine 3 mg, Riboflavin 1.25 mg, Pyridoxine hydrochloride 0.62 mg, D-Panthenol 1.25 mg, Vit B$_{12}$ 6.25 mcg, Choline chloride 5 mg, Niacinamide 37.5 mg, L-Lysine 5 mg, L-Methionine 5 mg, | To improve weight gain and production | 10-20 ml / 100 birds |
| 44 | VENTRI BEE-PLUS POWDER (Venky's) | Each g contains : Vit B$_1$ 4 mg, Vit B$_6$ 8 mg, Vit B$_{12}$ 40 mcg, Vit E 40 mg, Calcium D-Pantothenate 40 mg, Niacin 60 mg | * For better growth and production <br> * Improves metabolism and FCR | 200 g / tonne of feed 300 g / tonne of feed in summer |
| 45 | VENTRIPLEX-M LIQUID (Venky's) | Each 5 ml contains : Vit B$_2$ 1.25 mg, Vit B$_6$ 0.62 mg, Vit B$_{12}$ 6.25 mcg, Niacin 37.5 mg DL-Methionine 5 mg, D-Pantothenol 1.25 mg | * For better metabolism, growth and production <br> * For normal development and feathering | **Chicks up to 2 weeks:** 15 ml / 100 chicks daily **Chicks above 2 weeks:** 20 ml / 100 chicks daily |
| 46 | VETSOL B COMPLEX RECONSTITUTED LIQUID (Vets Farma) | Each 5 ml contains : Vit B$_{12}$ 6.25 mcg, Vit B$_1$ 3.75 mg, Vit B$_2$ 1.25 mg, Vit B$_6$ 0.62 mg, Calcium pantothenate 1.25 mg, Nicotinamide 36.5 mg | * For better health <br> * To increase productivity in chicks, growers, layers and breeders | 15-20 ml / 100 birds daily in drinking water |
| 47 | VISOL-B FEED SUPPLEMENT (Pfizer) | Each 5 ml contains : Vit. B$_2$ 1.2 mg, Vit B$_6$ 0.62 mg, D-Panthenol 1.25 mg, Niacina- | * For better health <br> * To increase productivity in chicks, growers, | 15-20 ml / 100 birds daily in drinking water |

| S. No. | Trade Name & Company | Composition | Indications | Dosage / Administration |
|---|---|---|---|---|
| | | mide 37.5 mg, Vit B$_{12}$ 6.25 mcg, Choline chloride 5 mg, L-Lysine 5 mg, DL-Methionine 5 mg | layers and breeders | |
| 48 | VITA-B-PLEX LIQUID (Qualitat) | Each 15 ml contains: Vit B1 – 15 mg, Vit B2 - 3.75 mg, Vit B6 – 1.86 mg, Vit B12 – 30 mcg, Vit C – 15 mg, Cal. Pantothenate – 3.75 mg, Niacinamide – 112.5 mg, Folic acid – 0.6 mg | * Better digestion and metabolism<br>* Better FCR<br>* Faster recovery after disease | 10 - 20 ml / 100 layers or 1000 chicks |
| 49 | VITA B PLEX POWDER (Qualitat) | Each 10 g contains: Vitamin B1 15 mg, Vitamin B2 3.75 mg, Vitamin B6 2 mg, Vit B12 25 mcg, Vit C 15 mg, Vit E 40 mg, Calcium pantothenate 3.75 mg, Niacinamide 110 mg, Folic acid 1 mg | * Better digestion and metabolism<br>* Better FCR<br>* Faster recovery after disease | 200 – 250 g / tonne of feed |

# VITAMIN B$_{12}$

| S. No. | Trade Name & Company | Composition | Indications | Dosage / Administration |
|---|---|---|---|---|
| 1 | CYNACO 100 POWDER (Avian Remedies) | Each Kg contains: Vit B$_{12}$ activity 100 mg, (as cyanocobalamin) carrier q.s. | * For improved growth in broilers and increased production in layers<br>* For better development and feed utilization in poultry<br>* Increases the biological value of proteins of plant origin | **Broilers / Replacements:** 220 g / tonne of feed<br>**Layers:** 100 g / tonne of feed<br>**Breeders:** 150 g / tonne of feed |
| 2 | MERIVITE 100 POWDER (Wockhardt) | Each Kg contains: Vitamin B$_{12}$ 100 mg | * Improves weight gain and feed conversion in broilers<br>* Improves growth and productivity in replacements<br>* Improves feed conversion in layers<br>* Improves hatchability in breeders | **Broilers / Replacement:** 220 g / tonne of feed<br>**Layers:** 100 g / tonne of feed<br>**Breeders:** 150 g / tonne of feed |
| 3 | NICOMIX-B$_{12}$ (DS) POWDER (Nicholas Piramal) | Each Kg contains : Vit B$_{12}$ 200 mg | * Improves the overall quality of feed<br>* Improves weight gain<br>* Maximizes egg production<br>* Ensures quality performance from breeders<br>* Reduces mortality | **Broilers:** 110 g / tonne of feed<br>**Layers:** 50 g / tonne of feed<br>**Breeders:** 75 g / tonne of feed |
| 4 | OSCO B$_{12}$ POWDER (Osco) | Each Kg contains : Vit B$_{12}$ 100 mg | * Improves growth and productivity<br>* Improves weight gain and feed conversion<br>* Improves egg production and hatchability | **Broilers / Replacements:** 220 g / tonne of feed<br>**Layers:** 100 g / tonne of feed<br>**Breeders:** 150 g / tonne of feed |

| S. No. | Trade Name & Company | Composition | Indications | Dosage / Administration |
|---|---|---|---|---|
| 5 | ULTRA-$B_{12}$-FS POWDER (Neospark) | Each Kg contains : Vit $B_{12}$ 100 mg, Elemental cobalt 100 mg, Elemental calcium 22.5%, Protein hydrolysate 50 ppm | For increased productivity in broilers, layers and breeders | **Broilers / Replacements:** 220 g / tonne of feed **Layers:** 100 g / tonne of feed **Breeders:** 150 g / tonne of feed |

# VITAMIN C

| S. No. | Trade Name & Company | Composition | Indications | Dosage / Administration |
|---|---|---|---|---|
| 1 | ASCOSOL-C POWDER (Neospark) | Each g contains: Ascorbic acid (coated Vit C) 500 mg, Casein protein 500 ppm, Elemental sodium 8.20 mg | * Debility, weakness<br>* Off feed, stress<br>* Vitamin C deficiency conditions | 10 g / 15 litres of water |
| 2 | AYUCEE (Ayurvet) | Natural vitamin C with bioflavonoids | * For reduction in mortality and losses due to heat stress<br>* For proper growth and production in chicks, growers, broilers, layers and breeders during summer stress<br>* For maintaining immunity and enhancing stress threshold as well as livability | 100 gm / ton of feed |
| 3 | HERBAL- C LIQUID (Indian Herbs) | A herbal preparation | * To meet higher requirements of Vit C during summer<br>* To prevent stress-induced depletion of Vit C and immune suppression<br>* For enhancing bioavailability of essential minerals and utilization of nutrients to improve FCR and productivity | **Feed Inclusion Rate:** 1: 1 Replacement of synthetic Vit C **Water Inclusion Rate:** Broilers and Layers: 10 – 20 ml / 1000 birds |
| 4 | HI-CEE (Hitha) | Each g contains: Vit 'C' (coated): 500 mg, base q.s. | * To boost immune system<br>* To improve eggshell thickness<br>* To increase absorption of calcium<br>* Important intercellular antioxidant | **Chicks:** 5 g / 1000 birds **Growers:** 10 g / 1000 birds **Layers / Broilers** : 15-20 g / 1000 birds **Feed Additive:** 150-200 g / tonne of feed |

| S. No. | Trade Name & Company | Composition | Indications | Dosage / Administration |
|---|---|---|---|---|
| 5 | HIM C (Himalaya) | Provides vitamin C in natural form. 6.7 mg of natural vit-C is equivalent to 100 mg of synthetic C | * It helps scavenge free radicals<br>* It helps cope with temperature related stress<br>* It helps improve better metabolic profile<br>* It helps in maintaining feed intake, growth, production, and semen quality | 100 g / tonne of feed |
| 6 | NATURAL – C (Natural Herbs) | It is a natural form of Vit C with many antioxidants | * Improves protein biosynthesis<br>* Enhances glucose metabolism<br>* Helps to optimize metabolic rate<br>* Protects from damaging effects of free radicals | 100 g / tonne of feed |
| 7 | PHYTOCEE (Natural Remedies) | Herbal poultry feed supplement for replacing synthetic vitamin C | * To optimize body resistance<br>* To enhance egg production and shell quality in layers<br>* To enhance fertility and hatchability in breeders<br>* To optimize overall performance of birds | 1:1 Replacement of synthetic Vitamin C, or as directed by the nutritionist |
| 8 | POL – C (Polchem) | Each g contains: 500 mg of ascorbic acid (coated vitamin – C) in water-soluble base | * Relieves heat stress by helping in secretion of anti-stress hormones<br>* Enhances immune response by suppressing synthesis of cortical hormones<br>* Ensures better body weight in broilers<br>* Reduces losses due to thin-shelled and | **Chicks:** 5 g / 1000 birds<br>**Growers:** 10 g / 1000 birds<br>**Adult Birds / Breeders:** 15 to 20 g / 1000 birds<br>**Poultry feed additive:** 150 – 200 g / tonne of feed |

| S. No. | Trade Name & Company | Composition | Indications | Dosage / Administration |
|---|---|---|---|---|
| | | | broken eggs<br>* Improves semen volume and sperm quality in breeder males<br>* Detoxifies mycotoxins | |
| 9 | PROCEE (Venky's) | Protein hydrolysate 4%, Vit C 40% | * Stress or disease conditions<br>* Growth phase in broilers and peak production in layers<br>* Early chick nutrition to stimulate development of intestinal tract for f<br>* aster growth of digestive system<br>* To support bone and eggshell formation<br>* To detoxify harmful substances<br>* To bridge the gap between the rate of biosynthesis of Vit C and its requirement | 2 g / litre of water or 200 g / tonne of feed |

## VITAMINS + MINERALS

| S. No. | Trade Name & Company | Composition | Indications | Dosage / Administration |
|---|---|---|---|---|
| 1 | AFFOMIN FORTE (Qualitat) | Each Kg contains: Vit A – 20, 00,000 IU, Vit D3 – 4,000,00 IU, Vit B6 – 200 mg, Vit B2 – 1g, Vit E – 300 mg, Vit K – 0.4 mg, Vit B12 – 4 mcg, Niacin 6 g, Cal. Pantothenate – 2 g, Choline chloride – 120 g, Manganese – 11 g, Iron – 3 g, Copper – 0.8 g, Zinc – 6 g, Cobalt – 0.18 g, Iodine – 0.4 g | * For better growth<br>* To improve resistance against infections | 2.5 Kg / tonne of feed |
| 2 | ALVITE-M POWDER (Alembic) | Each 250 g contains: Vit A 5,00,000 IU, Vit D3 1,02,500 IU, Vit B2 0.13 g, Vit E 87.5 IU, Vit K 0.1 g, Vit B12 0.75 g, Calcium pantothenate 0.25 g, Manganese 2.75 g, Iodine 0.1 g, Zinc 1.5 g, Iron 0.75 g, Copper 0.2 g, Cobalt 0.045 g, Choline chloride 6% w/w, Calcium 85 g, Antioxidant added | * Helps to combat stress<br>* Improves egg production<br>* Ensures excellent weight gain<br>* Improves FCR | **Broilers (Starters / Finishers) and Breeders:** 250 g / 50 Kg of feed or 5 Kg / tonne of feed<br>**Layers :** 250 g / 100 Kg of feed or 2.5 Kg / tonne of feed |
| 3 | AQUA - CAL - PHOS - D Liquid Feed Supplement (Harshvardhan's Lab) | Each 5 ml contains: Calcium – 100 mg, Phosphorus – 50 mg, Vit D3 – 400 IU, Vit B12 – 5 mcg, Aqueous base – q. s. | * Provides high concentration of Ca and P in ionic form. *Improves absorption and assimilation<br>* Enhances growth, weight gain, and egg production<br>* Reduces leg weakness, broken eggs, prolapse, and cage layer fatigue | **Chicks / Broilers:** 10 ml / 100 birds / day<br>**Growers:** 20 ml / 100 birds / day<br>**Layers / Breeders:** 50 ml / 100birds / day |

| S. No. | Trade Name & Company | Composition | Indications | Dosage / Administration |
|---|---|---|---|---|
| 4 | AYUMIN V POWDER (Ayurvet) | A mixture of vitamins and minerals | * Prevents vitamin and mineral deficiencies<br>* Improves growth rate, body weight and productivity | **Growers / Layers:** 2.5 Kg / tonne of feed<br>**Starters / Finishers / Breeders:** 5 Kg / tonne of feed |
| 5 | BIOVITE-M POWDER (Indo Biocare) | Each 500 g contains : Vit A 10,00,000 IU, Vit $D_3$ 2,00,000 IU, Vit $B_2$ 260 mg, Vit $B_{12}$ 1.5 mg, Vit E 175 units, Vit K 200 mg, Calcium di-pantothenate 500 mg, Nicotinamide 2 g, Choline chloride 30 g, Manganese 5.5 g, Iodine 200 mg, Zinc 3 g, Iron 1.5 g, Copper 400 mg, Cobalt 90 mg, Selenium 10 mg | * Improves feed efficiency<br>* Increases egg production in layers<br>* Enhances weight gain in broilers<br>* Prevents nutritional disorders and stress | **Starters / Broilers / Breeders:** 5 Kg / tonne of feed<br>**Layers:** 2.5 Kg / tonne of feed |
| 6 | CEKAY FORTE POWDER (Elpe) | Each 20 g contains : Vit C 150 mg, Vit K 30 mg, Zinc 300 mg, Manganese 300 mg | * Acute haemorrhagical conditions<br>* Stresses<br>* Leg-weakness<br>* Retarded growth and feather development<br>* After continued use of sulpha drugs<br>* Vitamin K afflictions | **Chicks / Growers:** 20 g / 100 birds<br>**During stress or haemorrhagic conditions:** 40 g / 100 birds<br>**Layers:** 20 g / 1000 birds |
| 7 | CHELAMIN-B LIQUID (Premium) | Each 15 ml contains : Protein hydrolysate 1.5 g, Calcium 45 mg, Iron 1.5 mg, Magnesium 24 mg, Manganese 11.55 mg, Copper 4.5 mg, Cobalt 1 mg, Vit $B_1$ 1.6 mg, Vit $B_2$ 4.5 mg, Cobalt 1 mg, Vit $B_1$ 1.6 mg, Vit | Vitamin and mineral deficiency conditions, stress, poor eggshell quality | **Chicks:** 15 ml / 100 birds<br>**Broilers / Growers:** 20 ml / 100 birds<br>**Layers:** 30 ml / 100 birds |

| S. No. | Trade Name & Company | Composition | Indications | Dosage / Administration |
|---|---|---|---|---|
| | | $B_2$ 4.5 mg,  Vit $B_6$ 2.23 mg, Vit $B_{12}$ 22.5 mg, Pantothenic acid 4.5 mg, Niacinamide 135 mg, Folic acid 720 mg, Sodium 30 mg, Potassium 10 mg | | |
| 8 | CHIKVIT POWDER (Intervet) | Each g contains : Vit A 8,000 IU, Vit $B_2$ 2.8 mg, Vit $B_{12}$ 5 mcg, Vit $D_3$ 1500 IU, Vit E 5 mg, Vit $K_3$ 5 mg, Vit PP 12.5 mg, D-calcium pantothenate 5 mg, Copper sulphate 0.7 mg, Zinc sulphate 2.5 mg, Ferrous sulphate 6.2 mg, Potassium iodide 0.4 mg, Manganese sulphate 3.8 mg, Sorbitol 20 mg | * Vitamin and mineral feed deficiencies <br> * Prevention of stress (transport)  and various infections <br> * Vitamin replacement after treatment <br> * Improvement of egg production | **Prophylactic:** **Broilers / Layers:** 0.5 g / litre of water for 3-7  days **Curative:** **Broilers:** 1 g / litre of water for 3-7 days **Layers:** 0-5 g / litre of water for 3-7 days |
| 9 | CHICK MIN-VIT POWDER (VM) | Each g contains : Vit A 10,000 IU, Vit $D_3$ 2,000 IU, Vit E 10 mg, Vit $B_2$ 3 mg, Vit $B_{12}$ 5 mcg, Vit K 10 mg, D-Calcium pantothenate7.5 mg, Copper  sulphate 2 mg, Zinc sulphate 2.5  mg, Ferrous sulphate 7 mg, Potassium iodide 0.4 mg,  Manganese sulphate 4 mg, Sorbitol 20 mg | * Stress, mineral / vitamin deficiencies, debility <br> * For better egg production,  weight gain and hatchability | **Chicks:** 0.5 - 1 g / litre of water **Broilers / Layers:** 1 g / litre of water |
| 10 | CONCIMIN POWDER FEED SUPPLEMENT (Concept) | Each 250 g contains : Vit A 5,00,000 IU, Vit $D_3$ 1,00,000 IU, Vit E 75 units, Vit K 100 mg, Vit $B_2$ 200 mg, Vit $B_{12}$ 600 mcg, Calcium pantothenate 250 mg, Choline chloride (50%) 15 g, Nicotinamide 1 g, | * Ensures better growth <br> * Stimulates egg production <br> * Improves hatchability <br> * Eliminates curled toe paralysis, slipped tendon and | 2.5 Kg / tonne of feed |

| S. No. | Trade Name & Company | Composition | Indications | Dosage / Administration |
|---|---|---|---|---|
| | | Calcium 70 g, Phosphorus 20 g, Iron 750 g, Manganese 2.75 g, Iodine 100 mg, Copper 200 mg, Zinc 1.5 g, Cobalt 45 mg | perosis<br>* Corrects fatty liver syndrome | |
| 11 | ENGROW (Varsha) | Each 100 ml contains: Methionine 25 mg, Lysine 30 mg, Arginine 5 mg, Cystine 2 mg, Choline 100 mg, Vit B1 10 mg, Vit B12 5 mg, Niacinamide 20 mg, Vit B6 15 mg, Manganese 100 mg, Magnesium 125 mg, Zinc 200 mg, Iron 150 mg, Copper 50 mg, Cobalt 150 mg, fortified with growth promoters | * Enhances body weight and FCR<br>* For better egg production<br>* Makes birds physically fit during lay | **Liquid:**<br>**Chicks:**<br>10 ml / 100 birds<br>**Broilers:**<br>10-15 ml / 100 birds in $2^{nd}$ and $4^{th}$ week for 5 days<br>**Growers:**<br>10-15 ml / 100 birds<br>**Layers:**<br>25 ml / 100 birds<br>**Premix:**<br>500 g – I Kg / tonne of feed |
| 12 | GROBLEND POWDER (Virbac) | Each 2 Kg contains : Vit A 50,00,000 IU, Vit $D_3$ 6,25,000 IU, Vit $B_2$ 2 g, Calcium pantothenate 4 g, Vit $B_6$ 400 mg, Vit $B_{12}$ 5600 mcg, Vit E 800 mg, Choline chloride 10 g, Copper 2 g, Manganese 27.5 g, Iron 7.5 g, Zinc 15 g, Iodine 1 g, Calcium 27.25%, Phosphorus 7.45% | * For better production<br>* For better utilization of feed<br>* To keep the flock healthy | 2 Kg / 1 - 1.5 tonne of feed |
| 13 | HI-LAY FEED SUPPLEMENT (For Layers) (Hitha) | Each 2.5 Kg. Contains: Vit A 82,50,000 IU, Vit $D_3$ 12,00,000 IU, Vit E 800 IU, Vit K 1 g, Vit $B_2$ 4.5 g, Vit $B_6$ 0.4 g, Vit $B_{12}$ 10 mg, Calcium pantothenate 6 g, Niacin 10 g, Choline chloride 50% 150g, Calcium 830 g, Cobalt | Poultry feed supplement for prevention of vitamin and mineral deficiencies | 2.5 Kg / tonne of feed |

| S. No. | Trade Name & Company | Composition | Indications | Dosage / Administration |
|---|---|---|---|---|
| | | 0.4 g, Copper 2 g, Iodine 1 g, Iron 7.5 g, Manganese 27.5 g, Zinc 15 g, Selenium 100 mg | | |
| 14 | HIVIT- MIN FEED SUPPLEMENT (For Broilers) (HITHA) | **VITAMINS:** Each Kg contains : Vit A 100,00,000 IU, Vit $D_3$ 20,00,000 IU, Vit $B_2$ 5.5 g, Vit $B_1$ 1.1 g, Vit $B_6$ 2 g, Vit $B_{12}$ 15 mg, Calcium pantothenate 9 g, Niacinamide 33 g, Vit C 7.5 g, Vit E 18 g, Vit K 3 g, Folic acid 0.6 g, Selenium 100 mg **MINERALS:** Each 2 Kg contains : Choline chloride 500 g, Manganese 95 g, Zinc 60 g, Iron 40 g, Copper 5 g, Iodine 1.2 g, Cobalt 0.5 g | * Poultry feed supplement for prevention of vitamin and mineral deficiencies<br>* Performance enhancer | 1 Kg of VIT and 2 Kg. of MIN to be added per tonne of feed |
| 15 | MINAMIL POWDER (Brihans) | Each 250 g contains : Vit A 5,00,000 IU, Vit $D_3$ 1,00,000 IU, Vit E 80 mg, Vit $K_3$ 0.1 g, Vit $B_2$ 0.3 g, Vit $B_6$ 0.1 mg, Vit $B_{12}$ 1 mg, Calcium pantothenate 0.3 g, Nicotinamide 2 g, Choline chloride 15 g, Calcium 80 g, Phosphorus 5 g, Manganese 3 g, Iodine 0.1 g, Iron 0.8 g, Zinc 2 g, Copper 0.25 g, Cobalt 0.05 g, Selenium 2.5 mg | * Provides all essential vitamins and minerals<br>* Improves feed conversion<br>* Stimulates growth and production | 20-50 g / 100 birds or 2-5 Kg / tonne of feed |
| 16 | NICOMIX-MIN (Nicholas Piramal) | Each Kg contains : Vit A 10,000,000 IU, Vit $D_3$ 15,00,000 IU, Vit $B_1$ 800 mg, Vit | For vitamin and mineral deficiency conditions | 1 Kg / tonne of feed |

| S. No. | Trade Name & Company | Composition | Indications | Dosage / Administration |
|---|---|---|---|---|
| | | B$_2$ 5,000 mg, Vit B$_6$ 1,600 mg, Vit B$_{12}$ 20.5 mcg, Niacin 12,000 mg, Calcium pantothenate 8,000 mg, Vit K 1,000 mg, Vit E 8,000 mg, Folic acid 800 mg, Manganese 70 g, Zinc 65 g, Iron 15 g, Copper 5 g, Cobalt 0.3 g, Iodine 0.5 g, Selenium 0.15 g, Molybdenum 1 g | | |
| 17 | NUTRI-BLEND VM (Harshvardhan's Lab) | Each 2.5 Kg contains Vit A 50,00,000 IU, Vit D$_3$ 10,00,000 IU, Vit B$_2$ 2 g, Vit E 750 IU, Vit K 1 g, Calcium pantothenate 2.5 g, Nicotinamide 10 g, Vit B$_{12}$ 6 mg, Choline chloride 150 g, Calcium 750 g, Manganese 27.5 g, Iodine 1g, Iron 7.5 g, Zinc 15 g, Copper 2 g, Cobalt 0.45 g, Selenium 100 mg, Molybdenum 1 g | * For prevention of vitamin and mineral deficiencies, particularly during periods of illness, convalescence, stress and general unfitness<br>* For better weight gain and productivity | **Growers / Layers:** 2.5 Kg / tonne of finished feed<br>**Broilers / Breeders:** 5 Kg / tonne of finished feeds |
| 18 | NUTRI LAY POWDER (Pfizer) | Each 2.5 Kg contains : Vit A 82,50,000 IU, Vit D3 12,00,000 IU, Vit E 800, Vit K 1 g, Vit B2 4.5 g, Vit B6 0.4 g, Vit B12 10 mg, Calcium pantothenate 6 g, Nicotinamide 10 mg, Choline chloride 50% 150 g, Calcium 830 g, Cobalt 0.4 g, Copper 2 g, Iodine 1 g, Iron 7.5 g, Manganese 27.5 g, Selenium 100 mg, Zinc 15 g | * To promote growth rate<br>* To increase weight gain<br>* To improve egg production<br>* To prevent laying slumps in layers and breeders | 1.5-2.5 Kg / tonne of feed |

| S. No. | Trade Name & Company | Composition | Indications | Dosage / Administration |
|---|---|---|---|---|
| 19 | SUPPLEVITE-M POWDER (Sarabhai Zydus) | Each 250 g contains : Vit A 5,00,000 IU, Vit D$_3$ 1,00,000 IU, Vit B$_2$ 0.2 g, Vit E 75 units, Vit K 0.1 g, Calcium pantothenate 0.25 g, Nicotinamide 1 g, Vit B$_{12}$ 0.6 mg, Choline chloride 15 g, Calcium 75 g, Manganese 2.75 g, Iodine 0.1 g, Iron 0.75 g, Zinc 1.5 g, Copper 0.2 g, Cobalt 0.045 g | * Prevents nutritional imbalances and deficiency diseases<br>* Improves feed utilization and feed conversion efficiency<br>* Ensures adequate weight gain in broilers and increased egg production in layers<br>* Helps to build resistance to diseases and stress<br>* Prevents fatty liver disease | **Starters/ Finishers/ Broilers / Breeders:** 1 Kg / 200 Kg feed or 5 Kg / tonne of feed<br>**Layers:** 1 Kg / 400 Kg feed or 2.5 Kg / tonne of feed |
| 20 | TATA VITE FORTE POWDER (Rallis) | Each 2.5 Kg contains : Vit A 100 lac IU, Vit D$_3$ 20 lac IU, Vit B$_2$ 2 g, Vit E 750 IU, Vit K 1 g, Calcium pantothenate 2.5 g, Niacinamide 10 g, Vit B$_{12}$ 8 mg, Choline chloride 200 g, Zinc 15 g, Iodine 1 g, Manganese 27.5 g, Copper 2 g, Iron 7.5 g, Cobalt 450 mg, Calcium 750 g, Selenium 2 g | For better performance, growth and production | 2-2.5 Kg / tonne of feed |
| 21 | TRIBLEND POWDER (Trichem) | Each 2.5 Kg contains : Vit A 82.5 lac IU, Vit D$_3$ 16 lac IU, Vit B$_2$ 2 mg, Vit B$_{12}$ 10 mg, Vit K 10 g, Vit E 750 IU, Calcium pantothenate 2.5 g, Niacin 10 g, Calcium 750 g, Manganese 27.5 g, Iodine 1 g, Iron 7.5 g, Zinc 15 g, Copper 2 g, Cobalt 100 mg, Choline chloride 150 g | For vitamin and mineral deficiency conditions | **Broilers / Breeders** : 5 Kg / tonne of feed<br>**Layers / Growers:** 2.5 Kg / tonne of feed |

| S. No. | Trade Name & Company | Composition | Indications | Dosage / Administration |
|---|---|---|---|---|
| 22 | ULTRAVITE-M POWDER (Neospark) | Each 2.5 Kg contains : Vit A 80 lac IU, Vit D$_3$ 16 lac IU, Vit B$_2$ 5 g, Vit B$_{12}$ 15 mg, Vit E 750 IU, Vit K 1 g, Niacinamide 10 g, Calcium pantothenate 2.5 g, Choline chloride 300 g, Calcium 760 g, Copper 2 g, Iodine 2 g, Iron 20 g, Manganese 55 g, Zinc 52 g, Cobalt 100 mg | To meet the requirements of vitamins and trace minerals of poultry | **Chicks / Growers / Layers:** 2.5 Kg / tonne of feed **Broilers / Breeders:** 5 Kg / tonne of feed |
| 23 | VENTRIMIN-17 POWDER (Venky's) | Vitamins, Minerals Feed concentrate with macro and micro minerals | * Provides essential vitamins and minerals * For balanced nutrition | **Starters / Broilers / Breeders:** 250 g / 50 Kg of feed **Layers:** 250 g / 100 Kg of feed |
| 24 | VIMINTA Z POWDER (Prime) | Each 2.5 Kg contains : Vit A 50,00,000 IU, Vit D$_3$ 12,50,000 IU, Vit B$_1$ 0.4 g, Vit B$_2$ 3.5 g, Vit B$_6$ 0.5 g, Vit B$_{12}$ 10 mg, Vit E 1,500 IU, Vit K 1 g, Folic acid 0.5 g, Niacin 10 g, Calcium pantothenate 5 g, Choline chloride 50% 150 g, Biotin 5 mg, Copper 3 g, Cobalt 0.5 g, Iodine 1 g, Iron 8 g, Manganese 27.5 g, Selenium 100 mg, Zinc 30 g | * Improves growth and egg production * To build resistance against diseases * To enhance feed conversion ratio * To prevent perosis, rickets, curled toe paralysis * To prevent encephalomalacia, exudative diathesis | **As a source of vitamins and minerals:** 2.5 Kg / 1000 Kg of feed **As a supplementation:** 1-1.5 Kg / tonne of feed |

# VITAMINS + AMINO ACIDS

| S. No. | Trade Name & Company | Composition | Indications | Dosage / Administration |
|---|---|---|---|---|
| 1 | AV-MIN LIQUID (AVR) | Each 500 ml contains: Methionine – 118 g, Lysine – 62 g, Choline chloride – 62 g, Sodium - 450 mg, Phosphorus – 150 mg, Magnesium – 575 mg, Zinc – 210 mg, Calcium – 900 mg, Iron – 220 mg, Copper – 155 mg, Cobalt – 200 mg, Manganese – 380 mg | * To improve the growth and for better weight gain<br>* To overcome leg weakness<br>* To minimize the loss of body weight during summer stress<br>* To make up mineral and amino acid deficiency<br>* To improve egg production | **Broilers:** 5 – 10 ml / 100 birds<br>**Layers and Breeders:** 20 ml / 100 birds |
| 2 | BIOMEX LIQUID (Indo Biocare) | Each 5 ml contains : Choline chloride 5 mg, Vit $B_2$ 1.25 mg, Vit $B_6$ 0.62 mg, Niacinamide 37.5 mg, DL-Panthenol 1.25 mg, Vit $B_{12}$ 6.25 mcg, Methionine 5 mg, Lysine 5 mg | Anorexia, debility, liver disorders, deficiency conditions | 10-20 ml / 100 birds daily in drinking water |
| 3 | CHEMVIT-A POWDER (Trichem) | Each 100 g contains : Vit A 5 lac IU, Vit D 29,000 IU, Vit E 200 mg, Vit $B_2$ 300 mg, Vit B6 60 mg, Vit $B_{12}$ 400 mg, Vit K 40 mg, Niacinamide 1.32 g, Calcium pantothenate 440 mg, Folic acid 10 mg, Choline chloride 100 mg, L-Lysine 1 g, L-Methionine 2 g, L-Tryptophan 200 mg | To improve growth and production | 1 g / litre of water |
| 4 | CHOLYMBI POWDER (Lyka) | Each 50 g contains : Choline chloride 10 g, L-Lysine hydrochloride 10 g, DL-Methionine 10 g, D-Biotin 1 mg, Vit $B_{12}$ 1.5 mg | * Aflatoxicosis, deficiency disease conditions<br>* To improve growth and egg production | **Prevention:** 1 g / litre of water for 7 days<br>**Curative:** 5 g / litre of water, or 250-500 g / tonne of feed |
| 5 | ENGROW Liquid and Premix (Varsha Group) | Each 100 ml contains: Methionine – 25 mg, Lysine – 30 mg, Arginine – 5 mg, Cystine – 2 mg, Choline – | * To enhance body weight and FCR<br>* To overcome mineral and amino | **Liquid:** Chicks – 10 ml / 100 birds<br>**Broilers:** |

| S. No. | Trade Name & Company | Composition | Indications | Dosage / Administration |
|---|---|---|---|---|
| | | 100 mg, Vit B1 – 10 mg, Vit B2 – 5 mg, Niacinamide – 20 mg, Vit B6 – 15 mg, Manganese – 100 mg, Magnesium – 125 mg, Zinc – 200 mg, Iron – 150 mg, Copper – 50 mg, Cobalt – 150 mg. Fortified with growth promoters | acid deficiencies <br> * For better egg production, and to sustain peak and minimize fluctuations <br> * To make the bird physically fit during lay | 10 to 15 ml / 100 birds in 2$^{nd}$ and 4$^{th}$ week for 5 days <br> **Growers:** <br> 10 to 15 ml / 100 birds <br> **Layers:** <br> 25 ml / 100 birds <br> **Premix:** <br> 500 g / tonne of feed |
| 6 | FARMVIT POWDER (AVR) | Each 100 g contains: Vit A – 5 lac IU, Vit D3 1 lac, Vit E – 200 mg, Vit B2 – 300 mg, Vit B6 – 60 mg, Vit B12 – 40 mcg, Niacinamide – 1.32 g, Calcium pantothenate 440mg, Folic acid – 10 mg, Choline chloride – 150 mg, L-lysine – 1 g, L-methionine – 2 g, L-tryptophan – 20 mg, | * Improves growth rate, hatchability, fertility an egg production <br> * Improves resistance to infections <br> * Provides all vitamins and essential amino acids | **Normal:** <br> 10 g / 25 litres of water <br> **During stress:** <br> 10 g / 10 litres of water <br> **In feed:** <br> 1 Kg / tonne of feed |
| 7 | PROTOSOL LIQUID (Vesper) | Each 5 ml contains: Arginine – 0.9%, Tryptophan 0.11%, Phenylalanine 0.7%, Glycine – 1.1%, Lysine – 0.8%, Methionine 0.6%, Pyridoxine – 4 mg, Niacinamide – 15 mg, Cyanocobalamin – 15 mcg, Protein hydrolysate – 50 mg, Selenium – 2ppm, Biotin – 2ppm | For better feed consumption, growth and production | 10 ml / 100 birds |
| 8 | SIMPLEX – LIQUID (Vetline) | Each 5 ml contains: Vit B1 3.5 mg, Vit B2 1.25 mg, Vit B6 0.62 mg, Niacinamide 37.5 mg, Di-panthenol 1.25 mg, Vit B12 6.25 mcg, Methionine 5 mg, Lysine 5 mg, | * For the maintenance of high egg production in layers <br> * For better weight gain in broilers | **Broilers and Layers:** <br> 10 – 20 ml daily / 100 birds in drinking water |
| 9 | SIMPLEX PLUS – LIQUID | Each 5 ml contains: Vit B1 7 mg, Vit B2 2.5 | Liquid formula with essential | **For 100 birds:** <br> Chicks: 5-6 ml |

| S. No. | Trade Name & Company | Composition | Indications | Dosage / Administration |
|---|---|---|---|---|
| | (Vetline) | mg, Vit B6 1 mg, Vit B12 12.5 mg, Biotin 25 mcg, Calcium pantothenate 2.5 mg, Niacin 75 mg, Choline chloride 10 mg, Methionine 10 mg, Lysine 20 mg | amino acids, B-vitamins, choline, and biotin | **Broilers / Growers:** 8-10 ml |
| 10 | UNIVIT (Vetmed) | Each 100 g contains: Vit A 5,00, 000 IU, Vit D3 29,000 IU, Vit E 200 mg, Vit B2 300 mg, Vit B6 60 mg, Vit B12 400 mcg, Vit K3 40 mg, Niacinamide 1.32 g, Calcium pantothenate 440 mg, Folic acid 10 mg, Choline chloride 150 mg, L-lysine 1 g, D-L methionine 2 g, L-tryptophane 20 g, | To reduce the general stress at the time of pneumonia, coccidiosis, vaccination, and plane of nutrition | **In water:** 1 g / litre of water once daily, in stress condition twice daily **In feed:** 20 g / 20 Kg of feed |
| 11 | VISELAM LIQUID (Brihans) | Each 5 ml contains: Vit A – 60000 IU, Vit D3 – 30000 IU, Vit E – 150 mg, Vit B12 – 25 mcg, Folic acid – 2.5 mg, Vit C – 100 mg, L-lysine – 25 mg, DL-methionine – 12.5 mg, L-tryptophan – 5 mg, Selenium – 100 mcg | * Ensures growth and reproduction<br>* Increases hatchability, production and prevents early chick mortality<br>* Increases weight gain and quality of eggs<br>* Helps in increasing absorption of calcium and phosphorus | **Chicks:** 5 ml / 100 birds **Broilers / Growers:** 7.5 ml / 100 birds **Layers:** 10 ml / 100 birds for 7 – 10 days every month |
| 12 | VITATONE-LM LIQUID (Sarabhai Zydus) | Each 5 ml contains : Vit A 2,50,000 IU, Vit D3 25,000 IU, Vit C 500 mg, Vit E acetate 150 mg, Lysine hydrochloride 25 mg, DL-Methionine 10 mg | * Prevents stress<br>* Removes weakness and debility<br>* Prevents crazy chick disease<br>* For better egg production, body resistance and weight gain<br>* Improves fertility and hatchability | 2-5 ml / 100 birds daily |

## 32. WATER CONDITIONER

| S. No. | Trade Name & Company | Composition | Indications | Dosage / Administration |
|---|---|---|---|---|
| 1 | O₂ (Avians) | A bag containing oxidizing material | * Effective as an antimicrobial even in the presence of organic matter<br>* Effective for 30 days<br>* Stops algae formation in the water tank<br>* Is a broad-spectrum antimicrobial and antiviral agent<br>* Is effective in all types of pH, hardness, and temperature of water | This bag has to be hanged in the water tanks. In water, it slowly releases nascent oxygen, which has tremendous antimicrobial property<br><br>**Presentation:** 2000 litres capacity tank bag |

## 33. WATER SANITIZERS

| S. No. | Trade Name & Company | Composition | Indications | Dosage / Administration |
|---|---|---|---|---|
| 1 | AQUA-TREAT [+ Water Acidifier] (Harshvardhan's Lab) | Lactic acid, Citric acid, Propionic acid and Ammonium salt | * Stops proliferation of harmful bacteria in water, such as *E. coli*, and salmonella<br>* Improves growth and feed conversion<br>* Improves absorption of nutrients<br>* Stimulates the activity of digestive enzymes | *1 ml / 10 litres of water on a continuous basis<br>*Up to 4 ml / 10 litres of water for periodic use so as to correct the pH of water and for better performance |
| 2 | AVITECH (Avians) | Chlorine dioxide | * Broad-spectrum antibacterial<br>* Effective over a wide pH range<br>* Rapid antimicrobial kill<br>* Effective at very low dosage | **Water sanitation:** 1 ml in 10 litres of water<br>**Flushing of water pipelines:** 2% for 15 to 30 minutes |
| 3 | BIO-QUAT 20 (+ Disinfectant) (Venky's) | Alkyl (C12-40%, C14-50%, C16- 10%) dimethyl benzyl, Ammonium chloride 20%, Inert ingredients q.s. | * Bactericidal, fungicidal, virucidal<br>* Effective substitute for chlorine for water sanitation<br>* Useful in food processing industries and table eggshell sanitation | **Surface disinfection:** 4 ml / litre of water **Table egg sanitation:** 1 ml / litre of warm water **Food surface sanitation:** 1 ml / litre of water **Sanitation of water:** 1 ml / 40 litres of water |
| 4 | CLEANTAB - 2000 (Stallen) | Each tablet contains 5g Sodium di-chloroisocyanurate (NaDCC) activity in an effervescent highly soluble formulation | * Broad-spectrum efficacy against the major groups of pathogenic microorganisms<br>* Has extremely rapid action<br>* Is powerful water sanitizer<br>* Is stable and ready-to-use solutions retain prolonged activity | **Normal purification:** 1 tablet / 600 litres of water<br>**Slight to moderate contamination:** 1 tablet / 300 litres of water<br>**Foot dip / vehicle cleaning / pipe cleaning / biofilm:** 1 tablet / 5 litres of water |

| S. No. | Trade Name & Company | Composition | Indications | Dosage / Administration |
|---|---|---|---|---|
| | | | * Is environmentally-friendly | |
| 5 | CLODOX (Neospark) | Each litre contains: Chlorine dioxide 40,000 ppm with suitable activators stabilizers | * Potent oxidizing biocide, disinfectant, cleaner, deodorant<br>* Water sanitizer, odour control | **Water sanitation:** 0.125 ml / litre of water **Empty shed / foot baths:** 25 ml / litre of water **Hand washing as antiseptic** 1 ml / litre of water |
| 6 | DISCLOR (Polchem) | Sodium hypochlorite, above 5% available chlorine | Used for sanitization of water | 1 ml / 10 litres of water |
| 7 | ENZOTAB (Vetnex) | Sodium dichloroisocyanurate (NaDCC) Each 9 g tablet contains NaDCC - 5 g Effervescent base – q. s. | * Active against bacteria, virus, fungi, and spores of all kinds<br>* Stable in organic debris and hardness in water | **In drinking water as sanitizer:** 1 tab / 600 litres of water **In contamination and disease outbreak:** 1 tab / 300 litres of water |
| 8 | pH-SIX (+ Water Acidifier) (Polchem) | Propionic acid, Acetic acid, Citric acid, Tartaric acid, Sodium acetate, Sodium citrate, Buffers and Stabilizers | * To control multiplication of *E.coli* and salmonella<br>* To favour colonization of useful bacteria like lactobacilli and streptococci within small intestine<br>* To facilitate absorption of calcium and antibiotics through the intestine | 1-2 ml / 5-10 litres of drinking water depending upon the pH and hardness of water |
| 9 | SANODRINK (Fort Dodge) | 1 litre contains : Didecyldimethyl ammonium chloride 22.5 g, Dioctyldimethyl ammonium chloride | * Prevents growth of bacteria and algae in waterers and water pipelines<br>* Effectively reduces cross- | 0.1 ml / litre of water |

| S. No. | Trade Name & Company | Composition | Indications | Dosage / Administration |
|---|---|---|---|---|
| | | 22.5 g, Octyldecyldimethyl ammonium chloride 45 g, Alkyldimethyl ammonium chloride 60 g, Azorubine 30 g, Total quaternary ammonium chloride 150 g | contamination through water * Highly bactericidal even in presence of organic matter | |
| 10 | SOKRENA-WS LIQUID (Virbac) | Each 100 ml contains : Didecyldimethyl ammonium chloride 7 g | Sanitization of drinking water to prevent water borne diseases of bacterial, viral and fungal origin | 0.5-1 ml / 10 litres of drinking water or 500 ml / 5000 litres of drinking water daily |
| 11 | VIGOROX (Avians) | Contains PAA, $H_2O_2$, organic acids, and stabilizer | **Drinking water sanitization:** 1 ml in 10 litres of water **Drinking water pipe lines flushing:** 20 ml in 1 litre of water **Shoe bath:** 10 ml in 1 litre of water **Sanitization and cleaning of poultry farms, and hatchery setters, spray, mopping:** 20 ml in 1 litre of water **Poultry equipment dip:** 10 to 20 ml in one litre of water **Spray in cases of bacterial and viral outbreaks:** 5 to 10 ml in one litre of water | |
| 12 | ZYSEPT (Sarabhai Zydus) | Didecyl-dimethyl ammonium chloride (DDAC) – 15 % | Water sanitizer | 1 ml / 20 litres of water |

# B.
# VACCINES

# 1. AVIAN COLIBACILLOSIS VACCINE

| S. No. | Trade Name & Company | Composition | Indications | Dosage / Administration | Regimen |
|---|---|---|---|---|---|
| 1 | NOBILIS *E. COLI* [KILLED VACCINE] (Intervet) | An inactivated vaccine, containing 100 mcg F11 antigen and 100 mcg FT- antigen of *Escherichia coli* per dose in - oil emulsion. The vaccine contains 0.05% w/v, formaldehyde as a preservative | Passive immunization against colibacillosis in broiler chickens by vaccination of broiler breeders | Inject 0.5 ml / bird by S/C route into back of the neck or I/M route into the breast muscle | **Broiler Breeder hens: Primary vaccina-tion:** 6-12 weeks **Revaccinati on:** 14-18 weeks. Interval between vaccinations has to be at least 6 weeks |

## 2. AVIAN ENCEPHALOMYELITIS (AE) VACCINES

| S. No. | Trade Name & Company | Composition | Indications | Dosage / Administration | Regimen |
|---|---|---|---|---|---|
| 1 | AE VAC [LIVE VACCINE] (Fort Dodge) | Avian encephalomyelitis vaccine | For controlling infectious avian encephalomyelitis in chickens | Information not available. Refer to company's literature | Information not available. Refer to company's literature |
| 2 | NOBILIS AE 1143 VACCINE [LIVE VACCINE] (Intervet) | Live virus of avian encephalomyelitis. Each dose of freeze-dried vaccine contains at least $10^3$ $EID_{50}$ A.E. virus, strain Calnek 1143 | For vaccination of future layers and breeding stock against avian encephalomyelitis | Oral administration in drinking water | Birds should be vaccinated between 8 and 16 weeks of age. It must be carried out at least one month before the onset of lay. |
| 3 | AE VACCINE [LIVE VACCINE] (Ventri) | Living, modified (attenuated) infectious avian encephalomyelitis (AE) virus strain | For controlling infectious avian encephalomyelitis in chickens | In drinking water | Only in broiler / layer breeders at 10-12 weeks of age |

## 3. CHICKEN INFECTIOUS ANAEMIA VACCINE

| S. No. | Trade Name & Company | Composition | Indications | Dosage / Administration | Regimen |
|---|---|---|---|---|---|
| 1 | NOBILIS CAV - P4 VACCINE (LIVE VACCINE) (Intervet) | Live attenuated freeze-dried vaccine against chicken anaemia virus. Each dose contains live CAV virus strain 26 P4 $10^3$. | Vaccination of chickens against chicken infectious anaemia | 0.2 ml per bird by intramuscular or subcutaneous injection | * The vaccine can be given to chickens from 6 weeks of age onwards<br>* The breeding stock should be vaccinated at least 6 weeks before the onset of lay |

## 4. COCCIDIOSIS VACCINE (LIVE)

| S. No. | Trade Name & Company | Composition | Indications | Dosage / Administration | Regimen |
|---|---|---|---|---|---|
| 1 | IMMUCOX II [LIVE VACCINE] (Fort Dodge) | Live coccidiosis vaccine against 5 **Eimeria** spp | For protection against coccidiosis | Information not available. Refer to company's literature | Information not available. Refer to company's literature |

## COCCIDIOSIS VACCINE (KILLED)

| S. No. | Trade Name & Company | Composition | Indications | Dosage / Administration | Regimen |
|---|---|---|---|---|---|
| 1 | COX-ABIC [KILLED VACCINE] (Sarabhai Zydus) | This vaccine contains purified antigen isolated from the gametocyte stage of Eimeria parasites in oil emulsion | To prevent coccidiosis in broiler breeders caused by different types of common **Eimeria** parasites. Passive immunity is obtained by revaccination of broiler breeders before point of lay. | Inject 0.5 ml by I/M route into the breast muscle of broiler breeders | Vaccinate hens twice just before laying between 18-22 weeks at an interval of 4-8 weeks |

# 5. COMBINED VACCINES (LIVE)

| S. No. | Trade Name & Company | Composition | Indications | Dosage / Administration | Regimen |
|---|---|---|---|---|---|
| 1 | LAS-MA [LIVE-VACCINE] (Hester) | Lyophilized vaccine of chick embryo origin containing LaSota strain of Newcastle disease virus and Massachusetts strain of infectious bronchitis virus | For protection against Ranikhet disease and infectious bronchitis | Given through drinking water, or by intra-ocular method | Use at two weeks of age or older. A **second dose** should be given 4-6 weeks later. **Booster** for growers between 16 and 18 weeks of age. |
| 2 | AE-POXINE [LIVE VACCINE] (Fort Dodge) | Live virus vaccine against avian encephalomyelitis and fowl pox | For protection against avian encephalomyelitis and fowl pox | Information not available. Refer to company's literature | Information not available. Refer to company's literature |
| 3 | BIO-VAC LS-H120 [LIVE VACCINE] (Stallen) | Freeze-dried live vaccine against Newcastle disease and infectious bronchitis. One dose of vaccine contains LaSota strain of NDV : not less than $10^{6.5}$ $EID_{50}$, and H120 strain of infectious bronchitis virus : not less than $10^{3.5}$ $EID_{50}$ | Prophylaxis of Ranikhet disease and infectious bronchitis | Oculo-nasal route / Drinking water | **Broilers/Layers: Previous vaccination**: At 4-8 days **Booster dose:** 3 weeks after the first administration. **In Layers** a third vaccination is necessary before the beginning of the laying period, i.e. between $15^{th}$-$20^{th}$ week, and then at an interval of |

| S. No. | Trade Name & Company | Composition | Indications | Dosage / Administration | Regimen |
|---|---|---|---|---|---|
| | | | | | about 4 months. |
| 4 | BRONKI - F [LIVE VACCINE] (Indovax) | Freeze-dried Lentogenic **F strain** of Newcastle disease virus and Massachusetts type high passage strain of IB virus cultivated in SPF chick embryo. Newcastle disease virus $10^6$ $EID_{50}$ per dose. Infectious bronchitis virus $10^{3.5}$ $EID_{50}$ per dose | For protection against infectious bronchitis and Ranikhet disease, recommended as primary vaccination | Intra-ocular (oculo-nasal drop) / Oral drop / Drinking water route. For details refer to company's literature | **Age of administration**: Chicks of 0-3 days of age |
| 5 | BRONKI - L [LIVE VACCINE] (Indovax) | Freeze-dried LaSota strain of Newcastle disease virus and Massachusetts type high passage strain of IB virus cultivated in SPF chick embryo | For protection against IB and ND, recommended as primary vaccination | Oral drop / Intra-ocular / Drinking water. For details refer to company's literature | **Primary vaccination:** 9-14 days **Booster dose :** 28-40 days |
| 6 | COMBINED LIVE VACCINE (LaSota + IB) [LIVE VACCINE] (Ventri) | Viruses of LaSota strain of Ranikhet disease + Mass type strain of infectious bronchitis. Vaccine is produced by mixing the above strains of chick embryo origin and lyophilized | Protects against both Ranikhet disease and infectious bronchitis | Intra-ocular route / Drinking water | 3-4 weeks of age (1000 dose / 10 litres of water and 500 dose / 5 litres) |
| 7 | LIVE B1-M48 LIVE VACCINE (Hester) | Live B1-M48 is a live CEO virus vaccine. It contains | This vaccine is recommended for vaccination of chicken | Drinking water and Intra-ocular method. | This vaccine is recommended for use at |

| S. No. | Trade Name & Company | Composition | Indications | Dosage / Administration | Regimen |
|---|---|---|---|---|---|
| | | Newcastle disease virus type B1, and infectious bronchitis strain B1 Massachussetts type | against Newcastle disease and infectious bronchitis, Massachusetts type for both initial and revaccination | For details, see company's literature. | one day of age or older. **A second dose** should be given at 2 week of age. For replacement pullets a **booster vaccination** should be given between 14 and 16 weeks of age. |
| 8 | ND LASOTA + IBD STANDARD VACCINE [LIVE] (Ventri) | Each dose of vaccine contains not less than $10^3$ $EID_{50}$ / dose of IBD (inter-mediate strain) virus and not less than $10^8$ $EID_{50}$ of ND (LaSota strain) virus | For protection against Ranikhet and infectious bursal disease | Eye drop method Through drinking water | At 6-7 days of age. At 14 days (2 weeks) and above. |
| 9 | ND+IB [LIVE VACCINE] (Fort Dodge) | Live virus vaccine against Newcastle disease (with LaSota strain antigen) and infectious bronchitis virus (Mass type M 41) | For protection against Ranikhet disease and infectious bronchitis | Information not available. Refer to company's literature | Information not available. Refer to company's literature |
| 10 | NOBILIS AE+POX [LIVE VACCINE] (Intervet) | Live freeze-dried vaccine against encephalomyelitis and fowl pox in chickens. Each dose contains at least $10^{2.5}$ $EID_{50}$ A.E. virus, strain Calnek 1143 and | Active immunization of healthy chickens (layer and breeder replacement pullets) against avian encephalomyeli | By wing-web method | **Primary vaccina-tion:** 8-16 weeks **Revaccinati-on:** During moulting period. (Do not |

| S. No. | Trade Name & Company | Composition | Indications | Dosage / Administration | Regimen |
|---|---|---|---|---|---|
| | | $10^{2.8}$ EID$_{50}$ fowl pox virus, strain Gibbs | -tis and fowl pox | | vaccinate 28 days before the laying period or during lay, and also in chickens younger than 8 weeks of age) |
| 11 | NOBILIS IB + ND (Ma 5 + CLONE 30) [LIVE VACCINE] (Intervet) | Live, freeze-dried vaccine against infectious bronchitis and Newcastle disease in chickens. Each dose of vaccine contains at least $10^{3.5}$ EID$_{50}$ of the IB strain MA5 (serotype Massachusetts) and $10^6$ EID$_{50}$ of the ND strain Clone 30 | Immunization of healthy chickens against the Massachusetts type or serologically related types of infectious bronchitis and against Ranikhet disease | Intra-ocular/Intra-nasal/Spray/ Drinking water One dose per bird | **Primary vaccination:** From one day of age onward **Revaccination:** If ND is endemic revaccination with clone 30 at 4 weeks |
| 12 | NOBILIS SG 9R (Intervet) | *Salmonella gallinarum* strain 9R > 5 x $10^7$ viable bacteria | For active immunization of chickens as an aid in the control of *S. gallinarum* and *S. enteritidis* infections | 0.2 ml / bird subcutaneous injection | **Initial vaccination** should be carried out at 6 weeks of age. **Revaccination** at intervals of 12 weeks |

# COMBINED VACCINES (KILLED)

| S. No. | Trade Name & Company | Composition | Indications | Dosage / Administration | Regimen |
|---|---|---|---|---|---|
| 1 | BURSINE NK [KILLED VACCINE] (Fort Dodge) | IBD (Bursine 2) + NDV (Kimber) | For protection against infectious bursal and Ranikhet disease | Information not available. Refer to company's literature | Information not available. Refer to company's literature |
| 2 | COMBINED INACTI-VATED VACCINE (ND+IBD) [KILLED VACCINE] (Ventri) | LaSota strain and / or $R_2B$ strain Newcastle disease virus and infectious bursal disease intermediate *(Gainsville Tribio strain)* virus, both of SPF chick embryo origin and chemically inactivated and blended suitably in stable emulsion using powerful adjuvants | * Prevention against Ranikhet disease and infectious bursal disease <br> * Vaccine is especially used for breeders vaccination programme to avoid handling <br> * Vaccine is chemically inactivated and blended suitably in stable emulsion using powerful adjuvants. | Inject 0.5 ml by S/C route in the lower neck region or I/M route in the breast muscle | **Layer and Broiler Breeders:** 16th-20th week and mid-lay age (45th-50th week) |
| 3 | FOWL CHOLERA + INFECTIOUS CORYZA INACTIVATED VACCINE [KILLED VACCINE] (Ventri) | Killed vaccine made from local selected strains of fowl cholera (Avian *Pasteurella multocida)* and infectious coryza *(Haemophilus gallinarum)* | Immunity studies show that vaccine administered as per schedule protects for about 1 year | Inject 0.5 ml by S/C route | At 8 weeks or older and repeat after around 6 weeks later |
| 4 | G-OLVAC (ND+IBD) [KILLED VACCINE] (Stallen) | One dose of vaccine contains: Inactivated Newcastle disease virus; not less than $10^{8.5}$ | Prophylaxis of Ranikhet disease and infectious bursal disease | Inject 0.5 ml by S/C route (in the back of the neck) or by I/M route (in the breast) | **Breeders:** At the age of 18 weeks. For details, refer to company's |

| S. No. | Trade Name & Company | Composition | Indications | Dosage / Administration | Regimen |
|---|---|---|---|---|---|
| | | $EID_{50}$, and Inactivated IBD virus; not less than $10^{5.5}$ $EID_{50}$ | | | literature |
| 5 | GUMBIN (IBD+ND) [KILLED VACCINE] (Sarabhai Zydus) | Inactivated Gumboro (IBD MB) virus and inactivated Newcastle disease (ND VH) virus in oil emulsion | For immunization of chickens against Gumboro and Ranikhet disease, particularly with the aim of conferring passive immunity to the offspring of breeder flocks | Inject 0.5 ml by S/C or I/M route | **Breeders:** Two weeks and above once or twice prior to point of lay |
| 6 | IB-OLVAC [KILLED VACCINE] (Stallen) | One dose of vaccine contains inactivated Newcastle disease virus not less than $10^{8.5}$ $EID_{50}$, and inactivated infectious bronchitis virus not less than $3\times10^{7.5}EID_{50}$ each. | Prophylaxis of Ranikhet disease and infectious bronchitis | Inject 0.5 ml by S/C route (in the back of the neck) or I/M (in the breast) route | **Layers /Breeder hens:** At the age of 18 weeks. For details, refer to company's literature |
| 7 | NOBILIS REO + IB + G + ND (Intervet) | Inactivated Reo virus strains 1733 and 2408; Inactivated IB strain M41; Inactivated Gumboro strain D78; Inactivated ND strain Clone 30. Water-in-oil emulsion | It is an inactivated combined vaccine for the immunization of chickens against reovirus infection, infectious bronchitis (serotype Massachusetts), Gumboro | The vaccine should be given to birds not less than 4 weeks before the expected onset of lay. Dose 0.5 ml / bird by intramuscular or subcutaneous injection. For details, see company's literature. | |

| S. No. | Trade Name & Company | Composition | Indications | Dosage / Administration | Regimen |
|---|---|---|---|---|---|
| | | | disease and Newcastle disease | | |
| 8. | NOBILIS SALENVAC-T (Intervet) | Inactivated cells of *Salmonella enteritidis* PT 4 and *Salmonella typhimurium* DT 104. Vaccine contains aluminium hydroxide as an adjuvant and thiomersal as a preservative | Indicated for the vaccination of breeders and layers type chickens against *S. enteritidis* and *S. typhimurium* infection | **Normal vaccination:** 0.5 ml / bird by intramuscular route. **For High Risk of early infection: Primary:** 0.1ml/bird at day one of age **1st booster:** 0.5ml / bird at 4 weeks later **2nd booster:** 0.5ml / bird at 14-18 weeks of age | **Normal vaccination schedule:** Two vaccinations with a minimum interval of 6 weeks. The recommended age of vaccination is 10-12 weeks for the first and 14-18 weeks for the second vaccination. **For high risk of early infection:** Vaccinate at one day and repeat the dose 4 weeks later. This is followed by **a booster dose** at 14 – 18 weeks of age. |
| 9 | INACTI / VAC IBD-ND [KILLED VACCINE] (Hester) | Killed virus vaccine contain-ing Newcastle disease and standard type 1 strain of infectious bursal disease virus in | For protection against Ranikhet and infectious bursal disease in breeder hens | Inject 0.5 ml by S/C injection | *First, **'prime'** with live virus vaccines for IBD and ND at least 4 weeks before the |

| S. No. | Trade Name & Company | Composition | Indications | Dosage / Administration | Regimen |
|---|---|---|---|---|---|
| | | stable oil emulsion | | | use of this vaccine. *Vaccinate with killed IBD-ND between 16 and 20 weeks of age. |
| 10 | INACTI / VAC IBD+ ND [KILLED VACCINE] (Hester) | Quadrivalent infectious bursal disease vaccine containing the Delaware variants A & E and the Maryland isolates and standard type 1 infectious bursal disease virus with strains of Newcastle disease virus in stable oil emulsion | For protection against infectious bursal disease and Ranikhet disease in breeder hens | Inject 0.5 ml by S/C route | *First, **'prime'** birds with live virus vaccines for IBD and ND at least 4 weeks before the use of this vaccine. *Vaccinate with this vaccine between 16 and 20 weeks of age. |
| 11 | INACTI/VAC IBD, ND, EDS (Hester) | It contains high titering strains of infectious bursal disease (IBD), Newcastle disease, and EDS 76 virus suspended in stable oil emulsion | Gives protection from infectious bursal disease, Newcastle disease, and egg drop syndrome virus | 0.5 ml / bird | Information not available. See company's literature. |
| 12 | INACTI / VAC IBD+ ND, IB+ [KILLED VACCINE] (Hester) | Vaccine containing killed Newcastle disease virus, Massachusetts and Arkansas strains of IB | For protection against Ranikhet disease, infectious bronchitis and infectious | Inject 0.5 ml S/C per bird | *First, **'prime'** birds with live virus ND-IB vaccine at 10 to 14 days |

| S. No. | Trade Name & Company | Composition | Indications | Dosage / Administration | Regimen |
|---|---|---|---|---|---|
| | | virus, standard type 1 strain, Delaware variant A & E and Maryland strains of infectious bursal disease virus | bursal disease | | and at 12 weeks of age and with mild or intermediate strain of live virus IBD vaccine at 21 days and 12 weeks of age. *Vaccinate with this vaccine between 16 and 20 weeks of age. |
| 13 | INACTI/VAC IBD, REO (Hester) | Standard type 1 infectious bursal disease virus & avian reovirus. It contains two strains of reovirus: the S1133 strain of reovirus (a tenosynovitis pathotype) and the strain 1733 strain (a malabsorption syndrome pathotype) | Effective against infectious bursal disease and reovirus infection | Information not available. See company's literature | Information not available. See company's literature. |
| 14 | INACTI/ VAC IBD, ND, REO (Hester) | It contains high titering strain of infectious bursal disease virus (standard type 1) and Newcastle disease and two strains of reovirus: S1133 and 1733 strain. | It gives protection from Gumboro disease, Ranikhet disease, and reo virus infection | By using virus concentration, large amounts of all the antigens are provided in a 0.5 ml dose /bird | Information not available. See company's literature |

| S. No. | Trade Name & Company | Composition | Indications | Dosage / Administration | Regimen |
|---|---|---|---|---|---|
| 15 | INACTI/VAC IBD, ND, IB, EDS (Hester) | It contains infectious bursal disease(IBD), Newcastle disease, infectious bronchitis (IB) virus (Massachusetts type), and egg drop syndrome (EDS 76) virus | It gives protection from Gumboro disease, Ranikhet disease, infectious bronchitis, and egg drop syndrome virus | 0.5 ml / bird given by S/C route | Information not available. See company's literature. |
| 16 | INACTI / VAC IBD, ND IB+REO [KILLED VACCINE] (Hester) | Killed virus vaccine containing strains of Newcastle disease virus, Massachusetts and Arkansas strains of IB virus, and S1133 and 1733 strains of reovirus. It also contains one IB strain - standard type 1 strain. | For protection against IBD, Ranikhet disease, infectious bronchitis, and reovirus infection | 0.5 ml by S/C injection | Information not available. See company's literature. |
| 17 | INACTI/VAC IBD+, ND, IB+, REO (Hester) | Inactivated killed virus of Newcastle disease and Massachusetts and Arkansas strains of infectious bronchitis, two reovirus strains- S1133 strain (a tenosynovitis pathotype) and the strain 1733 (a malabsorption syndrome pathotype). It | For broad-spectrum protection against IBD, ND, IB, and REO virus for breeder hens and replacement pullets. | Birds should be **'primed'** with live virus Newcastle-Bronchitis vaccine at 10-14 days and at 12 weeks of age. **Prime** with attenuated live virus tenosynovitis vaccine at 7 days and at 12 weeks of age. Dosage is 0.5 ml subcutaneously in lower neck region | Vaccinate with IBD+, ND, IB+, REO between 16 and 20 weeks of age |

| S. No. | Trade Name & Company | Composition | Indications | Dosage / Administration | Regimen |
|---|---|---|---|---|---|
| | | also contains four IBD strains - standard type 1, the Delaware variant A and E (BTO) and Maryland strains | | | |
| 18 | INACTI/VAC ND, IB+ (Hester) | It contains Newcastle disease virus strain and two strains of infectious bronchitis, Massachusetts and Arkansas | Protects from Newcastle disease and infectious bronchitis. Developed for breeders and layers. | 0.5 ml by S/C injection. | *First, **'prime'** birds with live virus vaccines for ND and IB at least 4 weeks prior to the use of this vaccine. *Vaccinate with this vaccine between 16 and 20 weeks. |
| 19 | INACT/VAC ND, IB (Hester) | Vaccine contains high titering strain of Newcastle disease and Massachusetts strain of IB virus | Gives protection from Newcastle disease and infectious bronchitis virus. When injected in emulsion, it controls the absorption of the virus and greatly enhances the development of high levels of immunity | Information not available. See company's literature. | Information not available. See company's literature. |
| 20 | ND + IBH [KILLED VACCINE] (Ventri) | Inactivated and emulsified viruses with oil adjuvants to get | For controlling inclusion body hepatitis hydro-pericardium | **Commercial chicks / Breeder flocks:** Inject 0.2 ml / chick by S/C | **Primary vaccination: Commercial chicks /** |

| S. No. | Trade Name & Company | Composition | Indications | Dosage / Administration | Regimen |
|---|---|---|---|---|---|
| | | stable oil emulsion. The vaccine dose contains litre of $10^5$ $CID_{50}$ IBH / HPS virus and $10^8$ $EID_{50}$ LaSota virus. The IBH / HPS isolate is grown in the SPF chicks whereas the LaSota virus is grown in the SPF eggs | syndrome and Ranikhet disease in chicks in the early age; and for breeder birds for developing good immunity and transfer of maternal immunity to the progeny chicks | route (in the back of the neck) or I/M (in the breast muscle) route **Booster dose: 0.5 ml / bird** | **Breeder flocks:** 1-3 day or 10 day old chicks **Booster dose: Breeder flocks:** $16^{th}$-$18^{th}$ week $20^{th}$-$22^{nd}$ week $35^{th}$-$40^{th}$ week (mid lay) |
| 21 | NEW BRONZ [KILLED VACCINE] (Fort Dodge) | Killed virus vaccine against Newcastle disease (Kimber) and infectious bronchitis | For protection against Ranikhet disease and infectious bronchitis | Given either by S/C or I/M injection. Details not available. Refer to company's literature. | Injection is given at least 4 weeks prior to the onset of egg production. Details not available. Refer to company's literature. |
| 22 | NOBILIS G+ND [KILLED VACCINE] (Intervet) | Inactivated combined vaccine against Gumboro and Newcastle disease (Ranikhet disease). Contains ND virus strain Clone 30 and Gumboro virus strain D78. Water-in-oil emulsion. | For protection against Gumboro and Ranikhet disease | 0.5 ml per bird by I/M or S/C injection | Should be given to birds not less than 4 weeks before the expected onset of lay. For best results, give 6 or more weeks after **priming** with live vaccine. |
| 23 | NOBILIS IB+G+ND [KILLED VACCINE] (Intervet) | Combined inactivated vaccine against infectious bronchitis | For protection against infectious bronchitis, Gumboro and | 0.5 ml per bird by I/M or S/C injection | Should be given to birds not less than 4 weeks before the |

| S. No. | Trade Name & Company | Composition | Indications | Dosage / Administration | Regimen |
|---|---|---|---|---|---|
| | | (Massachusetts serotype), Gumboro disease and Newcastle disease (Ranikhet disease). Contains IB strain M 41, Gumboro strain – D78 and ND strain Clone 30 | Ranikhet disease | | expected onset of lay. For best results, give 6 or more weeks after priming with live vaccine. |
| 24 | NOBILIS IB+ND [KILLED VACCINE] (Intervet) | Combined inactivated vaccine against infectious bronchitis (Massachusetts serotype M 41) and Newcastle disease (Ranikhet disease) Clone 30 virus | For protection against infectious bronchitis and Ranikhet disease | 0.5 ml per bird by I/M or S/C injection | Should be given to birds not less than 4 weeks before the expected onset of lay. For best results, give 6 or more weeks after priming with live vaccine. |
| 25 | NOBILIS REO + IB + G + ND [KILLED VACCINE] (Intervet) | Combined inactivated vaccine against reovirus infections (strains 1733 and 2408), infectious bronchitis (Massachusetts serotype M41), Gumboro disease (strain D 78) and Newcastle disease (Ranikhet disease) Clone 30 | For protection against reovirus infection, infectious bronchitis, Gumboro and Ranikhet disease | 0.5 ml per bird by I/M or S/C injection | *The vaccine is recommende-d for the booster vaccination of breeding stock. *Should be given to birds not less than 4 weeks before the expected onset of lay. For best results, give 6 or more |

| S. No. | Trade Name & Company | Composition | Indications | Dosage / Administration | Regimen |
|---|---|---|---|---|---|
| | | | | | weeks after **priming** with live vaccine. |
| 26 | OL-VAC B + G [KILLED VACCINE] (Stallen) | One dose of vaccine contains: Inactivated Newcastle disease virus not less than $10^{8.5}$ $EID_{50}$, and inactivated infectious bronchitis virus not less than $3 \times 10^{7.5}$ $EID_{50}$ each strain. Also, inactivated infectious bursal disease virus not less than $10^{5.5}$ $EID_{50}$ | Prophylaxis of Ranikhet disease, infectious bronchitis, and infectious bursal disease | Inject 0.5 ml by S/C route (in the back of the neck) or I/M route (in the breast) | **Breeders:** At the age of 18 weeks. |
| 27 | PM-OLVAC [KILLED VACCINE] (Stallen) | Inactivated vaccine against Newcastle disease and fowl cholera. One dose of vaccine contains: Inactivated *Pasteurella multocida* : not less than 100 $PD_{50}$, inactivated Newcastle disease virus : not less than 100 $PD_{50}$ | Prophylaxis of Ranikhet disease and fowl cholera in chickens | Inject 0.5 ml by S/C route in the back of the neck | **Primary vaccination:** At 3-5 weeks of age. **Booster dose:** 4 weeks later |
| 28 | PROVAC-3 [KILLED VACCINE] (Fort Dodge) | NDV (Kimber) + IBV (M 41) + IBDV (Bursine 2) | For protection against Ranikhet disease, infectious bronchitis, and | Information not available. Refer to company's literature. | Information not available. Refer to company's literature. |

| S. No. | Trade Name & Company | Composition | Indications | Dosage / Administration | Regimen |
|---|---|---|---|---|---|
| | | | infectious bursal disease | | |
| 29 | PROVAC-4 [KILLED VACCINE] (Fort Dodge) | NDV (Kimber) + IBV (M 41) + IBDV (Bursine 2) + Reovirus (1733 & 2408) | For protection against Ranikhet disease, infectious bronchitis, infectious bursal disease and reovirus infection | Information not available. Refer to company's literature. | Information not available. Refer to company's literature. |
| 30 | QUADRACTIN ND + IBD + IB + REO [KILLED VACCINE] (Sarabhai Zydus) | Combined inactivated oil emulsion vaccine containing Newcastle disease (VH strain), infectious bursal disease (MB strain), infectious bronchitis (M 41 strain) and reo virus (S1133 strain) | The vaccine is indicated for use against Ranikhet disease, infectious bursal disease, infectious bronchitis and viral arthritis infections | Inject 0.5 ml / bird by S/C or I/M route | **Breeders**: Before point of lay (Pre-vaccination with corresponding live virus vaccine is essential) **Precautions**: Do not vaccinate during laying or 21 days or less prior to slaughter |
| 31 | TRIPLE INACTIVATED VACCINE (ND+IBD+IB) [KILLED VACCINE] (Ventri) | Killed virus vaccine against Newcastle disease, infectious bursal disease and infectious bronchitis | For protection against Ranikhet disease, Gumboro disease, and infectious bronchitis | Inject 1 ml by S/C route in the neck region or I/M in the breast muscle | **Layer & Broiler breeders:** 16-24 weeks |

## 6. EGG DROP SYNDROME VACCINES

| S. No. | Trade Name & Company | Composition | Indications | Dosage / Administration | Regimen |
|---|---|---|---|---|---|
| 1 | INACTI / VAC EDS [KILLED VACCINE] (Hester) | Killed virus vaccine containing high concentration of EDS 76 virus in stable oil emulsion | For protection against egg drop syndrome in breeder hens and commercial layers | Inject 0.5 ml by S/C route | **Breeders and Layers:** Vaccinate between 12 and 18 weeks of age |
| 2 | NOBI-VAC EDS 76 [KILLED VACCINE] (Intervet) | Inactivated BC 14 adenovirus strain in aqueous phase of an oil adjuvant emulsion. Each dose contains at least 1000 haemagglutinating units of the BC 14 virus strain | For the protection of breeding and parent stock against egg drop syndrome 76 throughout the laying period | Inject 0.5 ml by S/C route | **Vaccination** : At the point of lay (18-20 weeks of age) |
| 3 | PROLOCK [KILLED VACCINE] (Indovax) | High concentration of inactivated EDS virus strain 127 in a stable oil emulsion | For immunization of breeding / laying hens against egg drop syndrome | Inject 0.5 ml / bird by S/C route or I/M route | **Age of administrati -on** is between 14 to 20 weeks (before point of lay) |

# 7. FOWL CHOLERA VACCINES

| S. No. | Trade Name & Company | Composition | Indications | Dosage / Administration | Regimen |
|---|---|---|---|---|---|
| 1 | CHOLERIN TRIPLE [KILLED VACCINE] (Sarabhai Zydus) | Inactivated *Pasteurella multocida* antigen (serotypes 1,3 and 4) in oil adjuvant emulsion | For active immunization of chickens against fowl cholera caused by *Pasteurella multocida* serotypes 1,3 and 4 | Inject 0.5 ml / bird by S/C route | **Pullets: Primary Vaccination:** 8-12 weeks of age **Revaccination** : 15-18 weeks |
| 2 | FC VAX [KILLED VACCINE] (Indovax) | Oil based emulsion of inactivated *Pasteurella multocida* | For protection against fowl cholera | Inject 0.5 ml / bird by S/C route | **Breeder parents: Primary Vaccination:** 6-9 weeks **Booster:** 25 weeks |
| 3 | FOWL CHOLERA [KILLED VACCINE] (Ventri) | Killed *Pasteurella multocida* bacterin | For protection against fowl cholera | Inject 0.5 ml by S/C route | **Primary Vaccination:** Chickens 8 weeks or older **Revaccination** : After 6 weeks |
| 4 | INACTI / VAC FC-3 [KILLED VACCINE] (Hester) | Oil emulsion of *Pasteurella multocida* bacterin, avian isolates, types 1,3 and 4 | For protection against fowl cholera | **Layers / Breeders** : Inject 0.5 ml by S/C route | **Primary Vaccination:** 12 to 16 weeks **Revaccination** : 4 to 6 weeks later |
| 5 | NOBI-VAC FC [KILLED VACCINE] (Intervet) | Inactivated *Pasteurella multocida* antigen (serotypes 1, 3 and 4) in an oil adjuvant emulsion | Protection of chickens against fowl cholera | Inject 0.5 ml by S/C route | **Primary vaccination:** 8-10 weeks **Revaccination** : 16-17 weeks later |
| 6 | PABAC [KILLED VACCINE] (Fort Dodge) | *Pasteurella multocida* (1, 3 and 4) | For protection against fowl cholera | Information not available. Refer to company's literature | **Early vaccination:** 10-12 weeks of age. **Second vaccination:** 14-16 weeks of age |

# 8. FOWL POX VACCINES

| S. No. | Trade Name & Company | Composition | Indications | Dosage / Administration | Regimen |
|---|---|---|---|---|---|
| 1 | ACTI / VAC FP [LIVE VACCINE] (Hester) | Lyophilized vaccine of tissue culture origin | For protection against fowl pox | Given by wing web method | **Primary vaccination:** Use at 6 weeks of age or older. **Revaccination:** 6 to 8 weeks later. Vaccinate pullets at least 4 weeks prior to onset of laying |
| 2 | FOWL POX VACCINE [LIVE VACCINE] (Bio-Med) | Live attenuated, ('BM') strain, freeze-dried | For protection against fowl pox | Inject 0.5 ml by S/C or I/M route into thigh region of chicks | **Primary vaccination:** At 4-5 weeks **Revaccination:** At 14-15 weeks |
| 3 | FOWL POX VACCINE [LIVE VACCINE] (Indovax) | Freeze dried. Fowl pox virus cultivated in SPF chick embryos, having virus $10^2$ $EID_{50}$ per field dose | For protection against fowl pox. Recommended as primary (initial) vaccination and revaccination | 0.2 ml / bird in the thigh muscle by I/M route | **Primary vaccination:** 6 weeks and older **Booster dose:** $16^{th}$-$18^{th}$ weeks |
| 4 | FOWL POX VACCINE [LIVE VACCINE] (Sarabhai Zydus) | Lyophilized freeze-dried mild, live vaccine propagated in SPF embryonated eggs for use in chickens | For the immunization of birds of all ages, from one day onwards, against fowl pox. Not recommended to vaccinate laying birds | Mix the vaccine with the diluent and single dose is given by piercing the wing web using needle applicator | **Day old chicks:** Single dose in the skin between leg and abdomen using needle-applicator **Replacement flocks:** Single dose at wing web |
| 5 | FOWL POX VACCINE [LIVE VACCINE] (Ventri) | Highly immunogenic local field strain produced by growing the virus on chicken embryo cell culture from SPF eggs | For protection against fowl pox | By prick method, by wing web method using lancet and by I/M injection. Reconstitute the vaccine with the diluent and inject by I/M route | **Primary vaccination:** At $6^{th}$-$7^{th}$ week **Booster dose:** $10^{th}$-$11^{th}$ week. In endemic areas apparently healthy birds may be vaccinated at |

| S. No. | Trade Name & Company | Composition | Indications | Dosage / Administration | Regimen |
|---|---|---|---|---|---|
| | | | | | $18^{th}$-$20^{th}$ week as booster dosing |
| 6 | OVO-DIPHTHERIN [LIVE VACCINE] (Intervet) | Live freeze-dried vaccine against fowl pox. Each dose contains live fowl pox strain $10^{3.7}$ EID$_{50}$ | For the immunization of chickens against fowl pox | By the wing web method | **Layers/Breeders:** $10^{th}$ week and after the moulting period |
| 7 | POXINE [LIVE VACCINE] (Fort Dodge) | Avian fowl pox virus | For protection against fowl pox | Information not available. Refer to company's literature. | Information not available. Refer to company's literature. |
| 8 | VAIOL-VAC [LIVE VACCINE] (Stallen) | One dose of vaccine contains not less than $10^{3.2}$ EID$_{50}$ | Prophylaxis of fowl pox | Mix the vaccine with the diluent. Pour a small quantity of the ready-to-use vaccine into the plastic container in the box. Administer by piercing the wing web using needle applicator | **Primary vaccination:** $5^{th}$-$6^{th}$ weeks **Revaccination: Layers/Breeders:** Before the beginning of the laying period |

# 9. FOWL TYPHOID VACCINE

| S. No. | Trade Name & Company | Composition | Indications | Dosage / Administration | Regimen |
|---|---|---|---|---|---|
| 1 | NOBILIS SG 9R (LIVE VACCINE) (Intervet) | Live freeze-dried vaccine, containing 9R strain of *Salmonella gallinarum,* with a stabilizer. The vaccine contains at least $2 \times 10^7$ viable bacteria per dose | Immunization of all classes of healthy chicken against *Salmonella gallinarum* (fowl typhoid) and *Salmonella enteritidis* infections | The freeze-dried vaccine should be reconstituted in the diluent. Give 0.2 ml by S/C injection into the back of the neck | **Primary vaccination:** 6 weeks of age **Revaccination:** 16 weeks **Subsequent vaccination:** At 12 weeks interval |

# 10. GUMBORO DISEASE (INFECTIOUS BURSAL DISEASE) LIVE VACCINES

| S. No. | Trade Name & Company | Composition | Indications | Dosage / Administration | Regimen |
|---|---|---|---|---|---|
| 1 | BUR 706 [LIVE VACCINE] (Virbac) | Freeze-dried modified live vaccine containing S-706 strain of infectious bursal disease virus | For protection against Gumboro disease | Intra-ocular / Intra-nasal route 1 drop in one eye / nose / bird. Oral: In drinking water | **Primary vaccination: Broilers:** 12th-14th day **Layers/ Breeders:** 14th day **Booster: Broilers:** 22nd-24th day **Layers/ Breeders:** 28th day |
| 2 | BURSA B$_2$ K [LIVE VACCINE] (Indovax) | Freeze-dried IBD virus-invasive intermediate strain (B$_2$K) cultivated in SPF chick embryo. Titre of $10^{2.9}$ EID$_{50}$ per dose | Recommended in broilers for protection against Gumboro disease | Oral drop / Intra-ocular / Drinking water. 15-20 litres of water for 1000 doses contain 45-60 g of skimmed milk powder | **Age of birds:** 10-14 days |
| 3 | BURSINE-2 [LIVE VACCINE] (Fort Dodge) | Modified live virus vaccine (Bursine 2 intermediate) against infectious bursal disease | For protection against Gumboro disease | Orally : In drinking water | 7 days of age or above |
| 4 | BURSINE PLUS [LIVE VACCINE] (Fort Dodge) | Live virus vaccine contain-ing bursine 2 intermediate plus strain against infectious bursal disease | For protection against Gumboro disease | Information not available. Refer to company's literature | Information not available. Refer to company's literature |
| 5 | BURSA PLUS V 877 VACCINE STRAIN V 877 [LIVE VACCINE] | This vaccine contains live, non-cloned low passage serotype 1 variant virus which has been | For protection against Gumboro disease | For use in chickens from 10 days of age by eye drop / drinking water method | **Broilers:** Between 7-14 days of age depending upon the level of maternal |

**841**

| S. No. | Trade Name & Company | Composition | Indications | Dosage / Administration | Regimen |
|---|---|---|---|---|---|
| | (Fort Dodge) | shown to be very effective against v v IBD | | | antibodies **Layer pullets** : 14 days of age because maternal antibodies decline slowly in layers |
| 6 | GEORGIA STRAIN [LIVE VACCINE] (Indovax) | Freeze-dried. Infectious bursal disease virus-intermediate strain (Georgia) cultivated in primary chick embryo fibroblast cultures derived from SPF chick embryo. The vaccine has a titre of at least $10^{2.9}$ PFU per dose | Recommended as primary (initial) vaccination and revaccination | Intra-ocular / Intra-nasal route/ Intra-ocular/Intra-nasal route. Oral in drinking water with skimmed milk powder @ 3 g / litre as stabilizer. For 1000 doses, dissolve in 15-20 litres of water containing 45g of skimmed milk powder | **Vaccination: Age of birds: Vaccination: Age of birds:** 10 days to 4 weeks |
| 7 | GUMBORO DISEASE VACCINE LIVE (Bio-Med) | Vaccine contains live attenuated Gumboro disease intermediate strain virus propagated in SPF chicken embryo fibroblast cell culture. Vaccine contains at least $> 10^3$ EID$_{50}$ of virus per dose | For prevention of Gumboro disease | Drinking water method. For details, see company's literature. | Chicks should be vaccinated at 10-12 days of age and repeated at 4 weeks of age by oral route |
| 8 | GUMBORO I [LIVE VACCINE] (Hester) | Lyophilized vaccine of chick embryo origin containing intermediate strain of standard type I of | For protection against Gumboro disease | Given through drinking water and also by intra-ocular route | **Primary vaccination:** One week of age or older **Revaccination** Given 10 to 14 days later |

| S. No. | Trade Name & Company | Composition | Indications | Dosage / Administration | Regimen |
|---|---|---|---|---|---|
| | | infectious bursal disease virus | | | **Booster:** Given in breeders between 8 and 14 weeks |
| 9 | GUMBORO M-1 (Hester) | It contains lyophilized vaccine of chick embryo origin. M1 is a mild strain of standard type 1 IBD virus | It gives protection from IBD virus | Suitable for primary vaccination of chicks with low or negligible levels of maternal antibody | Information not available. Refer to company's literature |
| 10 | GUMBORO I+ (Hester) | Lyophilized vaccine of infectious bursal disease, standard type 1, intermediate invasive strain | It protects from infectious bursal disease. It is recommended for both initial vaccination with maternal antibody and for revaccination | **Drinking water method:** Drinking water vaccination should be done during the cooler part of the day. Remove any disinfectant or sanitizer from water for 24 hours, prior to vaccination, to allow the birds get thirsty. Mix vaccine in water according to the schedule mentioned in the pack. **Intra-ocular method:** Rehydrate the vaccine with diluent provided. Place the dropper over the vial containing the rehydrated vaccine on the chick with one | **First dose:** Vaccine is recommended for use at 12 to 14 days of age or older in chickens with low or variable levels of maternal antibody, where early challenge exists. **Second dose** should be given 10 to 14 days later **For breeders:** A booster dose is given between 3 to 6 weeks prior to the use of inactivated vaccine. |

| S. No. | Trade Name & Company | Composition | Indications | Dosage / Administration | Regimen |
|---|---|---|---|---|---|
| | | | | eye turned up. Then, put one drop of vaccine into the open eye and hold until bird swallows. | |
| 11 | IBA-VAC [LIVE VACCINE] (Stallen) | Freeze-dried live vaccine against infectious bursal disease. One dose of vaccine contains not less than $10^3$ $EID_{50}$ | Prophylaxis of infectious bursal disease | Dissolve the contents of the vial in a small quantity of water deemed necessary for administration. Carefully mix the vaccinal water before distribution | At 12-15 days of age (usually 3$^{rd}$ week of age) |
| 12 | IBD-BLEN BURSAL DISEASE VACCINE [LIVE VACCINE] (Virbac) | Freeze-dried live vaccine against infectious bursal disease. IBD virus, W2512 strain, at least $10^{2.0}$ $EID_{50}$, excipient q.s. one dose | The vaccine is recommended for the protection of healthy chickens against IBD as well as v v IBD | By drinking water | Initial vaccination of healthy meat-type chickens is carried out between 7-14 days of age |
| 13 | INFECTIOUS BURSAL DISEASE VACCINE LIVING (LUKERT STRAIN) [LIVE VACCINE] (Ventri) | Mild Lukert type strain (live) of Gumboro (IBD) disease virus of SPF chick embryo origin and then lyophilized | * Prevents very virulent form of clinical Gumboro disease <br> * Also prevents subclinical IBD causing immuno-suppression | Intra-ocular | **For early priming of grower chicks** : between 3-7 days |
| 14 | INFECTIOUS BURSAL DISEASE VACCINE LIVING (INTERMEDIA TE STRAIN ) [LIVE | Tribio Gainsville intermediate strain of IBD virus, SPF chick embryo origin and then lyophilized | * Prevents very virulent form of clinical Gumboro disease <br> * Also prevents subclinical IBD causing | Intra-ocular / Drinking water | **By intra-ocular method** on 14$^{th}$-18$^{th}$ day for booster vaccination after priming with Gumboro |

| S. No. | Trade Name & Company | Composition | Indications | Dosage / Administration | Regimen |
|---|---|---|---|---|---|
| | VACCINE] (Ventri) | | immuno-suppression | | disease vaccine (Lukert type) between 3$^{rd}$ - 7$^{th}$ day |
| 15 | INFECTIOUS BURSAL DISEASE VACCINE LIVING (INTERMEDIATE PLUS STRAIN) [LIVE VACCINE] (Ventri) | This vaccine contains an intermediate plus type strain of infectious bursal disease virus of chicken embryo origin | This vaccine is to be used in the chicks with adequate maternal immunity and it should be withdrawn after the elimination of the persistent vv IBD infection on the farm and shift to the 2 vaccines of intermediate standard regularly | Information not available. Refer to company's literature. | Information not available. Refer to company's literature. |
| 16 | INFECTIOUS BURSAL DISEASE VACCINE MB "INTERMEDIATE" STRAIN [LIVE VACCINE] (Sarabhai Zydus) | The MB "Intermediate" strain vaccine is a lyophilized (freeze-dried) live strain of IBD virus, propagated in SPF embryonated eggs | For immunization of chicks and chickens against Gumboro disease of the new virulent field isolates | Add 5 g of skimmed milk powder or 50 ml of milk to one litre of water before adding the vaccine. **Broiler chicks: In drinking water: 4 days of age:** 1000 doses in 8 litres of water + milk. **10-12 days** :1000 doses in 10 litres of water + milk. **17-18 days** :1000 doses in 20 litres of water + milk. **Eye drop method:** One | **Broiler chicks with known immunity:** Single vaccination: 10-12 days **Broiler chicks of unknown origin:** Primary vaccination: 4 days. **Booster dose:** 17-18 days |

| S. No. | Trade Name & Company | Composition | Indications | Dosage / Administration | Regimen |
|---|---|---|---|---|---|
| | | | | drop of vaccine into one eye of each chick | |
| 17 | IV 95 STRAIN INFECTIOUS BURSAL DISEASE VACCINE, LIVING [LIVE VACCINE] (Indovax) | Freeze-dried vaccine containing invasive intermediate strain (IV 95) of infectious bursal disease virus cultivated in SPF chick embryos | Recommended for protection against Gumboro disease, as revaccination | Oral (in drinking water with skimmed milk powder @ 3g / litre of water) 15 to 20 litres of water for 1000 doses having 45g of skimmed milk powder | Age of birds 10 days to 4 weeks |
| 18 | NOBILIS GUMBORO D78 (INTERMEDIATE) [LIVE VACCINE] (Intervet) | Live freeze-dried vaccine containing D 78 strain of infectious bursal disease virus. It contains at least $10^4$ PFU $TCID_{50}$ per bird dose | Active immunization of chickens against Gumboro disease | Through drinking water / oculo-nasal / spraying One dose per bird | **Vaccination** Birds of 7-28 days of age: |
| 19 | NOBILIS GUMBORO 228 E (INTERMEDIA-TE PLUS) [LIVE VACCINE] (Intervet) | A live freeze-dried vaccine against infectious bursal disease, grown on embryonated eggs. Each dose contains at least $10^4$ $EID_{50}$ of the Gumboro vaccine strain 228 E | Live virus vaccine for the active immunization of chickens against infectious bursal disease | Drinking water | **Vaccinations: Broilers:** In parents vaccinated with live vaccine - 7-14 days. In parents vaccinated with killed vaccine -14-21 days. **Layers:** In parents vaccinated with live vaccine - 14-21 days. In parents vaccinated with killed vaccine 21-28 days |

| S. No. | Trade Name & Company | Composition | Indications | Dosage / Administration | Regimen |
|---|---|---|---|---|---|
| 20 | POULVAC BURSA F [LIVE VACCINE] (Fort Dodge) | Infectious bursal disease virus (V877 intermediate plus) | For protection against infectious bursal disease | Information not available. Refer to company's literature | Information not available Refer to company's literature |

# GUMBORO DISEASE (INFECTIOUS BURSAL DISEASE) KILLED VACCINES

| S. No. | Trade Name & Company | Composition | Indications | Dosage / Administration | Regimen |
|---|---|---|---|---|---|
| 1 | BURSINE K [KILLED VACCINE] (Fort Dodge) | Killed virus vaccine (Bursine 2) against infectious bursal disease | For protection against Gumboro disease | Inject 0.5 ml by S/C or I/M route | **Primary vaccination:** 16-22 weeks **Revaccination:** During moulting period |
| 2 | BURVAX [KILLED VACCINE] (Indovax) | High concentration of highly antigenic inactivated infectious bursal disease vaccine strain in oil emulsion | Recommended as revaccination in breeder flocks after priming with live vaccine to provide high level of maternal antibodies in progeny | Inject 0.5 ml per bird by S/C or I/M route | **Primary vaccination:** 18-22 weeks **Revaccination:** 40-45 weeks |
| 3 | GAMB-VAC [KILLED VACCINE] (Stallen) | One dose of vaccine contains inactivated infectious bursal disease virus not less than $10^{5.5}$ $EID_{50}$ | Prophylaxis of infectious bursal disease | Inject 0.5 ml by S/C route (neck) or I/M route (in the breast) | **Breeders/ Layers:** 18 weeks of age |
| 4 | GUMBORO DISEASE VACCINE (INACTIVATED) KILLED (Bio-Med) | The vaccine contains inactivated intermediate strain virus of Gumboro disease. It is adjuvanted with aluminium hydroxide gel. Minimum titre per dose (before inactivation ) is kept at $>10^{6.5}$ $CCID_{50}$ of Gumboro disease 'Intermediate' | * It gives protection from Gumboro disease * It induces long lasting high-grade immunity in chicks already vaccinated with live Gumboro disease 'intermediate | 0.5ml/ chick subcutaneous injection in the lower neck region | The vaccine is recommended for use in layers and breeders at the age of 16-17 weeks |

| S. No. | Trade Name & Company | Composition | Indications | Dosage / Administration | Regimen |
|---|---|---|---|---|---|
| | | strain virus | ' strain vaccine. | | |
| 5 | INACTI / VAC IBD [KILLED VACCINE] (Hester) | Vaccine containing killed strain of standard type-1 infectious bursal disease virus in oil emulsion | For protection against Gumboro disease in breeder hens | Inject 0.5 ml by S/C route | *Prime birds with mild or intermediate strain of live virus IBD vaccine 4 weeks before the use of this vaccine. *Vaccinate with killed IBD vaccine between 18 and 20 weeks of age |
| 6 | INACTI / VAC IBD+ [KILLED VACCINE] (Hester) | Quadrivalent killed virus vaccine containing the Delaware variant A & E, Maryland isolates and standard type-1 infectious bursal disease virus in oil emulsion | For protection against Gumboro disease in breeder hens | Inject 0.5 ml by S/C route | *Prime birds with mild or intermediate strain of live virus IBD vaccine 4 weeks before the use of this vaccine. *Vaccinate with killed IBD+ between 16 and 20 weeks of age |
| 7 | INFECTIOUS BURSAL DISEASE INACTIVATED VACCINE [KILLED VACCINE] (Ventri) | Highly immunogenic strain produced from selected strains of IBD virus, grown on chick embryo cell culture derived from SPF eggs, inactivated chemically and emulsified with high grade adjuvants | * Prevents very virulent form of clinical Gumboro disease<br>* Also prevents subclinical IBD causing immuno-suppression | Inject 0.5 ml by S/C injection in the back of neck or I/M in the breast muscle | **Layer and Broiler breeders:** At $16^{th}$-$24^{th}$ week and mid lay ($45^{th}$- $50^{th}$ week) This vaccine can be used simul-taneously with either Gumboro disease mild Lukert type vaccine (I/O route) from $3^{rd}$ to $7^{th}$ day or with IBD intermediate strain vaccine |

| S. No. | Trade Name & Company | Composition | Indications | Dosage / Administration | Regimen |
|---|---|---|---|---|---|
| | | | | | (Tribio Gainsville strain) on 14th to 18th day as per local situation |
| 8 | INFECTIOUS BURSAL DISEASE VACCINE MB "INTERMEDIATE" STRAIN [KILLED VACCINE] (Sarabhai Zydus) | The MB oil emulsion vaccine has been developed for booster vaccination in chickens, especially breeders | For immunization of chicks and chickens against Gumboro disease of the new virulent field isolates | By S/C or I/M injection. For details refer to company's literature | After use of the live MB "Intermediate" strain, this vaccine can be used for replacement laying and breeding pullets at 6-10 weeks of age and at point-of lay. |
| 9 | NOBILIS GUMBORO INACTIVATED [KILLED VACCINE] (Intervet) | Immunogenic virus strain of Gumboro disease, inactivated with formalin and suspended in the aqueous phase of an oil adjuvant emulsion. Each dose of vaccine contains at least $10^{6.6}$ TCID$_{50}$ of the Gumboro virus strain D78 | For the vaccination of breeding and parent stock. The offspring of vaccinated birds will be protected against Gumboro disease by maternal antibodies for at least the first 4 weeks of life | Information not available. Refer to company's literature | Information not available. Refer to company's literature |

# 11. INFECTIOUS BRONCHITIS VACCINES (LIVE)

| S. No. | Trade Name & Company | Composition | Indications | Dosage / Administration | Regimen |
|---|---|---|---|---|---|
| 1 | ACTI / VAC M 48 [LIVE VACCINE] (Hester) | Lyophilized vaccine of chick embryo origin containing Massachusetts strain of infectious bronchitis virus | For protection against infectious bronchitis | Through drinking water/intra-ocular route, and by coarse-spray method | **Primary vaccination:** One day of age or older. **Second dose:** At 2 weeks of age or older **Booster:** In growers between 16 and 18 weeks of age |
| 2 | AVIAN INFECTIOUS BRONCHITIS VACCINE LIVING (MASS TYPE) [LIVE VACCINE] (Ventri) | Contains Mass type of live infectious bronchitis vaccine virus strain produced by growing virus on SPF eggs | For protection against avian infectious bronchitis | **Primary dose :** Intra-ocular or beak dipping method **Booster dose:** Drinking water method | **Primary vaccination:** **Broilers:** 4-5 days of age **Layers:** 2 weeks of age **Booster dose:** 10-12 weeks of age |
| 3 | BIORAL H 120 VACCINE [LIVE VACCINE] (Virbac) | Freeze-dried vaccine containing modified live H 120 strain of infectious bronchitis virus | For protection against infectious bronchitis | Intra-ocular route / Intra-nasal route - one drop into one eye or nose / bird. Oral - Through drinking water Spray method | **Layers/Breeders: Primary vaccination:** 32 days **Revaccination:** $1^{st}$ booster : $9^{th}$-$10^{th}$ week (both) $2^{nd}$ booster (in Breeders) - $15^{th}$-$16^{th}$ week |
| 4 | BI-VAC 1 [LIVE VACCINE] (Stallen) | Freeze-dried live vaccine. One dose of vaccine contains not less than $10^4$ $EID_{50}$ of Massachusetts H120 | Prophylaxis of infectious bronchitis | Through drinking water. For details see company's literature | **Primary vaccination:** 2-4 weeks **Revaccination:** 8-12 weeks |
| 5 | BRON MASS [LIVE VACCINE] (Fort Dodge) | Live attenuated freeze-dried vaccine against infectious bronchitis (Massachusetts type M 41) | For protection against infectious bronchitis | Intra-ocular (with diluent) In drinking water (without diluent) | Information not available. See company's literature. |

| S. No. | Trade Name & Company | Composition | Indications | Dosage / Administration | Regimen |
|---|---|---|---|---|---|
| 6 | BRONKICHIC K [LIVE VACCINE] (Indovax) | Freeze-dried high passage Massachusetts type avian infectious bronchitis virus strain, cultivated in SPF chick embryos $10^3$ $EID_{50}$ per field dose | Recommen-ded as primary (initial) vaccination and revaccination | Through drinking water **Note:** Do not administer LaSota for 10 days following infectious bronchitis live vaccination | **Primary vaccination:** 0-9 days **Booster dose:** 28-40 days |
| 7 | NOBILIS IB H-120 VACCINE [LIVE VACCINE] (Intervet) | Live freeze-dried vaccine. Each dose of vaccine contains at least $10^{3.5}$ $EID_{50}$ of the infectious bronchitis virus strain H 120 | For revaccination of future layers and breeding stock against the Massachusetts type of infectious bronchitis | By intra-ocular/ intra-nasal/ coarse spray/ drinking water One dose per bird | The vaccine is safe for use from one day of age onwards |
| 8 | INFECTIOUS BRONCHITIS VACCINE [LIVE VACCINE] (Bio-Med) | Freeze-dried vaccine containing live attenuated Massachusetts strain of infectious bronchitis virus | For protection against infectious bronchitis | Through drinking water | **Primary vaccination:** 3-4 weeks **Booster dose:** 13-15 weeks |
| 9 | INFECTIOUS BRONCHITIS VACCINE [LIVE VACCINE] (Sarabhai Zydus) | Lyophilized (freeze-dried) vaccine containing mild live virus (attenuated H-120 strain), propagated in SPF embryonated eggs | For the immunization of fowls against infectious bronchitis | Through Drinking water/ Spray/ Ocular/ Nasal drop method **Second vaccination** may be used in flocks immunized by primary vaccination. For details, refer to company's literature | **Broilers/Layers/ Breeding flock: Primary vaccination:** At one day of age **Booster dose:** At 10-18 days **Revaccination: Breeders:** At 4-5 weeks . **Layers:** At 18-20 weeks (i.e. at the point of lay) |

| S. No. | Trade Name & Company | Composition | Indications | Dosage / Administration | Regimen |
|---|---|---|---|---|---|
| 10 | NOBILIS IB Ma 5 (LIVE VACCINE) (Intervet) | Live attenuated infectious bronchitis virus (strain Ma 5). One dose contains live IB strain $10^{3.5}$ $EID_{50}$ | For protection against infectious bronchitis | Intra-ocular, Intra-nasal, Coarse spray, Drinking water | The optimum time, method of the first administration and revaccination depend largely on the local situation. Therefore, seek advice of a veterinarian. |

# INFECTIOUS BRONCHITIS VACCINES (KILLED)

| S. No. | Trade Name & Company | Composition | Indications | Dosage / Administration | Regimen |
|---|---|---|---|---|---|
| 1 | INFECTIOUS BRONCHITIS INACTIVA-TED VACCINE [KILLED VACCINE] (Ventri) | Highly immunogenic infectious bronchitis virus (Mass type) strain, grown on SPF eggs, inactivated chemically and emulsified with high grade adjuvants | For protection against infectious bronchitis | Through injection. Further details not available | **Broiler and Layer Breeder flock:** At 15th-20th week. *Vaccinate after 14th week after 2 primings with live infectious bronchitis vaccine at 2nd and 10th week *Live infectious bronchitis vaccine should not be used after 14th week, only killed infectious bronchitis vaccine should be used in this case. |
| 2 | INACTI/VAC IB (Hester) | It contains infectious bronchitis killed virus Massachusetts type | It gives protection from infectious bronchitis | 0.5 ml / bird injected by S/C route | Information not available. See company 's literature |
| 3 | INACTI/VAC IB+ (FOR BREEDER HENS) (Hester) | It contains two strains of infectious bronchitis Massachusetts and Arkansas type | It gives broad protection against different strains of bronchitis virus | 0.5 ml / bird by S/C injection in the lower neck region using aseptic technique | **Breeder hens and commercial layers** should be **'primed'** with mild or intermediate strains of live virus bronchitis vaccine at least 4 weeks prior to the use of this vaccine. Vaccinate with inactivated IB+ between 16 and 20 weeks of age . |

| S. No. | Trade Name & Company | Composition | Indications | Dosage / Administration | Regimen |
|---|---|---|---|---|---|
| 4 | NOBI-VAC IB [KILLED VACCINE] (Intervet) | Immunogenic virus strain of the Massachusetts type of infectious bronchitis virus, inactivated with formalin and suspended in the aqueous phase of an oil adjuvant emulsion. Each dose of vaccine contains at least the equivalent of $10^{6.6}$ $EID_{50}$ of the infectious bronchitis virus strain M 41 | For protection of breeding and parent stock against infectious bronchitis | For details refer to company's literature | The H-52 vaccination at 16 weeks of age can be replaced by the use of inactivated vaccine against infectious bronchitis to achieve a long lasting protection throughout the laying period |

## 12. INFECTIOUS CORYZA VACCINES

| S. No. | Trade Name & Company | Composition | Indications | Dosage / Administration | Regimen |
|---|---|---|---|---|---|
| 1 | CEVAC CORYZA K (Vetnex) | A and C strains of *Haemophilus paragallinarum* | For prevention of infectious coryza | 0.5 ml by S/C or I/M injection | **Layers and Breeders:** 0.5 ml per layer/breeder by S/C or I/M injection |
| 2 | CORYVAX [KILLED VACCINE] (Indovax) | Infectious coryza vaccine, *Haemophilus paragallinarum* bacterin, containing standard serotype A, C and indigenous strains cross-reacting with types A, B and C | For protection against infectious coryza | Inject 0.5 ml / bird by S/C route | To be decided in consultation with a veterinarian **Booster dose:** After 2-4 weeks |
| 3 | CORYZA OIL 3 [KILLED VACCINE] (Fort Dodge) | *Haemophilus paragallinarum* (A, B and C) | For protection against infectious coryza | Inject 0.5 ml per bird by S/C route | Given when birds are 5 or 6 weeks or older. Repeat 3 to 4 weeks later |
| 4 | CORYZA-VAC [KILLED VACCINE] (Fort Dodge) | *Haemophilus paragallinarum* (inactivated) A, and C strain | For protection against infectious coryza | Inject 0.5 ml by S/C route at 6 weeks | Information not available. Refer to company's literature |
| 5 | HAEMOVAX [KILLED VACCINE] (Virbac) | Adjuvanted inactivated vaccine | For protection against infectious coryza | **Layers / Breeders** : Inject 0.3 ml / bird by S/C or I/M route | **Primary vaccination: Layers:** 4th-6th week. **Breeders:** 6th-8th week **Revaccination : Layers:** 12th-14th week |
| 6 | HG-GEL-VAC 3 [KILLED VACCINE] (Stallen) | One dose of vaccine contains : Inactivated *Haemophilus paragallinarum* | For vaccination of chickens against infectious | Inject 0.5 ml by S/C route in the dorsal region of neck | **Primary vaccination:** 6th-8th weeks **Revaccination** : 16th-18th |

| S. No. | Trade Name & Company | Composition | Indications | Dosage / Administration | Regimen |
|---|---|---|---|---|---|
| | | serotype A,B,C : not less than $3 \times 10^9$ CFU of each serotype | coryza | | week, before the start of laying |
| 7 | INACTI / VAC CORYZA [KILLED VACCINE] (Hester) | Oil based emulsion containing *Haemophilus paragallinarum* bacterin, serotype A, strain 221 and serotype C | For protection against infectious coryza in breeders and layers | Layers / Breeders : Inject 0.5 ml by S/C route | **Layers/Breeders:** Between10th-14th weeks of age. **Revaccinate 4 to 6 weeks later** |
| 8 | INFECTIOUS CORYZA BACTERIN [KILLED VACCINE] (Sarabhai Zydus) | Inactivated, water-in-oil emulsion bacterin containing strains W, 221 and Modesto (serotypes A & C) of *Haemophilus paragallinarum* | For immuniza-tion of chickens against infectious coryza | Inject 0.5 ml / chicken by S/C route into lower third of back of the neck region | **Primary vaccination:** One month before expected natural outbreak of disease in the area **Booster dose:** 4 weeks later |
| 9 | INFECTIOUS CORYZA INACTIVATED VACCINE [KILLED VACCINE] (Ventri) | Inactivated *Haemophilus paragallinarum* organisms emulsified with adjuvants | For prevention of infectious coryza | **Early age group:** Inject 0.25 ml/bird by S/C route Inject 0.4 ml / bird by S/C route **Booster dose:** 0.5 ml / bird **Normal Schedule A.** 0.5 ml 0.5 ml **B.** 0.5 ml 0.5 ml **Booster dose:** 0.5 ml | **Early age group:** At 4-5 weeks At 7-8 weeks **Booster dose:** (If required) **Normal Schedule A.** 8 weeks 11 weeks **B.** 17 wks onwards 21 wks onwards **Booster dose:** (If necessary) |
| 10 | NOBILIS CORYZA [KILLED VACCINE] (Intervet) | An inactivated vaccine containing three different serotypes (A, B and C) of *Haemophilus* | For protection against infectious coryza | Inject 0.5 ml by S/C route in the lower part of the back of the neck | Inject chickens between 5 and 10 weeks of age. Chickens are vaccinated twice. |

| S. No. | Trade Name & Company | Composition | Indications | Dosage / Administration | Regimen |
|---|---|---|---|---|---|
| | | *paragallinarum.* Each dose contains strain 083 of serotype A, Spross strain of serotype B, and H-18 of serotype C | | | **Revaccinate** not later than 4-6 weeks before the onset of lay. |
| 11 | POULVAC CORYZA OIL-3 ABC [KILLED VACCINE] (Fort Dodge) | *Haemophilus paragallinarum* (A, B and C) | For protection against infectious coryza | Inject 0.5 ml by S/C route | Given when the birds are 5 or 6 weeks older and repeated 3 to 6 weeks later |

## 13. LEECHI DISEASE (INCLUSION BODY HEPATITIS)

| S. No. | Trade Name & Company | Composition | Indications | Dosage / Administration | Regimen |
|---|---|---|---|---|---|
| 1 | H P VAX [KILLED VACCINE] (Indovax) | Oil based emulsion of inactivated suspension of hepatic tissue obtained from chickens infected with inclusion body hepatitis / hydropericardium | Recommended for protection of broiler chicks against hydro-pericardium-hepatitis syndrome (HHS) | Inject 0.2 ml / bird by S/C route | **Age of vaccination:** 7 days |
| 2 | NOBILIS FAV [KILLED VACCINE] (ANGARA / LEECHI) (Intervet) | Inactivated vaccine containing fowl adenovirus 4 | For protection against Leechi disease (Angara or Hydropericardium- hepatitis syndrome) | **In Broilers:** Inject 0.5 ml by S/C or I/M route. **In Layers:** Inject 0.5 ml by S/C or I/M route. **In Breeders:** Inject 0.5 ml by S/C or I/M route | **In Broilers:** Between 8-15 days of age **In Layers:** At the age of 16-22 weeks, but not less than 4 weeks before the onset of lay **In Breeders:** At the age of 8-10 weeks, and a second dose at 16-18 weeks of age. |
| 3 | INCLUSION BODY HEPATITIS [KILLED VACCINE] (Ventri) | IBH inactivated vaccine. Chemically inactivated and emulsified with adjuvants to ensure stable oil emulsion | For protection against inclusion body hepatitis (Leechi disease) | **Chicks:** Inject 0.2 ml by S/C route **Parents:** Inject 0.5 ml by S/C route | **Chicks:** Up to 4 weeks **Parents:** Pre/mid-lay |

# 14. MAREK'S DISEASE VACCINES

| S. No. | Trade Name & Company | Composition | Indications | Dosage / Administration | Regimen |
|---|---|---|---|---|---|
| 1 | BIO-MAREK HVT [LIVE VACCINE] (Stallen) | Freeze-dried live vaccine. Prepared from FC-126 strain of turkey herpesvirus. One dose of vaccine contains not less than 1500 PFU | Prophylaxis of Marek's disease | Inject 0.2 ml by I/M route in the breast, using an automatic syringe | At 1-2 days of age |
| 2 | HVT + SB1 CELL ASSOCIATE-D VACCINE (Merial Select, Inc) (Marketed by Hester) | The vaccine has a minimum titre of **8000 PFU** for the HVT and **4000 PFU** for the SB1 | For protection against Marek's disease | Inject 0.2 ml / chick by S/C route | For best results vaccinate at one day of age |
| 3 | MAREK'S DISEASE VACCINE [LIVE VACCINE] (Bio-Med) | Live attenuated freeze-dried vaccine containing HVT virus. Each dose contains $>10^3$ PFU of virus | For protection against Marek's disease | Inject 0.2 ml by S/C route in the neck region | **Primary vaccination** : Day-old chicks |
| 4 | MAREK'S DISEASE VACCINE [LIVE VACCINE] (Hester) | Lyophilized vaccine contain-ing serotype 3, FC-126 strain of HVT-live virus | For protection against Marek's disease | Inject 0.2 ml by S/C route | Suitable for vaccination in one-day-old chicks |
| 5 | MAREK'S DISEASE VACCINE [LIVE VACCINE] [CELL-FREE] (Indovax) | Freeze-dried cell-free, Marek's disease turkey herpervirus (FC 126) cultivated in primary chick embryo fibroblast cultures derived from SPF chick embryos containing 1500 PFU of HTV FC 126 virus | This vaccine is recommended for use in healthy one-day old chicks (at hatchery) for protection against Marek's disease | Inject 0.2 ml / chick by S/C route | Day-old chicks. Site-back of the neck. |
| 6 | MAREK'S DISEASE | Frozen, cell-associated Marek's | This vaccine is recommended for | Inject 0.2 ml / chick by S/C | Day-old chicks. Site- |

| S. No. | Trade Name & Company | Composition | Indications | Dosage / Administration | Regimen |
|---|---|---|---|---|---|
| | VACCINE [LIVE VACCINE] [CELL-ASSOCIATED] (Indovax) | disease virus vaccine containing turkey herpesvirus (FC 126) cultivated in primary chick embryo fibroblast cultures derived from SPF chick embryos. Hermetically sealed ampoules contain 1000 doses of vaccine stored in liquid nitrogen | use in healthy one-day old chicks (at hatchery) for protection against Marek's disease | route | back of the neck. |
| 7 | MAREK'S DISEASE VACCINE [CELL-FREE] [LIVE VACCINE] (Sarabhai Zydus) | Chick embryo adapted live virus cell-free vaccine containing serotype 3 (FC-126 strain) of HVT virus. The Marek's disease vaccine is produced in SPF chick embryo origin cell cultures, containing Marek's disease virus serotype 3 (FC-126 strain) | The vaccine has been developed to protect against Marek's disease caused by Marek's disease virus, including very virulent strains of the virus | Inject 0.2 ml / chick by S/C route in the back of the neck or by I/M route in the leg | Day-old chicks |
| 8 | MAREK'S DISEASE VACCINE HVT, FC-126 [LIVE VACCINE] [CELL-FREE] (Ventri) | Freeze-dried vaccine. FC-126 strain of turkey herpesvirus (serotype 3) grown on cell culture derived from SPF eggs and then released from cell by cell rupture (cell free virus) | For protection against Marek's disease | Inject 0.2 ml by S/C route in the back of the neck | Day-old commercial / breeder and broiler chicks at hatchery |

| S. No. | Trade Name & Company | Composition | Indications | Dosage / Administration | Regimen |
|---|---|---|---|---|---|
| | | and freeze-dried | | | |
| 9 | MAREK'S DISEASE VACCINE - HVT, FC-126 [LIVE VACCINE] [CELL - ASSOCIATED] (Ventri) | FC-126 strain of turkey herpesvirus, grown on cell culture derived from SPF eggs. The cells so infected are suspended in suitable buffer and programme-freezed and stored and transported in liquid nitrogen containers | * Prevents Marek's disease<br>* Generally used in grand parents and parents and in pure line breeder flocks especially where there are high levels of MD maternal antibodies present in day-old chicks | Inject 0.2 ml by S/C route in the back of the neck | Day-old parent chicks at hatchery |
| 10 | MAREK'S DISEASE VACCINE STRAIN SB-1 [LIVE VACCINE] [CELL-ASSOCIATED] (Ventri) | SB-1 strain of Marek's disease vaccine of serotype -2 grown on cell cultures derived from SPF eggs. The cells so infected are suspended in a suitable buffer and programme-freezed, and stored and transported in liquid nitrogen containers | * Prevents Marek's disease<br>* Generally used in grand- parents and parents and in pure line breeder flocks especially where there are high levels of MD maternal antibodies present in day-old chicks<br>* SB-1 strain is recommended especially when problems of late Marek's disease and very virulent Marek's disease occur. In such cases vaccine can be mixed with cell-associated HVT vaccine and given simultaneously | Inject 0.2 ml by S/C route in the back of the neck | Day-old parent chicks at hatchery |
| 11 | MAREK'S HVT 8000 + SB-1 4000 | 8000 HVT and 4000 SB-1 Marek's PFU | For prophylaxis of Marek's disease | Inject 0.2 ml / bird by S/C route | Day-old chicks at hatchery and |

| S. No. | Trade Name & Company | Composition | Indications | Dosage / Administration | Regimen |
|---|---|---|---|---|---|
| | PFU [LIVE VACCINE] (Virbac) | levels | | | on 18th-20th day |
| 12 | MD VAC CFL (LYO) [LIVE VACCINE] (Fort Dodge) | Cell-free lyophilized vaccine containing FC-126 strain of HVT virus | For protection against Marek's disease | Inject 0.2 ml / bird by S/C route | Day-old chick. Site back of neck |
| 13 | NOBILIS MAREK VACCINE Lyo STRAIN THV [LIVE VACCINE] [CELL-FREE] (Intervet) | It is a stable freeze-dried culture of turkey herpesvirus propagated on chick embryo fibroblasts. It contains at least 1000 PFU of the virus strain PB-THV 1 (Serotype 3) per bird dose | Immunization of chickens against Marek's disease | Inject 0.2 ml by I/M or S/C injection | **Primary vaccination** : Day-old chicks |
| 14 | NOBILIS MAREK THV + SB1 [LIVE VACCINE] [CELL-FREE] (Intervet) | Live freeze-dried vaccine containing HVT strain serotype 3, and Marek's disease virus strain SB1 serotype 2 | Immunization of chickens against Marek's disease | Information not available. Refer to company's literature | Information not available. Refer to company's literature |
| 15 | NOBILIS MAREXINE CA 126 + SB1 [LIVE VACCINE] [CELL-ASSOCIATED] (Intervet) | Frozen vaccine containing HVT strain FC 126 serotype 3  $10^3$ PFU and Marek's disease virus strain SB1  serotype 2 $10^{2.88}$ PFU | Immunization of chickens against Marek's disease For use when very virulent strain of MDV (vv MDV) are prevalent | 0.2 ml per bird by I/M or S/C injection | Day-old chicks |
| 16 | VVMD-VAC [LIVE VACCINE] (Fort Dodge) | Cell-associated live virus vaccine containing HVT FC-126 and 301 B/1 strain of Marek's disease virus | For protection against Marek's disease | Inject 0.2 ml by S/C or I/M route | Day-old chicks. Site back of neck |

# 15. MYCOPLASMA VACCINES (LIVE)

| S. No. | Trade Name & Company | Composition | Indications | Dosage / Administration | Regimen |
|---|---|---|---|---|---|
| 1 | VAXSAFE MG TS 11 VACCINE [LIVE VACCINE] (Fort Dodge) | Live *Mycoplasma gallisepticum* (strain TS-11) | Prophylaxis of *Mycoplasma gallisepticum* infection | Eye drop route | **Laying birds:** 3-14 weeks Vaccination should be done 3-4 weeks prior to expected exposure to virulent MG |
| 2 | NOBILIS MG 6/85 [LIVE VACCINE] (Intervet) | It is a live vaccine, prepared from 6/85 strain of *Mycoplasma gallisepticum* in a freeze dried preparation sealed under vacuum | Prophylaxis of *Mycoplasma gallisepticum* infection | By fine aerosol spray | Chickens of 6 weeks of age or older |

## MYCOPLASMA VACCINES (KILLED)

| S. No. | Trade Name & Company | Composition | Indications | Dosage / Administration | Regimen |
|---|---|---|---|---|---|
| 1 | MG BAC [KILLED VACCINE] (Fort Dodge) | *Mycoplasma gallisepticum* bacterin | For protection against *Mycoplasma gallisepticum* infection | Information not available. Refer to company's literature | Information not available. Refer to company's literature |
| 2 | MYC-VAC [KILLED VACCINE] (Stallen) | One dose of vaccine contains: Inactivated *Mycoplasma gallisepticum* : not less than $3 \times 10^{10}$ CFU | Prophylaxis of *Mycoplasma gallisepticum* infection in chickens | **Layers / Breeders:** Inject 0.5 ml by S/C route in the back of the neck | **First vaccination:** At 10-12 weeks. **Booster dose:** 4 weeks before laying |
| 3 | NOBILIS MG [KILLED VACCINE] (Intervet) | Inactivated virus strain S6 in an emulsion developed for the enhancement of immune response | For the protection of layers and breeders against *Mycoplasma galliseptium* infection | Inject 0.5 ml / bird by S/C route into the lower, back part of the neck or I/M route into the breast muscle | Chickens can be vaccinated from 3 weeks of age onwards and healthy birds at least 3-4 weeks before production starts |

## 16. RANIKHET DISEASE VACCINES (LIVE)

| S. No. | Trade Name & Company | Composition | Indications | Dosage / Administration | Regimen |
|---|---|---|---|---|---|
| 1 | ACTI / VAC B1 [LIVE VACCINE] (Hester) | Lyophilized vaccine of chick embryo origin containing B1 strain of Newcastle disease virus | For protection against Ranikhet disease | Through drinking water/intra-ocular/intra-nasal/and coarse spray method. See company's literature | **Primary vaccination** at one day of age or older. **Second dose** at 2 weeks or older. **Booster dose** in growers between 16 and 18 weeks of age |
| 2 | ACTI / VAC LAS [LIVE VACCINE] (Hester) | Lyophilized vaccine of chick embryo origin containing LaSota strain of Newcastle disease virus | For protection against Ranikhet disease | Through drinking water/intra-ocular/intra-nasal/and coarse spray method. See company's literature | **Primary vaccination:** 5 days of age or older **Revaccination:** 3-6 weeks later, after the use of B1 strain **Booster dose** in growers between 16 and 18 weeks of age |
| 3 | ACTI / VAC $R_2$ B [LIVE VACCINE] (Hester) | Lyophilized vaccine of chick embryo origin containing $R_2B$ Mukteshwar strain of Newcastle disease virus | For protection against Ranikhet disease | Given by I/M or S/C injection | **Primary vaccination:** 6 weeks or older **Booster:** After the use of B1/LaSota vaccine, in growers given between 16 and 18 weeks of age |
| 4 | AVINEW [LIVE VACCINE] (Virbac) | Live modified freeze-dried vaccine against Newcastle disease containing VG/GA strain | For protection against Ranikhet disease | Intra-ocular / Intra-nasal / Oral (in drinking water) (after 4 days of age) / spray | **Primary vaccination:** **Broilers:** 4th-5th day **Layers/Breeders** : 5th-6th day 1st **Booster:** **Broilers:** 24th-25th day **Layers/Breeders** : 24th day 2nd **Booster:** |

| S. No. | Trade Name & Company | Composition | Indications | Dosage / Administration | Regimen |
|---|---|---|---|---|---|
| | | | | | **Layers/Breeders** : $7^{th}$-$8^{th}$ week $3^{rd}$ **Booster: Layers:** $16^{th}$-$17^{th}$ week **Breeders:** $22^{nd}$-$28^{th}$ week |
| 5 | BIO-VAC B1 [LIVE VACCINE] (Stallen) | Freeze-dried **B1 (Hitchner)** vaccine. One dose of vaccine contains not less than $10^{6.5}$ $EID_{50}$ | Prophylaxis of Ranikhet disease | Oculo-nasal route and through drinking water | **Primary vaccination: Broilers / Layers:** 4-8 days **Booster dose:** 3 weeks after the primary vaccination. **In layers:** A third vaccination is necessary before the beginning of the laying period, i.e. between $15^{th}$- $20^{th}$ week and then at an interval of about 4 months |
| 6 | BIO-VAC LASOTA [LIVE VACCINE] (Stallen) | Freeze-dried vaccine. This vaccine is prepared using the attenuated LaSota strain of Newcastle disease virus. One dose of vaccine contains not less than $10^{6.5}$ $EID_{50}$ | Prophylaxis of Ranikhet disease | Through drinking water. Dissolve the contents of the vial in a small quantity of water, then pour it into the quantity of drinking water deemed necessary for administration | **Broilers / Layers: Primary vaccination:** 4-8 days **Booster dose:** 3 weeks after the primary vaccination. **In layers:** A third vaccination is necessary before the beginning of the laying period i.e. between $15^{th}$-$20^{th}$ week and then at an interval of about 4 months |
| 7 | BIO-VAC NDV 6/10 [LIVE VACCINE] | Freeze-dried vaccine. This vaccine is | Vaccinal prophylaxis of Ranikhet | Oculo-nasal route / through drinking water / | **Broilers / Layers / Breeders: Primary** |

| S. No. | Trade Name & Company | Composition | Indications | Dosage / Administration | Regimen |
|---|---|---|---|---|---|
| | (Stallen) | prepared with Newcastle disease virus strain NDV 6/10. One dose of vaccine contains not less than $10^{6.5}$ $EID_{50}$ | disease in chickens | spray method | **vaccination:** 4-8 days **Booster dose:** 3 weeks after the primary vaccination. **In Layers and Breeders:** A third vaccination is necessary before laying. Vaccination must be carried out every 3 months thereafter. |
| 8 | F STRAIN [LIVE VACCINE] (Indovax) | Freeze-dried vaccine. Lentogenic F (mild) strain cultivated in SPF chick embryos | For primary (initial) vaccination of healthy chickens for the preven- tion of Ranikhet disease | Intra-ocular / Intra-nasal | **Primary vaccination:** 0-7 days |
| 9 | LASOTA STRAIN [LIVE VACCINE] (Indovax) | Freeze-dried vaccine. Lentogenic LaSota strain cultivated in SPF chick embryos. The vaccine contains $10^6$ $EID_{50}$ of virus per field dose | Recommended for revaccination of chickens against Ranikhet disease at 2 weeks of age and above. 9-14 days if used as primary | Intra-ocular / Intra-nasal / Oral (in drinking water with skimmed milk powder @ 3 g / litre) as stabilizer | **Age of birds 4-8 weeks-** 20 litres of water / 1000 doses (60 g skimmed milk powder) **9-10 weeks** - 30 litres of water / 1000 doses (90 g skimmed milk powder) **11-20 weeks** - 35 litres of water / 1000 doses (105 g skimmed milk powder) |
| 10 | MUKTESHWAR STRAIN ($R_2B$) [LIVE VACCINE] (Indovax) | Live freeze-dried mesogenic Mukteshwar $R_2B$ strain cultivated in SPF chick | Recommended as revaccination against Ranikhet | Inject 0.2 ml / bird by SC / IM route | **Primary vaccination:** 6-8 weeks **Booster dose:** 16 weeks |

| S. No. | Trade Name & Company | Composition | Indications | Dosage / Administration | Regimen |
|---|---|---|---|---|---|
| | | embryos. The vaccine contains at least $10^5$ EID$_{50}$ of virus per field dose | disease for birds previously primed with the lentogenic strain | | |
| 11 | NOBILIS ND CLONE 30 [LIVE VACCINE] (Intervet) | Live freeze-dried vaccine against Newcastle disease. Each dose contains at least $10^6$ EID$_{50}$ of ND virus strain Clone 30 | For active immunization of chickens against Ranikhet disease. A high immunogenicity paired with a mild reaction. Therefore it is specifically suited to protect chickens relatively susceptible to bacterial and viral stresses | Intra-ocular / Intra-nasal / Spray / Drinking water | From one day of age onwards |
| 12 | NOBILIS ND LASOTA [LIVE VACCINE] (Intervet) | Live freeze-dried vaccine containing Newcastle disease virus (LaSota strain). Each dose contains at least $10^6$ EID$_{50}$ of the strain LaSota | Immunization of healthy chickens against Ranikhet disease | Intra-ocular/Intra-nasal/Spray/ Drinking water | Vaccination is safe to use from one day onward (Previously vaccinated with Clone 30) |
| 13 | NEWCASTLE B1 [LIVE VACCINE] (Fort Dodge) | Live vaccine containing B1 strain of Newcastle disease virus | For protection against Ranikhet disease | Intra-ocular / Intra-nasal | Information not available. Refer to company's literature |
| 14 | NEWCASTLE DISEASE VACCINE LIVING (B1 STRAIN) [LIVE | Live vaccine containing B1 strain of Newcastle disease virus | This vaccine is suitable for the priming of chicks against Ranikhet | Intra-ocular / Intra-nasal / Drinking water For details refer to company's | For details refer to company's literature |

| S. No. | Trade Name & Company | Composition | Indications | Dosage / Administration | Regimen |
|---|---|---|---|---|---|
| | VACCINE] (Ventri) | | disease during the first week of life | literature | |
| 15 | NEWCASTLE DISEASE VACCINE LIVING (LASOTA STRAIN) [LIVE VACCINE] (Ventri) | LaSota strain of Ranikhet disease virus. It is produced by growing live virus in SPF eggs and then lyophilized | For protection against Ranikhet disease | Intra-ocular / Intra-nasal drop/ In drinking water - | **Primary vaccination:** 4-10 days **Booster dose:** 4-5 weeks **2nd Booster dose:** 15-16 weeks |
| 16 | NEWCASTLE DISEASE VACCINE LIVING (R₂B STRAIN) [LIVE VACCINE] (Ventri) | $R_2B$ strain (Mukteshwar strain) vaccine is produced by growing virus on SPF eggs and then lyophilized | For protection against Ranikhet disease | Inject 0.5 ml by S/C or I/M injection | **Breeders/Pullets:** 8-10 weeks **Booster dose:** (for commercial layers) : 17 weeks |
| 17 | NEWCASTLE LASOTA [LIVE VACCINE] (Fort Dodge) | Live virus vaccine (LaSota strain) against Newcastle disease | For protection against Ranikhet disease | | Information not available. Refer to company's literature |
| 18 | NEWCASTLE DISEASE CLONE VACCINE [LIVE VACCINE] (VH-STRAIN) (Sarabhai Zydus) | Live freeze-dried mild strain (VH) of Newcastle disease virus propagated in fertile eggs from SPF flocks certified to be free from Marek's disease, leukosis and other avian pathogens | For immunization of poultry against Ranikhet disease | **Oral:** In drinking water, add 5 g skimmed milk powder or 50 ml of skimmed milk / litre of water. Then add vaccine. **Oculo-nasal:** (1000 dose in 30-50 ml of sterile water). One drop into one nose / eye. **Beak Dip:** 1000 dose in 100 ml sterile water | **Oral: 4 days to 3 weeks:** 5-10 litres / 1000 doses **4-8 weeks;** 20 litres/ 1000 doses. **8 weeks and above:** 40 litres / 1000 doses |
| 19 | POULVAC NDW [LIVE STRAIN VACCINE] (Fort Dodge) | An attenuated freeze-dried, live vaccine containing Newcastle disease | For protection against Ranikhet disease | Eye drop / Coarse spray / **Booster vaccination:** Eye drop / | **Broilers / Layers / Breeders:** one day of age **Booster vaccination:** For |

| S. No. | Trade Name & Company | Composition | Indications | Dosage / Administration | Regimen |
|---|---|---|---|---|---|
| | | virus (Strain NDW) | | Drinking water | this information refer to company's literature |
| 20 | RANIKHET DISEASE LIVE VACCINE 'F' STRAIN (Bio-Med) | It contains Ranikhet disease 'F' strain. It is a lentogenic strain I.P. (VET) | For prevention of Ranikhet disease. It is the least stress causing vaccine virus strain in this class.<br>* The vaccine is prepared by propagating the vaccine strain in SPF eggs.<br>* The vaccine contains >$10^6$ $EID_{50}$ of Ranikhet disease 'F' strain virus per dose | Administer orally reconstituted vaccine to the chick in drinking water. For further information, see company literature. | **Primary vaccination:** It is recommended for use in 1-7 days old tender chicks. |
| 21 | RANIKHET DISEASE LIVE VACCINE (LASOTA STRAIN) (Bio-Med) | It contains live LaSota strain of Ranikhet disease virus. It is a lentogenic strain (I.P.) and is slightly more invasive than the 'F' strain | For Ranikhet disease prevention. It confers quite good immunity lasting for 6 weeks. It contains >$10^6$ units of Ranikhet disease LaSota strain virus per dose propagated in SPF eggs | Administer one drop of reconstituted vaccine orally to the chick in drinking water. Use cold non-sanitized drinking water stabilized with 2 g skimmed milk powder /litre of water. For 1000 chicks use one litre per day of age, e.g., for 10 days old chicks use 10 litres of | **Chicks:** Between 1-3 weeks of age **Booster vaccination** can be given at any age when the pullets & layers are threatened by the outbreak of Ranikhet disease in nearby areas. |

| S. No. | Trade Name & Company | Composition | Indications | Dosage / Administration | Regimen |
|---|---|---|---|---|---|
| | | | | water which chicks can drink in one to 2 hours. | |
| 22 | RANIKHET DISEASE VACCINE LIVE 'RB' STRAIN (Bio-Med) | Vaccine contains live attenuated RB strain virus propagated in SPF chicken eggs . Contains > $10^6$ E.I.D$_{50}$ virus per dose | * For prevention of Ranikhet disease <br> * This vaccine does not cause any stress, lameness, and mortality, which was a usual feature of R$_2$B strain vaccine | 0.5ml I/M into thigh region of each chick | **Broilers:** 3-4 weeks of age. See company's literature for more information |

# RANIKHET DISEASE VACCINES (KILLED)

| S. No. | Trade Name & Company | Composition | Indications | Dosage / Administration | Regimen |
|---|---|---|---|---|---|
| 1 | CEVAC NEW K (Vetnex) | LaSota strain | For prevention of Ranikhet disease | 0.5 ml by S/C or I/M injection | **Layers/Breeders:** 0.5 ml by S/C or I/M injection |
| 2 | ENCIVAX [KILLED VACCINE] (Indovax) | High concentration of inactivated Newcastle disease virus in a stable oil emulsion. Each dose of vaccine contains efficacy of at least 50 $PD_{50}$ per field dose | Recommended for layers and breeders to boost the immunity of flocks against Ranikhet disease previously vaccinated with live vaccines | Inject 0.5 ml / bird by S/C (site-neck region) or I/M (site- thigh) | **Primary vaccination:** Point of lay **Revaccination:** Middle of laying cycle |
| 3 | INACTI / VAC CHICK ND [KILLED VACCINE] (Hester) | Killed virus vaccine in oil emulsion | For protection of baby chicks against Ranikhet disease | **Chicks:** Inject 0.1 ml by S/C route per one-day old chick. Vaccine is used with B1 strain of live ND virus. | One-day-old chicks |
| 4 | INACTI / VAC ND [KILLED VACCINE] (Hester) | Killed virus vaccine in oil emulsion | For protection against Ranikhet disease | Inject 0.5 ml by S/C route | Birds should be **'primed'** with live virus ND vaccine 4 weeks before the use of this vaccine. Vaccinate with killed ND at 16 to 20 weeks of age |
| 5 | INACTI / VAC PULLET ND (KILLED VACCINE) (Hester) | Killed virus vaccine in oil emulsion | For protection against Ranikhet disease | Pullets : Inject 0.25 ml by S/C route | Information not available |
| 6 | NECTIV [KILLED VACCINE] (Sarabhai Zydus) | Inactivated lentogenic VH strain of Newcastle disease virus in an oil emulsion | For immunization of chickens of all ages against Ranikhet disease | **Broilers:** Inject 0.2 ml by S/C or I/M (in the thigh) **Layers / Breeders:** Inject 0.5 ml by S/C (in the neck) or I/M | **Primary vaccination: Broilers (Day old):** 0.2 ml by SC/IM and simultaneously live ND vaccine |

872

| S. No. | Trade Name & Company | Composition | Indications | Dosage / Administration | Regimen |
|---|---|---|---|---|---|
| | | | | (in the breast muscle) after priming with a live vaccine | via oculo-nasal / spray / drinking water **Layers/Breeders**: Vaccinate during growing period and before point of lay |
| 7 | NEWCASTLE DISEASE INACTIVATED VACCINE [KILLED VACCINE] (Ventri) | Contains: LaSota strain virus and / or Mukteshwar (R$_2$B) strain virus in inactivated form. Produced with high titering strain of Newcastle disease virus suspended in stable emulsion | For protection against Ranikhet disease | **Breeders:** Inject 0.5 ml by S/C (in the lower neck region) or I/M (in the breast muscle) | **Breeders:** 16-20 weeks and mid lay (45$^{th}$-50$^{th}$ week) |
| 8 | NEWCASTLE K [KILLED VACCINE] (Fort Dodge) | Chick embryo adapted killed Newcastle disease virus vaccine (Kimber strain) in an oil emulsion | For protection against Ranikhet disease | Inject 0.5 ml by S/C (site- neck region) injection | **Primary vaccination:** 3-10 weeks |
| 9 | NOBILIS NEWCAVAC [KILLED VACCINE] (Intervet) | Immunogenic virus strain of Newcastle disease, inactivated with formalin and suspended in the aqueous phase of an oil adjuvant emulsion. Each dose of vaccine contains at least 10$^3$ haemagglutinating units of the Newcastle disease virus strain Clone 30 | For protection of breeding and parent stock against Ranikhet disease throughout the laying period | 0.5 ml per bird by I/M or S/C injection | To be given as a booster, not less than 4 weeks before the onset of lay. For best results give this vaccine six weeks after priming the bird with a live vaccine |

| S. No. | Trade Name & Company | Composition | Indications | Dosage / Administration | Regimen |
|---|---|---|---|---|---|
| 10 | NOBILIS ND BROILER [KILLED VACCINE] (Intervet) | ND virus Clone 30 - water-in-oil emulsion | For the vaccination of day-old chicks against Ranikhet disease in areas where RD is endemic | 0.1 ml / broiler by S/C injection (into the back of the neck) or I/M injection (into the thigh muscle) | At day-old, in combination with live ND vaccine e.g. Nobilis clone 30, administered by spray or the oculo / nasal route |
| 11 | OL-VAC [KILLED VACCINE] (Stallen) | One dose of vaccine contains inactivated Newcastle disease virus not less than 100 PD / 50 | Prophylaxis of Ranikhet disease | Inject 0.5 ml by S/C (in the neck) or I/M (in the breast) | **Primary vaccination:** At 18-20 days **Booster dose:** At 18-20 weeks. For further details, refer to company's literature |
| 12 | RANIKHET DISEASE VACCINE (KILLED ) (Bio-Med) | It is prepared by treating Ranikhet 'LaSota' strain virus with formalin and stabilizers. It is adjuvanted with aluminium hydroxide gel (2 mg aluminum per dose). Minimum titer per dose is kept at $> 10^{8.6}$ $EID_{50}$ of Ranikhet disease LaSota strain virus. | For prevention of Ranikhet disease in layers and breeders at the age of 16-17 weeks. It induces long lasting (one full laying period) high-grade immunity in chicks already vaccinated with live Ranikhet disease vaccine, e. g. LaSota and/or 'RB' strain vaccines . | 0.5ml/ bird intramuscularly in thigh region. Younger chicks (4-5 days-old ) suffering from respiratory disease can be given 0.25ml/chick | **For Layers and Breeders:** Recommended at 16-17 weeks of age |

## 17. REOVIRUS VACCINE (LIVE)

| S. No. | Trade Name & Company | Composition | Indications | Dosage / Administration | Regimen |
|---|---|---|---|---|---|
| 1 | NOBILIS, REO STRAIN 1133 [LIVE VACCINE] (Intervet) | Live, freeze-dried vaccine containing $10^{3.1}$ $TCID_{50}$ per dose of the temperature sensitive, highly attenuated strain 1133 of Reovirus | The vaccine is intended for the prevention of tenosynovitis (viral arthritis) in chickens of 7 days or older. It is also intended for priming of breeders replacement stock | Inject 0.2 ml per bird by S/C route into the back of the neck or by I/M route | **In areas of high exposure: Primary vaccination:** At 7th day **Revaccination:** At 5-7 weeks and again 9-11 weeks. **In areas of lesser exposure:** At 5-7 weeks and again 9-11 weeks. (To complete this programme for breeding birds, an inactivated reovirus vaccine is recommended between 18th and 22nd weeks) |

## REOVIRUS VACCINES (KILLED)

| S. No. | Trade Name & Company | Composition | Indications | Dosage / Administration | Regimen |
|---|---|---|---|---|---|
| 1 | REO [KILLED VACCINE] (Sarabhai Zydus) | The vaccine contains high levels of inactivated Reovirus (S1133 strain) in an oil emulsion | The vaccine is indicated for use against viral arthritis in breeders for the induction of passive protection of their chicks | Inject 0.5 ml / bird by S/C or I/M route | **Primary vaccination:** 12 weeks **Booster dose:** 20 weeks |

| S. No. | Trade Name & Company | Composition | Indications | Dosage / Administration | Regimen |
|---|---|---|---|---|---|
| 2 | NOBILIS REO INAC. (Intervet) | Inactivated Reovirus strains 1733 and 2408 water-in-oil emulsion | * For the immunization of chickens against reovirus infections (tenosynovitis)<br>* For the booster vaccination of breeding stock against reovirus to protect their offspring | 0.5 ml / bird by intramuscular or subcutaneous injection | *Should be given to birds not less than 4 weeks before the expected onset of lay<br>*For best results, give this vaccine six weeks after priming with a live vaccine |
| 3 | TRI-REO [KILLED VACCINE] (Fort Dodge) | Three strains of Reoviruses 1133, 2408, 3005 in an inactivated form, suspended in an oil emulsion adjuvant | Protection against reovirus infections | 0.5 ml / bird by S/C or I/M route | **Early vaccination:** Between 7 to 10 days to provide initial protection **Additional vaccination:** Between 5 to 6 weeks if needed to protect the breeder birds. **Priming prior to ProVac vaccine:** Give 4 to 6 weeks prior to ProVac vaccine to prime the inactivated product **ProVac Reo vaccine:** Give 4 weeks prior to the onset of egg production |

# C.
# DIAGNOSTIC ANTIGENS

# DIAGNOSTIC ANTIGENS

| S. No. | Trade Name & Company | Composition | Indications | Dosage / Administration | Regimen |
|---|---|---|---|---|---|
| 1 | NOBILIS MG ANTIGEN (Intervet) | The antigen is a suspension of killed and coloured *Mycoplasma gallisepticum* organisms, strain S6 of Alder (U.S.A.) | For detection of *Mycoplasma gallisepticum* infection in chickens | For performance of the test, refer to company's literature | Positive reactions show within 2 minutes and are characterized by blue coloured flocculation |
| 2 | NOBILIS MS ANTIGEN (Intervet) | The antigen is a suspension of killed and coloured *Mycoplasma synoviae* organisms, strain WVU- 1853 (A.T.C.C.) | For detection of *Mycoplasma synoviae* infection in chickens | For performance of the test, refer to company's literature | Positive reactions show within 2 minutes and are characterized by blue coloured flocculation |
| 3 | NOBILIS SP ANTIGEN (Intervet) | Pullorum antigen | For detection of *Salmonella pullorum* infection in chickens | For performance of the test, refer to company's literature | A positive reaction is indicated by agglutination within 2 minutes after mixing |
| 4 | *SALMONEL- LA PULLORUM* COLOURED ANTIGEN (Ventri) | Suspension of *Salmonella pullorum* organisms in 1% formol saline and stained suitably | This antigen is used for detection of Salmonella positive carriers and control of infection in poultry | Refer to company's . literature | If a clump formation occurs within one minute after mixing, the bird under test is to be treated as a positive reactor. If no such clumping occurs, the bird can be treated as negative |

# Comments on the First Edition (2004) of this Book from Four Reputed International Journals, published from England, namely:

(1) World's Poultry Science Journal, (2) Poultry Internationl, (3) International Poultry Production, and (4) International Hatchery Practice

## 1. World's Poultry Science Journal (2004), Volume 60, September Issue, Number 3, page 398

**This book on poultry diseases is the first of its kind ever written for Indian farmers and poultry professionals. The theme: effective disease diagnosis, treatment and control. The objective: prevention of losses, more profits and better economics.**

The book has five sections, divided into 43 chapters. The first section deals with infectious, nutritional and metabolic diseases as well as miscellaneous conditions. The second section tackles various aspects of disease diagnosis. The third section is on treatment and prevention of disease. Apart from providing a comprehensive list of commercial medicines and vaccines, this section also gives an account of antibiotic growth promoters, probiotics, mould inhibitors, toxin binders, enzymes, oligosaccharides, osmoregulators, methyl donors, acidifiers, and biosurfactants. Section four discusses disease control and has chapters on biosecurity, disinfection and sanitization. This

Section also discusses nature of the bird's immune system, ways and means to boost the immune response, properties of vaccines and various vaccination schedules. The last section that of 'tips on rearing and management' has been tackled with the firm belief that origin of more than 80% of the poultry health problems lies in poor management, and that a high standard of rearing and management is half the battle.

**The comprehensive coverage of poultry diseases, discussed from various angles, will certainly prove valuable to the farmers in minimizing losses from sickness and deaths.** This, in turn, would make the poultry farming a profitable enterprise. **Though the book is written to meet requirements of poultry farmers, it will be equally useful to poultry consultants, diagnostic laboratories, and feed and pharmaceutical professionals. In addition, the book will acquaint the veterinary students and teaching community with practical aspects of poultry health management.**

## 2. Poultry International (2004) Volume 43, November issue, Number 12, page 42

**A consultant with the Phoenix Group in Jabalpur, India, Dr. J. L. Vegad has made a thorough compilation of material on poultry diseases and management**

**for farmers and poultry professionals.** The 800-page book starts with the main groups of disease-causing organisms. For each condition, there are descriptions of the causes, methods of transmission, symptoms, treatment and control, together with appropriate black-and-white pictures showing particularly the most important features in diagnosis. Section 2, 3 and 4 of the book cover general aspect of disease diagnosis, treatment and prevention, and control, respectively. The final section, covering nearly 350 pages, is called 'Tips on rearing and management'. **This gives a helpful guide to the practical aspects of rearing chicks, broilers and laying hens, as well as a great deal of information on feeding and nutrition. Finally, there are substantial listings of the medications, feed additives and vaccines available for poultry in India.**

## 3. International Poultry Production (2005) Volume 13, Number 1, page 36

This tome of over 800 pages is divided into five sections. These sections focus on diseases, disease diagnosis, disease treatment/prevention, disease control and tips on rearing and management.

**This is the first ever such book to be written for an Indian audience (although it is just as valuable to readers virtually anywhere else in the world)** and its objective is the prevention of losses, and the creation of more profits and better economics.

Although the text is relatively devoid of tables, diagrams and pictures it is not that heavy to read because **it is carefully broken down into logical sections** and bold text is liberally used to highlight key words and phrases.

Central to the book is a 'table' that covers some 275 pages that provides a comprehensive review of antibiotics, feed additives, vaccines and anything else that can be given to a bird!

For every substance four columns entitled 'trade name and company', 'composition', 'indications', and 'dosage/administration' ensure that **this is probably the most comprehensive table of this type that the reviewer has ever seen.**

**The book has a unique blend of technical information and its practical application. This is a real credit to its author as it is a reflection of his real and lasting input into veterinary education in India for over 50 years.**

If one has a criticism of this tome it is **'why did the publishers put such a useful text, that will be constantly referred to by the reader, in a paperback?**

Surely this must be an indication that they expect to publish a second edition in a couple of years time!

## 4. International Hatchery Practice (2005) Volume 19, Number 3, page 31

This tome of over 800 pages is divided into five sections. These sections focus on diseases, disease diagnosis, disease treatment/prevention, disease control and tips on rearing and management.

**This is the first ever such book to be written for an Indian audience (although it is just as valuable to readers virtually anywhere else in the world)** and its objective is the prevention of losses, and the creation of more profits and better economics.

Although the text is relatively devoid of tables, diagrams and pictures it is not that heavy to read because **it is carefully broken down into logical sections** and bold text is liberally used to highlight key words and phrases.

Central to the book is a 'table' that covers some 275 pages that provides a comprehensive review of antibiotics, feed additives, vaccines and anything else that can be given to a bird!

For every substance four columns entitled 'trade name and company', 'composition', 'indications', and 'dosage/administration' ensure that **this is probably the most comprehensive table of this type that the reviewer has ever seen.**

**The book has a unique blend of technical information and its practical application. This is a real credit to its author as it is a reflection of his real and lasting input into veterinary education in India for over 50 years.**

If one has a criticism of this tome it is **'why did the publishers put such a useful text, that will be constantly referred to by the reader, in a paperback?**

Surely this must be an indication that they expect to publish a second edition in a couple of years time!

# Index